A CENTURY
OF PSYCHIATRY

A CENTURY
OF PSYCHIATRY

edited by Hugh Freeman

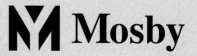

PROJECT MANAGER
Elisabeth Lawrence

PUBLISHER
Cathy Peck

SENIOR BUSINESS DEVELOPMENT MANAGER
Christine Oram

DESIGN AND LAYOUT
Gisli Thor
Judith Campbell

COVER DESIGN
Deborah Gyan for The Designers Collective

PICTURE RESEARCH
Elisabeth Lawrence

PROOF READING
Roderick Crews

INDEX
Jan Ross

EDITORIAL ASSISTANCE
Frances Cook
Morag Hughes

PRODUCTION
Yolanta Motylinska

ISBN 0 7234 3174 4

British Library Cataloguing in Publication Data
A catalogue record for this book is available from the British Library

Library of Congress Cataloging in Publication Data
A catalog record for this book is available from the Library of Congress

Published by Mosby–Wolfe Medical Communications, an imprint of Harcourt Publishers Limited.
Lynton House, 7–12 Tavistock Square, London WC1H 9LB, England.

Printed in Barcelona, Spain by Grafos SA, Arte Sobre Papel, 1999.

FOREWORD

A hundred years is a moment in the history of mankind: for psychiatry the past century contains almost all of its history. True, over the past several millennia there were individuals whose work was of capital importance for the development of our discipline: the past century however excels in terms of quality and quantity of innovations in psychiatry and in the numbers of revolutionary upheavals in our discipline.

In the past hundred years knowledge about the structure of the brain and about the manner in which it functions has expanded beyond all expectations. Neurosciences are hailed as the most important and most promising branch of scientific enquiry. Techniques of assessment of psychiatric disorders and of their treatment have helped to make psychiatry an accepted medical discipline similar to, if not the same as, all the others. Techniques of rehabilitation have been defined and proven to work. The profession has become conscious of the ethical imperatives that should govern work in this field and defined deontological principles for its practitioners.

There were also dark periods in the history of psychiatry over the past ten decades. Abuses of psychiatry for political purposes, mishandling, sterilisation and extermination of people who suffered from a mental illness or impairment, abuses and misuses of the privileged relationships between patients and psychiatrists, economic exploitation of the mentally ill and retarded have happened: they have been condemned by the profession and taught us much about ways to prevent such events from happening ever again. It is up to us and those who will be practising psychiatry in the future centuries to remember how easily things can go wrong and how important it is to remain alert and watchful concerning the behaviour of mental health workers.

The book before us presents an experienced editor's choice of issues that characterised psychiatry over the past hundred years. The book does not aim to be comprehensive: rather, it describes the events and developments in psychiatry highlighting some of them and leaving others outside of the limelight. The authors of the chapters composing the book have been selected with care and deal with their chapters with remarkable authority and competence.

I am delighted to see this book in print and applaud what I believe the chief intention of books about history should be — to help us to live the future using the best of the traditions of the past, thinking about the psychiatry of the past while building an even better and more helpful discipline for the future.

Norman Sartorius
President, World Psychiatric Association
Geneva, May 1999

PREFACE

The end of the twentieth century — and also of the second millennium — is a time for re-assessing almost every sphere of human life. In this process, the discipline of psychiatry will certainly need to be included, not least because of the enormous changes it has experienced in all its aspects, particularly during the last 50 years. In this, it is no different from the rest of medicine, so far as clinical advances and scientific knowledge are concerned; but where it is unique is in psychiatry's deep relationships with social, cultural, and political aspects of society. This volume has tried to acknowledge all the complex interplays between the professional management of psychiatric disorder and the general evolution of life, between about 1895 and the present day.

The book's purpose is essentially to inform people in the mental health professions and others interested in psychiatry, throughout the world, about the recent historical background to their work, and to do so in an interesting way.

I hope that it may be possible to avoid any misunderstanding by making clear at the outset what it has, and has not set out to do:

- This is not an academic work of historical scholarship; there are no references in the text, but only a guide to further reading for each section.
- It has not attempted to give a comprehensive account of every aspect of psychiatry during the century. Rather, it has selected a number of themes in each period which are believed to be significant, but has inevitably had to leave others out.
- The organisation of the text is partly chronological and partly thematic, so that readers can more easily use it selectively; this means that there is a certain amount of necessary repetition.
- Readers are assumed to have a basic knowledge of the subject, but detailed technicalities and jargon have been avoided as much as possible. The fact that many readers will not have English as their first language has been kept in mind.

The contributors are a diverse group. They are men and women from many different countries and varied disciplines — psychiatry, psychology, nursing, psychoanalysis, history, epidemiology, social administration, and sociology. In this way, it is hoped that a wide range of viewpoints has been represented, and rigid orthodoxy or dogma of any kind avoided. At the same time, they share the values of humane concern for people troubled by mental disorder and of a commitment to scientific truth (so far as that can be established at any time). This has been a truly international effort, reflecting the worldwide cooperation which is so essential to the progress of scientific knowledge.

Just as psychiatry has evolved through the century, so has the history of the subject. For many years, though, it was anything but an exciting area of scholarship; in fact, it attracted relatively little interest worldwide until the 1960s. At that point, as the political and cultural upheavals or *événements* of the time erupted in many countries, the history of psychiatry became a rather surprising focus for bitter ideological disputes. What had been a fairly neglected backwater of the evolution of science was now the setting of a veritable *kulturkampf*.

New voices — particularly that of Michel Foucault — denounced conventional historical accounts as 'whiggish', in that they portrayed a steady progress from states of ignorance and barbarism to relative enlightenment. This condemnation was directed both at the social administration tradition of describing how mental health services had developed, and at more technical accounts of improved scientific knowledge. Psychoanalysts who saw progress only in terms of a growing acceptance of Freudian theory were equally anathema to the 'revisionists'. Their view was largely a Marxist one, interpreting developments in psychiatry mainly in terms of social class and power relationships.

Yet theoretical construction of psychiatry and of mental disorder itself in such primarily political terms has been marked most particularly by a lack of clinical understanding. The most overwhelming feature of the psychoses and dementias is that they cause chronic disability in very large numbers of people, and that up to now this disability has been mostly untreatable. This situation exists in every human population, in the same way that troublesome symptoms of anxiety and depression are very common amongst all of them. Furthermore, bodily disease, malnutrition, ageing, and the toxic effects of drugs often complicate the clinical picture of psychiatric disorders, but have rarely featured in sociological explanations.

Now is the time, though, to leave behind these ideological struggles and accept whatever legitimate contribution can be made to the story by each one of the disciplines involved. I will not try to summarise the wealth of information and opinion that the many distinguished contributors have provided here; they speak for themselves. But the theme is essentially an optimistic one, in that present-day knowledge and methods of treatment offer the best hope there has ever been for the relief of mental suffering. Psychiatry's next task is to make these available to many more of the world's population than have been able to benefit from them up to now.

Acknowledgements

It is a pleasure to acknowledge the unfailing help I have received from the staff of Mosby-Wolfe — Alison Taylor, Christine Oram, and Elisabeth Lawrence — and from the freelance editor, Cathy Peck. I would also like to thank the Neuroscience department of Servier International, Mike Sumpter, Bertrand de Lavenne, and Emmanuel Caillaud. As in all things, I am grateful for the loving support of my wife, Professor Joan Freeman.

Hugh Freeman
London, April 1999

CONTRIBUTORS

Arie, Tom CBE, MA, BM(Oxon), FRCP(Lond), FRCPsych, FFPHM, is Foundation Professor Emeritus of Health Care of the Elderly, University of Nottingham. He trained in Oxford and at the Maudsley and Royal London Hospitals. One of the early psychogeriatricians, he has been Vice-President of the Royal College of Psychiatrists and Chairman of its Old Age Section, and Chairman of the World Psychiatric Association's Geriatric Psychiatry Section. Involved in education and public policy he writes and travels, and has been Visiting Professor or adviser in many countries. He is Vice-Chairman of RSAS-AgeCare, one of the oldest UK medical charities.

Berner, Peter Univ. Prof., Dr. med. His education and study of medicine were in Vienna. After graduation, he was appointed to the Psychiatric Neurological University Clinic of Vienna, and in 1966 promoted to Dozent (university lecturer). In 1971, he was nominated Professor of Psychiatry and Director of the Psychiatric University Clinic of Vienna, Emeritus since September 1991. His positions have included: Mental Health Adviser to the United Nations High Commissioner for Refugees in Geneva; Visiting Professor at the University of Lausanne; Secretary General of the World Psychiatric Association; Visiting Professor at the University of Paris V.

Berridge, Virginia BA, PhD, is Professor of History, London School of Hygiene and Tropical Medicine, University of London and Head of the history group there. She is author of several books on the history of drug policy, on AIDS and British health policy. Recent titles are, *Opium and the People; Opiate Use and Drug Control Policy in 19th and early 20th Century England* (expanded edition, 1999); and *Health and Society in Britain Since 1939* (1999).

Birley, James Leatham Tennant FRCPsych, FRCP, is Emeritus Psychiatrist, Bethlem Royal and Maudsley Hospitals. He trained and worked at the Maudsley Hospital, London. His main interest, both in research and practice, has been social psychiatry and the provision of services for people with long-standing psychiatric problems. Since retiring, he has helped to set up a training programme for community psychiatric nurses working in this field, and has assisted the revival of psychiatry in Eastern Europe, through the Geneva Initiative on Psychiatry, of which he is Chairman. He is a Past President of the Royal College of Psychiatrists and of the British Medical Association, and a Distinguished Fellow of the American Psychiatric Association.

Brown, Paul MB BS, MRCPsych, FRANZCP, trained at the London Hospital, and was Director of Psychiatric Residency Training at the Hebrew University, Jerusalem. He specialised in management of psychological trauma, and was awarded the Milton Erikson Prize. From the 1990s, he has lived in Melbourne, Australia. His RANZ College activities have included commissioning its history, membership of the Editorial Board of the *ANZ Journal of Psychiatry*, and Chair of the Special Interest Group on Psychological Trauma. In 1997, he founded the Pierre Janet Centre, which conducts teaching and research into trauma, dissociation, and the contribution of Janet.

Buhl, Katharina is a medical student. She was born in Düsseldorf, Germany, where she attended school. She started her medical studies at the Rheinische-Friedrich-Wilhelms University, Bonn, and in 1996 transferred to the Christian-Albrechts University, Kiel.

Burti, Lorenzo MD, is Specialist in Psychiatry, Neurology and Medical Statistics, Associate Professor at the University of Verona Medical School, and Associate Clinical Director South-Verona Community Mental Health Service. He has been on the Faculty of the Institute of Psychiatry of the University of Verona since 1973, and was appointed Associate Professor in 1992. He has been clinical coordinator of one of the community teams of the Institute, and since 1996, has been responsible for the residential and semi-residential facilities. He has authored or co-authored more than 100 publications and three volumes on community mental health, rehabilitation, and related research. He was the founding President of the Italian Association of Psychological Rehabilitation.

Cahn, Charles H MD, Associate Professor of Psychiatry, McGill University, Montreal, Canada, and Psychiatrist, Douglas Hospital, Montreal, was born in Berlin. He studied medicine in Oxford and Toronto, and his postgraduate studies in psychiatry were in London and Montreal. He has been Chair of the History of Psychiatry Section of the World Psychiatric Association since 1993, and is a life member of the Canadian Psychiatric Association and life fellow of the American Psychiatric Association. He is the author of *History of Douglas Hospital — 100 Years of Progress* (1981), and *A Window on European Psychiatry* (1985).

Campbell, Karen MA, has worked in the field of mental health user development since 1991, first as Development Worker for User Participation based at Fulbourn Hospital, Cambridge, moving to the Manic Depression Fellowship (MDF) in 1993, as the first full-time Self-Help Group Development Officer. She has personal experience of using services and has been involved for several years with user organisations such as Survivors Speak Out. In 1998, she was appointed as Chief Executive of MDF and is a founder member of the UK support network for Survivor Workers.

Cardno, Alastair G MB ChB, MRCPsych, MMedSc, is a Medical Research Council Clinical Training Fellow, Division of Psychological Medicine, University of Wales College of Medicine, Cardiff. He qualified in medicine from Dundee University in 1986, and had psychiatric training in North Yorkshire and South Wales. His main research interest is in the genetic basis of clinical variation in psychotic illnesses.

Carvajal, César MD, is Professor of Psychiatry, Faculty of Medicine, University of Los Andes and Clinical Psychiatrist at the Hospital del Trabajador (Santiago, Chile). He graduated in medicine from the Pontificia Universidad Católica de Chile, Santiago, obtained his postgraduate specialisation in psychiatry there, and went on to train at the University of Navarra, Spain, and at FORENAP (For Applied Neuroscience Research in Psychiatry), Rouffach, France. He is the Psychiatric Editor of *Revista Chilena de Neuro-Psiquiatría* and on the Editorial Board of *Revista de Psiquiatría Clínica*. He was the President of the Chilean Society of Biological Psychiatry (1995–1997). His clinical research and publications are in PTSD, depression, and psychoendocrinology.

Cooper, John E BA(Oxon), BM, BCh, FRCP, FRCPsych, is Emeritus Foundation Professor of Psychiatry, University of Nottingham, and was formerly Consultant Psychiatrist and Vice-Dean, Bethlem Royal and Maudsley Hospitals and Institute of Psychiatry, London, and UK Director of the US–UK Diagnostic Project. His research interests include the development of standardised interviews and rating scales, the diagnostic process, psychiatric classifications, and cross-cultural epidemiology. He is a consultant to WHO Geneva in the design of international collaborative studies on schizophrenia, the development of standardised interviewing and rating scales, and the development of ICD–8, ICD–9, and ICD–10. He is also a member of WHO Expert Panel on Mental Health.

Crammer, John L MA, MRCS, FRCPsych, is Reader Emeritus in Biological Psychiatry, Institute of Psychiatry, University of London. He was formerly a Senior Lecturer and Consultant Psychiatrist, Maudsley Hospital, London, Assistant Editor of the *British Medical Journal*, and Editor of the *British Journal of Psychiatry*. He has published on periodic psychoses, drug use and metabolism, asylum history, and is writing a history of insulin coma.

Cunningham Owens, David Griffith MD(Hons), FRCP, FRCPsych, is Reader in Psychiatry and Honorary Consultant Psychiatrist, University of Edinburgh, and Royal Edinburgh Hospital. After training in general medicine and neurology, he moved to the Medical Research Council's Clinical Research Centre at Northwick Park Hospital, becoming a member of the scientific staff and Consultant Psychiatrist. His research interests lie in the biology of major psychiatric disorders, particularly schizophrenia, and in antipsychotic psychopharmacology. He has been active in the field of structural brain imaging in psychoses since the 1970s and is currently involved in MRI studies of the precursors of psychotic illness in patients at high risk of developing schizophrenia.

Dally, Ann Gwendolen MA(Oxon), MD, DObstRCOG, has degrees in history, medicine, and in the history of medicine. On retirement from clinical practice in psychiatry, she went to the Wellcome Institute for the History of Medicine as Research Fellow. Her last published books are *A Doctor's Story* (1990), *Women under the Knife* (1991), and *Fantasy Surgery* (1996).

Donnelly, Michael AB, PhD, is Professor and Chair of Sociology, University of New Hampshire, USA. Professor Donnelly taught previously at Harvard University, and has held visiting appointments at the European University Institute, the University of London, and the University of Trento. His publications include *Managing the Mind: Medical Psychology in Early c19 Britain* (1983), and *The Politics of Mental Health in Italy* (1992).

Eaton, William W PhD, Professor in the School of Public Health, Johns Hopkins University, Baltimore, directs the Training Program in Psychiatric Epidemiology in the Department of Mental Hygiene, where he also teaches and conducts research. He was previously Assistant Chief, Center for Epidemiologic Studies, National Institute of Mental Health, where he coordinated the methodology of the Epidemiologic Catchment Area Program. He has published over 100 scientific articles in the field of psychiatric epidemiology, and edited several monographs in the area, including *Epidemiologic Field Methods in Psychiatry: the NIMH Epidemiologic Catchment Area Program*, with Larry G Kessler. The third edition of his text, *The Sociology of Mental Disorders*, is expected in 1999.

Engstrom, Eric J BA, MA, PhD, is a lecturer in the Department of History, Humboldt University of Berlin. Dr Engstrom studied at Lewis and Clark College, University of Munich, and the University of North Carolina at Chapel Hill. He has been a Fulbright Fellow and a Fellow of the Carolina Society of Fellows. He has published several articles on Emil Kraepelin, and is currently completing a study on the history of university psychiatric clinics in Germany as well as preparing a conference on the history of the Charité hospital in Berlin.

Fenton, George W MB, FRCP(Ed), FRCP(Lond), FRCPsych, is Emeritus Professor, University of Dundee, having been Head of Psychiatry there from 1983 to 1996, and formerly Professor and Head of the Department of Mental Health, the Queen's University of Belfast. Previously, he was a Consultant Psychiatrist and Neurophysiologist at the Maudsley Hospital and a Senior Lecturer at the Institute of Psychiatry, University of London. His special interests include neuropsychiatry, clinical neurophysiology, and neurosurgery for mental disorder.

Fink, Max MD, is Professor of Psychiatry and Neurology Emeritus, SUNY at Stony Brook, and Professor of Psychiatry, Albert Einstein College of Medicine. Dr Fink graduated from New York University College of Medicine and is certified in neurology, psychiatry, and psychoanalysis. In January 1952, he first administered electroshock and developed a lifelong interest in its use, mechanism of action, and teaching. His principal publications include the edited volume *Psychobiology of Convulsive Therapy* (1974), the textbook *Convulsive Therapy: Theory and Practice* (1979), the videotape *Informed ECT for Patients and their Families* (1986), and the trade book *Restoring the Mind: The Promise of Electroshock* (1999). He established the journal *Convulsive Therapy* (1985), and has published more than 250 scientific articles.

Freeman, Hugh DM(Oxon), MSc, MA, Hon FRCPsych, FFPHM, studied psychology and medicine at Oxford and then trained at the Institute of Psychiatry, London. He was a clinician and university teacher in Manchester, developing interests particularly in community psychiatry, epidemiology, psychopharmacology, and the relationship of mental health to the environment. For ten years, he was Editor of the *British Journal of Psychiatry* and also founded *Current Opinion in Psychiatry*. He has written and edited major works on community psychiatry, the history of British psychiatry, and environmental aspects of mental health. He has been a consultant to the World Health Organization and is currently Honorary Visiting Fellow at Green College, Oxford, Honorary Consultant Psychiatrist,

Salford Mental Health Trust, and Honorary Professor at the University of Salford. He is Chairman of the Section on Psychiatry and Public Policy, World Psychiatric Association and a Corresponding Fellow of the American Psychiatric Association. He is also an Honorary Member of five national Psychiatric Associations and has been a Visiting Professor in four countries.

Garfinkel, Paul E MD, FRCP(C), is Professor and Chair, Department of Psychiatry, University of Toronto, and President and CEO of the Centre for Addiction and Mental Health. He obtained his medical degree from the University of Manitoba and did a psychiatric residency at the University of Toronto, where he later joined the staff of the Clarke Institute of Psychiatry. In 1982, he was appointed Psychiatrist-in-Chief of the Toronto General Hospital and then of The Toronto Hospital. He is a Fellow of the Royal Society of Canada and has served as Visiting Professor in England, Ireland, Italy, and the United States. He is a researcher, particularly in the field of eating disorders, as well as a clinician and administrator.

Gelder, Michael DM(Oxon), FRCP, FRCPsych, is Emeritus Professor of Psychiatry, University of Oxford. He is a fellow of Merton College Oxford, a member of the Association of Physicians of Great Britain, a fellow of the Academy of Medical Sciences, and formerly a member of the Medical Research Council. He was Chairman, Oxford University Department of Psychiatry 1969–1997, and Joint Editor of the *Oxford Textbook of Psychiatry*.

Grob, Gerald N BSS, MA, PhD, is the Henry E Sigerist Professor of the History of Medicine, Rutgers University in New Brunswick, NJ. His speciality is the history of mental health policy. He has written more than 50 articles and has authored or edited more than a dozen volumes. His major work is a three-volume history of mental health policy [*Mental Institutions in America: Social Policy to 1875* (1973); *Mental Illness and American Society 1875–1940* (1983); and *From Asylum to Community: Mental Health Policy in Modern America* (1991)]. More recently, he published a one-volume comprehensive history entitled *The Mad Among Us: A History of the Care of America's Mentally Ill* (1994). He is an elected member of the Institute of Medicine of the National Academy of Sciences, and has held Guggenheim and other fellowships, as well as NIMH research grants.

Harris, Brian BSc, MB BS, FRCPsych, is Senior Lecturer and Consultant in General Psychiatry at the University of Wales College of Medicine, Cardiff. His main interest has been the hormonal associations of mood disorders, particularly those associated with the peripartum period. He has published major works concerning steroid hormones in saliva, and he has established associations between changes in progesterone and maternity blues. Current work includes continued validation of questionnaires for the detection of postnatal depression, particularly in the context of women who are positive for thyroid antibody status.

Healy, David MD, FRCPsych, is a Reader in Psychological Medicine and Director of the North Wales Department of Psychological Medicine, University of Wales College of Medicine. He is a clinical psychiatrist who has training in pharmacology and in research on monoamine reuptake systems. He is a former secretary of the British Association for Psychopharmacology, and has an established interest in the history of neuropsychopharmacology. He has published two volumes of interviews with eminent psychopharmacologists and scientists from the pharmaceutical industry, in addition to *The Antidepressant Era*, which is at present the only history of the antidepressants.

Henderson, John H MB ChB, FRCPsych, FFPHM, has been a Consultant Psychiatrist, Regional Officer for mental health, WHO Regional Office for Europe, and Regional Advisor for mental health, WHO South-East Asia Region. He is a member of the WHO Expert Panel on Mental Health. He was formerly Director of the European Commission Independent Team of Experts in Mental Health, and of Grants and Projects, for the Mental Health Foundation, UK.

Jackson, Mark BSc, MB BS, PhD, is Senior Lecturer, Centre for Medical History, University of Exeter. He trained in medicine in London, and then completed his doctoral dissertation on the history of infanticide in the eighteenth century. He was a Research Fellow at the Wellcome Unit for the History of Medicine in Manchester, before moving to the University of Exeter in 1998. He is the author of *Newborn Child Murder: Women, Illegitimacy and the Courts in Eighteenth-Century England* (1996) and numerous articles on infanticide. His recent research on the history of learning difficulties has produced articles, two edited volumes, and a monograph, *The Borderland of Imbecility: Medicine, Society, and the Fabrication of the Feeble Mind in Late Victorian and Edwardian England,* to be published in 2000.

Jolley, David MSc, MB BS, FRCPsych, is Consultant Psychiatrist and Medical Director for Wolverhampton Health Care NHS Trust and Professor of Old Age Psychiatry at Wolverhampton University. Qualifying from Guy's Hospital, London, he obtained postgraduate training in psychiatry in Manchester and established the first psychogeriatric service in the north-west of England. Generations of doctors and other health care workers learned the principles and joys of psychogeriatrics in that service and went on to create others. His move to Wolverhampton in 1995 was to redevelop community health services, including psychiatry and health care of the elderly, and postgraduate education. His research includes service delivery and evaluation, residential care, depression in late life, suicide, and other modes of death in old age.

Jones, Kathleen BA, PhD, Hon FRCPsych, is Emeritus Professor of Social Policy, University of York. She was the Head of the Department of Social Policy and Social Work, University of York, from 1965 to 1987. She is the author of *A History of the Mental Health Services* (1972); *Ideas on Institutions* (with AJ Fowles, 1984); *Experience in Mental Health* (1988); *The Making of Social Policy* (1991); and *Asylums and After* (1993).

Klein, Rachel G PhD, is Professor of Clinical Psychology (in Psychiatry), Columbia University, College of Physicians and Surgeons, and Director of Clinical Psychology, New York State Psychiatric Institute. She has undertaken research on childhood psychopathology and the clinical efficacy of psychotherapeutic and psychopharmacological interventions in children and adolescents. Her therapeutics research has spanned psychopathology, attention deficit hyperactivity disorder, conduct disorder, learning disorders, anxiety disorders, and major depression. Her interest in developmental psychopathology has led to longitudinal studies of children with separation anxiety disorder, and ADHD.

Lewis, Melvin MB BS, DCH, FRCPsych, is Professor of Child Psychiatry and Pediatrics, Yale Child Study Center, Yale University. He graduated from Guy's Hospital Medical School, London, and completed his psychiatric and child psychiatry training at Yale. He is also trained in psychoanalysis and joined the Yale faculty in 1961. He was Editor of the *Journal of the American Academy of Child and Adolescent Psychiatry* from 1975 to 1987, and is Editor of *Child and Adolescent Psychiatry: A Comprehensive Textbook,* now in its second edition (1996). He is also the Consulting Editor for *Child and Adolescent Psychiatric Clinics of North America* and co-author of *Clinical Aspects of Child and Adolescent Development* (1971), with Fred Volkmar, now in its third edition (1990).

Lieh Mak, Felice MD, FRCPsych, FRANZCP, FHKAM(Psych), FAPA, CBE, is Head and Chair Professor, Department of Psychiatry, The University of Hong Kong. She received her training in psychiatry in the UK. She has published widely on the cross-cultural aspects of child psychiatry and on schizophrenia. She was President of the World Psychiatric Association from 1993 to 1996. During her term, she strengthened the educational role of the Association and mobilised member societies in defence of the rights of the mentally ill. She was made an Honorary Fellow of the Royal College of Psychiatrists (UK) in 1994 and appointed Commander of the Order of the British Empire in 1997.

Likierman, Meira BA, PhD, PGCE, is a Senior Child Psychotherapist at the Tavistock Clinic, and an adult psychotherapist in private practice. She has taught psychoanalytic theory extensively in the UK and abroad, both on psychotherapy trainings and on university courses. She is currently spending a year designing and establishing an intensive psychotherapy module on the Psychodynamic Masters programme at the University of Oxford. She has published in major journals including the *International Journal of Psychoanalysis, International Review of Psychoanalysis, Journal of Child Psychotherapy,* and *British Journal of Psychotherapy.* She is currently completing a book on the development of Melanie Klein's thought for the Tavistock Clinic Book Series.

Lôo, Henri MD, is Head of the University Department of Mental Health and Therapeutics, Sainte-Anne Hospital and Professor of Psychiatry, University Paris V, Cochin Port-Royal Faculty of Medicine. He received his medical degree in Paris and was an interne des Hôpitaux de Paris and des Hôpitaux Psychiatriques de la Seine. He was appointed as an assistant to Professor Jean Delay and then Professor Pierre Deniker until becoming Associate Professor and then Professor of Psychiatry, focusing on drug addiction. With Deniker, he was amongst the first to elaborate the concept of pharmacopsychosis and the deficit syndrome of drug addicts. He has also worked in the field of psychopharmacology, particularly in the biology and clinical action of antidepressant drugs. He is the author of 15 books and many papers. He is an associate member of the Académie de Médecine and holder of the Légion d'Honneur.

McGuffin, Peter MB ChB, PhD, FRCP, FRCPsych, is Director of the Social Genetic and Developmental Psychiatry Research Centre, Institute of Psychiatry, London. He was previously Professor of Psychological Medicine at the University of Wales College of Medicine, Cardiff. He qualified in medicine at Leeds University and underwent postgraduate training in general medicine and psychiatry there before completing his psychiatric training at the Maudsley Hospital, London. He subsequently trained in genetics in London and at Washington University, St Louis, MO, USA.

Mayes, Linda C MD, is Arnold Gesell Associate Professor of Child Psychiatry, Pediatrics, and Psychology, and Coordinator of Early Childhood Services, Yale Child Study Center, Yale University. She is a graduate of the Western New England Institute for Psychoanalysis and principal investigator on a longitudinal study of high-risk children exposed prenatally to drugs.

Merskey, Harold DM(Oxon), FRCP, FRCPsych, FRCP(C), Professor Emeritus in Psychiatry at the University of Western Ontario, London, Canada, graduated at Oxford and trained principally at the University of Sheffield. He was Consultant Psychiatrist at the National Hospitals for Nervous Diseases, London (UK) and then at the London Psychiatric Hospital, London, Ontario. He has published widely on psychiatric and other aspects of chronic pain, and with N Bogduk, edited the *Classification of Chronic Pain Syndromes.* His interests in mind/body relationships led to the publication of *Analysis of Hysteria* (second edition, 1995). He serves on the Scientific Advisory Board of the False Memory Syndrome Foundation.

Millard, David W MA, MD, FRCPsych, is Emeritus Fellow, Green College, Oxford and Consultant in Old Age Psychiatry, Oxfordshire Mental Healthcare NHS Trust. Dr Millard qualified from the University of Birmingham and has been a Consultant Psychiatrist since 1966. For about 20 years, he was a lecturer in applied social studies at the University of Oxford. From 1983 to 1991, he edited the *International Journal of Therapeutic Communities.*

Mumford, David Bardwell MD, MPhil, MA, MRCPsych, is Consultant Psychiatrist, Senior Lecturer in Psychiatry, and Director of Medical Education, University of Bristol. He has published papers on somatic symptoms associated with anxiety and depression; on eating disorders in Pakistan and among Pakistanis in Britain; on culture shock among British volunteers working abroad; and on translation methods in cross-cultural studies. In collaboration with colleagues in Pakistan, Dr Mumford undertook a series of community-based epidemiological surveys of psychiatric morbidity — in mountain villages in the Hindu Kush, in rural Punjab, and in urban Rawalpindi. He is the principal author of the Bradford Somatic Inventory and of the Culture Shock Questionnaire.

Musto, David F MA, MD, is Professor of Child Psychiatry and History of Medicine, Yale Child Study Center, Yale University. He is a graduate of the University of Washington School of Medicine and completed his graduate work in history and residency in psychiatry at Yale. He later served as Special Assistant to the Director of the National Institute of Mental Health. In addition to the history of psychiatry, he is an authority on the history of drugs and alcohol, and is the author of *The American Disease: Origins of Narcotic Control* (1999), now in its third edition.

Newton, Jennifer BA, MA, PhD, is Senior Lecturer in Community Care, University of North London. Through the 1980s, she worked for MIND (the National Association for Mental Health), reviewing literature and practice relating to prevention, and publishing *Preventing Mental Illness* (1988) and *Preventing Mental Illness in Practice* (1992). She recently completed a multi-site evaluation of the implementation of community care policy in England on behalf of the Sainsbury Centre for Mental Health — *Care Management: Is It Working?* (1996), and an evaluation of a befriending scheme for people with serious mental health problems. She was Chair of the Good Practices in Mental Health Organisation for five years.

Nolan, Peter W PhD, MA, RMN, RGN, RNT, is Senior Lecturer, School of Health Sciences, University of Birmingham. He undertook psychiatric nursing training in London, and has subsequently worked throughout the UK and also in Sudan, Libya, and Egypt. He currently collaborates with psychiatric nurses in the USA, Ireland, Sweden, France, and Latvia. He has been studying the history of psychiatric nursing in different parts of the world for over 20 years and has written extensively on the subject. His present research interest focuses on observing the transition of psychiatric nursing from traditional mental health care settings into primary care.

O'Brien, Laurence Stephen MB ChB, MRCPsych, is Clinical Director of Mental Health Services, Aintree Hospitals (NHS) Trust, Liverpool. He trained in psychiatry with the British Armed Forces, developing a special interest in the effect of trauma on mental health. After running the British Army's principal Psychiatric Treatment Unit in Saudi Arabia during the Gulf War, he was in charge of the Army's principal In-Patient Treatment Unit and responsible for its psychiatric training. Since leaving the Army, he has continued an interest in post-traumatic mental health problems and published a book on it. He is currently Clinical Director of a busy urban mental health service and consultant to a sub-regional alcohol treatment unit.

O'Dwyer, Anne-Marie MB, MRCPsych, MRCP, has worked in behavioural and cognitive psychotherapy, and is Consultant Psychiatrist at the Bethlem Royal and Maudsley Hospitals. Her clinical interests include obsessive–compulsive disorder and anxiety disorders, and her research interests span neurobiology and the psychotherapy of anxiety disorders.

Okasha, Ahmed MD, FRCP, FRCPsych, is Professor of Psychiatry, Founder and Chairman, Institute of Psychiatry, Ain Shams University, Cairo, Egypt. He is the Director of the WHO Collaborating Center for Mental Health in Cairo, a Member of the Executive Committee and Secretary for Sections of the World Psychiatric Association, the Chairman of the Ethics Committee of the WPA, and President of the Egyptian Psychiatric Association. He is a member of the editorial boards of many national and international psychiatry journals, and has published more than 200 original papers, and edited and contributed to 25 books in Arabic and English. His main interests are transcultural, epidemiological, and biological psychiatry.

Olié, Jean-Pierre MD, is Head of the Department of Psychiatry, Sainte-Anne Hospital and Medical School Cochin, Paris and Professor of Psychiatry at University Paris V. He was awarded the Prix Jocelyne Chedoudi by the Medical National Academy for research on mood disorders in 1985. He is a member of the Scientific Board of the Society Medico-Psychologique, and is Editor of *l'Encephale*.

Peters, Uwe Henrik MD, is Emeritus Professor of Psychiatry, University of Cologne.

Pichot, Pierre MD, is Honorary Professor of Psychiatry, Paris University Medical School, and a member of the French National Academy of Medicine. After completing his medical studies at the Paris Medical School and psychology studies at the Sorbonne, Professor Pichot worked from 1948 with Professor Delay at Sainte-Anne Hospital, Paris. In 1955 he became Associate Professor of Psychiatry, in 1965 was given a Chair of Medical Psychology, and in 1970, succeeded Professor Delay as Head of the Department of Psychiatry. From 1948 to 1968, he also had teaching positions in psychopathology at the Sorbonne. He is Doctor honoris causa of the Universities of Munich, Barcelona, and Thessaloniki, and of New York Medical College. He is also a corresponding or honorary member of numerous scientific societies and, from 1977 to 1983, was President of the World Psychiatric Association. His works include several books and numerous publications related to clinical psychology, psychopathology, psychopharmacology, and the history of psychiatry. His main research fields have been quantitative psychopathology techniques and statistical methods.

Pines, Malcolm MB ChB(Cantab), FRCP, FRCPsych, was formerly a Consultant Psychotherapist at several teaching hospitals in London, and is currently in private group analytic practice. His postgraduate training was at the Maudsley Hospital and at the London Institute of Psychoanalysis. At the Cassel Hospital, he developed an interest in in-patient psychotherapy and therapeutic community. Moving to St George's Hospital, he had the opportunity to introduce group psychotherapy to the in-patient unit and to begin working with large groups. He subsequently taught and supervised at the Maudsley Hospital and the Tavistock Clinic. He helped to found the Institute of Group Analysis, London, and to strengthen the work of the International Association of Group Psychotherapy, of which he is a past President. Currently, he is Editor of the *Journal of Group Analysis* and of *The International Library of Group Analysis*. He has published a book *Circular Reflections* (1998), and some collected papers as *Secular Reflections*.

Ritson, Bruce MD, FRCPsych, FRCP, is Consultant at the Alcohol Problems Clinic, Royal Edinburgh Hospital and Senior Lecturer, Department of Psychiatry, The University of Edinburgh. He is the current Chairman of the UK Medical Council on Alcoholism and Coordinator of the European WHO project concerning the community response to alcohol and related problems, and was the past Chair of the Faculty of Addiction Psychiatry at the Royal College of Psychiatrists. His work has included the development and evaluation of alcohol treatment services, and he is the author of numerous articles and books on the prevention and treatment of alcohol problems, and cross-national studies.

Scott, Jan MD, FRCPsych, has recently taken up the post of Professor and Head of Department of Psychiatry at the University of Glasgow. She has research interests into psychosocial interventions in severe mental disorders, particularly chronic depression and treatment-resistant bipolar disorders. She trained at the Cognitive Therapy Center in Philadelphia in 1984 and helped to establish the first British Diploma Course in Cognitive Therapy, at Newcastle upon Tyne. She is currently principal investigator on a multi-centre Medical Research Council clinical trial of cognitive therapy for people with bipolar disorders, and continues to explore integrated psychobiosocial models of causality of severe disorders.

Scull, Andrew BA, MA, PhD, is Professor of Sociology, University of California, San Diego. Born in Scotland, he was educated at Oxford and Princeton. He has been a Guggenheim Fellow and an American Council of Learned Societies Fellow, and served as President of the Society for the Social History of Medicine. His research has ranged widely over the history of Anglo-American psychiatry, from the eighteenth century to the present, and his many books include: *Museums of Madness* (1979); *Madhouses, Mad-Doctors and Madmen*

(1981, ed.); *Decarceration* (1977, and second edition 1984); *Social Order/Mental Disorder* (1989); *The Most Solitary of Afflictions: Madness and Society in Britain, 1700–1900* (1993); and *Masters of Bedlam: The Transformation of the Mad-Doctoring Trade* (1997, with Nicholas Hervey and Charlotte Mackenzie).

Sengoopta, Chandak MA, MB BS, MDPsych, PhD, is Medical Historian (Social History), Wellcome Institute for the History of Medicine, London. After qualifying in medicine and psychiatry, he trained in the history of science and medicine at Johns Hopkins University, USA. He currently teaches two courses on the history of psychiatry at the Wellcome Institute and University College London, and is writing a monograph on the cultural history of sexual and behavioural endocrinology. He has published widely on the historical links between medical and cultural concepts of masculinity and femininity, most recently in *History of Psychiatry* and *Isis*.

Shearer, Ann MA(Cantab), is a Jungian analyst in private practice. She is a member of the Independent Group of Analytical Psychologists, London, and has been Chairwoman of the International Association for Analytical Psychology. After reading history at Cambridge, she worked as a journalist on *The Guardian*, and as a freelancer; she was also an international consultant on social aspects of disability. Her books include: *Disability: Whose Handicap?* (1981), *Woman: Her Changing Image* (1987), *Athene: Image and Energy* (1996) and (co-edited with Jane Haynes) *When a Princess Dies* (1998), essays by Jungian analysts on reaction to the death of Diana, Princess of Wales.

Shephard, Ben BA, read History at Oxford University and has made numerous historical and scientific documentaries for television. Since turning to medical history, he has published papers on Maghull Hospital in the First World War (in *150 Years of British Psychiatry*, Volume 2. *The Aftermath*, 1996), 'shell-shock' on the Somme, British military psychiatry 1939–1945, and the rehabilitation of Prisoners of War after 1945. He also reviews for *The Times Literary Supplement*. His history of military psychiatry, provisionally entitled *Wounds of War*, will be published in 2000.

Shorter, Edward PhD, FRSC, has held the Hannah Chair in the History of Medicine at the University of Toronto's Faculty of Medicine since 1991. In 1996, he was cross-appointed as Professor of Psychiatry for his contributions as a historian of this discipline. His various research interests have culminated in the publication of over a dozen books, a two-volume history of psychosomatic medicine: *From Paralysis to Fatigue* (1992) and *From the Mind into the Body* (1994), and *A History of Psychiatry from the Era of the Asylum to the Age of Prozac* (1997). In 1995, in addition to being elected a Fellow of the Royal Society of Canada, he was awarded the Jason A Hannah Medal for *From Paralysis to Fatigue*. In 1997 he received a Humboldt Research Prize from the Humboldt Foundation in Bonn, Germany.

Snowden, Pete MB ChB, BSc, FRCPsych, is Consultant Forensic Psychiatrist to the Mental Health Services of Salford NHS Trust, and Honorary Clinical Lecturer in Forensic Psychiatry, University of Manchester. He qualified in medicine at the University of Liverpool, where he also obtained a degree in biochemistry. He then trained in forensic psychiatry in Manchester, where he is based at a medium-secure unit. He is currently Chair of the Forensic Faculty, Royal College of Psychiatrists. He was appointed to the Advisory Board on Restricted Patients in 1997, and is an adviser to the Department of Health on forensic psychiatry. His main interests are in service development, clinical risk assessment and management, and the history of forensic psychiatry.

Stanton, Martin DPhil(Oxon), BA, is a clinical staff member at the Tavistock Marital Studies Institute, and works in private practice as a psychoanalytic psychotherapist with individuals and couples. In 1985, he founded, and is the Director of the Centre for Psychoanalytic Studies at the University of Kent at Canterbury, and pioneered the first British MA course in psychoanalytic studies there. He chairs the Universities Association for Psychoanalytic Studies. His publications include *Outside the Dream* (1983), *Sandor Ferenczi* (1991), and *Out of Order: Clinical Work and Unconscious Process* (1998).

Tansella, Michele MD, is Specialist in Nervous and Mental Diseases, Professor of Psychiatry and Director of the Postgraduate School in Psychiatry, University of Verona. He is also Head of the South-Verona Community-Based Mental Health Service (WHO Collaborating Centre for Research and Training in Mental Health and Service Evaluation). He graduated in medicine at the University of Bari and then worked in the Section of Psychopharmacology at the Mario Negri Institute, Milan, and at the Institute of Psychiatry, London in the General Practice Research Unit. His main research interests are epidemiological psychiatry, including service evaluation, evaluation of outcome and costs of mental disorders, and mental disorders in primary care settings.

Tantam, Digby MA, MPH, PhD, FRCPsych, is Clinical Professor of Psychotherapy, and Director of the Centre for the Study of Violence, University of Sheffield, as well as Associate Medical Director of the School of Health and Related Research. He trained in behavioural sciences at Harvard University, has a degree in mathematics and philosophy, and has been a general psychiatrist with a special interest in rehabilitation and responsibility for the intensive care ward, a professor in a psychology department, the psychiatrist to the University of Warwick, and a consultant psychotherapist. He is a practising group analytic psychotherapist and a professional member of the American Group Psychotherapy Association. He has a special interest in Asperger syndrome, and has published widely.

Tomov, Toma MD, PhD, is Head of the Department of Psychiatry, Medical University, Sofia, and Co-Director of the Bulgarian Institute for Human Relations, New Bulgarian University, Sofia. He graduated from the Medical School in Sofia, and is now a family and group therapist. He was formerly a WHO consultant for the Tanzanian Mental Health programme for four years. He has published in both English and Bulgarian in the field of epidemiological and community psychiatry, psychiatric disability, and post-traumatic stress disorders. He has focussed on the adverse effects of paternalistic social arrangements on mental health, and total control social systems, with emphasis on the traumatic aspects of human interactions, which are guided by group and community norms derived from values instigated by parochialism, social isolation, ethnic hatred, and racism. He is a member of over a dozen professional and other bodies, including the Bulgarian Psychiatric Association, the Bulgarian Association of Social Workers, and the Bulgarian Association of Psychotherapy and Psychological Counselling.

Turner, Trevor Howard BA, MD, FRCPsych, DHMSA, is Consultant Psychiatrist and Clinical Director of R&D, Homerton and St Bartholomew's Hospitals, London. He is also Honorary Senior Lecturer, St Bartholomew's and the Royal London School of Medicine, Queen Mary and Westfield College, University of London. He completed a classics degree, before qualifying in medicine at St Bartholomew's Hospital. After psychiatric training at The Maudsley Hospital, including a research lectureship at the Institute of Psychiatry, he was appointed Consultant Psychiatrist at Barts and Hackney Hospitals, and then Medical Director of the City and Hackney Community Services NHS Trust. His MD thesis was based on a study of Victorian psychiatric casebooks. He is Chairman of the North Thames Division of the Royal College of Psychiatrists. His research interests include the history of psychiatry, the treatment of severe mental illness, the special problems of the inner city, and the development of community-orientated services.

Vaughn, Christine BA, MSc, PhD, is an attached worker and Consultant Research Psychologist at the Social Psychiatry Section, Institute of Psychiatry, London. She is an American born, London-based psychologist, educated at Stanford University and the University of London, who has had a long association with the MRC Social Psychiatry Unit. She has also held positions with the Salford Health Authority in Manchester (UK), the Clinical Research Center for the Study of Schizophrenia in Camarillo, California, and the University of California at Los Angeles. She has led residential training courses in the use of the Camberwell Family Interview and related expressed emotion scales, and to date has trained more than 400 clinicians and researchers from 35 countries. Currently, she is collaborating with Professor Robert Liberman on a family assessment interview manual for clinicians.

Weber, Matthias M MD, is Psychiatric Consultant and Head of the Historical Archives, Max-Planck-Institute of Psychiatry, Munich. He studied at the University of Munich. He has published several articles on the history of German psychiatry, and is currently preparing a research project on the life and work of Emil Kraepelin.

Whitrow, Magda BA, ALA, is Austrian by birth, but has lived in England for over 60 years. She is an honours graduate of the University of London. After a number of years in charge of special libraries and editing specialist periodicals, she became editor of the *Isis Cumulative Bibliography for the History of Science, Medicine and Technology* (1913–65) (published in six volumes from 1971 to 1984). In recognition of this, she was made an honorary member of the Académie Internationale d'Histoire des Sciences and received the Walford Award from the Library Association. She then took up research into the history of psychiatry and wrote a biography of Julius Wagner-Jauregg (1857–1940), published in 1993.

Wilkinson, David Gregor BSc, MB ChB, M Phil, FRCP, FRCPsych, is Professor of Liaison Psychiatry, and Honorary Consultant in Psychiatry, The University of Liverpool, where he has clinical responsibilities for patients, teaching medical students, training doctors, and undertaking research on mental health problems. He has undertaken research on medical aspects of civilian trauma. He is also an elected Officer of The Royal College of Psychiatrists, and edits the *British Journal of Psychiatry*. He has published a number of books and articles on stress and on various psychiatric topics, and is the joint Editor of a major British text book on general adult psychiatry, published in 1998.

Wing, John K CBE, MD, PhD, FRCPsych, spent much of his career as Director of the Medical Research Council's Social Psychiatry Research Unit at the Institute of Psychiatry in London. In 1989, he set up a new Research Unit for the Royal College of Psychiatrists. His work in social and epidemiological psychiatry included the International Pilot Study of Schizophrenia; cohort studies of hospitals and districts with different methods of care; use (with Lorna Wing) for epidemiological research of one of the first psychiatric district registers; detailed studies and tests of rehabilitation methods; creating a long series of pioneering instruments ranging from the Present State Examination (now expanded as 'SCAN' but with phenomenology intact) to the 12-item HoNOS. He is currently working on an epidemiologically-based needs assessment of psychiatric services in England.

Wing, Lorna MD, FRCPsych, is Consultant Psychiatrist, National Autistic Society. She was a member of the Medical Research Council's Social Psychiatry Unit from 1964 to 1990. She set up the Camberwell Register of psychiatric illness and learning disability for use in epidemiological studies, examined the effects on the residents of the closure of a hospital for adults with learning disabilities, and developed the concept of a spectrum of autistic disorders. She now works part-time at the Centre for Social and Communication Disorders and is developing methods of diagnosis and assessment of autistic and related disorders.

CONTENTS

1981–1990 Chapter 9 **New Scientific Paradigms** 287

The early *1900*s & before. . .

Chapter 1
The Century Begins

Major world events

1900 Inaugural airship flight by Ferdinand Von Zeppelin (Germany)
1901 Death of Queen Victoria (Great Britain)
1901 Hopkins (Great Britain) isolated the first amino acid
1903 Pierre et Marie Curie (France) received the Nobel Prize for Physics together with Henry Becquerel (France)
1905 Revolt on board the battleship Potemkin (Russia)
1907 Rudyard Kipling (Great Britain) received the Nobel Prize for Literature
1909 Selig (USA) produced *The Count of Monte-Cristo*, the first Hollywood film

Major events in psychiatry

1896 Emil Kraepelin initiated a series of monographs, *Psychologische Arbeiten*; nine volumes were subsequently to appear
1899 Sigmund Freud's *Die Traumdeutung (The Interpretation of Dreams)* published in Vienna
1900 Jung became an assistant at the Burghölzli mental hospital in Zurich, under Eugen Bleuler
1900 Karl Wernicke published his *Grundriss de Psychiatrie (Basic Psychiatry)* in Leipzig
1901 Sigmund Freud's *Zur psychopathologie des alltagslebens (The Psychopathology of Everyday Life)* first published in Vienna
1902 Charles Mercier published his *Textbook of Insanity* in London
1903 Barbituric acid, the original compound of the barbiturates, synthesised
1903 The first volume of *Archives of Neurology and Psychiatry* appeared in the USA
1904 Freud's *The Psychopathology of Everyday Life* published in Vienna
1905 The spirochaete organism causing syphilis was identified, but only isolated in cases of general paralysis of the insane in 1913
1905 Sigmund Freud's *Drie abhandlungen zur sexual theorie (Three Essays on the Theory of Sexuality)* published in Vienna
1905 Jung's *Word Diagnostic Association Studies* published in Zurich
1905 Wassermann developed his complement fixation test, and published it in 1906
1907 Alfred Adler's *Study of Organ Inferiority and its Psychical Compensation* published
1907 First International Congress of Psychiatry and Neurology in Amsterdam
1908 Eugen Bleuler coined the term 'schizophrenia'
1908 Clifford Beers, the earliest and possibly best known reformer this century, published *A Mind that Found Itself* in the USA
1909 The first Juvenile Psychopathic Clinic established in Chicago
1909 Freud published the case of *Little Hans*, in Vienna
1909 Serieux and Capgras, in Paris, described the "chronic interpretative delusional state" which "developed gradually in vulnerable individuals"
1910 Adolf Meyer became Professor of Psychiatry, Johns Hopkins University, USA
1910 Paul Ehrlich's 'Salvarsan' came into use in Germany
1910 Sigmund Freud's *Uber psychoanalyse (Five Lectures in Psychoanalysis)* published in Vienna

THE EARLY 1900s & BEFORE...

by Trevor Turner

"The position of the psychiatrist around 1900 was not a particularly happy one. Although he was better able to classify the psychoses and predict their outcome than his predecessors a century before, he still suffered from the same ignorance of the causes of mental illness and he still had to be content with the same miserable methods of treatment. If he worked in an institution or a clinic he saw only severe and hopeless psychoses, and although anatomy and physiology had been so helpful to his medical colleagues, they had failed to teach him anything about the nature of these illnesses except in the case of general paresis. His patients were prisoners, and in a way he himself was a prisoner caught up in the difficulties of the field in which he had chosen to work".

Thus wrote Erwin H Ackerknecht, in 1959, in his *Short History of Psychiatry*, in a chapter entitled 'From neurology to psychoanalysis', and the general perception of the 1900s, as outlined by most psychiatric historians, has been of a nadir leading to a renaissance. Alexander and Selesnick, in their 1966 *History of Psychiatry*, writing from "the vantage point of our present dynamic era", referred to "the Freudian age". Gregory Zilboorg (with George Henry) in 1941 had produced *A History of Medical Psychology* that trumpeted "the second psychiatric revolution". He also denounced "the psychology offered by descriptive psychiatry" as "not science", and described the era preceding the introduction of psychoanalysis as "brain mythology". To Zilboorg, "medical and psychological theories" around 1900 appeared to have become "more an intellectual pastime than a search for the practical solution of a problem", while therapy in psychiatry was "not even empirical, still less... causal". For him psychiatry was "in a rut of the past", that lagged far behind general medicine, in terms of intellectual zest or creative thinking, let alone scientific recognition or public respect.

Fin de siècle

Yet if one considers the richly documented world of the *fin de siècle*, as in Barbara Tuchman's 1966 *The Proud Tower*, it is a time almost legendary in its wealth of artistic and scientific changes. Tolstoy and Zola were still writing; Ibsen was introducing his 'new drama'; Oscar Wilde, George Bernard Shaw, and Henry James were to the forefront of the English-language tradition. Sherlock Holmes was emerging from the pen of Sir Arthur Conan Doyle, a canon of work full of psychological as well as medical insights, and there was even a psychiatrist as hero. This was Dr John Seward "the lunatic-asylum man, with the strong jaw and good forehead", to be found in Bram Stoker's novel, *Dracula* (1897), recording his diary on a phonograph and partaking in the final decapitation of the Count.

In 1895 came the death of Louis Pasteur, the leading light of the germ theory of infection, and emblematic of an extraordinary range of discoveries — Koch's postulates formalised in 1882 and, roughly speaking, a new 'germ' isolated every year for the past 20 years. This highlighted the failure to establish any definite pathogen for a mental illness. The spirochaete organism causing syphilis was identified in 1905, but only isolated in cases of GPI (general paralysis of the insane) in 1913. The continuing aetiological, diagnostic, and therapeutic dilemmas of the psychiatric profession, by contrast with the heroic advances in medicine and surgery, seemed dusty and repetitive.

Also in 1895, KW Röntgen (1845–1923) produced his X-ray machine, the Lumière brothers began showing moving pictures to the public in Paris, and Sigmund Freud (Chapter 2, p. 47) and Joseph Breuer (1842–1925) published their studies on hysteria. By 1910, a psychoanalytic circle in Vienna was well established, with Carl Gustav Jung (1875–1961) and Alfred Adler (1870–1937) still adherents. In other aspects of life, neon lights and electric washing machines were being introduced, and Marie Curie had published her treatise on radioactivity. The nuclear age may even be said to have begun since Ernest Rutherford (1871–1937) had presented his theory of the atom to a meeting of the Manchester Literary and Philosophical Society.

The psychiatric zeitgeist

While the first decade of the 1900s, therefore, has often been hidden between the high tide of late Victorian invention and expansion, and the new twentieth-century world created by the Great War, it is nevertheless illustrative of the organisation, problems, and potential of psychiatric practice. Faced with the rising numbers in asylums, fuelled by 'degeneration theory' and its offspring, eugenics, yet trying to embrace the rising demand for 'nerve clinics' and the fashionable speciality of neurology, psychiatry worked hard at developing an academic edge. This was particularly so in central Europe — in German and Austro-Hungarian universities — but research laboratories were also springing up in France, the UK, and the USA. Numerous textbooks and journals informed a better understanding of the speciality, while international congresses occurred almost every other year. A veritable century of psychology seemed to beckon.

To understand this period one must review the underlying zeitgeist, in terms of both the broader historical trends and the considerable social and scientific changes in the way people lived their lives. Only against this background is it possible to assess the central roles of, e.g. Emil Kraepelin (1856–1926) (Chapter 2, p. 49), Pierre Janet (1859–1947) (Chapter 4, p. 99), and (in a later decade), Julius Wagner-Jauregg (1857–1940) (Chapter 3, p. 74). The problem of dealing with 'nerves' should be considered in relation to the fashionable term 'neurasthenia', patients' perspectives, the ordinary doctor's understanding of psychological problems, and the rivalries (especially Anglo-German) in national approaches. These reflected the long period of peace that Europe had enjoyed, with only the brief eruption in Europe of the Franco-Prussian War (1870). Although scientific research was fundamental to the work of clinics and laboratories, the popularity of spiritualism and mysticism was, however, just as pronounced.

In a short story, *The Leather Funnel*, published in 1900, Sir Arthur Conan Doyle discussed "the psychology of dreams". One character denounces this as "a science of charlatans", but is met with the following answer. "The charlatan is always the pioneer. From the astrologer came the astronomer, from the alchemist the chemist, from the mesmerist the experimental psychologist. The quack of yesterday is the professor of tomorrow. Even such subtle and elusive things as dreams will in time be reduced to system and order. When the time comes the researches of our friends... will no longer be the amusement of the mystic but the foundations of a science". It is no surprise, therefore, that Sigmund Freud's *Interpretation of Dreams* (*Die Traumdeutung*), published in 1900, should have found a fertile soil in which to be recognised. It was widely and favourably reviewed over the next two years, despite needing six more years to sell its first print-run of 600 copies! In Freud's lifetime, there were to be eight variously revised editions. On the other hand, *Logische Untersuchungen* (1900–1) by Edmund Husserl (1854–1938), founder of the phenomenological school, had little impact at the time.

The historical background

Kraepelin in Britain

In his *Memoirs*, Emil Kraepelin (Chapter 2, p. 49) gives a fascinating description of his visits to Britain and France, and of the world of an academic psychiatrist just before the turn of the century. During the "long holidays" in 1889, he and his wife travelled from Dorpat in Estonia (where he was then professor), to Hamburg and Göttingen, before attending the annual meeting of German psychiatrists in Jena, where he lectured on "measurements of fatigue". They were then able to go on to Italy, visiting Lago di Guarda, Parma, Bologna, Ravenna, and Florence. They went on to Naples, Capri, and Sorrento, returned via Venice to Innsbruck, visiting brother-in-law and brother, and then back to Dorpat.

In the following summer (1890), Kraepelin visited England with a colleague. On the way, he attended a meeting of Eastern German psychiatrists, and Karl Kahlbaum (1828–1899) and Carl Wernicke (1848–1905) also appeared there. Travelling on via friends in Dresden, visiting the great psychologist Wundt in Leipzig and passing through Belgium, he then stayed in London. However, he "thoroughly disliked the city and the way of life with its endless, uniform rows of houses, its lack of beautiful buildings and views, its confusing masses of people, its dull air, monotonous, tasteless cuisine and bleak Sundays". He did enjoy the National Gallery and the British Museum, and was delighted to visit Sir Francis Galton (1822–1911), "a fine old gentleman, who had stimulated the field of psychology without having had any real contact with this particular branch of science".

Kraepelin then mentions that he attended a lecture given by Dr (later Sir) George Savage (1842–1921) — an eminent English alienist who in 1904 was to treat the novelist Virginia Woolf — at "the old mental asylum Bethlem, which I had visited only a short time previously". Kraepelin was rather negative about this, feeling that 'Bedlam' did not have much to offer, and that "our highly esteemed bed treatment was completely rejected here". More disapprovingly, he noted that Savage gave a lecture to students, in which "the most important symptoms were only briefly mentioned". It seems that Savage then "narrated his experiences with paralytics in a most amusing manner, but without especial emphasis on the clinical and medical aspects". Since Kraepelin also found the English theatre disappointing, and only the "somewhat gross and dominating boorish scenes were excellently acted" in Shakespeare plays, and that in England "the ridiculous is not considered the ridiculous", there was certainly a difference in cultural expectation. He contrasted this, however, with the behaviour of the French, "who are very sensitive in such matters".

Kraepelin in Europe

Subsequently, Kraepelin left "the noisy, foggy city of London", spent four days on a walking tour in North Wales, and then departed for France. He enjoyed his stay in Paris, noticing "a certain similarity between life here and life in the large Italian cities, although everything seemed to be more elegant and more cultivated in Paris". He then called on a number of professionals, obviously looking for a professorial chair (he mentions Heidelberg and Tübingen), and discussed the design of psychiatric clinics, noting that, "usually one or two rooms at the most were allotted for scientific activity in the psychiatric institution". He went on to an International Medical Congress in Berlin, "where I gave a lecture on the mental effects of alcohol and tea".

To Kraepelin, the French clinician Valentin Magnan (1835–1916), the leading contemporary theorist of degeneration, was "the most interesting person there"; his "talk on circular insanity" was particularly mentioned. When Kahlbaum "wanted to banish alcoholics to an island to keep them away from alcohol", the chairman Wilhelm Erb (1840–1921) (of 'Erb's paralysis' fame) asked whether "someone had an island for this purpose?". From such conversations with colleagues, Kraepelin also learned that "an appointment to Heidelberg was within the realms of possibility" — and so it proved to be.

Behind all this travel and networking, however, there was a world of illness. Kraepelin's second daughter died in February 1890, aged 18 months "within a couple of days, of nasal diphtheria"; he had to send his other daughter away "to protect her from infection". He was thus not unhappy to leave Dorpat, in 1891, but was delayed because his daughter then became ill with "a purulent inflammation of the ear". Held up from sea travel because of drift ice, they had to make "the long and cumbersome journey to Germany with the small children by train". His son then became ill, with glandular swellings on the back of his neck, which probably originated "from an earlier post-vaccinal infection". Sadly, the boy subsequently died "from a fast-developing septicaemia, which I also caught". Kraepelin reports, however, that "Heidelberg's magnificent landscape and the new, satisfying sphere of activity in Germany helped us slowly overcome the difficult beginning".

With regard to his work, he found his clinic in Heidelberg "splendidly equipped", but taking in large numbers of admissions. He enjoyed giving instruction, and was surrounded by "distinguished men". Since he did not have to examine students, had no private practice, and "did not do any hypnotism", "a lot of time was left over for my scientific work". Kraepelin also had to pay his respects to the Grand Duke Friedrich, and was impressed with the Duke's interest in psychiatry. He was less impressed, however, with his first assistant at the clinic in Heidelberg, a Dr Schoenthal, who apparently had "outstanding clinical talent, but unfortunately he was a psychopath and committed suicide, apparently because he was afraid of becoming mentally ill".

Nevertheless, Kraepelin carried on with his aim of classifying "the clinical pictures", keeping "Kahlbaum's and Hecker's ideas in mind", and differentiating between "dementia praecox, which essentially corresponded with hebephrenia, and dementia paranoides with hallucinations, which quickly developed into mental deficiency". He admitted that "a profuse group of all kinds of insanity was left over, and was simply characterised by the content and origin of the delusion". These were his conclusions, as summarised in the fourth edition of his textbook (September 1893), although his ideas were to change over succeeding editions during the early 1900s.

A world of new inventions

The world portrayed by Kraepelin is therefore one of a relatively small but established psychiatric profession, extending throughout Europe, with academic centres, annual meetings, over-crowded asylums, earnest students, and aspiring assistants. In terms of the relationships and day-to-day activities of the leading practitioners, it was perhaps not very different from the world of the late twentieth century. It was also a world dominated by the notion of 'progress', with a burgeoning scientific and industrial complex, and new drugs regularly coming on the market. Thus, Bayer Chemicals introduced their 'Aspirin' brand in 1899, and Paul Ehrlich's 'Salvarsan' came into use in 1910. In the USA, the 1906

Food and Drug Act (FDA) represented the introduction of State concern with new therapeutics, and thus initiated the licensing process that has become so well known to pharmaceutical companies in the modern era.

In terms of background science, apart from the isolation during the 1880s of the bacteria causing common diseases, such as tuberculosis, cholera, and diphtheria, there had been a phenomenal growth in applying chemistry to industry. This was especially the case in Germany, which took the lead in the development of pharmaceutical products. In other countries, JJ Thomson at Cambridge (1856–1940) discovered the electron in 1897, and in 1898, Martinus Beijerinck (1851–1931), working in Amsterdam, described a filterable virus as causing tobacco mosaic disease. In the same year, Marie Curie (1867–1934) and Pierre Curie (1859–1906) in Paris described radioactivity ('Uranium rays'), while a year later, Lord Rutherford described alpha and beta rays — two different forms of radioactivity.

The year 1900, considered by some medical writers as the last year of the old century rather than the first of the new, saw the deaths of influential figures as diverse as John Ruskin (1819–1900), Friedrich Nietzsche (1844–1900), and Oscar Wilde (1856–1900). JM Browning began manufacturing his revolver, Count von Zeppelin started flying his air machines, the first gramophone records were marketed, and there was a rediscovery, by accident, of the genetic work of the Moravian monk, Gregor Mendel (1822–1884). This work had originally been published in the 1850s and 1860s, but ignored then. Also, Max Planck (1858–1947) read his outline paper on quantum theory.

During the next 10 years, the hormone adrenaline was isolated, Guglielmo Marconi (1874–1937) transmitted telegraphic radio messages from Cornwall to Newfoundland, Ronald Ross (1857–1932) won the Nobel Prize for medicine for his work on malaria, Willem Einthoven (1860–1927) invented a form of electrocardiograph, and Albert Einstein (1879–1955) formulated the special theory of relativity (1905). More notoriously, 'Typhoid Mary' was found and incarcerated, the plastic age began with the first commercial manufacture of Bakelite, and Halley's comet returned (1910), with apparently a brisk sale of 'comet pills' in the USA to ward off the poisonous gases thought to be in the comet's tail.

New ideas, new movements

In terms of literature, the theatre, and arts, the first decade of the twentieth century continued to provide material of interest to the psychiatrist. Anton Chekhov (who was medically qualified) produced the plays *Uncle Vanya* (1900) and *Three Sisters* (1902), before dying in 1904. Joseph Conrad wrote *Lord Jim* (1900), *Youth* (1902), *Nostromo* (1904), and *The Secret Agent* (1907). Rudyard Kipling, Thomas Mann (e.g. *Buddenbrooks*, 1901), Strindberg, Wedekind, Maxim Gorki, Samuel Butler, Henry James, George Bernard Shaw, Theodore Herzl, Jack London, Herman Hesse, Edith Wharton, Anatole France, JM Synge, and Arthur Schnitzler were all writing and publishing. In painting, Picasso moved from his blue to his pink period, and artists as diverse as Paul Cézanne, Henri Matisse, Claude Monet, Edvard Munch, Pierre August Renoir, Henri Toulouse-Lautrec, Paul Gaugin, Henri Rousseau, John Singer Sargeant, Augustus John, Pierre Bonnard, Marc Chagall, Wassily Kandinsky, and Kasimir Malevich were all in their heyday. Composers were equally varied, with Edward Elgar, Richard Strauss, Leos Janacek, Giacomo Puccini, Jean Sibelius, Frederick Delius, Franz Lehar, Gustav Mahler, and Arnold Schoenberg (amongst of course many others) producing new works and new styles.

In 1900 the more thoughtful psychiatrist, interested in religion, philosophy, the humanities, and even education, would have welcomed — in addition to Freud's *Interpretation of Dreams* — Wilhelm Wundt's *Comparative Psychology*, Henri Bergson's *Le Rire*, and (perhaps) Bertrand Russell's *A Critical Exposition of the Philosophy of Leibniz*. He (and it was probably a 'he', although the first women psychiatrists were now starting to train), might have gone on to enjoy William James' *The Varieties of Religious Experience*, published in 1902, or even Max Weber's *The Protestant Ethic and the Birth of Capitalism*, of 1904. This psychiatrist may have mourned the death of the philosopher of science and social Darwinist, Herbert Spencer (1820–1903), in which case it is unlikely he would have done the same for the death of Mary Baker Eddy (1821–1910), founder of the Christian Science movement. Whether he would have read Freud's *The Psychopathology of Everyday Life* (1901), LT Hobhouse's *Mind and Evolution* (1906), or Alfred Adler's *Study of Organ Inferiority and its Psychical Compensation* (1907) would have depended on his linguistic skills and non-materialistic leanings.

If financially well off, this doctor might have had a telephone, a typewriter, and even a refrigerator, might have driven (if American) one of Henry T Ford's new cars, and might have bought one of the newly fashionable fountain pens. On a more practical note, he might have read the British Lunacy Commission's Report, for 1906 for example, identifying more than 121,000 persons certified as insane in England and Wales, a figure rising remorselessly throughout the decade. He may have preferred to think about childhood rather than the 'degenerate', ageing cohorts of his asylum, and visited the theatre in 1904 to see JM Barrie's *Peter Pan* (far crueller than Freud in its depiction of childhood psychology), or have mourned in 1907 the generation gap, as affectionately portrayed in Edmund Gosse's book *Father and Son*.

Assassins and 'Dreadnought' politics

If interested in 'forensic' events, our thoughtful psychiatrist may have tried to study reports of the mental state of the anarchist Leon Czolgosz (officially deemed sane, but viewed by some as "drifting towards dementia praecox") — who shot the US President McKinley in September 1901. Throughout the decade, he would have had every chance of developing such an interest. Notorious assassinations included the murder of Sipyagin, the Russian Minister of the Interior, in 1902, of the King (Alexander I) and Queen of Serbia in June 1903, of King Carlos I and the Crown Prince of Portugal in February 1908, and of Prince Ito of Japan in October 1909. An interest in international affairs would have seen him follow the strange case of Alfred Dreyfus, the (Jewish) French army officer falsely accused of treason, up to his pardon in the middle of the decade; the political success of Theodore Roosevelt, who succeeded McKinley and called for anarchists to be prohibited from immigrating to the United States; and the conclusions of the Boer War and Russo-Japanese War, with their hints of modern warfare in terms of 'concentration camps' and armament technology.

There was increasing unrest in Russia, exemplified by the mutiny on the battleship *Potemkin* and the abortive revolution of 1905. He might thus have felt anxious, or even neurasthenic, at the rising tide of strikes and organised labour, the Liberal landslide in the UK general election of 1906, the Entente Cordiale between Britain and France, and the imperial rivalries, exemplified by the scramble for colonies in Africa, that were developing between the great powers. In this fast changing world, the relative dullness of the asylum or the antiseptic quiet of the pathological laboratory may have been more attractive than we are able to understand. A correspondent at the 1900 Paris Exposition, viewing the new machine-guns and long-range cannon there exhibited, suggested that war had now become a science rather than a sport.

Cultural influences

Perhaps one of the most poignant summaries of that psychiatric world of *fin de siècle*, *gilded age*, or *belle epoque* can be found in Henry Ellenberger's 1979 *Discovery of the Unconscious*. This period, seen by Ellenberger as "the dawn of a *new* dynamic psychiatry", was against a background of a continuing predominance of classical culture and education, Latin remaining compulsory for some doctoral theses in France until 1900. Academic institutes were powerful, and harboured intense rivalries in both science and the arts. International meetings became larger and larger, that of psychology growing from 160 participants in 1886 to 503 in 1896. To attend these, one had to be able to understand French, German, English, and sometimes Italian. Pseudo-sciences such as astrology, homeopathy, and phrenology also did well, in a world that was male, authoritarian, royalist, imperialist, and based on servants, railways, and the notions of status and progress.

There was an underlying positivist ethic — i.e. knowledge based on observable facts rather than religious or speculative theories — as reflected in the work of Herbert Spencer (1820–1903) or John Stuart Mill (1806–1873). German language and research was dominant in scientific fields, but French concepts predominated in the world of the arts, music, and diplomacy. At the heart of Europe, the cities of Vienna, Prague, and Budapest represented the complex urban culture of the Austro-Hungarian monarchy, one of four empires to be destroyed by the Great War in the next decade.

One of the influences reacting to this positivist world was neo-romanticism. The Pre-Raphaelites in England, the Symbolists in France, and the Jugendstil movement in Austria and Germany were representative of this approach in philosophy, literature, and the arts. The celebration of Narcissus, the deity of self-admiration in Greek mythology, as well as renewed interest in hypnotism, somnambulism, and other psychical phenomena (the Society of Psychical Research was founded in Britain in 1882), was part of an increased movement towards attempting to understand the unconscious. This linked to a sense of the decadence of the modern world, and thus the popularity in psychiatry of degeneration theory, first expounded by Benedict Morel (1809–1873), and exemplified by the success of *Degeneration* by Max Nordau (1849–1923) published in 1892. In the same year, the British psychiatrist, Daniel Hack Tuke (1827–1895) edited *The Dictionary of Psychological Medicine*, a multi-author summation of the century's knowledge of psychiatry, in the broadest sense. These parallel traditions — the scientific/descriptive and the aesthetic/psychological — were antithetically representative of the time.

Psychiatric trends

Ellenberger has also pointed to further features of the *fin de siècle*. This included a sense of pessimism, related to the philosophy of Schopenhauer (1788–1860) and Nietzsche, an enjoyment of the eccentric and the luxurious, and cults of mysticism and eroticism, the latter often based on technical work published by writers such as Richard von Krafft-Ebing (1840–1902) and Havelock Ellis (1859–1939). By contrast, the dominant or 'official' psychiatric perspective came from the work of Wilhelm Griesinger (1817–1868), whose 1861 textbook had insisted on mental diseases being brain diseases, and since whose time neurology and psychiatry in Germany had been wholly combined. This was further developed in the work of Theodore Meynert in Vienna (1833–1892), who termed his own textbook of psychiatry a *Clinical Treatise on Diseases of the Forebrain* (1885), and of Karl Wernicke (1848–1905).

Wernicke, who had studied in Vienna under Meynert because of a shared interest in neuroanatomy, wrote his famous three-volume *Textbook of Diseases of the Brain* between 1881 and 1883, and produced his *Basic Psychiatry* (*Grundriss de Psychiatrie*) in 1900. Although this aimed to establish a direct relationship between psychopathology and brain function, it took little note of the newly developing psychological and dynamic ideas. His accidental death in 1905 may have significantly affected the decline of this neuropsychiatric approach. Such 'brain mythology' was partly countered by the work of Emil Kraepelin (1856–1926), who did include experimental psychology as well as neurology in his formulation of psychiatric disorder. He was also notably humane towards his patients, having written (1880) his first book as a plea against the death penalty, in contrast to his later Great War role as a leading advocate of unrestricted submarine warfare.

With regard to psychodynamic ideas other than Freud, the works of Auguste Forel (1848–1931) and of Eugen Bleuler (1857–1929) (Chapter 2, p. 52), one of Forel's students, were of considerable significance. Forel became Professor of Psychiatry at the University of Zurich, supervising the Burghölzli Mental Hospital. He developed an interest in hypnosis, visiting the much-admired expert in hypnotic suggestion Hippolyte-Marie Bernheim (1840–1919) at Nancy, and published a core work on sexual disorders (*Die Sexuelle Frage*) in 1905. Eugene Bleuler, coming from a politically active family, became interested in psychiatry as part of a reaction to the German professors brought in to Swiss hospitals (e.g. Griesinger, von Gudden, and Hitzig). Appointed as Medical Director to the Rheinau Mental Hospital in 1886, where he spent virtually all his time with his patients, he succeeded Forel at the Burgholzli in 1898.

Bleuler's work and lectures resulted in his famous 1911 textbook, *Dementia Praecox or the Group of Schizophrenias*, although he had already coined the term 'schizophrenia' in 1908 (see below). Taking his approach from both organic and dynamic influences (Carl Jung joined his staff in 1900), he felt that the psychotic condition called 'dementia praecox' (and named by him 'schizophrenia') had an organic basis, possibly toxic or hereditary, but also had secondary, psychogenic symptoms. He emphasised the loosening of associations, the loss of contact with reality via 'autism', and a generally wider notion of illness than that envisaged by Kraepelin. These concepts also led to a therapeutic strategy based on psychological/occupational approaches, which in turn engendered more optimism in treatment. The resulting tendency for him to attract famous patients (e.g. the dancer Nijinsky), may have been more of a burden than a benefit.

The rise of neurology

A further influence on the aspiring psychiatrist was the neurological work of John Hughlings Jackson (1835–1911) and his colleague William Gowers (1845–1915) at the National Hospital for Neurology, London. Using an approach defined as "receptive to evolutionary psychophysiology", Jackson outlined the organisation of the nervous system as occurring at different levels in an ascending hierarchy. He regarded the highest cerebral functions, which were to do with consciousness and thought, as no more than developed elaborations of the most basic sensory and motor reflexes. These higher levels overrode the lower ones, and were thus the first to be lost in disease, reducing individuals to lower levels of organisation. In his view, such a deficit could lead to epileptic attacks, or to a range of neuropsychiatric symptoms, even outbursts of mania, since "the increased action [results from] what, metaphorically speaking, is loss of control of lower centres by the higher centres".

Influential contemporaries on the British medical psychological scene were Henry Maudsley (1835–1918) and Charles Mercier (1852–1919). Maudsley's original, groundbreaking publication (*The Physiology and Pathology of Mind*, 1867) was succeeded by many other papers and books, but the third revision of his original work (*The Pathology of Mind*, 1895) was his last serious textbook. From then until his death in 1918, he became a retired, pessimistic figure, caring for his senile wife Ann (the daughter of the early nineteenth-century psychiatrist John Conolly), but wealthy enough to provide the funds to found the Maudsley Hospital in 1914. Mercier, a pupil of Hughlings Jackson, also published widely, his *Textbook of Insanity* (1902) being based on the notion that all life is teleological, aimed at the "continuation of the race to which the individual belongs". He had previously written on the organisation and management of lunatic asylums, lectured on nervous diseases at two London medical schools, and was a renowned medico-legal expert. To him the most important cause of insanity — which he considered a disorder of conduct rather than of mind — was "alteration in the composition of the blood by which the highest nerve regions are nourished". He was strongly opposed to what he called "Freudism", and in his later years became a forthright opponent of those believing in spiritualism and telepathy.

Early sexology

Two other areas of influence must be mentioned. Firstly, sexual problems came increasingly to the fore. They included pathology, fears of venereal disease, especially syphilis, and a stifling sexual code that belied a relatively discrete sexual freedom (mistresses such as Edward VII's Mrs Keppel were widely accepted) in high society. The suffragette movement and the notion of the 'new woman', who was now even able to go to work, along with increasing publications concerned with sexual conflicts, influenced both Freud's theory of the libido and a number of other more organic researchers. Perhaps most prominent in this respect was the work of Richard von Krafft-Ebing, who had trained as a psychiatrist in Germany and embraced Morel's theory of degeneration as a cause of criminality. He became Professor of Psychiatry in Graz and then in Vienna from 1892 to 1902. His *Lehrbuch der Psychiatrie* (1879) published in English in 1905 (*A Textbook of Insanity Based on Clinical Observation*) contained influential pre-Kraepelinian descriptions of delusional and mood disorders.

Von Krafft-Ebing's continuing fame, however, has rested on more specialist work, as outlined in his 1886 *Psychopathia Sexualis*. This contained some 50 alluring case histories of sexual perversions, and was an extraordinary publishing success, going into ten editions and enlarging to nearly 600 pages. The cases became more numerous and more detailed, the doctor's subjective feelings came into the discussion, and the book was received quite positively, particularly because of its helpfulness in terms of legal issues. Certainly, that was the tone of the *British Medical Journal* review in 1893, calling it a "purely legal book of German type".

It was also von Krafft-Ebing who coined the terms 'masochism' and 'sadism', in memory of the writers Leopold Sacher-Masoch (1836–1935) and the Marquis de Sade (1740–1814). Increasing numbers of studies appeared in this field, as well as the first specialised *Jährbuch* (including a current bibliography) in 1899, which by 1905 had quadrupled in length to over 1000 pages. While von Krafft-Ebing decided that most severe sexual perversions were hereditary or constitutional, it was not surprising that others increasingly attributed such behaviour to upbringing (e.g. corporal punishment), and various psychological causes. Although by the turn of the century the belief in masturbation as a significant cause of many forms of mental illness had largely receded, the recognition of a relationship between sexual function or repression, and mental illness became widely accepted.

The new science of sexology was magisterially outlined by Havelock Ellis (1859–1939) in the seven volumes of his *Studies in the Psychology of Sex*;

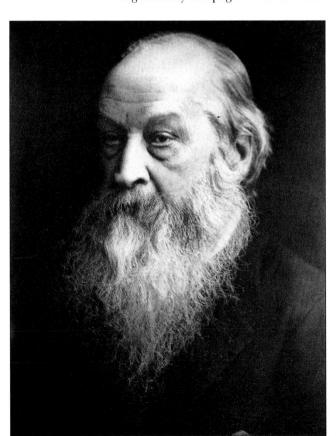

Dr Henry Maudsley (1835–1918), founder of the Maudsley Hospital, aged about 80. Reproduced with permission from the Bethlem Royal Hospital Archives and Museum.

Vol 1 *Sexual Inversion* was originally published in America in 1897, and Vol 7, also in America, in 1928. This work provided a background to Freud's sexual theories, but without really enabling them to be readily accepted by the public. Attempted publication of Ellis' first volume in the UK led to the successful prosecution of George Bedborough, the publisher, in 1898 for "obscene libel". Ellis became rather a reclusive sage therefore, increasingly admired for his theories and writings, despite having no clinical practice after 1893.

Background to 'the unconscious'

However, theories of dreams and notions of the unconscious had long been established, through a range of writers and researchers. The work of Herman Helmholtz (1821–1894), for example, especially on the principle of the conservation of energy (that ultimately, energy is never lost or gained, but only transformed), and on perception as a matter of learning to decode on the basis of experience, generated his notion of "unconscious inferences". These ideas, the word-association work of Francis Galton, and the famous clinical studies of hypnosis initiated by Jean Martin Charcot (1825–1893), provide much of the theoretical and clinical background to the rise of Freudian psychoanalysis. Since Pierre Janet's (1859–1947) key thesis, *L'Automatisme Psychologique*, was published in 1889 and had a considerable scientific impact, it is not surprising that, by 1900, there was a widespread sense of 'knowledge' about the unconscious (Chapter 4, p. 99).

This 'knowledge' has been interpreted by Ellenberger as showing the unconscious to have four types of functions. These were: (a) "conservative", such as memory, elicited via hypnotism; (b) "dissolutive", related to phenomena such as dissociation; (c) "creative", as emphasised by the romantic tradition; and (d) "mythopoetic". The latter was an area notably explored by Theodore Flournoy (1854–1920), who had studied psychology under Wilhelm Wundt in Leipzig and became Professor of Psychology in Geneva in 1891. In particular, he researched widely about mediums and reincarnation, as discussed in his popular book, *From India to Planet Mars* (1900). Other works on multiple personality, such as the study by Morton Prince (1854–1929) entitled *The Dissociation of a Personality* (1905), also created much public interest. Hopes for the future of this new knowledge were indeed immense, allied as they were to an assumption that the twentieth century would bring about a "synthesis of science and life", according to a popular science author, Ludwig Büchner. Enormous expectations as to the efficacy of psychological approaches in all forms of illness naturally followed.

Sigmund Freud and the rise of psychoanalysis

Of the major themes which are especially relevant to the psychiatry of this period, the life and work of Sigmund Freud has been analysed in numerous studies and biographies.

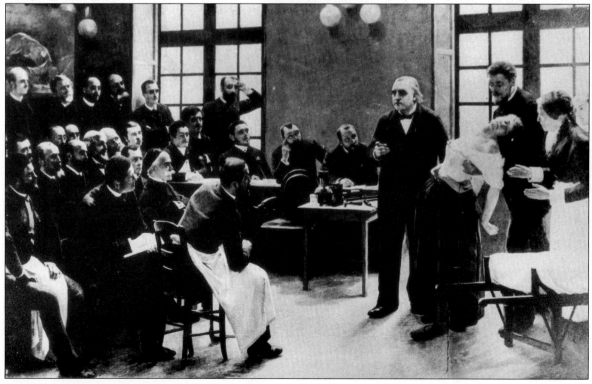

One of the founders of neurology in France, Jean-Martin Charcot is shown in this painting by Pierre-André Brouillet (c. 1887), demonstrating a patient with hysteria at the Salpêtrière. Courtesy of the National Library of Medicine, Bethesda.

These include *Sigmund Freud, Life and Work* by Ernest Jones, first published in three volumes between 1953 and 1957, and *Freud, Biologist of the Mind* by Frank J Sulloway (1979). During the period 1895–1910, Freud published a number of books and papers, the most outstanding of which are detailed in the table below.

Sulloway's bibliography records some 77 articles, papers, and books as written by Freud between 1877 and 1910, reflecting his creative and literary interests, and moving from neurological to psychological subjects. Entering medicine in 1873 and starting in private practice in Vienna as a neurologist in 1886, Freud experimented with the use of hypnosis before turning to free association. At the same time, the concepts of repression and the structure of the unconscious were being developed by his research. There followed his theories of child sexuality, the meetings of the 'Wednesday Society' (from 1902), and his appointment as a Professor Extraordinarius at the University of Vienna in the same year. More adherents joined, including Carl Jung and the 'Secret Ring' of Karl Abraham (1877–1925), Otto Rank (1884–1939), Sandor Ferenczi (1873–1933), Ernest Jones (1879–1958), Max Eitingon (1881–1943), and Hanns Sachs (1881–1947). The first international meeting of psychoanalysts was held at Salzburg in 1908.

By 1910, therefore, Freud's theories, his group of 'disciples', and his influence (particularly following a 1909 invited visit with Jung to the USA), were coming to full fruition. There was still considerable scepticism about his theories, not least amongst the established psychiatric and neurological figures. Ernest Jones in England had embarrassing problems resulting from some of his interviews with children, which resulted in him having to leave the UK for Toronto. The main features of Freudian psychology, however, were already in existence, including the ideas on infantile sexuality, the Oedipus and castration complexes, and the general dynamics of mental processes. The secessions of Adler and Jung were still to come.

Bernard Hart, then an assistant medical officer at Long Grove Asylum, outside London, read a paper entitled *The Psychology of Freud and his School* to the British Psychological Society at Oxford in 1910. It provided a thoughtful summary of the contemporary reaction to Freud from a relatively supportive point of view. Hart admitted that his task was one of "considerable difficulty", suggesting that parts of his paper would seem "confused and unconvincing". He emphasised that no attempt would be made "to demonstrate the accuracy of Freud's observations", preferring merely to "set forth general principles", and outlining Freud's meaning of "the unconscious", which he differentiated from the "subconscious of Janet and the French school". Hart accepted the "purely psychological method in the investigation of psychical facts", and summarised the notion of complexes, as an analogue of the conception of 'forces' in physics. Examples were given of the free association method, outlined by Jung, and of how symptoms arise thereby. A description of the process of psychoanalysis, bringing the repressed complex to the light of day but

---

Early publications of Sigmund Freud

Studies in Hysteria (Studien über hysterie), 1895. English translations by AA Brill were published in 1899 (part of the work) and fully in 1936.

The Interpretation of Dreams (Die Traumdeutung), 1900 (although issued in 1899). The first English translation, again by AA Brill, was published in 1913. Enlargements and revisions continued up to an eighth edition in 1930.

The Psychopathology of Everyday Life (Zur psychopathologie des alltagslebens), first published in 1901, in *Monatsschrift für Psychiatrie und Neurologie*. A revised reprint was published in 1904 in Berlin by Karger.

Jokes and their Relation to the Unconscious (Der witz und siene beziehung zum unbewussten). First German edition, 1905, and the first English translation in 1916 by AA Brill.

Three Essays on the Theory of Sexuality (Drie abhandlungen zur sexual theorie) 1905. The first English translation by AA Brill, was in 1910, for the *Journal of Nervous and Mental Diseases*.

Five Lectures on Psychoanalysis (Uber psychoanalyse), 1910. The first English translation, by HW Chase, was published as *The Origin and Development of Psychoanalysis* in the *American Journal of Psychology*.

resting "almost altogether upon an empirical basis", was accompanied by doubts about the theoretical aspects. According to Hart, however, "almost everyone who has taken the time and trouble to master Freud's technique — a task, by the way, of no mean difficulty — has confirmed his results in all their essential detail".

Discussing the role of dreams, Jung's work with psychotics, and the notion of "flight into the disease", Hart was careful about the "sex theories", admitting that they had been altered considerably, and that one "cannot feel assured that a similar fate will not await them in the future". He considered that Freud had developed the "first clear formulation of the principle that mind can be treated as phenomenon, capable of psychological explanation... certainly a notable departure in the history of science". Yet it was admitted that Freud had also "formulated wide-reaching generalisations from a comparatively small number of facts". In his subsequent treatise, *The Psychology of Insanity* (1912), Hart admitted his debt to a number of Freudian principles, but also described "the influence of Dr Jung of Zurich, Professor Janet of Paris, Professor Karl Pearson, and the late Professor von Krafft-Ebing". While Freud has dominated subsequent historical interest, therefore, it is important to recognise the influence of other contemporaries on psychiatric theory and practice during this period (Chapter 2, p. 41).

Emil Kraepelin (1856–1926)

Emil Kraepelin worked initially, between 1878 and 1882, in Munich, under Professor Bernard von Gudden (1824–1886), who subsequently died along with his patient, the 'mad' King Ludwig of Bavaria, by drowning in the Starnberg Lake. Kraepelin then moved to Leipzig, working with Paul Flechsig (1847–1929) and Wilhelm Erb (1840–1921). More importantly, he came under the influence of Wilhelm Wundt (1833–1920), who encouraged him to write his *Compendium of Psychiatry*, published in Leipzig in 1883. This was in fact the first of nine editions of his *Lehrbuch der Psychiatrie*, a work greatly influenced by an understanding of experimental psychology as a scientific endeavour. As a popular textbook, it became increasingly lengthy and attracted an almost legendary interest, new editions appearing every three or four years. His eighth edition (1909–1913) was in four volumes and had some 2500 pages. Nevertheless, in 1896, he also found time to initiate a series of monographs, *Psychologische Arbeiten*, some nine volumes of which were subsequently to appear.

English translations of his work also appeared at the beginning of the century. In 1902, A Ross Defendorf at Yale University produced *Clinical Psychiatry – a Textbook for Students and Physicians*, which he described as "abstracted and adapted" from the sixth German edition of Kraepelin's *Lehrbuch der Psychiatrie*. In England, Thomas Johnstone, of Leeds, produced a translation entitled *Lectures on Clinical Psychiatry (by Dr Emil Kraepelin)* in 1904, based on the second German edition. A preface by Kraepelin states that the aim of the lectures was "as a guide to the clinical investigation of the insane", while Johnstone described them as "eminently practical" and commented on the importance of "observing the periodicity of nervous diseases through a long period of time". The translation was very well received and published several times. The French reaction was more mixed, however. Deny and Roy (*La Démence Precoce*, 1903) admired his work, but others were more critical, on the grounds that the concept of dementia praecox was somewhat vague and that the condition did not always lead to a negative outcome.

Kraepelin was appointed to the professorial chair at Dorpat in 1885, from which he moved to Heidelberg in 1891. In 1903, he took up the Chair in Munich, where his new psychiatric clinic opened in 1904; it became internationally recognised and was often visited by both senior and aspiring psychiatrists. Co-workers included Alois Alzheimer (1864–1915), Franz Nissl (1860–1919), and August Paul von Wassermann (1866–1925), discoverer of the Wassermann test for syphilis in 1906.

The most important influences on Kraepelin were probably Karl Kahlbaum and Wilhelm Wundt. The former developed a clinically based body of research, the description of catatonia (1874) being the classic example of his nosology. Like Kahlbaum, Wundt was also critical of the vague speculation that passed for some psychological approaches, while stressing the importance of "apperception", whereby one is able to connect up personal knowledge with incoming data from the senses. His theories derived strongly from Immanuel Kant (1724–1804), and were profuse and complex. From them, however, Kraepelin was able to develop a process of empirical psychiatric research based on realism, psychophysical parallelism, and even (in part) an evolutionary approach. English commentators considered that Thomas Clouston (1840–1915), with his category of adolescent insanity (as outlined in an address in 1888), had in fact preceded Kraepelin's dementia praecox. Essentially, Kraepelin felt that psychosis could be classified into "natural disease units", which were derived from pathology, aetiology, and the clinical symptoms.

Kraepelin sought to link anatomical and psychological data, so as to establish disease groups. He also advocated a clinical approach, having become disillusioned with the difficulty of differentiating diseases via brain dissection — even the brain of a patient with general paralysis of the insane (GPI) — from a normal brain. He especially looked at patients' outward behaviour; the need for a translator (patients in Dorpat were Estonian and often didn't speak German) may have accustomed him to develop a particularly close form of observation. As he built up his clinical caseload and database, he gradually came to the conclusion that in whatever way patients presented — whether with mania, melancholia, or any other disorder — they tended to progress towards a dementia-type state. Increasingly, they began to resemble each other, and there was an accompanying "destruction of the personality". He introduced the term 'dementia praecox' in the fourth edition (1893) of his textbook, as a "subacute development of a peculiar, simple condition of mental weakness occurring at a youthful age".

From this, he moved on to his classic differentiation between manic–depressive disorder and dementia praecox, with accompanying forms such as dementia paranoides; the details and case examples developed increasingly over the years. His methodology of recording each case on special cards, which he regularly reviewed and sorted to try and find prognostic and defining features, provided the basis for his influential nosology.

After describing hebephrenic, catatonic, and paranoid forms of dementia praecox in 1899, he had developed some different subtypes by the eighth edition (1913). He made an assumption that the disorder was an organic problem, possibly related to personality, but considered "auto-intoxication" as one of the most likely processes. His limited interest in "degeneration" was in contrast to other theorists concerning this group of conditions. The influence of Kraepelin was essentially based on systematic clinical skills, observation over time, and the development of a coherent approach to prognosis. The elaboration by Bleuler from 1908 of the disease concept 'schizophrenia' introduced a less pessimistic and more overtly psychodynamic model of the illness.

An interesting footnote to the predominance of Kraepelin's theories can be found in AA Brill's introduction to the 1936 American edition of Jung's *The Psychology of Dementia Praecox* (1906). Brill describes how Adolf Meyer had given him a "thorough grounding in clinical psychiatry and neuropathology" in 1903, which was apparently "the beginning of the new era of modern psychiatry... wherein the name of Kraepelin shone resplendently". Brill went on to study neuropathology and then clinical psychiatry, soon feeling he was "well versed in the descriptive psychiatry of Kraepelin and his school". However "after a few years, this, too, became somewhat monotonous. I lost interest. I was bored by the busy routine of describing, diagnosing and leaving the rest to fate". Brill thus went to Switzerland, and became enamoured of the "new interpretative psychiatry".

These two themes, the descriptive and the interpretative, that have informed twentieth-century psychiatry, derive directly from the unique linking together of career pathways, asylum material, academic research, and psychological interest that arose out of the degenerationist European culture of the 1890s and 1900s. Though one of the conditions most frequently referred to in the contemporary volumes of the (British) *Journal of Mental Science* was the German concept of dementia praecox, the use of the term schizophrenia was gradually to replace it over the next 30 years. The extent to which the psychoanalytic viewpoint dominated those years remains controversial, yet Kraepelin's core dichotomy remained central to clinical practice (Chapter 2, p. 49).

Syphilis and degeneration

In his collection of short stories about medical life, *Round the Red Lamp* (1894), Sir Arthur Conan Doyle included *The Third Generation*. This describes the visit, on a rainy evening, of a young aristocrat to Dr Horace Selby, "a specialist who has a European reputation". The young man shows the doctor a lesion on his shin, and when asked to "account for it", insists that he has done "nothing in my life with which to reproach myself". The lesion is described as "serpiginous"; he is then asked to show his teeth ("at which the doctor again made the gentle clicking sound of sympathy and disapprobation"), and his eyes are examined. The doctor's "pleasure" after this, is described as the kind of enthusiasm "the botanist feels when he packs the rare plant into his tin knapsack".

The case is declared as "typical"; the patient is told that he has "interstitial keratitis" and that there are "indications of a strumous diathesis". It is considered that he has "a constitutional and hereditary taint" — the father and grandfather had a similar condition, the latter being "a notorious buck" of the 1830s. He had apparently "died horribly", and the doctor now considered that his deeds were "living, and rotting the blood in the veins of an innocent man". The patient recalls that his father wore gloves in the house, worried about "his throat, and then his legs", and that he was constantly fussing about his son's health.

When advised by the doctor that there were "many thousands who bear the same cross as you do", he bursts out with anger at the injustice of it all, and confesses he is soon to be married. They discuss ways in which he might postpone this event (such as an urgent visit to Australia), and various powders and ointments are prescribed. The next morning, the doctor wakes to read in the newspaper of "a deplorable accident". The young man had "slipped and fallen under a heavy carriage", and died before reaching hospital.

This young man, of course, had general paralysis of the insane (GPI), with the hereditary stigmata of Hutchinson's teeth and an Argyll-Robertson pupil. Such language and presentations reflected the rising number of diagnosed 'paretics' in the late nineteenth century, which had been a significant contributory factor to degeneration theory. This proposed that mental illnesses of a mild degree in the first generation, such as neurasthenia, would be passed on to successive generations with increasing severity, ending in dementia or complete idiocy. Consequences of this included the rise of the Eugenics Movement (the journal *Biometrika* was founded in Britain in 1902 by Francis Galton and Karl Pearson (1857–1936), and the Eugenics Education Society in 1907) as well as growing public concern as to the increasing numbers of 'feeble-minded'.

These fears resulted in widespread segregation of the feeble-minded, and even sterilisation (in the USA), under laws such as the Mental Deficiency Act of 1913 in the UK, which were designed to protect society from being 'infected' by 'degenerate seed' (Chapter 2, p. 55). For syphilis and GPI (also known as dementia paralytica), the increase varied from country to country. By the mid-1890s, Europe and North America were reporting the greatest number of cases; the Kommune Hospital, Copenhagen, had some 90 admissions in the period 1876–1880, but over 450 in 1911–1915. The Scottish Lunacy Commissioners' Report of 1907 described continued increases in the admission and death rates of GPI over the past 25 years. Also noted were the lower numbers in women (by the early 1900s, the ratio was about 2.5 male to 1 female), and the relative rarity of GPI in non-European populations — as reported by contemporary researchers, including Kraepelin. What is striking is its subsequent decline — prior to effective treatment — with death rates of over 2000 per year in England and Wales between 1901 and 1914, falling rapidly to under 1000 a year by the mid-1920s.

The debate as to the causes of GPI centred on life-style factors (e.g. alcohol or even cigar-smoking), with increasing epidemiological evidence towards the end of the nineteenth century that it was actually caused by syphilis. At the Moscow International Congress of Medicine of 1897, von Krafft-Ebing referred to "civilisation and syphilisation", and there were continuing concerns that the disease's increase was due to moral and physical decadence, associated with an increasing tendency to "premature and rapid racial decay". Given the high rates of syphilis in countries like Persia and Egypt, why should GPI be so uncommon there? When Kraepelin visited Java in 1904, he was unable to find a single case amongst the native population, but still maintained that syphilitic infection was essential for the development of GPI. In his *Clinical Lectures on Mental Diseases* (1904), Thomas Clouston of Edinburgh described it as "a disease of extraordinary interest physiologically, pathologically, and psychologically". There was "one cause above all others – predisposing or exciting – viz the syphilitic poison", with two "exciting causes", namely "sexual excess, especially if indulged in at or after middle life, and alcoholic intemperance, especially if impure and bad drinks are used".

Certainly, there were at this time clear difficulties in clinical diagnosis, as shown by the problem of what was termed 'pseudo paralysis', until the establishment of a definitive test. Given the importance of GPI as a disease, symbolising many doctors' views that mental illness was organically based, as well as its prevalence (in some mental institutions between 20 and 40% of male admissions had that diagnosis), the

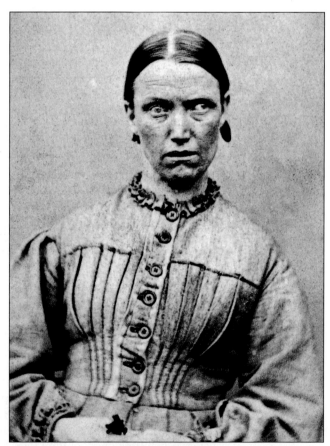

Albumen print of a female patient with 'general paralysis of the insane'; taken at the West Riding Lunatic Asylum, Wakefield, Yorks; attributed to Sir James Crichton-Browne, n.d. (c. 1869). Reproduced with permission from the Wellcome Institute Library, London.

ability to understand it and treat it became a benchmark of the progress of psychiatry during this period. Many desperate treatment approaches were used, including cold packs, mercury, and even trepanning of the skull (as well, of course, as leeching, venesection, and sexual abstinence). Even Paul Ehrlich's (1854–1915) discovery of Salvarsan (arsphenamine) in 1909 did not necessarily prevent the progression of the disease. Effective treatment was to await the research of Julius von Wagner-Jauregg, who had been trying a variety of fever treatments during the 1900s, with limited results until the development of malaria therapy in 1917 (Chapter 3, p. 64).

Nevertheless, the most important breakthrough of the decade was the discovery of the Wassermann complement fixation test, developed during 1905, and published in 1906. This was the first objective diagnostic test for a psychiatric condition, reinforcing strongly the neuropsychiatric orientation of the profession as a whole. The variety of mental and physical symptoms associated with GPI was so great that it was not helpful in the search for specific brain conditions associated with specific symptoms. It was relevant, though, in the differentiation of manic–depressive psychoses. Apart from Kraepelin, key studies for the understanding of GPI in the decade include those of Wagner (1902), Diefendorf (1906), and Mott (1908).

Neuropsychiatry

Increasing knowledge of localisation and the function of the nervous system had been developed in the work of Pierre Broca (1824–1880), Eduard Hitzig (1838–1907), Gustav Fritsch (1839–1891), and David Ferrier (1843–1928), as well as Hughlings Jackson and William Gowers. Much of this was centred around developments in the understanding of epilepsy — a condition mythologised as related to genius via the lives of such as Dostoievsky (1821–1881), Flaubert (1821–1880), Helmholtz (1821–1894), and Van Gogh (1853–1890). Why epilepsy should have been apparently so common in the late nineteenth century is not entirely clear, but the prevalence of syphilis and the obstetric complications due to nutritional disorders such as rickets may have been relevant.

More neurologically orientated journals had also become established, e.g. in Britain, the West Riding *Lunatic Asylum Reports* (1870–1876). This was succeeded by *Brain*, the journal founded in 1878 by James Crichton-Browne (1840–1938), Jackson, Ferrier, and John Bucknill (1817–1897). The relationship between fits and psychosis was especially interesting in terms of temporal lobe epilepsy, as described in the classic paper by Jackson and Stewart (1899) about the "dreamy state" (epileptic attacks with a warning of a crude sensation of smell and with the intellectual aura…). There was a general belief that the two states (epilepsy and mental illness) were related, with degeneration and alcohol theories put forward to explain this, the latter especially by Kraepelin.

Whether these phenomena arose by chance, or whether insanity and epilepsy weakened the brain towards susceptibility for each other were the subjects of an active debate in the early 1900s. There were important contributions from Ziehen in Leipzig (*Psychiatrie*, 1902), and Wernicke (*Grundriss der Psychiatrie*, 1900). Part of the problem was the general increase in the number of different types of insanity, related to different physical conditions, as particularly illustrated in Clouston's 1904 textbook. He included a detailed discussion of "epileptic insanity", but also differentiated conditions such as "hysterical insanity", "the insanity of masturbation", "the insanity of lactation", and "traumatic insanity", amongst others. He suggested that "morbid mental effects" associated with fits could occur in "six chief ways". These included: "after them", "before them", "instead of them" (*epilepsy larvée*, or masked epilepsy), progressive memory loss and mental "obscuration or twisting" (i.e. a dementia), as 'chronic insanity' instead of fits (which cease), and as a form of chronic insanity which develops into fits. Others suggested, however, that the concept of combined psychosis should be rejected, and such views reinforced those of Kraepelin. His long-standing attempt to bring together the myriad diagnoses (so current at the time) was based upon the natural history and prognosis of disorders, rather than individual clinical features.

Within the realms of neuropathology, however, the most striking development of the decade was the establishment of 'Alzheimer's' disease, together with the work of Arnold Pick (1851–1924). Alois Alzheimer (1864–1915) had developed an interest in neuropathology through contact with Franz Nissl (1860–1919) and his associates. He joined Kraepelin in Heidelberg in 1903, and moved with him and Nissl to Munich, attracted by the new 'royal' psychiatric unit that was due to open in the next year. A particular interest of the time was to separate out the different causes of dementia, using innovative histopathological methods that required meticulous preparation. His original presentation was at a meeting of South-West German psychiatrists, held in Tübingen in 1906, where he reported "a characteristic disease of the cerebral cortex".

Alzheimer described the course of illness of a 51-year-old woman, who started being extremely jealous towards her husband, and then developed memory impairment. She then started to scream because of fear of people wanting to kill her, and became increasingly helpless and perceptually impaired. She died after four years of illness, "completely apathetic in the end", and an autopsy showed "an evenly affected atrophic brain". There were characteristic changes in the neurofibrils, accumulating in dense bundles, as well as foci of deposition of a "peculiar substance in the cerebral cortex".

Further studies over the next few years confirmed his findings. Kraepelin summarised these in the eighth edition of his textbook, published in 1910, and Gaetano Perusine in the same year published a report on four cases entitled *Histology in Clinical Findings of Some Psychiatric Diseases of Older People*. Alzheimer himself published a classic description *On Certain Peculiar Diseases of Old Age* in the following year, and was actually surprised at having a disease named after him. His main interest had been to show that chronic states of cognitive decline (i.e. dementia) could occur in younger people. The brain plaques described by Alzheimer were already known to be quite typical of senile dementia.

In the same period, Arnold Pick, who trained with Meynert and Karl Westphal (1833–1890), was working as Professor of Neurology and Psychiatry in Prague. He published widely and was particularly interested in the relationship between localised cerebral abnormalities and specific symptoms. Thus, an 1892 paper linked atrophy of the temporal lobe with specific disorders of speech and movement, although modern 'Pick's disease' is defined as a combination of progressive dementia, frontal lobe features, and other behavioural manifestations. It was not in fact until 1906 that he published his paper on frontal atrophy, which was the fourth case of this neuropathological condition to be reported.

The English research tradition was best exemplified in the work of Frederick Mott (1853–1928). In the early 1880s, he studied in Vienna and Germany, and in 1895 was appointed Pathologist to the London County mental hospitals, as well as Director of the Pathological Laboratory at Claybury Asylum in Essex. Also a physician at Charing Cross Hospital, he became Lecturer in Medicine and Neurology in 1907. Before moving with the laboratory to the Maudsley Hospital in 1914 (when that institution opened), he studied the enormous range of clinical material created by the patients of Claybury Asylum. He also initiated the *Archives of Neurology and Psychiatry*, the first volume of which appeared in 1903, as a vehicle for the work of himself and his pupils.

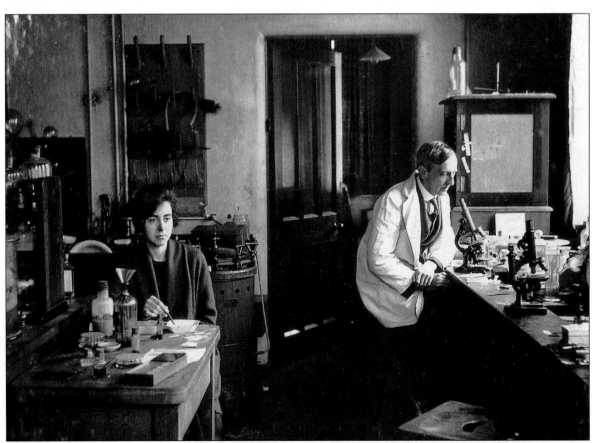

Sir Frederick Mott in the pathological laboratory of the Maudsley Hospital, 1918. Mott was the first pathologist of the London Country Asylums, moving his laboratory from Claybury Hospital to the Maudsley in 1916. Reproduced with permission from the Bethlem Royal Hospital Archives and Museum.

Working on cerebral localisation (with Maudsley and Sir Charles Sherrington) as well as on the degeneration and regeneration of peripheral nerves, he produced a number of original findings on the cyto-architecture of the cortex, and became increasingly interested in the role of 'internal secretions' in mental illness. His monograph on *Tabes* in 1902 demonstrated that GPI as well as tabes represented some kind of syphilitic disease of the nervous system, and this was based wholly on pathological and statistical methods. From a particular interest in the role of 'ductless glands' in dementia praecox, he became convinced that at least a part of the causation of mental disease was related to activity of the supra-renal (adrenal), thyroid, and sex glands. Mott was strongly supportive of the first group of women trainee psychiatrists (e.g. Helen Boyle 1869–1957, the first female President of the Royal Medico-Psychological Association), who were then just starting to come into the speciality.

In addition to Alzheimer, Pick, and Mott, many other influential individuals were at work at the time. Sir David Ferrier held the Chair of Neuropathology at King's College London, while Sir Victor Horsley (1857–1916) was a leading neurosurgeon at the National Hospital in London and a crusader for alcohol temperance. In France, Pierre Marie (1853–1940), Joseph Babinski (1857–1932), and Joseph Déjérine (1849–1917) were the leading figures, training amongst others the Portuguese future leucotomist Egas Moniz (1874–1955). Perhaps the most striking contributions of the period, however, were those made by Ivan Pavlov (1849–1936) and Sir Charles Sherrington (1857–1952). Essentially physiologists, they both received the Nobel Prize and concentrated their work on the nervous reflex.

Pavlov established the theory of conditional reflexes via his famous dogs, moving from the study of digestion to areas of higher nervous function. Methodologically rigorous and fascinated by natural science, he and his research group in St Petersburg developed this theory between 1902 and the 1930s. Sherrington, an equally dedicated physiologist, visited Pavlov and is reported to have commented — on one of the team's experiments on whether innate activity could be suppressed — that, "Now I understand the joy with which the Christian martyrs went to the stake". Sherrington's own masterwork *The Integrative Action of the Nervous System* (1906) developed a theory of behaviour based on an understanding of nervous integration. In particular, his experiments on reflexes allowed him to understand the control effected by higher brain centres. He conceived of the central nervous system as a synaptic network, and by linking anatomy, physiology, and general behaviour, formulated a sophisticated understanding of an organism in its environment.

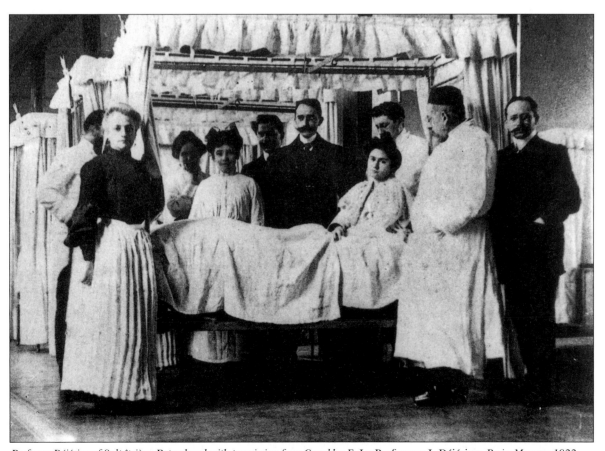

Professor Déjérine of Salpêtrière. Reproduced with permission from Gauckler E. Le Professeur J. Déjérine. *Paris: Masson; 1922.*

Although 'nerve specialists' (as neurologists were called) continued to be part of a broad sub-speciality dealing with psychiatric patients, the separation of neurology from psychiatry increased rapidly from this time. The German and Central European academic tradition tended to keep the two specialities together as one, but in Britain and America, psychiatrists were professionally being left behind in the asylums, while the nerve specialists became part of the élite of general medicine, both in the leading hospitals and in research work. Thus a patient such as Virginia Woolf, with a fluctuating manic–depressive disorder, saw a neurologist (Sir Henry Head, 1861–1940), and mainstream psychiatrists such as Sir George Savage (1842–1921), as well as spending time in a private nursing home. The rise of psychoanalysis enhanced this split, although Freud's original research had been very much neurological. This separation also prefigured the beginnings of other forms of specialisation, e.g. in alcoholism or mental retardation, and the differing worlds of the asylum, the private clinic, and private ('office') practice.

The relationship of psychiatry to neurology was discussed at an annual meeting of German psychiatrists in 1904. Professor Fürstner of Strasbourg (then part of Germany) accepted that many doctors were then opposed to the union, but insisted that the "separation of neurology and psychiatry is an artificial one". Consideration of the names of those attending the great international congresses on the care of the insane (the first in Antwerp in 1902, the second in Milan in 1906, the third in Vienna in 1908, and the fourth in Berlin in 1910) would see an admixture of the two groups. The fashion for specialist congresses, though, was growing, with the first 'Congress of Experimental Psychology' in 1904, and 'The International Committee for the Study of the Causes and Prophylaxes of Mental Diseases' in Amsterdam in 1907. Freud's first psychoanalytic congress in 1908 was part of such a schismatic trend.

Famous patients

Although the perception of psychiatry from the patient's point of view was not in vogue at the time, several famous cases became classics of popular interest. Best known in the English-speaking world was Clifford Beers, who wrote *A Mind that Found Itself* in 1908, and in 1909 founded a Mental Hygiene society. This was strongly supported by such luminaries as William James (1842–1910) and Adolf Meyer (1866–1950). The former had published his *Principles of Psychology* in 1890, a strongly physiological text, while his *Varieties of Religious Experience*, consisting of the Gifford Lectures delivered in Edinburgh in 1902, took a similarly pragmatic look at ethics and religion.

Meyer, born and medically trained in Switzerland, but then emigrating to America, became the dominant figure in American psychiatry, initially via his work at the New York Pathological Institute where he was appointed Director in 1901, and then as Professor at Johns Hopkins University. His support for the Mental Hygiene movement derived from his notion of 'psychobiology', and from his interest in the individual patient's social environment, in relation to the family and continuing follow-up (Chapter 4, p. 103). Meyer in fact met Clifford Beers, who had had at least three psychotic episodes and seems to have been quite badly treated in three separate mental hospitals. The US-based National Committee for Mental Hygiene developed into an International Committee by 1919, and claimed to be a significant factor in improving attitudes towards the mentally ill.

Equally famous, although for more theoretical reasons, was the case of Daniel Paul Schreber, whose *Memoirs of my Nervous Illness* was published in 1903. Little is actually known of Schreber (probable dates 1851–1911), but his illness seems to have been quite severe, with complex delusions and hallucinations, and in particular a conviction that his body was being transformed into that of a female. Since Schreber felt it was his duty to spread this knowledge as a kind of blessing to mankind, he went through considerable legal efforts to get himself discharged from the psychiatric clinic in Leipzig, where he had been admitted voluntarily in 1893. He eventually succeeded in 1902, although probably still unwell at the time of his release. Apart from providing an extraordinary picture of the effects of severe mental illness, Schreber came to prominence because Freud decided to use his memoirs to see if psychoanalysis could be helpful in understanding the basis for psychosis. Thus in 1911, Freud published *Psychoanalytic Notes upon an Autobiographical Account of a Case of Paranoia (dementia paranoides)*, having probably been attracted to Beers' book by Bleuler. Between 1909 and 1912, Freud, Bleuler, and Jung were co-editors of a biannual publication *Jahrbuch für Psychoanalytische und Psychopathologische forschungen*, and it was in this work that Freud's study of Schreber first appeared.

The essence of Freud's interpretation was that Schreber's illness was due to conflict over unconscious homosexuality, which was unacceptable to the patient because of an implied castration threat; the ensuing struggle generated the psychotic state. Bleuler was rather more sceptical, having much more practical knowledge of looking after patients with psychoses, but the subsequent history of psychoanalysis was to see this case taken up as exemplary of the basis of paranoia. Schreber thus became mentioned in many subsequent textbooks, although his memoirs were not actually translated into English until the 1950s.

A further patient of Freud's, Sergei Pankejeff (1887–1979) is also instructive, in that he links up many of the psychiatric approaches of the time. Troubled by obsessions even as a child, Sergei was admitted to a succession of private hospitals, where it seems he was usually treated as a case of manic–depressive illness. A particular episode of depression was associated with gonorrhoea, and when he was about 19, Sergei's only sister committed suicide. He sought treatment from a number of specialists, including the Russian neuropsychiatrist, Vladimir Bechterew (1857–1927) in St Petersburg, Emil Kraepelin in Munich, and Theodore Ziehen (1862–1950) in Berlin. The latter two felt that manic–depressive psychosis was the diagnosis, but in 1910 Sergei called on Sigmund Freud in Vienna, and was in therapy until discharged as 'cured' in 1914. Sergei was of course the 'Wolf Man', reported by Freud in 1918 as having a form of obsessional neurosis, and a significant contributor to the Freudian framework related to the 'primal scene'.

Less well known is the detailed *Analysis of a paranoid case as a paradigm*, reported by Jung in *The Psychology of Dementia Praecox* in 1906. The patient was a seamstress admitted in 1887 to the Burghölzli Hospital, Zurich, with chronic hallucinations (she referred the voices to invisible telephones), and manifesting active delusions. These included beliefs that she had a fortune in millions, was owner of the hospital, and owned "a seven-floored note factory with cold-raven-black windows", which signifies paralysis and starvation. She also complained of her spinal cord being torn out in the night, and of being tormented by hundreds of thousands of snakes. For some two years, Jung put her through a series of word association tests, since she was quite appropriate in her behaviour (she was a diligent worker), although tending to whisper "power words" to herself.

The details of these tests are given, with lists of "stimulus" word and her "reaction", as well as the reaction time. For example, when given the word "pupil", she replied, "now you may write Socrates". Jung described this as "quite a striking reaction for a seamstress". Some associations are quite obvious (e.g. "emperor" leading to "empress"), but others rather bizarre. Jung lists 80 in all, the final one being "head" leading to "wisdom", which he suggested belongs to "the complex of her extraordinary intelligence". He described the patient as speaking "as if in dreams", and felt that in contrast to a poet, she was thinking "without any directing idea". He commented that "the conscious psychic activity of the patient restricts itself to the creation of a systematic wish fulfilment, as it were, as an equivalent for a life of toil and deprivation and for the depressing experiences of an unhappy family milieu". The conclusion was that his analysis of this case of paranoid dementia confirmed "*in extenso* the theoretical hypotheses set forth in the antecedent chapters".

Rather more down to earth is a local newspaper's description of a lecture given, in October 1911, by an ex-patient on his "personal experiences in the Burntwood Asylum", a mental hospital in the English Midlands which by 1900 had over 800 patients. The lecturer told his audience that "to do justice to his subject he ought to have at least four hours", so as to detail the poor attention and treatment he had received, both in the 'poorhouse' and in the asylum. He went on to describe his experiences in the "padded room", but was complimentary to the Medical Superintendent, although complaining of a system of espionage in the dining-room and over the patients' letter-writing. The lecture seems to have lasted for about two hours, was described as "most extraordinary" by the reporter, and was characterised by the speaker regularly joining in the uproarious laughter of the audience. It represents a matter-of-fact acceptance in the popular press of institutionalisation and the absurdities often associated with its processes.

Treatment approaches

The treatment of mental patients around 1900 is usually regarded now as characterised by "therapeutic nihilism", yet the range of approaches — physical, pharmacological, occupational, and psychological — was really quite imaginative. Though the effectiveness of these treatments was less clearly defined, that did not prevent energetic methods being used. Thus, Sir John Batty Tuke, addressing the British Medical Association in 1898, insisted that "the extreme delicacy of the brain structure demands early and assiduous medical treatment in order to prevent disintegration and destruction of tissue". In his view, "if we exclude general paralysis and epileptic insanity from consideration, at least 80% of recent cases are amenable to treatment". Unfortunately, such treatment was costly since it involved "nursing, possible change of residence, and continuous medical attendance". By contrast, a Dr CG Hill, in his Presidential Address to the American Medico-Psychological Association in 1907, stated that "our therapeutics is simply a pile of rubbish".

Likewise, Silas Weir Mitchell (1829–1914), addressing the American Neurological Association in 1909, stated that "we have sadly to confess the absolute standstill of the therapy of insanity and the relative failure, as concerns diagnosis in mental maladies, of even that most capable diagnostician, the post-mortem surgeon". For Weir Mitchell to make such a pessimistic statement was especially striking, since his method of treatment, known as "Weir Mitchelling", and outlined in his classic exposition *Fat and Blood* (1877), was very highly regarded. The particular diagnosis for which it was meant to be most useful was "neurasthenia", first outlined as a distinctive entity by the New York neurologist and electrotherapist George M Beard (1839–1883) in 1869.

That diagnosis became particularly popular after Beard wrote *A Practical Treatise on Nervous Exhaustion (Neurasthenia): Its Symptoms and Nature etc.* in 1880. It encompassed a range of physical symptoms such as headaches, insomnia, menstrual problems, and dyspepsia, and provided a means of bridging the gap between psychological states and physical disorder. The book was soon translated into other languages, since neurasthenia had an alluring neurological tinge, being based on the notion of nerve fatigue, yet could embrace all sorts of presentations (anxious, depressive, hysterical, near-psychotic) that were so exasperating to practising doctors. The treatment for this became Weir Mitchell's 'cure', involving seclusion, rest, massage, electricity (in some cases), and a diet that was often just milk in various forms. This would go on for a number of weeks, under the complete control of the doctor, and was particularly suited to the rising number of 'nerve' clinics and general health sanatoria coming into fashion both in Europe and America.

On a more practical level, the treatment approaches to be found in different textbooks do not vary much. Those suggested by Charles Mercier in his 1902 *Textbook of Insanity* are probably representative of the typical organically orientated, practical doctor. Acutely disturbed states, described by him as "acute insanity", required food and sleep; the availability of a padded room was essential in case of disturbed behaviour, and a stomach tube could be used to give both nutrients and hypnotics. He would also give brandy with 'strychnia', and excessive amounts of food, particularly carbohydrates.

Drugs used included paraldehyde and barbiturates such as Sulphonal and Trional, and he welcomed the fact that "our choice of these has greatly extended of late years". Particularly useful he felt was hyoscine, given via a hypodermic needle or dissolved in a cup of tea or a glass of wine. This apparently allowed "a breathing time" to take the steps necessary to have the patient removed to an institution, which he deemed to be essential in every case of acute insanity, unless those responsible were "very wealthy", and could arrange for at least "three attendants and a medical man to reside in the house". A practical measure, in terms of home care, was to remove the patient to the ground floor, "bag and baggage, bed and bedding. Then if he jumps out of the window he can do himself little harm".

His views on the treatment of more chronic illnesses, such as "fixed delusion" or paranoia, were less positive. He regarded the latter as "an incurable and irrecoverable malady", requiring "restraint in an institution". He bemoaned the fact that "scarcely a week, and never a month, passes in which the newspapers do not report a murder committed by a person suffering from this form of insanity". For alcoholism, "the first thing... is to deprive the patient of his alcohol, and this can only be done by sending him to an institution". Even so, he suggested that in the first week, a dose of whisky and hot milk was good for their sleep, while "copious feeding, regular hours and fresh air" were the other components of the treatment programme. The treatment of GPI was based on "sufficient staff", institutional care, and sulphonal or paraldehyde to calm the patient, and if necessary rectal injections of chloral. He mentions trephining, paracentesis of the spinal canal, and blistering of the scalp, even though he did not think they were at all effective.

Such physical approaches were not, however, scorned. Given the concomitant widening in the range of surgery during this period, the notion of surgical treatment for mental illness was regularly considered. Theories of autoinfection, due to fermentation and putrefaction within the intestines, as well as concerns about infected teeth causing insanity, were to lead to heroic extractions and operations in the succeeding decades (Chapter 4, p. 79). A particular approach to patients of "a nervous disposition", with long-standing abdominal symptoms, especially pain, was surgery for the "floating kidney". A study of Glasgow Royal Infirmary records showed that 89% of such patients were women, usually middle-aged and multiparous, and while half were treated conservatively, about half underwent operation to fix the kidney by "nephrorrhaphy". Apparently, 96% of those treated in this way were deemed 'cured'. Whether this success rate was maintained out of the hospital (and follow-up was unusual in the early 1900s) is difficult to say.

In terms of general therapeutic approaches, the *British Medical Annual* for 1909 quoted extensive sources, from both America and Europe, and suggested a wide range of therapeutics. Thus *Bornyval*, a combination of borneol and valerianic acid, is recommended for neuroses of the stomach and bowels, hysteria, neurasthenia, insomnia, and in the menopause. Also mentioned is *Bromural*, easily soluble in water, and useful apparently as a nerve sedative and "mild" hypnotic. It was said to be most efficacious in all forms of nervous excitability and insomnia, especially those "frequently associated with mental overwork, financial worry, hysteria, mild alcoholism, excessive use of tobacco, etc.".

Other approaches to treatment included "*Cannabis americana*" (apparently as good as *Cannabis sativa*) and 'lecithin', given by intramuscular injection for locomotor ataxia and GPI. A general approach is summarised in the term 'opotherapy' (animal extracts) for a range of conditions, both physical and psychological; these included pituitary extracts, thyroid gland, pancreas, and 'neuriprin'. This latter was an extract of "cerebrum, preserved with bromine", and used in Italy as a "nervine" sedative. It was reported useful in "a severe case of spinal and cerebral neurasthenia".

Also, practical approaches were outlined for the management of alcohol problems, including "a healthy time-table", with atropine and strychnine given hypodermically in small doses. An essay on the management of delirium tremens concludes that a hot bath or hot pack is of great assistance, hyoscine hydrobromide is the best sedative, aperients are required for the bowels, and digitalis should be given for pneumonia if that intervenes.

On the management of hysteria, the book admitted that "special attention of recent years has been directed to psychical methods of treatment, and yet it is a truism to state that psychotherapeutics have been practised, consciously or unconsciously, not only by physicians but also by priests and by charlatans, ever since medicine was an art". Approaches suggested include hypnotic suggestion (regarded as less beneficial than suggestion in a waking state), direct suggestion, which was "most efficacious when it is made with quiet confidence, in moderate and temperate language", and psychoanalysis. In particular, an account is given of Freud's method of mental catharsis, "whereby the pent-up emotion is dislodged". The patient is advised that "before she start on her narrative it is impressed on her that she must relate everything that comes into her head", but the process is regarded as slow and tedious, and the "persistent and insistent questioning on sexual subjects" is deemed to be "unpleasant and revolting to the feelings both of the physician and of the patient".

Just as important in this overview is the range of advertisements for private asylums, mental hospitals, specialist hotels, and hydropathic establishments. Treatments at Matlock (in Derbyshire) included Nauheim baths, Schott exercises, Weir Mitchell treatment, Turkish baths, Russian baths, electric high frequency and X-rays, inhalations, massage, and Swedish exercises. Amongst the wide range of vaccines, serums, antitoxins, and tonics that were offered, one could buy Nepenthe. This preparation was derived "entirely from opium", was claimed to give more relief than any other form, apparently did not produce nausea, constipation, headache, or depression, and was such that "habitual use does not weaken its effects".

While all these resources had to be paid for, the treatment available in the standard pauper asylum was much more limited. Essentially it was shelter, some occupation, and sedation if a patient was very noisy. A section of the *Journal of Mental Science* in 1902 summarises treatment reports. A Dr Paris (from France) outlined the value of "rest in bed", suggesting that expenses were not increased by the extra staff, because it obviated "the cost of the destructiveness of the maniacal patient". There was also a reduced need for surgical treatments, because of fewer wounds and fractures. Another report from France complains at the refusal of the relatives of female patients to allow gynaecological examinations, since 59 out of the 61 patients that they had been allowed to examine showed considerable gynaecological troubles associated with the mental illness.

There was a plea from America for the "wider establishment of out-patient departments", since the current ones were so overcrowded that mental patients "cannot receive the attention they require. As it is, these sufferers have to content themselves with a dose of mistura alba or calomel, or perhaps a dose of bromide and some hasty words of reassurance, and then the 'next patient'". The use of exercise treatment, separate hospitals and asylums, villa colony asylums, and other structural arrangements are also mentioned, as are the drugs outlined above.

A particularly optimistic report of electrical 'faradisation' of the head for chronic insomnia and associated neuroses suggested that nearly 80% of cases showed cure or marked improvement. The method involved application of a current, via a large electrode, for about 15 minutes, applied to the brow and the nape of the neck. The importance of attention to detail, and the avoidance "of any loose connection" is stressed. It is suggested that there is "no remedial measure at present known to the profession, other than a prolonged holiday, which will give such immediate and more or less prolonged benefit".

An outside view of The City Lunatic Asylum, near Dartford, April 1866. Reproduced with permission from The Illustrated London News Picture Library.

Asylums

Behind the plethora of books, lectures, congresses, laboratory findings, and treatment approaches lay those ever-enlarging institutions, the asylums. These were variously considered as safe havens for the innocent victims of untreatable diseases, as disposal units for the degenerate and socially unwanted, or simply as "museums of madness" where alienists could indulge in interminable classification or bureaucratic somnolence. Nevertheless, the numbers they contained rose throughout the period in question. The debate as to the reasons for this has continued to this day, but there is no evidence of a specific increase in any disease. For example, the suggestion that schizophrenia was on the rise because of an infectious agent is not borne out by asylum statistics, particularly for younger admissions. On the other hand, the easier acceptance of asylum care for 'difficult' relatives, the widening definitions of insanity, and an increasingly elderly population could explain much of the process. Clouston advocated both these latter factors and quoted figures showing no rise in the admission rate of private patients, but only in that of the pauper classes. Organic conditions seem to have been significant, but it is difficult to avoid the conclusion that the asylums did in fact contain many individuals (at least 60–70%) with severe mental disorders.

A particular problem was the size of institutions. Originally designed, in the heyday of 'moral treatment', to have no more than one or two hundred patients, many now had 2000 or more. The largest institutions, with 5000 or more, were in the United States. They were highly standardised in their arrangements, in terms of food, activities, staffing, and treatment approaches; the

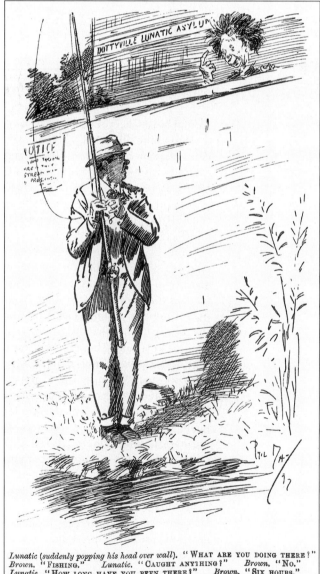

Lunatic (suddenly popping his head over wall). "WHAT ARE YOU DOING THERE?" Brown. "FISHING." Lunatic. "CAUGHT ANYTHING?" Brown. "No." Lunatic. "HOW LONG HAVE YOU BEEN THERE?" Brown. "SIX HOURS." Lunatic. "COME INSIDE!"

"Come Inside"; Punch cartoon, August 1897. Reproduced with permission from Punch.

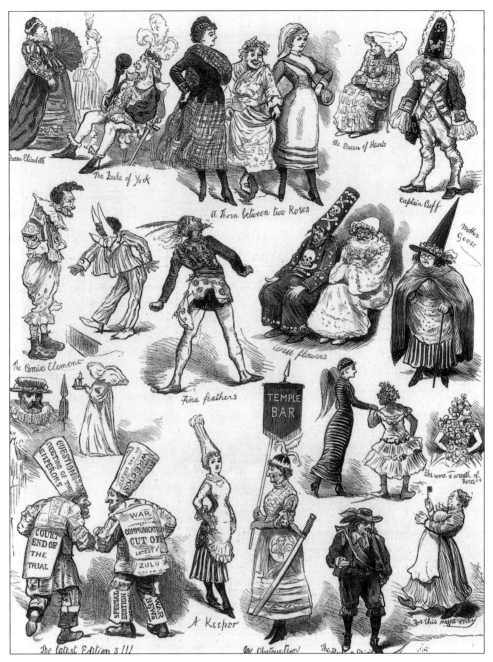

Fancy dress ball at the Brookwood Surrey Lunatic Asylum, January 1881. Reproduced with permission from The Illustrated London News Picture Library.

attendants or 'nurses' wore uniforms, keys were everywhere, and many relied upon patients' labour (in laundries, kitchens, or on farms) to ensure their financial stability. Sports, fêtes, the cinema (later), weekly dances, and a range of other activities took place, particularly in the private institutions, while high walls, distance from the local town, and long driveways kept patients and the public well apart. Wards would have up to 100 patients in, with special 'refractory' units for the more difficult ones.

In most countries, the system was stagnating and the reputation of psychiatrists amongst other doctors was third-rate. Ernest Jones described an English asylum superintendent who was desperate to employ an assistant medical officer and stated that qualifications did not matter too much, provided that the doctor could play cricket with the patients. Since half a dozen doctors (including the superintendent) were likely to be looking after 1500 to 2000 patients, the notion of providing any kind of 'therapy', as opposed to merely documenting and feeding, was difficult to sustain.

If there was any group of asylums that were properly run, it was those in Germany, thanks to more liberal funding from the individual German states and because of the tradition of associated scientific research, as illustrated by Kraepelin's career. Even so, the violence, agitation, and hopelessness of the average psychiatric in-patient unit is well documented.

In terms of statistics, the numerous asylum histories also record very similar patterns. Though admissions and numbers increased, the number discharged remained the same, so the number eventually dying in the asylum must have increased. Thus, the Buckinghamshire County Pauper Lunatic Asylum admitted 112 patients in 1901 and 198 in 1911; its population had increased from 514 to 676 in the same period. By the end of

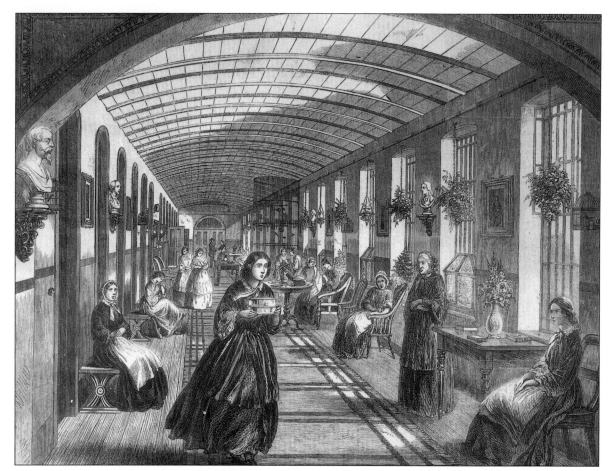

The Royal Hospital of Bethlem — The Gallery for Women, March 1860. Reproduced with permission from The Illustrated London News Picture Library.

1911, there were 699 in-patients, of whom 381 had a psychosis, 114 were mentally handicapped, 61 were epileptic, 21 were brain-damaged, and 33 had senile dementia. The English Commissioners in Lunacy, visiting Colney Hatch Asylum (in North London) in 1898, considered the care and staffing to be inadequate. They counted one attendant for every 13 males and one nurse for every 15 women. Specific examples included, "Number 2 ward, 39 patients under 3 attendants, 2 of the patients being epileptics, 4 in bed, and 18 so actively suicidal as to be always kept in sight", while "Number 19 [ward] has 58 patients under 4 nurses, 37 being epileptics, 5 in bed, and 1 actively suicidal".

These asylum reports also describe the nature of the environment. Thus in Leavesden Hospital for the mentally retarded, although radiators were installed in the corridors in 1901, near the entrance to each block, ward temperatures of barely 5°C were recorded in a cold January. A few years later, these conditions were accepted as being inadequate, but no action was taken to improve things. A typhoid outbreak in 1899 led to major repairs to the drainage and sewage works, but in 1904 a water sterilising plant had to be installed. On the more positive side, the asylum authorities in 1902 bought a gramophone player and records, while the year before, a special recreation room for male attendants was adapted "to keep the men from the

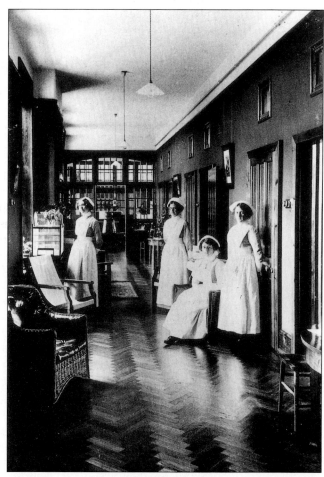

Nurses in a corridor, taken at Saxondale Mental Hospital, Nottingham (c. 1912). Reproduced with permission from the Wellcome Institute Library, London.

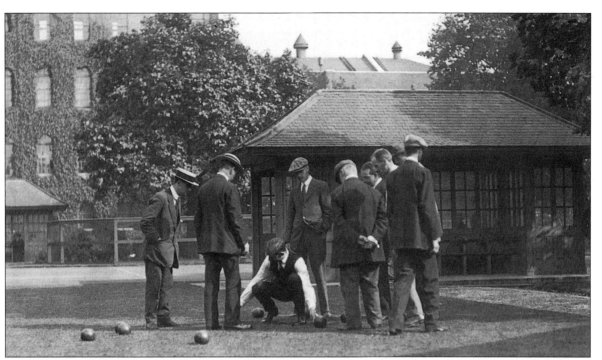

A game of bowls in the men's airing court of Bethlem Hospital, early twentieth century. Reproduced with permission from the Bethlem Royal Hospital Archives and Museum.

public houses". Neither attendants nor junior doctors could leave the hospital without permission, but a programme of regular staff football matches against other hospitals began around 1901, and a gymnasium club was opened in 1910.

Typical advertisements for staff represent the kind of qualifications required. In April 1900, Burntwood Asylum advertised for a male attendant "capable of playing cornet or clarinet". Wages of £30 per annum went along with board, lodging, washing, and an allowance in lieu of beer, as well as additional pay for playing in the band. However, previous asylum experience was not necessary, and applications needed to state only age, height, occupation, and whether married or single, and to provide references, if possible with a photograph. In fact, the routine use of photography, as part of the documentation of both patients and attendants, began during this time, but involved considerable debates as to its ethics. Many asylum casebooks nevertheless included photographs, primarily as a means of identification, although attempts at diagnostic classification were also made.

While the nature of large, publicly funded asylums is well recorded, less is known about the private clinics for psychiatric patients. By and large, however, their inmates were not particularly easy to manage, often having severe mental illnesses as well as the habits of superiority of the upper classes. By 1880, some 2700 "nervous" patients were to be found in 81 separate, private hospitals in Germany and Austro-Hungary, while by 1906, there were 8500 patients in some 140 private hospitals. A particular feature of these clinics was their ability to attract customers. By careful use of language — "nervous" rather than "insane" — they reduced the stigma of being admitted to what was, to all intents and purposes, a madhouse. While containing patients who were both voluntary and involuntary, many of the newer clinics remained largely 'open', i.e. voluntary. Psychotic patients would thus reside alongside alcoholics, obsessionals, hysterics, and neurasthenics. Treatment consisted of massages and baths, the Weir Mitchell approach, various distractions and occupational activities (appropriate to their class expectations such as concerts and tea parties), a range of sedatives and hypnotics (see above), and various forms of talking therapy.

One of the most systematic of these was "persuasion therapy", as outlined by Paul Charles Dubois (1848–1914), Professor of Neuropathology at Berne. Taking his view from the Romanticist tradition — that mental illness could be understood as a disorder of the soul and was amenable to psychological approaches — he suggested that the doctor's task was to convince the patient that their neurotic experiences were irrational. This could be seen as a form of re-education, and very much went against the Freudian viewpoint of the importance of the emotional interaction or transference, between patient and therapist. An important intermediary figure in this debate was Edouard Claparéde of Geneva (1873–1940), who considered that the process of thinking intervened when instinctive behaviour could not solve a problem. His research included studies with animals and children (e.g. *Psychology of the Child*, 1905), and he had a significant influence on Jean Piaget (1896–1980).

Miscellaneous influences

Although psychiatry was dominated by the German and French schools, significant contributions also came from other European countries. Thus in the Netherlands, Leendert Bouman (1869–1936), who had studied in Vienna under von Krafft-Ebing and Wagner-Jauregg, developed a psychological psychiatry that attempted to relate scientific research to a Calvinistic faith. Appointed Professor to the Free University of Amsterdam in 1907 and fully aware of modern research into the physiology of the brain, he felt that psychic factors remained essential to understanding psychotic illness. He urged the importance of "research into sleep, dream and hypnotic states", while acknowledging the pitfalls attending such an approach as outlined in the work of Freud and Jung. He thought that a synthesis of faith and science was possible, and thus opposed any separation of psychiatry and neurology. His subsequent career has been called "a search for the soul in psychiatry", and significantly affected the development of a very psychological psychiatry in the Netherlands.

Of equal importance in terms of the impact of experimental psychology on psychiatric practice was Theodule-Armand Ribot (1839–1916), who had studied under Herbert Spencer, Claude Bernard (1813–1878), and Jean-Martin Charcot. Founding in 1876 the journal *La Revue Philosophique*, he was appointed in 1888 to the Chair of Experimental Psychology at the Collége de France in Paris. His reputation was very much that of a popular writer on psychology, and his views on evolution had considerable influence on such as Pierre Janet. In particular, he considered that there was a psychological dimension to heredity, whereby one could inherit emotional and intellectual dispositions as well as physical ones. His key book was *L'Heredité Psychologique*, first published in 1873, and reaching its ninth edition by 1910.

Another influential figure, August Wimmer (1872–1937), was the leading theorist of a particular Danish psychiatric tradition. Graduating in 1897, his book *Degenererede Børn* (1909) strongly influenced child psychiatry in Denmark, although his key work, *Psychogenic Forms of Mental Diseases*, published in 1918, was on psychogenic reactions. Though he was a major figure in Scandinavian psychiatry, the lack of a translation into English of his major work until after the Second World War limited knowledge of his findings outside that area. Like Bouman and Ribot, Wimmer's significance is a reflection of the impact of the discipline of psychology on medical practice.

Progress in psychiatry

In 1901, the *Journal of Mental Science* published a number of communications under the title, 'Progress of psychiatry'. From America, a Dr Bannister reported on the difficulties of the New York Pathological Institute, and the appointment on to an advisory board there of representatives of "the related specialties of psychology and general biology" as well as pathologists and neurologists. He also reported on the examination of the assassin Czolgosz, admitting that "the psychology of the anarchist of the present day, is, in some respects, a problem". Dr Jules Morel, from Belgium, reported on an increase in the numbers of criminal lunatics, suggesting that some 80% should be deemed to be suffering from hereditary conditions, since such lunatics were "almost entirely recruited amongst the degenerates". He outlined the cost to the state of specific degenerate families, and quoted from comments made at recent congresses of psychology about the need for reform, if we "wish to defend society with pure consciences".

Dr A Friis from Denmark wrote about the increasing need for accommodation for incurable patients, but described the year under review as having been "rich in psychological literature", mentioning a work by a Dr Wurtzen, *Personal Responsibility (Psychological and Criminal)*. Similar emphasis on degeneracy comes from the report from Dr René Semelaigne of France, describing the case of a sequestrated woman (confined in an apartment for years, and found quite naked in bed and covered with "every kind of vermin"), a criminal assault to obtain morphia, and a "cocainomaniac" father with idiot children. He also reported on a thesis by a Dr Victor Parant on delusions resulting from jealousy, described as "hereditary degenerates, with stigmata and abnormalities of morals and of temperament".

More practically, Dr J Bresler from Germany described treatment of the insane without isolation, and the family care of patients, mentioning the notion of patients being boarded out. He even suggested that they should be "visited by inspectors specially trained in lunacy", a prediction almost of community care. A pathological report on functional psychoses, suggesting that "it was impossible to distinguish a sane from an insane brain", was also highlighted, as was the fact that psychiatry had just been made a compulsory subject in the medical curriculum in that country.

Dr FM Cowan from Holland reported on an International Congress of Criminal Anthropology in Amsterdam, concentrating on the problems of staffing in asylums. He quoted from a paper by Dr L Bouman (1869–1936) on twins who became insane at the same time, had a similar course, and were discharged cured at about the same time. Calls for more female attendants in asylums and considerations as to boarding out were also discussed, as were standardised forms for recording symptoms in patients who had fits. Concern was expressed that certain such questions could only be properly answered by doctors, and not by nurses or attendants.

Dr Giulio Ferrari from Italy mentioned the Fifth Congress of Criminal Anthropology, presided over by Professor Cesare Lombroso (1836–1909), architect of the notion of the "criminal type". He also made reference to malformations of the nails in cases of periodic insanity. There is a report of "an ideal goniometer for the measuring of the facial angle", as well as one on the psychological basis to graphology. Professor Henry Morselli (1852–1929), who coined the term "dysmorphophobia", was apparently preparing a volume on "the mediums" as well as a second edition of his treatise on psychiatry (*Trattati di semiologia psichiatria*), while the translation of William James' *Talks to Teachers on Psychology* was also being undertaken, since his *Principles of Psychology* had been a great success. From Norway, came a brief report from Dr M Holmboe, again emphasising the need for asylum accommodation, and the difficulties of "efficient nursing in private houses". It seems that farmers used to be happy to receive single lunatics on that basis, but now had "a higher appreciation of home life", and were thus less willing.

Alfred Binet (1857–1911)

Director of the Department of Physiological Psychology at the Sorbonne in Paris from 1892, the psychologist Alfred Binet initially worked on tests measuring sensori-motor abilities to assess intelligence. He concluded that certain intellectual faculties, e.g. the ability to abstract, could be measured and thus moved on to devise a test (at the request of the French Minister of Public Instruction) to differentiate between normal and subnormal children. Collaborating with the psychiatrist Theodore Simon (1873–1961), he produced in 1905 the Binet–Simon scale, which became the basis for all subsequent intellectual testing. The tests were revised in 1908 and 1911, and were soon widely accepted. By using a battery of test questions, rather than relying on anatomical, pathological, or other criteria, they established the notion of a mental age, by comparison with a child's peer group.

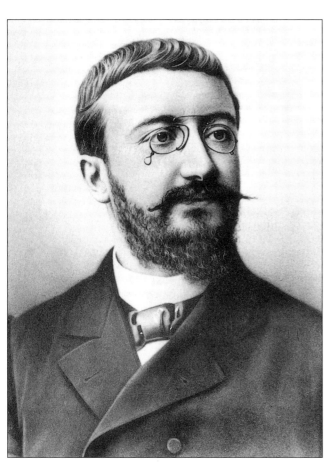

Alfred Binet. Photogravure by Synnberg Photo-gravure Co. Chicago. Reproduced with permission from the Wellcome Institute Library, London.

Binet also argued that his programme should be used as a means of training children who were behind the average attainment for their age, thus opposing concepts of degeneration and the notion that measured intelligence is something one is born with. Binet had been one of the co-founders of the journal *L'Année Psychologique* (in 1893), and prior to his work on intelligence scales, had published widely on psychology. One of his first pieces of research was, oddly enough, on the psychic life of micro-organisms, and he also wrote on sexual psychology and first coined the term fetishism. Binet was a prolific writer, although shy and retiring; his work became a paradigm of formal psychological testing, outliving in impact the writings of many more famous contemporaries.

Pierre Janet (1859–1947)

Although Janet can be regarded as one of the outstanding psychologists of his time, his work has been strangely neglected, especially in the English-speaking world. In part, this is due to his being overshadowed by Freud and psychoanalysis, and in part because he never developed a school of followers, so that some of his work has not been clearly understood. Born into an established professional family, he at first studied philosophy, became interested in hysteria, and wrote *L'Automatisme Psychologique* (1892) before training in medicine in Paris. He worked in experimental psychology, initially under Charcot and then at the Sorbonne, and was appointed Professor at the Collége de France in 1902 (Chapter 4, p. 99).

Janet's publications included *Les Obsessions et la Psychasthénie* (1903), *Les Nevroses* (1905), and a collection of lectures delivered at Harvard in 1907, *The Major Symptoms of Hysteria*. He coined the term 'psychasthenia', embracing what are roughly now the phobic anxiety states and obsessive–compulsive disorders, developed a classification of these conditions, and introduced the term 'dissociation'. He theorised that individuals had an integrated form of psychological functioning, arranged hierarchically from primitive reflexes up to the higher echelons of moral and logical thinking. His work greatly influenced Jung and Adler, particularly his notions of psychological tension and 'subconscious fixed ideas' with their pathogenic role. Janet deemed this material to be at the heart of hysteria, but unlike Freud, did not consider a cure to be created just by bringing such ideas into consciousness, which might merely make them obsessions. The task, as he saw it, was to get rid of them, replacing them via mental re-education of some form.

During the period 1900–1910, the approaches of Janet and Freud operated side-by-side, with the latter tending to gather more disciples as each year went by. A particular example of the polemics thus generated was the First International Congress of Psychiatry and Neurology in Amsterdam in September 1907, described by Ellenberger. There, Janet's prestige was confirmed, and little support obtained for Freud, particularly his sexual theory of the basis of neurotic symptoms. This was probably the high tide of Janet's influence, however, and increasingly the sheer volume of psychoanalytic literature, e.g. that dealing with myths and anthropology, began to dominate psychotherapeutic approaches.

In 1910, at a German psychiatric meeting, a Dr Hoche had spoken on "a psychic epidemic among physicians", concluding that the Freudian movement was "the return, in a modernised form of a magical medicine, a kind of secret teaching". In fact, numerous other conflicting psychotherapeutic schools were developing, although Janet continued to be held in high esteem. As memorably described by Ellenberger, "France, England and Germany were the prey of a nationalistic mass neurosis... and the expectation of war was reflected in the literature of the time and in the general outlook of the people's mentality".

Conclusion

The history of psychiatry from the 1890s to 1910 prefigures many of the events, theories, and practices that were to dominate the twentieth century. Although 'alienists' were an established profession, with a role in asylum management and brain research, the conflicting streams of neurology and neuropathology, as well as psychology and psychotherapy, could hardly be contained within the one speciality. The traditional journals, such as the *Annales Medico-psychologique* (founded 1843), *Allegemeine Bezeitschrift für Psychiatrie* (founded 1844), *The American Journal of Insanity* (founded 1844), and *The Journal of Mental Science* (founded 1853) could no longer contain the variety and detail of publications being produced.

Textbooks with numerous editions, such as those written by Kraepelin, Clouston, or von Krafft-Ebing, competed with a wide variety of specialist literature and numerous communications, meetings, and congresses. Varying treatments, whether pharmacological, physical, or psychotherapeutic, abounded in private nerve clinics and in the crowded public asylums. Like the airports of today, these were always adding new buildings, were becoming more and more dehumanised, and were often seen as actual hindrances to the search for health.

The most important contributions diagnostically were those of Wasserman, with his test for syphilis antibodies, and Binet and Simon with their intelligence testing. The neuroses continued to flounder in a sea of descriptive terms, and although Kraepelin's distinction between dementia praecox and manic–depressive insanity has been a foundation of our understanding of the psychoses, its success could be seen as due to the very untreatability of the asylum population. This sheer inefficacy, allied to a highly organised administrative system, enabled symptoms to be reviewed over long periods, without the interference of a therapeutic remission. Such a captive population was therefore useful, at least, for diagnostic research and the clarification of the course of disease — "They also serve who only stand and wait".

Nevertheless, it is probably true to say that the language of psychiatry by the end of the period had become more comprehensible, both to contemporaries and to historians looking back. The dilemmas and concerns of practitioners even seem to have a relatively modern ring. Thus, in a *Lancet* publication of 1912 on "early mental disease", Maurice Craig (1866–1935) could write that "we can sum up mental disorder as a reaction of the whole organism to those internal and external influences to which it is exposed". One might even suggest that Salvarsan, dynamic psychiatry, and the mental hygiene movement were the first representatives of today's notion of the bio-psycho-social approach to psychiatric disorders.

FURTHER READING

The early 1900s & before...

Secondary sources

Ackerknecht EH. *A Short History of Psychiatry* (trans. S Wolff). New York and London: Hafner; 1968.

Alexander FG, Selesnick TS. *The History of Psychiatry*. New York: Harper and Row; 1966.

Ellenberger H. *The Discovery of the Unconscious*. New York: Basic Books; 1979.

Hare EH. The origin and spread of dementia paralytica. *Journal of Mental Science*. 1959; **105**:594–626.

Hoff P. Kraepelin — clinical section part 1. In: Berrios G, Porter R, eds. *A History of Clinical Psychiatry*. London: Athlone Press; 1995: 261–279.

Kraepelin E. *Memoirs* (trans. C Wooding-Deane). Berlin and London: Springer-Verlag; 1987.

McWhinnie DL, Hamilton DNH. The rise and fall of surgery for the 'floating' kidney. *British Medical Journal*. 1984; **288**:845–847.

Shorter E. *A History of Psychiatry — From the Era of the Asylum to the Age of Prozac*. New York: John Wiley & Sons; 1997.

Tuchman B. *The Proud Tower*. London: Hamish Hamilton; 1966.

Zilboorg G, Henry GA. *History of Medical Psychology*. New York: Norton; 1941.

Contemporary texts/papers

Alzheimer A. A characteristic disease of the cerebral cortex. In: Schultze E, Snell O, eds. *Allgemeine Zeitschrift für Psychiatrie und Psychisch-Gerichtliche Medizin*, Vol. LXIV. Berlin: Georg Relmer; 1907: 146–148.

Alzheimer A. On certain peculiar diseases of old age. *Zeitschrift für die gesamte Neurologie und Psychiatrie*. 1911; **4**:356–385.

Binet A, Simon T. Sur la nécessité d'établir un diagnostic scientifique des états inferieurs de l'intelligence. *L'Année Psychologique*. 1905; **11**:163–190.

Clouston TS. *Clinical Lectures on Mental Diseases*. London: J and A Churchill; 1904.

Craig M. The early treatment of mental disorder in early mental disease — *The Lancet* Extra Numbers no.2. London: Wakley and Son; 1912: 191–194.

Diefendorf AR. The aetiology of dementia paralytica. *British Medical Journal*. 1906; *ii*:744–746.

Hart B. The psychology of Freud and his school. *Journal of Mental Science*. 1910; **56**:431–452.

Husserl E. *Logische Untersuchungen*. Halle: Niemeyer; 1900–1.

Jackson JH, Stewart JP. Epileptic attacks with a warning of a crude sensation of smell and with the intellectual aura (dreamy state). *Brain*. 1899; **22**:534–541.

Mercier C. *A Textbook of Insanity*. London: Swan Sonnenschein; 1902: 46.

Mott FW. Recent developments in our knowledge of syphilis in relation to diseases of the nervous system. *British Medical Journal*. 1908; *i*:10–14.

Pick A. Über einen weiterer Symptomenkomplex im Rahmen der Dementia senilis. *Monatschrift für Psychiatrie*. 1906; **19**:97–108.

Wagner CC. The comparative frequency of general paresis. *American Journal of Insanity*. 1902; **58**:587–596.

1911–1920

1911–1920 CHAPTER 2

Major world events

1911	First expedition to the South Pole, by a Norwegian team
1911	George Claude invented the neon tube in France
1912	Sinking of the Titanic
1912	Wegner developed a complete theory about the derivation of continents
1913	Charlie Chaplin (USA) directed his first short film
1914	Opening of the Panama Canal
1914	Assassination of the Archduke Franz Ferdinand in Sarajaevo
1914	First blood transfusion using collected blood samples in Belgium
1917	International Red Cross received the Nobel Peace Prize
1918	First postal air service established (USA)
1918	Germany signed armistice agreement
1919	American Senate voted for Prohibition, prohibiting the sale and manufacture of alcohol
1919	League of Nations established

Major events in psychiatry

1911	Eugen Bleuler published his textbook, *Dementia Praecox or the Group of Schizophrenias* in Leipzig
1912	*The Psychology of Insanity*, by Bernard Hart, published in London
1913	Jung resigned from the International Psychoanalytic Association, his post at Zurich University, and editorship of the *Jahrbuch*
1913	Mental Deficiency Act was passed in the UK
1914	The term 'shell-shock' coined by British soldiers
1914	Freud's *On the History of the Psychoanalytic Movement* was published in Vienna
1915	Emil Kraepelin established the German Psychiatric Research Institute (*Deutsche Forschungsanstalt für Psychiatrie*)
1917	Giuseppe Epifanio, psychiatrist at the university psychiatric hospital, Turin, used barbiturates to put patients with major illnesses into prolonged sleep
1917	Julius Wagner-Jauregg, Professor of Psychiatry at the University of Vienna, discovered a method of arresting the progress of neurosyphilis by infecting the patients with malaria
1917	*Freud's Mourning and Melancholia* published in Vienna
1918	The first attempt to visualise brain structure by pneumoencephalography introduced by the American, Dandy
1919	Publication, in Paris, of Pierre Janet's magnum opus, *Les Médications Psychologiques,* translated as *Psychological Healing* (1925)
1920	In Britain, control legislation was passed in the Dangerous Drugs Act
1920	Hugh Crichton-Miller founded the psychoanalytically orientated Tavistock Clinic, London
1920	First out-patient clinic for training psychoanalysts founded in Berlin
1920	Melanie Klein, in Berlin, was the first to conceptualise the developmental theory and uses of play in the psychoanalytic treatment of children
1920	Freud's *Beyond the Pleasure Principle* published in Vienna

SHELL-SHOCK

by Ben Shephard

The term 'shell-shock' was coined by British soldiers in 1914 and taken up by medicine and the Army soon after. By 1916, though, it had ceased to be medically respectable and it was banned completely by the Army two years later. After the war, the British government set up a special committee to bury it for ever. Yet 'shell-shock' has remained in the language, as shorthand for the psychological problems which soldiers developed during the First World War.

The significance of 'shell-shock' in the history of psychiatry remains a matter of argument. This chapter will review the psychiatric debates provoked by 'shell-shock' and look at the medico-military phenomonon that it represented.

Phase 1: initial bewilderment

In understanding and treating 'shell-shock', the French, Germans, and British passed through more or less the same four stages, though not at the same time. First, there was a phase of bewilderment at the scale of the problem and its bizarre symptomatology, coupled with a feeling of therapeutic impotence in tackling it. "I wish you could be here", Sir William Osler wrote to an American friend in July 1915, "in this orgie of neuroses and psychoses and gaits and paralyses. I cannot imagine what has got into the central nervous system of the men and I see it is as bad in Germany. Hysterical dumbness, deafness, blindness, anaesthesia galore. I suppose it was the shock and the strain, but I wonder if it was ever thus in previous wars".

British bomb-throwers in action. The Sphere, April 1915. Reproduced with permission from The Illustrated London News Picture Library.

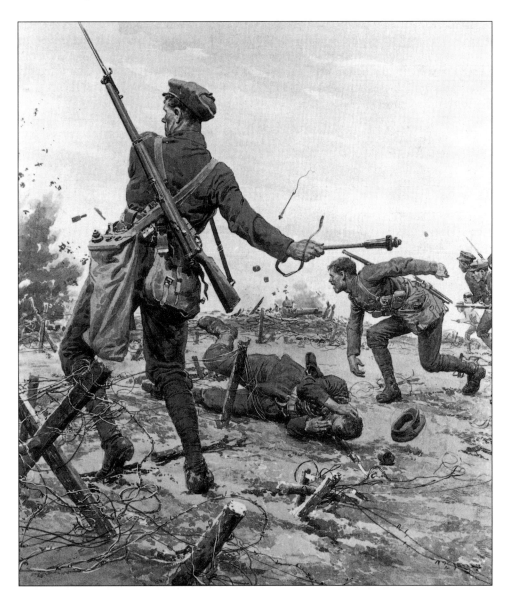

By then, psychiatrists across Europe were speculating about the effects of modern artillery fire on conscript armies in fixed trenches. It was quite natural that attention should focus first on the shellfire itself. Most of the early cases showed breakdown after shelling (many had been buried by explosions); knowledge of the physical and physiological effects of high explosive (e.g. how localised its blast was) remained fairly rudimentary. Moreover, few doctors suggested that the effects were entirely physical. The British neuropathologist FW Mott, for example, argued in 1917 that tiny particles of shells produced microscopic lesions in the brain, though he had earlier acknowledged that psychological factors, morale, and physical exhaustion were all intermingled.

In Germany, there were those who favoured the idea of *Granatkonkussion* or bomb concussion — an "injury due to the effects of an explosion but without an overt lesion, as a result of shaking or the pressure of air or gases". Prominent amongst these was the Berlin neurologist, Hermann Oppenheim, who revived the hypothesis which he had first put forward in the 1890s, of a 'traumatic neurosis' brought about by undetectable microscopic changes in the brain. Indeed, the wartime German debate was initially a re-run of the pre-war argument over industrial accidents. In this, Oppenheim's notion of a 'traumatic neurosis' had been rejected in favour of the alternative explanation, which interpreted the symptoms following traumatic accidents as manifestations of hysteria. Thus in the German context, the medical historian Paul Lerner has argued, male hysteria had become an acceptable diagnosis before the war because, "by attributing the disease to the patient's psyche", it "made trauma patients ineligible for pensions and mandated their return to work". In this way, says Lerner, "a powerful — and uniquely German — opposition between hysteria and work was formed which…displaced the traditional femininity of the disease". Given their pre-war experience, German doctors tended to see the war "as an industrial accident writ large".

In France too, there were advocates for the view that symptoms were physically caused; but the dominant voice was that of Joseph Babinski. While his pre-war attempts to dismantle Charcot — to argue that hysteria did not belong in neurology and was purely the product of suggestion — had not been altogether successful, his moralistic approach now matched the "stoic and belligerent climate of war", with male not female patients. Babinski insisted that symptoms were brought about not by the trauma of war itself, but either by unintentional suggestion from doctors or by the patient's auto-suggestion and imitation. He made no distinction between hysteria and malingering, arguing that forceful, authoritarian methods of treatment, using to the full the moral authority of the doctor, would restore men to the Army. This view found official favour.

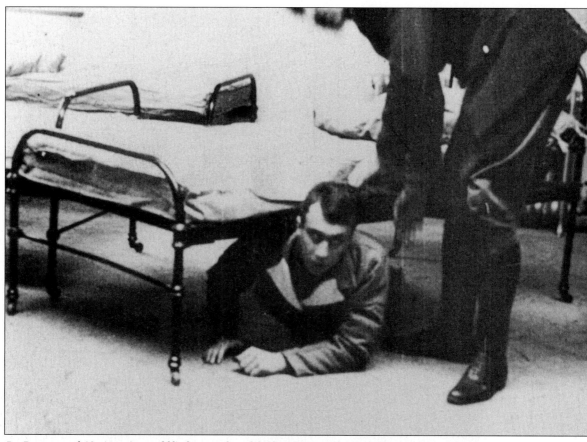

Pte Preston, aged 19. Amnesia, word blindness, and word deafness except to the word "Bombs!". His response is then to quickly get under his bed. From AF Hurst's film 'War Neuroses', 1918. Reproduced with permission from British Pathe plc.

Phase 2: miracle workers

About a year into the war, physical explanations of 'shell-shock' began to be discredited. Studies showed that its symptoms were not found in appreciable numbers amongst prisoners-of-war or wounded men — even when they had been exposed to heavy shellfire — but were present in some soldiers who had never been in battle.

That 'shell-shock' was more often 'emotional' than 'commotional' was confirmed by front-line reports. "In most cases of shell-shock the immediate cause of the nervous collapse is to be found in some sudden psychic shock", wrote Dr Harold Wiltshire in *The Lancet* in June 1916. Many of the cases he had treated in France had indeed been blown up, but the real causes of their breakdowns, he believed, were "horrible sights, losses, fright from an explosion, or sounds". Several patients had seen friends blown up or had had to clear up "the fragments of the killed".

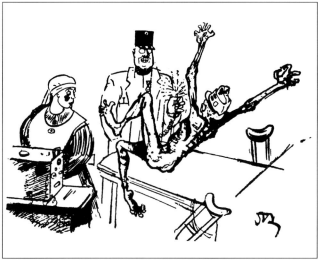

An Austrian cartoon based on the Kaufmann-Kur. By A. Stadler, reproduced in M. Hirschfeld and A. Gaspar (eds) Sittengeschichte des Erstens Weltkrieges *(Verlag für Sexualwissenschaft, Schneider and Co, Leipzig and Wein, 1930).*

"I can see it all, where we lost 30 or 40 men, they screamed and moaned, some with their arms blown off", one told Dr Wiltshire. Traumatic amnesia and disturbed dreams were common.

The implications of the new evidence were debated in medical meetings across Europe. In Munich, in September 1916, Oppenheim's hypothesis of organic causation was decisively rejected in favour of 'psychological' explanations advanced by Robert Gaupp, Karl Bonhoeffer, and Max Nonne. Their view was that, far from being anything new, the soldiers' strange symptoms were just the 'functional' disorders of peacetime — hysteria and neurasthenia — and could be quickly removed by skilful and confident therapists. Such 'miracle workers' had by then already begun to appear, usually doctors with pre-war experience in treating hysteria with suggestion and persuasion. Of these, the Hamburg neurologist Max Nonne was the most celebrated and

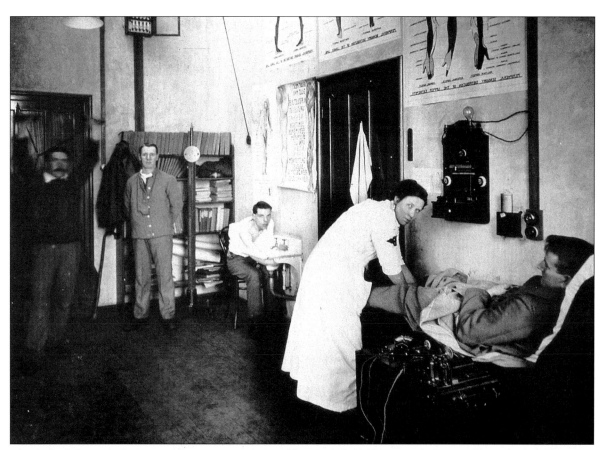

Electric shock therapy in the Treatment Department at the Maudsley Hospital, 1918. During the First World War the Maudsley was requisitioned for use as a military hospital treating 'shell-shock' cases. Reproduced with permission from the Bethlem Royal Hospital Archives and Museum.

successful, treating some 1600 patients during the war. As a young man, Nonne had spent time with both Charcot at the Salpêtrière and Bernheim at Nancy, before making his name with organic neurological research. The three necessary conditions for successful treatment of soldiers were, he wrote, "First, unfailing self-confidence; second, feelings of obedience on the patient's part; third [the creation of] an atmosphere of healing".

But not everyone had Nonne's skill. For others, the alternative tool was "plain speaking backed up by faradic current" (as the English physiologist ED Adrian put it) — or electricity as a prop for cure by suggestion. Lewis Yealland's dramatic account of 'curing' hysterical dumbness and paralysis at the neurological hospital at Queen Square, London, has been much quoted (for instance by Pat Barker in her novel, *Regeneration*), but Yealland was only a minor player in this league. The real maestros were Fritz Kaufmann of Mannheim, deviser of the 'Kaufmann cure', and Clovis Vincent of Tours, described as "France's most ruthless neurological matador" by the historian Roudebush. Both used 'torpillage', or electrical therapy. It was not however, always necessary to inflict pain. Many successful techniques involved deception, isolation, or simple ritual 'cures'.

For all their miraculous properties, these 'active treatments' ran into some public opposition and generated bad publicity. The 'Kaufmann cure' killed some 20 patients, while, in France, an attempt to prosecute a soldier who had punched Dr Vincent when the latter advanced on him with poised electrodes led to press condemnation of his methods. In Britain, the Army's use of the death penalty was criticised, but not its methods of treating 'shell-shock'. The one issue which did persistently inflame public opinion was the use of existing asylums for the treatment of psychotic military patients. 'Wrecked soldiers' were felt to deserve better than "what was good enough for the pauper patients".

Public opposition apart, there was by late 1916 growing evidence that simply removing symptoms was not always enough. Many 'cured' patients had relapses. There were, too, the beginnings of a shift in symptomatology away from hysteria towards 'anxiety neurosis' (as neurasthenia was increasingly called). All these factors helped to usher in a third phase, in which psychological models of the war neuroses and 'psychological' methods of treatment became more fashionable.

Phase 3: analytic methods

Throughout the war, doctors had distinguished between 'hysteria'— said to be found mainly in men — and 'neurasthenia', the officers' disorder. Men escaped into illness, developing hysterical blindness, deafness, or paralyses; whereas officers, with a greater sense of responsibility, had to stick it out, torn — so the argument went — by a conflict between the instinct of self-preservation, which urged them to flee, and their sense of duty and social position, which required that they stay at their post. Their symptoms were more complex — sweating palms, insomnia, irritability, startle responses.

Distinctions of class went beyond symptoms. Officers and men were sent to separate hospitals. Psychiatrists seldom used brutal, authoritarian, or magical techniques of treatment with officers or more intelligent patients (the Viennese professor of psychiatry, Wagner-Jauregg, was brought before a commission of enquiry in 1920 largely because his hospital *had* employed such methods on a middle-class patient; after ambiguous 'expert' testimony by Freud, Wagner-Jauregg was exonerated). In hospitals for officers, gentler, more analytic methods were preferred almost from the start of the war. Also, the generally backward state of British psychiatry and the reluctance of many British neurologists to handle 'functional nervous disorders' gave an important role in the treatment of 'shell-shock' to a small group of medically trained academic psychologists who were more receptive to the writings of Déjérine and Janet than the latters' French colleagues. They were allowed to experiment with simple analytic psychotherapy at several base hospitals, notably Maghull near Liverpool and Craiglockhart outside Edinburgh. One of them, the psychologist-cum-anthropologist William Rivers, also made some use of Freudian ideas of repression, while emphasising that the war had decisively disproved the idea of the sexual aetiology of neurosis.

Freud himself claimed in 1920 that only the abrupt end of the war had prevented the German, Austrian, and Hungarian armies from introducing the "purely psychological treatment of war neuroses". This was wishful thinking; while the German authorities had been sufficiently impressed by the work of Ernst Simmel in Posen to send observers to the Psychoanalytic Conference in Budapest in 1918, there is no evidence that they were planning such a wholesale conversion.

Phase 4: the psychosomatic approach

That there was a fourth phase in the literature of the war neuroses is perhaps more apparent now than it was at the time. It derived partly from the appearance of a new type of patient: one who had been at war for years and whose symptoms had a chronicity, which resisted both the quick miracle cure and the gentler probings of psychotherapy. "Two years ago", the French neurologist Grasset wrote in 1917, (we) "always concluded our reports on psychoneurotics by declaring them 'rapidly and definitely curable'. Soon we omitted 'rapidly'; then we omitted 'definitely'; then we omitted 'curable'. Now we are content to write 'do not seem curable'".

It derived also from pre-war work on the effects of emotion on the endocrine and nervous systems — of which WB Cannon's *Bodily Changes* was the most notable example — and from work by Pavlov and Sherrington on the reflexes.

The writing which emerged is small in volume and very diverse, but interesting in its attempt to combine the physiological with the psychological. Some modern preoccupations — for example, with what is now called neuroendocrinology — are anticipated. WH Rivers, after flirting with Freud, ultimately came up with a 'biological' account of 'shell-shock', which drew on John Hughlings Jackson's ideas of evolutionary 'levels'. He argued that being shell-shocked deprived the soldier of the use of the later, more sophisticated levels of his nervous system and caused him to revert to more primitive functions. (As a young doctor, Rivers had been Jackson's house physician at the London neurological hospital in Queen Square.) Freud, too, went back into neurology. In *Beyond the Pleasure Principle*, he ignored the tortuous attempts of his disciples to reconcile 'shell-shock' with the libido principle, and instead came up with the completely new idea of a traumatically produced 'compulsion to repeat'.

A medico-military phenomenon

The clinical literature of 'shell-shock' is overwhelmingly derived from chronic cases seen in base hospitals. Yet that is only half the story. 'Shell-shock' was as much a practical and disciplinary problem as a clinical and theoretical one; many doctors, like Lord Moran, regarded the term as simply "a respectable name for fear". What, then, was the reality on the ground? Little has been written about the handling of 'shell-shock' in the field by the French and German armies, but the British Shellshock Commission of 1922 published important evidence from front-line doctors.

Their general view was that the British had made a huge mistake in allowing the concept of 'shell-shock' to become reified in the public mind. One witness doubted whether there would have been a problem "if the name had not been invented…We should have been bound to have men breaking down in the line but we should not have had the same quantity".

'Shell-shock' was an early example of a common modern phenomenon: a medical debate, hedged with scientific qualifications, but taken up by public opinion and the media in an oversimplified way. Several of the 1922 witnesses felt that its "vivid terse name" had aroused public interest and that "this class of case excited more general interest, attention, and sympathy than any other". This was probably because many patients were officers and most British doctors were used to dealing with private patients, whereas their French and German equivalents were more likely to have worked for the State, and to have treated public patients.

How 'shell-shock' was presented in the popular press remains unclear, but *The Times* took it up almost from the start of the war, and Lord Northcliffe's brother lent his house in Kensington as a hospital for 'war-shocked officers'. In May 1915, an article on 'Battle shock. The wounded mind and its cure' explained that

> "The effects of severe shell fire are very complicated; but…they tend to show themselves in a dazed state which may on the one hand be developed into complete unconsciousness, on the other lightened till a condition comparable to neurasthenia is observed. The soldier having passed into this state of lessened control becomes a prey to his primitive instincts. He may be so affected that changes occur in his sense perceptions; he may become blind or deaf or lose the sense of smell or taste. He is cut off from his normal self and the associations that go to make up that self. Like a carriage which has lost its driver he is liable to all manner of accidents. At night insomnia troubles him and such sleep as he gets is full of visions; past experiences on the battlefield are recalled vividly; the will that can brace a man against fear is lacking".

Some British doctors in France felt that "two years of vivid journalese in the home papers had prepared the mind" of soldiers coming to the front to the point where they "develop the belief that a bursting shell produce[s] mysterious changes in the nervous system which destroy their self-control". They were said to "prepare to become a case of shell-shock almost before the first shell drops near them".

Army policy, it was argued, further exacerbated the problem. No First World War army (except the American) gave its troops effective medical examination, let alone psychological testing, but the situation was particularly bad in Britain. In 1914, "the whole country was simply seething with recruits. They were medically examined... in the most haphazard manner". Despite some improvement later in the war, no attempt was made to eliminate 'mental defectives' or those whose pre-war histories suggested they might be psychologically vulnerable.

Then there was the whole question of labelling. Traditionally, the British Army had never acknowledged the existence of what is now called 'battle shock'. Anyone who broke down in battle without being wounded was, officially, either mad or a coward. But the Army's historian, Sir John Fortescue, acknowledged in 1922 that "numbers of men went out of their minds in the old campaigns, as they still do", and that "even the bravest man [could] not endure to be under fire for more than a certain number of consecutive days". "Tried old soldiers in former wars", Fortescue explained, used mysteriously to disappear for periods of rest and recovery from the nervous strains of battle.

The phenomenon of 'shell-shock', however, forced the British War Office to recognise a grey area between madness and cowardice. In 1915, even as some shell-shocked soldiers were being shot for cowardice or desertion, two new diagnostic labels were cre-

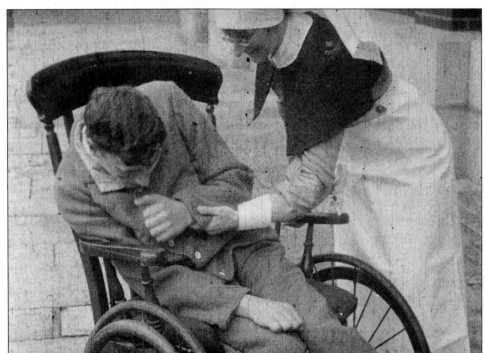

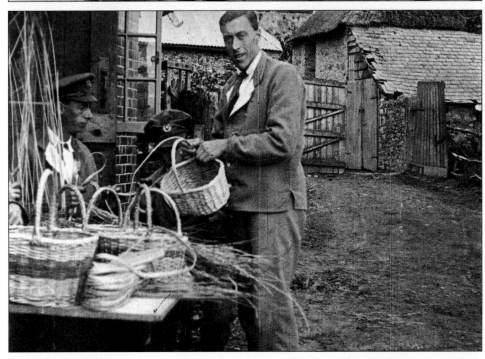

(Top) Pte Meek, aged 23, Seale Hayne Military Hospital. February 1917, complete retrograde amnesia, hysterical paralysis, contractures, mutism, and universal anaesthesia, dating from February 1916. (Bottom) Sudden recovery of memory, November 1917 with gradual recovery of body functions. June 1918, teaching basket-making, his peacetime job. From AF Hurst's film 'War Neuroses', 1918. Reproduced with permission from British Pathe plc.

ated. 'Shellshock-wounded' meant that the soldier had been blown up by an enemy shell and was entitled to be treated as 'wounded', with a wound stripe and a pension; 'shell-shock S' (for sickness) meant that he was simply suffering from nervous collapse. Most of these cases were evacuated to England, for the British were slow to follow the French example and create treatment centres near the front. The traditional British view was that "we can't be encumbered with lunatics in Army areas".

The overall effect of British policy is summed up by the Australian historian, AG Butler. "The idea and the name of 'shell-shock', though propounded in good faith as a helpful medical hypothesis [had become] through military and social exploitation and mass-sug-gestion — a devastating menace". This became clear during the battle of the Somme, between July and December 1916, when there were 16,139 cases of 'shell-shock wound-ed' alone. Many of these casualties were caused by extended artillery barrages and units

Hysterical pseudo-pseudohypertrophic muscular paralysis; (Top, middle) before treatment, (Bottom) after treatment, Netley Hospital, Southampton. From AF Hurst's film 'War Neuroses', 1918. Reproduced with permission from British Pathe plc.

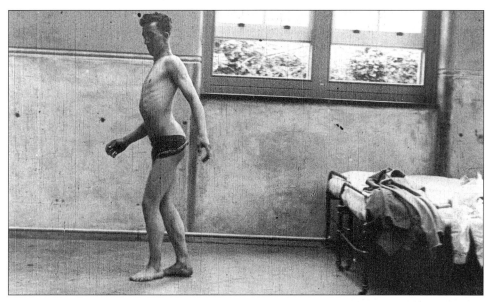

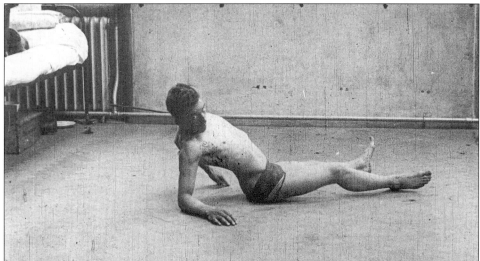

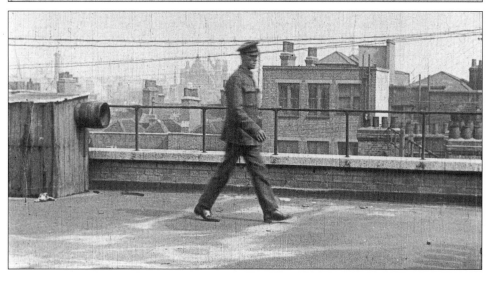

being kept in the line too long, but the knowledge that there was an honourable means of escape was thought to have helped swell the numbers. At the end of 1916, the British changed their policy. Forward treatment centres were created near the front and evacuation back to England discouraged. As a result, there were, according to official figures, only 7048 cases of 'shell-shock' in 1917 — the year of Passchendaele, the battle which is usually regarded as "the culmination of horror".

It would be a mistake to read too much into such figures. None the less, whether the steps taken by the French to deter psychiatric casualties — the provision of facilities for treatment near the front line from early on in the war, the denial of secondary gain by making sure all patients stayed in the military system as long as possible, the refusal to pay pensions to psychiatric casualties — had much effect is an interesting question. Unfortunately, while recent accounts suggest that both the British and the Germans had approximately 200,000 psychiatric casualties, there are no statistics at all for the French.

Certainly, many British and American doctors approved of the tough French policy and later advocated emulating it. For example, the London psychiatrist Bernard Hart, mainly remembered today as a fervent evangelist of Janet and Freud in his pre-war book *The Psychology of Insanity*, took a tough, Babinskian line in his evidence to the War Office Shell-Shock Committee in l922. He later applied it as Consultant to the Emergency Medical Services in the Second World War.

The American experience remains a puzzle. Entering the war late in 1917, they had had three years to observe and profit from the mistakes of others, as well as a wise and experienced administrator in Thomas W Salmon (who had learnt his psychiatry the hard way, at the Ellis Island immigration station and as Medical Director of the National Committee for Mental Hygiene). In theory, they did everything right. Psychologists tested their troops; in Europe, Salmon worked energetically to create a three-tier system of treatment (at division, Army, and base levels), which has remained ever since the model of military psychiatry. Yet even at that time, many cynics were sceptical about these arrangements and Salmon's policy did not eliminate the neuropsychiatric pensioner. Indeed, the fairly brief American involvement in the war produced some 69,394 neuropsychiatric casualties. As late as l927, there were some 68,727 American ex-servicemen of the First World War with neuro-psychiatric disorders in veterans' hospitals (over 45% of all patients in these hospitals).

Conclusion

"The war" Grafton Elliot Smith and TH Pear wrote in 1917, "has shown us one indisputable fact, that a psychoneurosis may be produced in almost anyone if only his environment be made difficult enough for him. It has warned us that the pessimistic, helpless appeal to heredity, so common in the case of insanity [is no longer adequate]. In the causation of the psychoneuroses, heredity undoubtedly counts, but social and material environment count infinitely more".

In the Anglo-Saxon countries, 'shell-shock' did produce a shifting of the psychiatric ground. The social environment of psychiatry changed because in the war respectable people — men of 'good character' — appeared to go mad, and a new kind of psychiatrist emerged to treat them. Society was forced to take madness more seriously and to redraw the line between that condition and sanity. Subsequent wars have further redefined the social role of psychiatry — the Second World War bringing community psychiatry, social psychiatry, group psychotherapy, the Therapeutic Community — and much else — in its wake; Vietnam brought post-traumatic stress disorder (Chapter 8, p. 248).

Whether this happened in France and Germany, however, is unclear. To Sandor Ferenczi in 1917, the pathology of the war simply seemed a "veritable museum of hysterical symptoms". More recently, Etienne Trillat has described the war as "a bloody interlude which provoked in the domain of psychological medicine, what one can call a regression.... Of all the writings in this epoch, only those of the Anglo-Saxons have a future, and this future will be psychosomatic medicine".

In German history, the legacy of 'shell-shock' was obscured by political and social upheaval. A generation of German psychiatrists, led by Karl Bonhoeffer and Robert Gaupp, emerged from war and revolution in 1918 convinced that the Germans' policy of sending military psychiatric cases back home for treatment had contributed to the "stab in the back", which they blamed for military defeat and political disaster. Soon after Hitler came to power, they began to lecture the Wehrmacht on what to do in the next war. As a result, the German Army treated war neurosis between l939 and l945 as a disciplinary, not a medical problem, and over 15,000 people were executed.

THE EMERGENCE OF PSYCHOANALYSIS

by Martin Stanton

Psychoanalysis originated in the late 1890s through a number of relatively informal exchanges between a small group of psychiatrists, neurologists, writers, lawyers, and sociologists in France, Germany, and Central Europe. It stemmed first and foremost from the Austrian neurologist Sigmund Freud's visit to France between October 1885 and March 1886, in which he imbibed the treatment methods of Charcot and Bernheim, and subsequently translated them for the German-speaking public. The nature of this lineage has remained controversial ever since, particularly with respect to parallels between Freud and Pierre Janet (Chapter 4, p. 102), another of Charcot's pupils, who developed his own suggestive techniques with neurotic patients. Even as late as August 1913, Janet presented a commissioned report on 'psychoanalysis' to the Seventh International Congress of Medicine in London, in which he accused Freud of virtual plagiarism. Ironically, the 'psychoanalytic defence', presented on that occasion by Carl Gustav Jung (Chapter 3, p. 71) — also a former Janet pupil — was equally critical of Freud.

Psychoanalysis generated an initial sense of identity through extensive personal correspondence around Freud's scientific papers and work in the early 1890s; particularly important in this respect was his 'self-analysis' — the term he gave to his correspondence with his close friend Wilhelm Fliess, an ear, nose, and throat specialist in Berlin. This prompted Freud's first overview of "psychology for neurologists", the *Project for a Scientific Psychology* in 1895. In October 1902, Freud started a regular Wednesday night meeting (the *Mittwochsgesellschaft*) at his house, 19 Berggasse, in Vienna, which was attended by five doctors and four 'interested laymen' — an event sometimes inflatedly referred to as the "foundation of the psychoanalytic movement". These occasions were complemented by shared holidays in several Central European spas and Italian resorts, where personal and scientific agendas were agreeably mixed.

Freud originally coined the term 'psychoanalysis' in 1896, and clearly intended it to apply to both a technique of working with mental disorders, and to an interpretative method that could be applied widely in both social and human sciences. If a preference had to be expressed between these two applications, Freud confessed that he had "never been a therapeutic enthusiast". It is significant in this respect that both of his main early innovatory books, *The Interpretation of Dreams* in 1900 and *The Psychopathology of Everyday Life* in 1902, were intended as metapsychological works addressing the specific form and function of unconscious process, rather than expositions of clinical experience. Similarly, in 1915, in his *Introductory Lectures on Psychoanalysis*, presented to a general rather than specialist audience at the University of Vienna, Freud dedicated his first semester to metapsychological themes, and only moved on to specific clinical aspects in the second part. Even when he did choose to consider psychoanalysis directly as a form of treatment for mental disorder, he remained both flexible and open to revision (amply illustrated in his frequent addition of footnotes to new editions of clinical papers). In this respect, it is significant that his first published account of a psychoanalytic case history — the *Fragment of an Analysis of a Case of Hysteria* in 1901 and 1905, or the Dora Case, as it is more popularly known — was a self-declared failure. The patient had walked out on Freud's treatment because he himself (in his own account) had failed to recognise and work with the issue of transference — the patient's projection of undigested psychic material onto the doctor. The case indeed encapsulates the tentative and experimental nature of early psychoanalysis, its capacity and tolerance of self-critique, and its prodigious conceptual creativity.

International recognition of psychoanalysis

The international recognition of psychoanalysis was secured in September 1909, when Freud, accompanied by two younger leading figures in the field, Carl Gustav Jung and Sandor Ferenczi, travelled to the USA to give a lecture series at Clark University, in Worcester, Massachusetts. These lectures were widely publicised and reviewed in medical journals. Jung's lecture series, in particular, on "Psychoanalysis and the Word Association Test", was particularly commended for its advances in the diagnosis of the *form* of any given mental disorder. At the Burghölzli Hospital near Zurich, Jung pioneered a treatment system in which a series of words were presented to a patient, and following each word, the individual was asked to provide the first association that came to mind. He measured the time it took for the patient to provide a response, and identified the words that commanded the longest response: these, he suggested, concealed a "complex" — an amalgam of deeply repressed unconscious material. Jung also selected those word associations which seemed to have no obvious or logical connection, again suggesting here that unconscious "displacements" or "condensations" at work merited further attention later in analysis. The great advantage of this method was that it conferred on psychoanalysis an empirical framework in which the "talking cure" could be mapped out and measured; and it also furnished a key concept — the complex — which could be represented in free-associative word-structures (Chapter 1, p. 19).

Foundation of an International Psychoanalytical Association

The great success of the American trip prompted the Hungarian psychoanalyst Ferenczi — with Freud and Jung's support — to propose the foundation of an International Psychoanalytical Association (IPA) at the Nuremberg Congress in 1910: "The psychoanalytically trained", he argued, "are surely best adapted to found an organisation which would combine the greatest personal liberty with the advantages of family organization. It would be a family in which the father enjoyed no dogmatic authority, but only that to which he was entitled by reason of his abilities and labours". Ferenczi's idealism and optimism about psychoanalysis, harked back to earlier, more open and cooperative days, since in fact, the future of the IPA proved to be riven with conflict and secession.

Indeed, Freud's initial decision not to stand as first President of the IPA, and instead to support Jung's canditature, immediately provoked division within the new organisation. Two Viennese medical psychoanalysts, Alfred Adler and Wilhelm Stekel, vocally expressed their opposition to Jung's nomination, and used the opportunity to elaborate on their own differences from what they perceived to be "mainstream" Freudian orthodoxy. Adler, who resigned from the Vienna Psychoanalytical Society and the IPA in May 1911, focused on Freud's underestimation of the role of social and economic factors in the aetiology of mental disorder. He advocated that psychoanalysis should develop an active role in primary care and education — a position that led him to stand as a socialist candidate in the Vienna city council elections in 1919 and to establish a psychoanalytic component in Austrian teacher training during the First Republic

(a tradition which survives and flourishes to this day). Stekel resigned in November 1912, ostensibly over a number of minor disputes including the ownership of a psychoanalytic publication, the *Zentrallblatt für Psychoanalyse*, of which he was the editor. He also demanded his right (which was refused) to reply in writing in the journal to public criticism from his colleague, Viktor Tausk — though Stekel later used the event to promote his own view that psychoanalysis should develop much shorter and more 'active' medical (as opposed to 'lay') approaches.

Introduction of the Oedipus complex

On the Zurich side of the schism, Jung found himself increasingly at odds with Freud's elaboration of the notion of the 'complex', particularly with the introduction of the Oedipus Complex in 1910, and its rapid promotion to the status of fundamental or 'nuclear' complex (*Kernkomplex*) by 1912. Jung first discretely explored the implicit prioritisation of sexual factors in the Freudian account of the development of neuroses in *Wandlungen und Symbole der Libido* (Symbols of Transformation), which was published in January 1912. Later in the year, he moved into a more boldly expressed and widely publicised critical position of the Freudian conception of the complex, in a series of lectures at

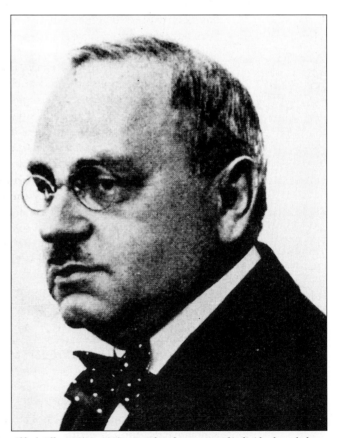

Alfred Adler (1870–1937). Developed a concept of individual psychology following a break with Freud in 1912. MD Medical Newsmagazine, *1961, 5th October, Page 148. Reproduced with permission from the Wellcome Institute Library, London.*

Fordham University, New York. The ensuing open conflict led him to resign from the IPA in April 1914.

In this context, therefore, it is hardly surprising that Freud's work during this emergent period of psychoanalysis from 1912 to 1919 mingled didacticism and polemicism. His early, if not premature *On the History of the Psychoanalytic Movement* of 1914 was written predominantly in the first person singular, and did not miss an opportunity to mark out emphatically the irrefutable nature of his own discoveries: "Every analysis conducted in a proper manner, and in particular every analysis of a child, strengthens the convictions upon which the theory of psychoanalysis is founded, and rebuts the re-interpretations made by both Jung's and Adler's systems". To support this position didactically, Freud wrote two series of papers in tandem: the *Papers on Metapsychology* in 1915, which provided extensive explorations of his key concepts of 'Instincts/Drives', 'Repression', and 'the Unconscious'; and the *Papers on Technique* of 1911–1915, which provided succinct if brief indications of the clinical methods employed in psychoanalysis. In particular, those related to: (a) opening and concluding treatment; (b) the use of free-association and dream interpretation; (c) the handling in sessions of the patient's unconscious reproduction of unresolved childhood conflicts (typically relating to parental intercourse or sibling rivalry for parental love); and (d) work in the transference — a term Freud applied to the unconscious parental figures who underlie the patient's ambivalent feelings and communications to the doctor in the session. In transference, the patient projects difficult and unresolved feelings for their parents onto the analyst: idealised and loving feelings generate a 'positive' transference, and envy and aggression precipitate a 'negative' one.

A third text — *On Narcissism: An Introduction* of 1914 — is now standardly added to these two complementary sets of papers, since for Freud, narcissism came to occupy a unique and problematic position between the metapsychological and the clinical. Freud made a distinction between two types of narcissim. Firstly, *normal* narcissism, evident in the general acquisition of ego-function (where "an original libidinal investment in the ego fundamentally persists, and is structurally related to all subsequent libidinal investment by the ego in objects in inner and outer worlds"). Secondly, *pathological* narcissism, displayed in narcissistic disorders and perversions, particularly homosexuality (where "young men take themselves as their sexual object, and look for a young man who resembles them and whom they may love as their mother loved them"). This tentative distinction between two modes of narcissism powerfully illustrates the tensions involved in extending a treatment method designed for specific neurotic pathologies into a general psychology of mental life.

Fundamental changes to clinical psychoanalysis

Although the main items in Freud's 1914–1915 general survey of principal ideas remain central to psychoanalytic work today, clinical practice is now significantly different. Clinical psychoanalysis underwent some fundamental changes during this initial experimental stage. First of all, the length of treatment altered radically. Initially, it rarely lasted more than a few months: Ferenczi's analysis with Freud, for example, took only three weeks in the autumn of 1914. Later treatments lengthened. This change was prompted particularly by work with psychotic and borderline patients (which Freud himself advised against), and by the stringent demands of training analyses, where thorough and in-depth work was deemed necessary to protect future analysts from the dangers of their profession.

Freud himself came to view the purposes of analysis as increasingly complex in themselves. He had already noted, somewhat ruefully, at the close of his analysis with Ernst Lanzer (otherwise known as the "Rat Man"), that although Lanzer's obsessive compulsions and prohibitions had disappeared, the exploration of the associative range of the rat delirium was far from complete (*Notes Upon a Case of Obsessional Neurosis* of 1909). In other words, the curative function of analysis may well have been completed, but the analyst's curiosity and research into the structure of the patient's obsessions certainly was not. Following this case, Freud's sense of the relative and diverse achievements of analysis became increasingly marked.

Analysis of the 'Wolf Man'

This is nowhere better illustrated than in his various accounts of his analysis of Sergei Constantinovitch Pankeiev (otherwise known as the 'Wolf Man') which began in 1910, and ended in midsummer 1914. Freud noted many years later that: "In these last months of his treatment, he (the Wolf Man) was able to reproduce all the memories and to discover all the connections which seemed necessary for the understanding of his early neurosis and mastering his present one.... I believed that his cure was radical and permanent". Yet indeed, the Wolf Man returned to Vienna in 1919 with the very same symptoms that had tortured him prior to his analysis. Freud then referred him on to his pupil, Ruth Mack Brunswick, who continued to see him for a number of years, though the case inspired many Freudian reflections on the complexities of the treatment. In later years, Freud standardly used this case to pose the question, "Is there such a thing as a natural end to an analysis?". To this, he provided a characteristically open-ended reply in *Analysis Terminable and Interminable* of 1937: "Two conditions must be approximately fulfilled — first, that the patient shall no longer be suffering from his symptoms and shall have overcome his anxieties and inhibitions; and secondly, that the analyst shall judge that so much repressed material has been made conscious, so much that was unintelligible has been explained, and so much internal resistance has been conquered, that there is no need to fear a repetition of the pathological processes concerned. If one is prevented by external difficulties from reaching this goal, it is better to speak of an incomplete analysis rather than of an unfinished one".

In short, for Freud, the consulting room remained always potentially open to reconsider issues of completion and completeness — open both for the patient in the context of their symptoms, and for the analyst in the context of their scientific reflections. Later, Nicholas Abraham and Maria Torok researched the associations in Russian (Pankeiev's mother-tongue) of the switchwords in the Wolf Man's famous dream of the six wolves. They discovered new linguistic links between symbolic motifs that had eluded Freud — notably the link between the 'six' motif (*shiestiero*) and the little sister (*siestorka*). This in turn they used to further substantiate Freud's diagnosis of the abusive impact of the sister's sexual intrusiveness in the aetiology of the Wolf Man's neurosis.

Post-First World War clients

By the end of the First World War, however, social pressures strongly militated against viewing psychoanalysis as a long-term and complex clinical treatment. First of all, the demand for psychoanalysis was much greater than had appeared to be the case when the principal client group was ostensibly formed by hysterics. The massive and multifaceted trauma of the War itself generated a huge demand for psychological therapies (this chapter, p. 40). Ferenczi in particular was instrumental in adapting psychoanalytic methods for the treatment of combat-related post-traumatic stress disorders (then diagnosed in Austria–Hungary as "war hysteria"). He widely publicised the observation that some occurrences of 'shell-shock' symptoms, including loss of the use of limbs, or loss of sight, were of somatoform rather than organic origin. He added that 'shell-shock' victims did not simply describe or hallucinate the events of battle, but also produced infantile and intimate material from their family lives. His work with these patients gained considerable official support for psychoanalytic approaches to war hysteria. A number of European government officials attended the Fifth International Psychoanalytical Association (IPA) Congress in Budapest in September 1918 with the specific intent of becoming updated on proposed new psychoanalytic treatment programmes. Ferenczi announced plans for the establishment of free psychoanalytic clinics for 'shell-shock' victims in all the main European capitals, where they would receive a new 'active' and brief form of psychoanalytic psychotherapy from specially trained psychoanalysts. He also proposed to explore possible group forms of psychoanalysis for all ex-servicemen.

The problem for the IPA with these proposals was neither need for the official enthusiasm, nor the potential presence of thousands of new patients, but rather the need for general acceptance of the new 'active' technique, and the training of thousands of new analysts to provide it. Ferenczi's notion of 'active technique' initially implied directing the patient's attention towards family and relationship issues — asking direct questions, for example, about fathers, mothers, and siblings, rather than following the 'fundamental rule' of free association, as well as time-limiting the treatment to a maximum of 15 sessions. In 1924, Ferenczi and Otto Rank attempted to proselytise this position in *The Development of Psychoanalysis*, but their radical proposals to impose strict time-limits and to direct sessions to specific issues encountered fierce resistance, not least from Freud himself. Ferenczi found himself under suspicion, and never regained his former closeness to Freud, while Rank resigned from the IPA later that year.

Psychoanalysis for children

Another new post-war potential client group for psychoanalysis was children. Freud's 'academic' interest in children — displayed first theoretically in 1905 in his *Three Essays on the*

Theory of Sexuality, and then further substantiated in *Analysis of a Phobia of a Five-Year-Old Boy* of 1909 — the Herbert Graf or 'Little Hans' Case — was soon developed into a separate form of clinical practice. In this area too, Ferenczi was instrumental in pioneering new play-based methods of child psychoanalysis, which he described in a number of crucial publications in 1913. These methods were later substantially developed in different ways by two of his pupils: Melanie Klein in first Germany and then the United Kingdom, and Margaret Mahler in the United States. A separate school of child psychoanalysis developed in Vienna from 1918 around the kindergarten work of Anna Freud (Sigmund Freud's daughter), Dorothy Burlingham, and later, Siegfried Bernfeld and Erik Erikson.

Patients' resistance to psychoanalysis

Faced with its own schisms, in the midst of turbulent, revolutionary times, it is hardly surprising that psychoanalysts attempted to use psychoanalytic methods to enquire why psychoanalysis might produce such conflict between its own proponents, and why indeed it encountered such vociferous public opposition. In the forefront of this enquiry was Karl Abraham, President of the Berlin Psychoanalytical Society from its foundation in 1910 to his untimely death at the age of 48 on Christmas Day 1925. Abraham was particularly concerned with the phenomenon of resistance to psychoanalysis, both within and without the consulting room, which he primarily related to the persistence of early infantile and narcissistic forms of relating, which he called "character". Notable in this respect were hate and envy, which, according to Abraham, derived primarily from dependence on the mother. If these emotions were not successfully integrated into ego-function, they developed a rigid defensive character structure, which remained unamenable to interpretation or any form of reasonable negotiation. Instead, these aspects of character would become increasingly immobile or melancholic in their thoughts and affects.

Possibly prior even to Freud's classic paper *Mourning and Melancholia* of 1917, Abraham argued that mourning embodied a fundamental psychic process. In this, the human subject acquired the ability to accept and process loss, but any substantial and pathological narcissistic defence against loss would result in melancholia. The patient's psychoanalytic experience in sessions could therefore be viewed as a form of mourning, but any resistance to such progress could be related to narcissistic character formation that blocked out real change. In such cases, according to Abraham, the main aim of analytic interpretations must be to identify and break down the resistance to them, and to puncture the subject's rigid character structure. Abraham's insights subsequently inspired a new technical focus in psychoanalytic clinical work: all dream, fantasy, and associative material within sessions could potentially be directly related to the analytic context itself. This con-

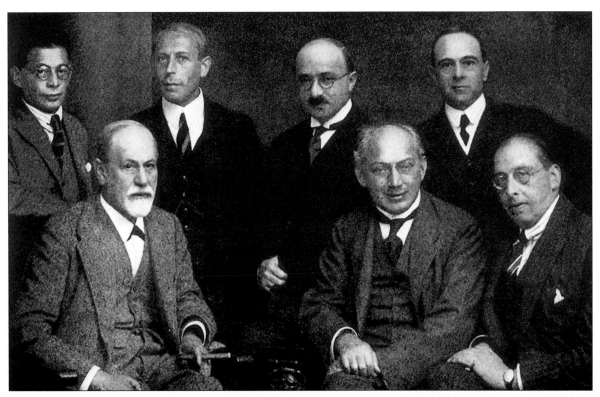

The 'Secret' Committee in 1922. (Sitting, from left to right) Sigmund Freud, Sandor Ferenczi, Hanns Sachs. (Standing, from left to right) Otto Rank, Karl Abraham, Max Eitingon, Ernest Jones. Reproduced from Zilboorg G. A History of Medical Psychology. New York: Norton; 1941. Photo courtesy of the Wellcome Institute Library, London.

text included both feelings about the analyst, and the restrictions of the method, and could consequently be interpreted in terms of resistance. Particularly important here was the work of Melanie Klein (Abraham's analysand and pupil), which she began in Berlin in 1919, and then refined and developed in London from 1926.

After Abraham's death, members of the Berlin School like Karen Horney and Wilhelm Reich further developed this notion of character into more socially and politically relevant categories. Horney introduced the notion of a "neurotic personality" — one which is haunted by self-doubt, recoils from competition, and is addicted to any form of analgesic in the vain attempt to eradicate psychic pain. Reich defined 'character' as *Panzierung* (armouring), after *Panzer* (a tank), to emphasise the tense and rigid structure he felt was articulated somatically through the subject's musculature. In November 1919, during the political upheavals, Reich significantly argued in numerous political broadsheets that 'character' was the crucial unconscious agent of all social control. He wryly supported this argument by observing that even the 'revolutionary' masses were vitally constricted in their protest by a very specific and unconscious form of character 'armouring'. The crowds in the Tiergarten in Berlin were easily restrained and obstructed in their aim to storm government buildings, because their 'character' constrained them to obey dutifully the many signs ordering them not to walk on the grass!

It is important to note just how radically psychoanalysis had distanced itself by 1919 from its early informal and experimental roots. First of all, it developed an institutional structure, with an international organisation (the IPA), national societies, and affiliated groups in many major Western cities. It also had a formalised training structure for analysts, including the requirement that all trainees should undergo personal analysis themselves.

Conclusion

The question whether all applicants needed to be medically qualified remained an open and controversial one. While most American IPA analysts argued that they should, many Europeans, following Freud, suggested that there was an important role for 'lay' (non-medical) analysts. Analysis also began to have a formal presence in universities: Ferenczi was elected the first Professor of a Department of Psychoanalysis at the University of Budapest in 1919. This was a trend he successfully exported to the United States in 1926 with his lecture series at the New School for Social Research in New York. To this day, that institution has fostered an ardent commitment to psychoanalysis.

In clinical terms, psychoanalysis had moved from its specific focus on hysterical and neurotic disorders to wider areas of mental health. Controversially, a small group of psychoanalysts, led initially by Jung and Bleuler, pioneered psychoanalytic treatment methods for schizophrenic disorders. Freud himself, though, remained convinced that psychoanalysis was inappropriate for this kind of work, because of the difficult or non-existent transference situations that arose with this category of patient. Partly in response to these shifts of clinical concern and partly in reaction to the Adler and Jung schisms, psychoanalysis developed a wide range of differing clinical approaches. Adler and Jung, for example, abandoned the couch for face-to-face work, and questioned Freud's method of dream interpretation. The Berlin School, and later the Kleinian School in London, placed particular emphasis on the analysis of resistance in analysis. They focused predominantly on transference and counter-transference issues as these arose in the specific context of the session, as opposed to concern for the detail of recollection of past events. Psychoanalytic work with children also raised new basic questions around the 'neutrality' and 'non-involvement' of the analyst — notably how play technique with children, such as Moreno's 1919 experiments in psychodrama, might be applied to creative therapeutic work with children. Finally, the pressures of providing psychotherapy for ex-combatants and 'shell-shock' victims provoked pioneering attempts to apply psychoanalytic methods to groups.

By 1919, psychoanalysis had emerged and established itself not only as a potential treatment for a wide range of mental disorders, but also as a lively and creative social and cultural force. It already had a strong presence in education, and an important influence too in the creative arts. Its researches into unconscious mental process and dreams, for example, provided a crucial new reference for both established academic disciplines, and emergent intellectual and cultural movements like dadaism and surrealism. Psychoanalysts themselves left the consulting room to play formative roles in other spheres and disciplines. For example: Otto Gross, anarchist and psychoanalyst, who had been analysed himself by both Jung and Stekel, became a seminal figure in the dadaist Cabaret Voltaire in Zurich in 1919; Andre Breton and Louis Aragon, both doctors engaged in psychotherapy with 'shell-shock' victims, contacted Freud and opened a mutually beneficial dialogue between surrealism and psychoanalysis — a dialogue later fruitfully developed by the creative collaboration of Spanish artist Salvador Dali and French psychoanalyst Jacques Lacan; finally, WH Rivers, (recently fictionally featured in Pat Barker's novel *The Ghost Road*) moved directly from anthropological research in Melanesia, to pioneer psychological treatments of shell-shock in the United Kingdom. At the same time, he was also elected the first chair of the newly formed medical section of the British Psychological Society.

In emerging from the Great War, psychoanalysis lost all trace of its original small-scale and marginal identity, and became a major innovative force in a wide range of fields spreading from medicine to the study of religion. The resultant loss of a special or exclusive clinical focus inevitably increased tensions both within the psychoanalytic movement itself, where schisms proliferated, and within the reception of psychoanalysis in general health care, where it began to be perceived as an exotic luxury for the rich or educated classes. Conversely, its new broad cultural presence inspired major changes in the perception of mental life — and particularly unconscious process — in various scientific and artistic fields of endeavour. It is in this broad perspective that its main lasting achievements are likely to be appraised, rather than in the efficacy or otherwise of Freud's early clinical experiments.

SIGMUND FREUD (1856–1939)

by Martin Stanton

Sigmund Freud was born in Freiberg, Moravia (now Pribor in the Czech Republic) on 6 May 1856. His father, Jacob Freud, was a Jewish wool merchant, who struggled most of his life with financial difficulties, while his mother, Amalia Natanson, was Jacob's third wife and 20 years younger than him. Sigmund had two half-brothers, Emanuel, who was married with children of his own, and was older than his stepmother, and Philipp, who was single, and a year younger than her. Freud's upbringing in this unusual family context was troubled and deeply confusing. He had marked conflicts with his brother Philipp, who became intimately involved with Amalia and made her pregnant. During Amalia's absence to give birth to Sigmund's sister Anna, Philipp conspired to have Sigmund's favourite nursemaid arrested for petty theft and sent to prison. Freud later frequently speculated that his personal insights into the Oedipus Complex and the sexual aetiology of the neuroses derived from these early family experiences. The family moved to Vienna, which was his mother's home, during Freud's later childhood; they were always financially precarious and without the help of one of his teachers, he might not have been able to complete his studies at the *gymnasium*.

Freud's university studies in Vienna progressed in an original way from philosophy and law to zoology and medicine. In 1883, he joined Theodor Meynert's Department of Psychiatry, but found that great brain anatomist "full of crochets and delusions". Freud soon developed very specific disagreements with the Meynert school, firstly in connection with his controversial involvement with the discovery of cocaine. Freud had advocated its use as a cure for morphine addiction and to increase 'vitality' in a paper of 1884, and did not acknowledge its addictive properties until three years later. At this time, Freud also believed that cocaine might be a 'wonder drug' that could cure severe depressive disorders, and experimented with it himself. He had also noticed that it caused numbness of the lips, mouth, and eyes, mentioning this to a younger colleague, Karl Koller. It was Koller alone, though, who developed its use as a local anaesthetic for eye operations.

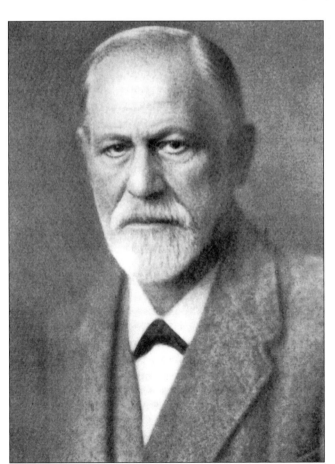

Sigmund Freud. Photo courtesy of The Royal College of Psychiatrists, London.

Freud also became centrally involved with Jean-Martin Charcot's use of hypnosis as a treatment for hysteria, having visited Paris between the autumn of 1885 and Easter 1886. Charcot's views were heavily derided in Austrian and German medical circles — and particularly by Meynert — so that Freud's adoption as the German 'disciple' and translator of this work placed him in an even more difficult position in the Vienna University Medical School.

Freud's 'discovery' of psychoanalysis progressed through a number of stages in the 1890s. Firstly, his experiences in Paris — particularly his autopsy research with Brouardel at the Paris morgue — led him to believe that severe sexual abuse of children directly contributed to the development of mental disorder in later life. This hypothesis has subsequently been called his 'Seduction Theory' — a term Freud himself never used. His cooperation with a Viennese physician, Josef Breuer, in evolving a 'talking cure' with hysterical patients led him to refine and qualify this view. In 1895, the two jointly published *Studies in Hysteria*, but later were estranged. Freud became increasingly aware of the function of 'fantasy' in the memory recall of abusive childhood events, and by September 1897, declared to his friend Wilhelm Fliess that he had 'abandoned' his original thesis, now maintaining that "there is no indication of reality in the unconscious". This particular *volte face* has attracted a great deal of critical attention in recent years, but careful historical research and careful reading of Freud's texts has revealed that his views on the relationship between sexual abuse and mental disorder remained complex. He never denied some causal link between the two, but suggested that unconscious repression and fantasy elaboration of traumatic scenes rendered the issue of proof problematic.

Freud's personal life offered some stability during this period of turbulent professional creativity. He became engaged to Martha Bernays two months after meeting her in 1882, and they eventually married in 1886, after a long and intense courtship that was often entirely dependent on correspondence. They had six children, but there is some speculation that the marriage proved not as fulfilling as Freud originally expected. Martha has frequently been described as a model *Hausfrau*, who shared little in common with her husband, and there has even been some speculation (based largely on correspondence with Jung and Ferenczi) that Freud engaged in a long-term affair with his sister-in-law, Minna Bernays, who moved permanently into the Freud household in the mid-1890s. It is certainly true that Freud regarded Minna as his 'treasure' and 'closest confidante', and shared both his new ideas and his love of cards with her. It is also clear from correspondence with Fliess that Freud suffered from frequent 'death deliria', chest pains, and arrhythmia, and that sexual relations with Martha ceased during this period.

Freud set out the main theoretical foundations of psychoanalysis in *The Interpretation of Dreams* in 1900 and *The Psychopathology of Everyday Life* in 1901. In these works, he proposed fundamental hypotheses on the structure and function of unconscious mental processes, and, in many ways, his subsequent work may be viewed as a critical review and refinement of these. Freud indicated two main sites in which to study and work clinically with unconscious processes. Firstly, the dream — whose recall in analytical sessions displayed various hidden meanings which were encrypted in the verbal or visual form of the patient's account. Secondly, there was the *parapraxis* — or Freudian slip — where bungled actions, the forgetting of familiar words, and the 'chance' substitution of one word for another, indicated repressed ideas that were either unbearable (such as thoughts of death) or socially unacceptable (such as sexual fantasies). There can be no doubt that Freud's work in these areas was substantially advanced by his meeting with Carl-Gustav Jung in early 1907. Jung's *Word Diagnostic Association Studies* of 1905 enabled an important critical refinement of Freudian thinking, notably around Jung's term the *complex*. For both men, complexes came to denote the basic unconscious structures that all individuals had to confront in their adaption to reality. In 1912, Freud claimed to have discovered the 'nuclear complex' — the Oedipus Complex — through which all children negotiated issues of incestuous attachment to their parents. However, Jung disagreed with the exclusive emphasis this placed on sexuality in the development of psychic life, and, after an extended acrimonious exchange with Freud, left the psychoanalytic movement. Here too, historians and critics have suggested that unresolved personal issues underlay the schism between the two — notably issues of repressed homosexuality between the two, as well as racism in Jung's more or less repressed anti-Semitism.

Like all his generation, Freud's personal and professional world was radically transformed by the First World War of 1914–1918. His sons Ernst and Martin were conscripted, and he saw the effects of shell-shock, severe poverty, and rationing loom large in his clinical practice. In the aftermath of the War, Freud attempted to introduce a new model of mental functioning to accommodate both his discovery of the role and function of unconscious process in shell-shock, and his reassessment of the place of aggression and destructiveness in human thought and behaviour. This new model is now traditionally referred to as the 'structural theory', though again, this term was not employed by Freud himself. The emergence of the structural theory is usually identified with the publication of *Beyond the Pleasure Principle* in 1920, but in fact major changes were already visible in his earlier papers on narcissism. They were also seen in his crucial text *Mourning and Melancholia* in 1917, where he suggests for the first time that mourning is a fundamental psychic process through which everyone has to negotiate their own and others' aggressive, destructive, and envious attacks.

Freud's clinical work on the 'death drive' also had a tragic personal dimension. In February 1923, he was diagnosed as having a leukoplastic growth on his jaw and palate, which at first was believed to be benign, but later found to be malignant. Freud subsequently underwent a series of operations to remove malignant tissue, which obliged him to wear a prosthesis from 1924 on, making it painful for him to talk. He also suffered from constant auditory disturbances, and gradually became almost deaf in his right ear. These symptoms obviously made it increasingly difficult for him to practise psychoanalysis. Following the *Anschluss*, the Nazi take-over of Austria in 1938, Freud's position in Vienna became increasingly precarious, and Ernest Jones managed to persuade the family to leave their home in the *Berggasse* and flee to London. In his new home in Maresfield Gardens, Hampstead (now the Freud Museum in London), Freud managed to finish his last great work, *Moses and Monotheism*, in 1939. In this, he explored the 'historical fantasy' that the Jewish people had murdered the original visionary Moses, and hidden the crime by substituting another more staid and legalistic figure. The book still provokes fierce critical controversy over how it should be read. Some argue that it is a playful semi-autobiography, with Freud clearly identifiable as the original Moses. Others suggest rather that it represents the final chapter of Freud's exploration of the death-drive, which he controversially located both in the Jews' own murder of their leader, and in the 'aetiology' of anti-Semitism. Whether either or both are the case, Freud finished the book in great pain. The ulcerated cancer wound was so foetid that even Freud's favourite chow dog *Jofi* would not go near him. Freud eventually arranged for his physician, Max Schur, to give him a fatal dose of morphine, and he died peacefully at home on 23 September 1939.

EMIL KRAEPELIN (1856–1926)

by Eric J Engstrom & Matthias M Weber

Biography

Emil Wilhelm Magnus Georg Kraepelin was born in 1856 in the north-German town of Neustrelitz (Grand Duchy of Mecklenburg). He was the son of middle-class parents struggling to maintain the outward appearances of bourgeois respectability. His father, Karl, was an actor, opera singer, and music teacher who, after falling on hard times, had changed careers to become a travelling story-teller of some repute. Rarely at home, often taking to drink, and chronically short of money, Karl's marriage to his wife Emilie soon floundered, leaving her to raise their children largely on her own. While Emil's relationship to his mother remained close throughout his life, the news of his father's death in 1882 was received indifferently, like that of a "foreigner" whose ties to the family had become little more than "sterile piety". When, later in his life, Emil Kraepelin had become convinced of the degenerative influence of alcohol and campaigned avidly on behalf of abolitionist causes, his admonitions lent voice not only to concerns for psychiatric patients and the health of the German nation as a whole, but also to worries about his own lineage.

Kraepelin attended the universities of Würzburg, Munich, and Leipzig. In Leipzig, he studied under Wilhelm Wundt (1832–1920), whose influence on Kraepelin was deep and long lasting. It was at Wundt's behest that in 1883 he drafted the first of nine versions of his famous textbook, although at the time Kraepelin wished instead to pursue work in the fields of criminology and experimental psychology. From the mid-1880s, Kraepelin's career took off in spectacular fashion. In 1885 he was appointed Professor of Psychiatry at the University of Dorpat in Estonia. It was here, on the very fringe of German academic life, that Kraepelin's psychiatric research agenda took shape and his sense of national identity came to prominence. Being confronted with Estonian patients whose language he did not understand, Kraepelin placed little emphasis on doctor–patient communication and clinical investigation, focusing his attention instead on experimental laboratory research. Furthermore, with Imperial Russian administrators intensifying their efforts to impose the Russian language on Estonian institutions, Kraepelin and his German colleagues came to see themselves manning an outpost of German culture and science on the fringe of European civilisation.

He then moved to Heidelberg in 1891. It was here that his clinical research began in earnest, leading ultimately to the formulation of his classic distinction between manic-depressive psychosis and dementia praecox. Twelve years later, he was named director of the university psychiatric clinic in Munich, where his attention turned increasingly to theories of degeneration, alcoholism, and mental hygiene. In the midst of the First World War and thanks to an intricate and far reaching web of contacts to prominent bankers, politicians, and philanthropists, such as James Loeb (1867–1933), Kraepelin founded the German Research Institute for Psychiatry, a forerunner of today's Max–Planck Institute for Psychiatry. After retiring from his university post in 1922, he devoted his energies to the development of the research institute up until his death in 1926.

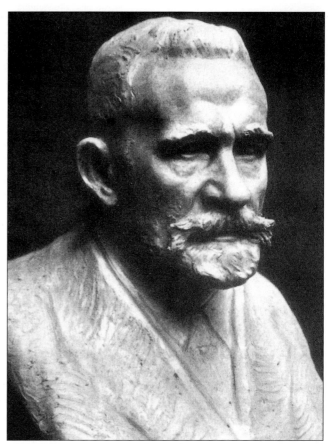

Emil Kraepelin. Photo courtesy of The Royal College of Psychiatrists, London.

Kraepelin's nosology and research agenda

Kraepelin's nosology evolved in response both to Griesinger's unitary psychosis theory and to the causal speculations of contemporary cerebral pathologists. In the 1860s, Griesinger was Germany's most prominent psychiatrist: he founded the university psychiatric clinic in Berlin and had been instrumental in reorientating German psychiatric thought and practice toward an understanding of mental illness as brain disease. However, the unitary psychosis theory of Griesinger — i.e. his belief that all psychiatric symptoms were, at root, manifestations of one single disease — had become increasingly untenable as a growing number of studies pointed to the existence of several distinct forms of mental illness (especially monomania, catatonia, and hebephrenia). Since clinical experience had not substantiated Griesinger's theory, Kraepelin decided to reject it and began constructing individual disease categories amidst the systemic vacuum of diverse and incompatible psychiatric theories. On the other hand, Kraepelin equally rejected the convoluted theories of the cerebral pathologists. In his opinion, what psychiatry needed in its efforts to establish a causal link between cerebral function and mental disease was less 'speculative' theory and more basic laboratory research into mental processes.

Holding fast to the postulate of somatic aetiology, Kraepelin thus turned to Wundtian experimental psychology. Trying to apply its methods to psychiatry, he undertook research using stimulus–reaction experiments to explore the effects of drugs, alcohol, and fatigue on psychological functioning. He hoped to be able to measure deviations from psychological norms and on the basis of these measurements, to isolate discrete disease categories. Throughout his entire career, Kraepelin devised experiments in an effort to quantify and demarcate psychological processes. In these experiments, he was careful to distinguish sharply between organic and psychological spheres, which he believed needed to be investigated separately. Ultimately, however, Kraepelin failed to bring these two spheres together: his conception of mental processes remained that of a psychosomatic parallelist, i.e. someone who believed that identifiable scientific laws governed respective phenomena *within* the mind and the body, but who simultaneously refrained from postulating causal links *between* mind and body. Furthermore, he investigated psychological symptoms not for their own sake, but rather as windows into deeper somatic causes, which he believed lay at the root of all psychiatric disorders.

Alongside his experimental investigations, Kraepelin also embarked on an ambitious clinical research project in the early 1890s. Strongly influenced by the work of Karl Kahlbaum (a psychiatrist in Görlitz) and Ewald Hecker (scientific pupil of Kahlbaum and head of the Johannisberg Clinic in Wiesbaden), he began to explore the longitudinal development of his patients' afflictions. He believed that by examining the entire course of an illness he could expose unique characteristics of natural disease entities. Thus, throughout the 1890s and indeed for the rest of his life, he meticulously catalogued the histories of hundreds of patients. In the process, he developed elaborate institutional strategies and diagnostic tools including his famous *Zählkarten*. The *Zählkarten* were cards used to collect, sort, and compare clinical information on his patients; they were designed specifically to observe and document patients' illnesses over extended periods of time. Today, it remains a matter of historical debate just to what degree Kraepelin's nosology was the product of this empirically based research or to what extent that research was merely the *post hoc* verification of his own preconceived categories of mental illness.

In any event, the fruits of his labours were harvested in the fifth edition of his textbook in 1896. There, he presented a system of classification which subordinated disease categories based on outward symptoms to those emphasising the origin, course, and termination of disease. It was in the context of this shift from a static synchronic, symptomatic perspective to a temporal or diachronic, clinical perspective that he constructed his two-part model of the endogenous psychoses. Initially, this classificatory model was received with reserve by his professional colleagues. Friedrich Jolly, Director of the Psychiatric University Clinic in Strasbourg, disputed Kraepelin's inclusion of the prognostic criteria in the construction of his clinical categories. Alfred Hoche, director of the Psychiatric University Clinic in Freiburg, was a tenacious critic of Kraepelin's concept of disease entities, arguing that psychiatry needed first to concentrate on establishing clearly defined syndromes before proceeding to speak about diseases. Yet in spite of these and other critics, by the time the seventh edition of his textbook appeared in 1903–1904, Kraepelin's bipolar nosology had gained widespread acceptance in German psychiatric thought and practice.

Politics

Having established his reputation as one of the foremost authorities in his discipline, in the decade prior to the First World War Kraepelin began to apply his psychiatric expertise toward the resolution of socio-political problems plaguing German society. He revisited his long-standing interest in criminal psychology in an article on 'Crime as a Social Disease', in which he proposed legal and penal reforms which would give professional psychiatrists a greater say in the extent and nature of the sentences passed on convicted criminals. He intensified his efforts to combat alcoholism by publicly criticising breweries, by delivering public lectures on the dangers of drink, and by coordinating efforts to establish sanatoria for recovering alcoholics. Kraepelin also warned of the urgent threat posed by syphilis and homosexuality to the vitality of the German people. In all of these fields of socio-political engagement, the somatic bent of Kraepelin's psychiatric thinking led him to interpret social problems in biological and social-Darwinist terms. For him, many social ills were the expression of degenerative forces which hobbled the nation in its "struggle for survival" (*Kampf ums Dasein*). Similarly, the 'cure' for these degenerative ills lay in their prevention and, ultimately, in aspirations of a biologically engineered populace. Accordingly, Kraepelin was an advocate of eugenic policies.

With the arrival of the First World War, the dangers of alcohol and syphilis loomed ever larger in Kraepelin's mind. For him scientific research now needed to go to battle against these internal enemies, which endangered public health and the collective national body, i.e. the *Volkskörper*. The defense of the *Volkskörper* became a personal, professional, scientific, and national imperative. Hence, it is hardly surprising that Kraepelin's conception of the origins and goals of the German Research Institute for Psychiatry, which he founded in 1917, reflected this inter-penetration of science and national mental hygiene. For him, the Institute was a home of rigorous science, and indeed, it became a centre of international research which brought together psychiatrists from around the globe. At the same time, it was designed to "serve the nation's health and to work toward healing the deep wounds which bitter fate has inflicted upon our fatherland".

Legacy

Kraepelin's legacy is a mixed one. His bipolar model became enormously influential in the early twentieth century and continues to shape the operational diagnostic systems DSM–IV and ICD–10. At the time, the model's success was due largely to the clinical utility of its prognostic orientation. Furthermore, its appearance was extremely auspicious in a profession casting about for reliable diagnostic criteria, struggling to develop a teachable canon of disease categories, and striving to mimic the spectacular successes of neighbouring disciplines such as bacteriology.

However, Kraepelin found it difficult to translate the results of his research agenda into effective therapeutic tools. Both his blind faith in the impartiality of scientific observations and his uncritical acceptance of those observations as objective 'facts' revealed the deep-seated positivist convictions guiding his psychiatric research. His instrumental rationality, with its inherent rejection of an inter-subjective approach to psychiatric therapy, helped produce a therapeutic vacuum which threatened to be filled by values and norms external to the subjective well-being of the patient. His psychiatry became vulnerable to the importation and adoption of normative criteria and ideologies drawn from the wider socio-political context. In early twentieth-century Germany, one such ideology was nationalism and it distracted Kraepelin's therapeutic attention away from the individual patient toward a larger *Volkskörper*.

EUGEN BLEULER (1857–1939)

by John K Wing

Eugen Bleuler was born in 1857 in the small Swiss village of Zollikon and took his medical degree in nearby Zurich. Apart from periods with Charcot in Paris, von Gudden in Munich and, briefly, studying neuropathology in London, he spent most of his life in Switzerland. He was Director of the Rheinan Hospital, 1886–1898 and then Professor of Psychiatry and Director of the Burghölzli in Zurich until 1927. He was responsible for a series of editions of an influential textbook, carried on after his death in 1939, by his son Manfred. Undoubtedly, the work with which his name is most associated is his monograph on 'dementia praecox', in which he re-worked Kraepelin's concept and re-named it *schizophrenia* (this chapter, p. 49). A link to another section in this series is his introduction of the term *autism* (Chapter 5, p. 139) to describe a key symptom in the new concept.

Bleuler's predecessors

Up to the middle of the nineteenth century, there was no concept corresponding to dementia praecox. A sort of orthodoxy was based on one aspect of Griesinger's teaching that only what we would now call 'affective' and 'schizoaffective' disorders constituted a 'primary' disease process. It was thought that what are currently described as chronic schizophrenic impairments could develop secondarily, but only after earlier affective episodes. Griesinger, who was Professor of Psychiatry in Berlin in the 1860s and thought that mental disease was essentially brain disease, eventually came to agree that there could be a primary psychosis even in the absence of these preliminary episodes. He thereby abandoned the classification system of mental disorders that had been traditional for him and his time. It was not until the publication of the fifth edition of Kraepelin's textbook (1896, 1987) that a firm line of demarcation was drawn between dementia praecox and affective psychosis, and a sort of consensus again achieved.

Both Griesinger's and Kraepelin's concepts were couched in terms of disease entities, following the lines of successful developments in medicine at that time. The anatomical and physiological concomitants of a number of

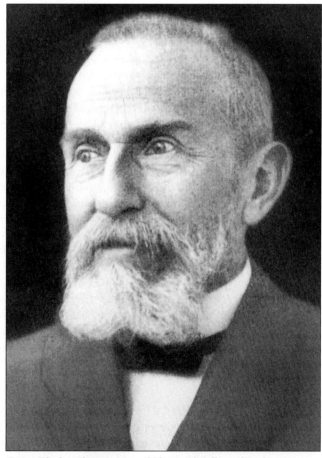

Eugen Bleuler. Photo courtesy of The Royal College of Psychiatrists, London.

important clinically identified syndromes had been discovered, often with a 'natural' history and a pathology, and sometimes with what appeared to be a single causal agent such as the tubercle bacillus or the cholera vibrio. These examples proved irresistible to contemporary neuro-psychiatrists, who were similarly carving more specific syndromes out of the global concepts of dementia, delirium, and insanity that preceded them. Since the causes of these disorders were unknown, though variously postulated, their classification depended largely on the course and outcome of groups of symptoms.

Kraepelin had introduced a simple distinction between two groups of disorders. On the one hand, were conditions characterised by mental deterioration, such as the catatonia and hebephrenia described by his contemporary Kahlbaum. With paranoid deterioration, these became sub-divisions of the disease dementia praecox. On the other hand, periodic forms of mania and melancholia, such as the *folie circulaire* of the French psychiatrist Falret were regarded as separate entities. Kraepelin's follow-up data suggested a mental state profile for dementia praecox that was recognisable at the time of presentation, and a generally regular and progressive course. The chief symptoms were auditory and tactile hallucinations, delusions thought disorder, incoherence, blunted affect, negativism, stereotypies, and lack of insight. These phenomena were expressed as psychological rather than physical abnormalities; catatonic symptoms, for example, were described in terms of disorders of the will. Paranoia was regarded as a separate disorder, characterised by incorrigible delusions often circumscribed in subject matter, a general absence of hallucinations, and a chronic but non-deteriorating course.

A sympathetic and illuminating account of the development of Kraepelin's ideas up to 1913 was provided by Berrios and Hauser in 1988. They point out that his concept was neither as simple nor as rigid as is generally assumed and that it continued to develop. Indeed, in 1920, Kraepelin eventually came to agree that dementia praecox and manic–depressive psychosis could co-exist and, thus, that a form of unitary psychosis could not be ruled out (Chapter 1, p. 13).

Bleuler's contribution

The term 'schizophrenia' stems from Eugen Bleuler who, in his preface to his work of 1911, acknowledged his indebtedness to Kraepelin's "grouping and description of the separate symptoms" and to Freud, whose ideas Bleuler used to "advance and enlarge the concepts of psychopathology". He did not accept the term 'dementia' as a valid description of the end-state, but did retain the separation from manic–depressive psychosis. At the same time he pointed out that affective symptoms could co-exist, which was an early example of comorbidity. His concept was based on an assumption that the manifold external clinical manifestations masked an inner clinical unity that "clearly marked [them] off from other types of disease". Moreover, he argued that "each case nevertheless reveals some significant residual symptoms common to all". The end-results were identical, not quantitatively but qualitatively. In a paper of 1908, he stated: "Personally I have never treated a patient who has proved on close examination to be entirely free from signs of the illness".

Bleuler's primary symptom was cognitive: a form of 'thought disorder', with loosening of the associations. It provided links to Kraepelin's 'dementia' and to the biological origins of the disease, but also, through 'psychic complexes' to ambivalence, autism, and disorders of affect, attention, and will. In his view, these essential symptoms could be observed in every case. Catatonia, delusions, hallucinations, and behavioural problems he regarded as accessory psychological reactions, not caused by the biological process or processes. Bleuler also won great renown for transplanting Freud's theories of the unconscious into orthodox psychiatry.

A substantial subgroup of the whole disorder was designated as 'simple schizophrenia', in which no accessory symptoms (the most easy to recognise) need be present. Diem, who worked with Bleuler, gave a description of two cases that he thought were due to simple dementing forms of dementia praecox. Both patients apparently normal as children, but as young men, began inexplicably to lose volition and purpose, ending as vagrants. Delusions and hallucinations were absent. Although no early developmental history was available, these two people certainly became severely impaired in psychological and personal functioning, and fitted Bleuler's description of simple schizophrenia. Bleuler's own examples are less easy to recognise. Amongst the lower classes, they "vegetate as day labourers, peddlars, even as servants". At higher levels, "the most common type is the wife..., who is unbearable, constantly scolding, nagging, always making demands but never recognising duties". Beyond this simple form, the largest subgroup was labelled 'latent schizophrenia'. These were "irritable, odd, moody, withdrawn or exaggeratedly punctual people". Bleuler thought it "not necessary to give a detailed description" of the mani-festations in this group, but it clearly merges with subsequent concepts of schizoid and schizotypal personality.

This is in contrast to Kraepelin, whose account even of the 'mild' form of the course of illness sounds severe. Thus, although Bleuler separated those with the disease from those without, the concept was in effect dimensional. While accepting much of Kraepelin's formulation, Bleuler substantially widened the concept, though continuing to describe his version as a disease entity. The simple and latent forms, whose vaguely defined pri-mary symptoms could be elaborated through psychic complexes, were thus able to carry the power of a widely recognised diagnosis.

In 1910, Freud, together with Bleuler, Jung, and Ferenczi founded the International Psychoanalytic Association, though Bleuler's contribution did not last long. Under the influence of contrasting types of theory, one psychoanalytical, the other biological, Bleuler's least differentiated sub-groups came to be used, in the USA, to label people with few or no clear-cut symptoms, while in the USSR, they resulted in 'sluggish schizophre-nia' — a psychotic diagnosis used to subdue political dissent.

Bleuler followed another line of development using ideas both from Kahlbaum, who had been the first to describe hebephrenia and catatonia, and Kraepelin, who included catatonia as a form of dementia praecox. Bleuler gave a detailed description of cataton-ic signs but regarded them as 'accessory' phenomena and tended to interpret them in psy-choanalytical terms.

On the other hand, he singled out autism as one of the fundamental features of schiz-ophrenia; this was regarded as an active withdrawal from contact with reality, in order to live in an inner world of fantasy. Gruhle pointed out that it was just as likely to be forced on the patient by the cognitive disorder. Kanner (1943) recognised, in a flash of genius, a syndrome in children that should be separated from the then amorphous mass of mental subnormality and childhood psychosis. His observations were exact and brilliant. However, by adopting the much less exact term 'early infantile autism' to describe it, he linked it inappropriately to Bleuler's concept of schizophrenia (Chapter 5, p. 139). At virtually the same time, Asperger described, with similar precision, an 'autistic psychopathy in child-hood' that is clearly part of the same spectrum as Kanner's syndrome because it shares a similar developmental history.

Operational criteria for classification

Whether the disorders recognised by applying the criteria laid down in DSM–III and its successors, and now in ICD–10, can be described as 'concepts' is a moot point. Certainly, the rules for schizophrenia in the *Diagnostic Criteria for Research* in sub-chapter F20 of ICD–10 are far from describing a disease concept. They do list most of the symptoms described by Kraepelin and Bleuler, but do not include a particular long-term course or outcome, or refer to a pathology or a cause. The distinction between schizoaffective and bipolar disorder is limited to a clinical judgement as to which type of symptom occurs first. Schizophrenia in ICD–10 is not a disease but a disorder. The introduction explains that this terminology is adopted "so as to avoid even greater problems inherent in the use of terms such as 'disease' and 'illness'. 'Disorder' is not an exact term, but it is used here to imply the existence of a clinically recognisable set of symptoms or behaviour that in most cases is associated with distress and with interference with functions". Flaum and Andreason, in *Schizophrenia Bulletin* illustrate the position clearly. They listed DSM–III–R and ICD–10 criteria, together with three further versions under consideration for DSM–IV. It is unlikely, in fact, that a disease concept will change its nature by choosing two of one kind of item and three of another, rather than three of the first kind and two of the second.

Conclusion

This review began with Griesinger and Kahlbaum, from whom Kraepelin and Bleuler gained their inspiration. The symptoms complained of by their patients have not much changed, but theories that were inconceivable during Bleuler's lifetime will generate different disease concepts. Since contemporary computerised systems provide for reliable rating of symptoms according to differential definitions, we can make concepts compete against each other in a way that would have been inconceivable to these pioneers. The more precisely the concepts and the predictions that follow from them are stated, the more easily they can be refuted if they are wrong, and the more solid the evidence if they are confirmed.

MENTAL RETARDATION

by Mark Jackson

The 1910s constituted a critical decade in the management of both adults and children who were referred to at that time in English-speaking countries as being 'mentally defective' or 'feeble-minded'. In Britain in 1913, for example, after extensive debates amongst doctors, social reformers, eugenists, teachers, and politicians, the passage of the Mental Deficiency Act obliged every local authority to establish a "committee for the care of the mentally defective". This committee was responsible for ascertaining the number of defectives in the area and for providing suitable care for them either in special institutions or under guardianship with families. The following year, the Elementary Education (Defective and Epileptic Children) Act similarly obliged British local education authorities to determine the number of defective children in the area and to make suitable provision for their education in special schools or classes. Under both Acts, a diagnosis of mental deficiency was to be made by a "duly qualified medical practitioner".

In subsequent decades, local authorities around Britain, individual states in America, and local and State authorities in mainland Europe all began to build new institutions for mental defectives or to send others to established institutions. The ideology of segregation manifested in this international process set the agenda for the treatment of mental deficiency on both sides of the Atlantic for much of the twentieth century.

Social context

The social and cognitive roots of these legislative and institutional developments were complex, and can be located in late nineteenth- and early twentieth-century concerns about law and order, morality, poverty, and the maintenance of national strength and racial purity.

Prior to the mid-nineteenth century, people referred to in English as 'idiots' or 'imbeciles' were generally cared for at home, in asylums for the insane, or in workhouses for the poor. However, from the middle of that century, humanitarian philanthropists began to establish purpose-built 'idiot asylums'. Drawing on contemporary optimism about the treatment of insanity and deficiency and on the pioneering educational work of Edward Seguin in both France and America, the aim of these asylums was to provide a suitable environment for the education and training of the mentally retarded.

In the later decades of the nineteenth century, extensive medical interest in an expanding asylum population contributed to more sophisticated classifications of mental defectives, in particular according to the degree of deficiency. In Britain, mental deficiency was increasingly understood to range from 'idiocy' (the most severe form), through 'imbecility', to 'feeble-mindedness'. In North America around the turn of this century, a slightly different terminology was adopted: the 'feeble-minded' constituted a general category, further sub-divided into 'idiots', 'imbeciles', and 'morons'.

At the same time, debates about mental defectives became increasingly pessimistic. Concern about the ways in which asylums, schools, prisons, and workhouses were 'overflowing' with defectives, together with gradual acknowledgement of the failure of educational and therapeutic approaches, led many commentators to regard mental defectives as permanently and incurably diseased. More critically, those in the highest grade — the feeble-minded or morons — were construed as the root cause of many social problems. They were seen as unable to find employment and maintain themselves, the perpetrators of crimes, the incubators of diseases (such as tuberculosis), and a source of poverty, alcoholism, and sexual promiscuity, as well as being the parents of hordes of illegitimate and defective children. On this basis, the feeble-minded were scapegoated as the prime cause of racial and imperial decline. Significantly, this bleak approach took hold in Britain, North America, and in many European countries.

In the early twentieth century, mental deficiency was understood to be a pressing social problem, which required urgent medical and administrative solutions. Doctors and social reformers advocated in particular the establishment of purpose-built schools and colonies that would enable mental defectives to be cared for throughout their lives. In the absence of State provision in most countries at that time, many reformers founded charities and established special schools and residential institutions, or set up after-care facilities, to ensure the effective control of the dangers thought to be associated with mental defectives.

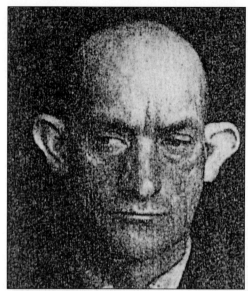
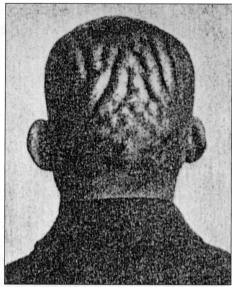
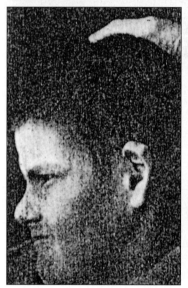
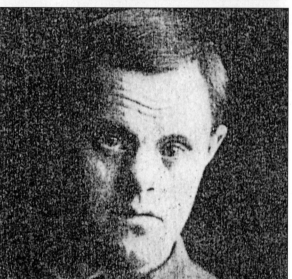

Defects in development: (Top, left) Misshapen "morel" ears: congenital; (Top, right) Congenital imbecile with convoluted scalp; (Bottom, left) Ear showing Darwinian Tubercle; (Bottom, right) Mongolian imbecile showing frontal corrugation. Reproduced from *Shuttleworth GE, Potts WA.* Mentally Deficient Children: Their Treatment and Training. *London: HK Lewis and Co.; 1916. Facing p. 12.*

This programme to segregate mental defectives received substantial impetus from a number of quarters. In Britain, large surveys of school children and institutional populations, anxieties about the fitness of recruits for the Boer War, the results of an Interdepartmental Committee on Physical Deterioration in 1904, the report of the Royal Commission on the Care and Control of the Feeble-Minded in 1908, and prevalent eugenic concerns about the effects of an unfit population on the health and wealth of the nation led to increasingly strident calls for more effective State intervention.

In the 1910s, these reforming efforts finally bore fruit in Britain. After extensive public and parliamentary debate, the Mental Deficiency Act was passed in the summer of 1913. Although there was opposition on the grounds that the medical science on which it was based was unproven and that it was designed essentially to curtail the liberty of the working classes, the Act received widespread support from all political parties, and from doctors, teachers, charity workers, eugenists, and an emergent group of social workers. In North America, similar social concerns and the results of numerous surveys by asylum superintendents were used to legitimate specific State intervention, particularly in the management of feeble-minded criminals, referred to as 'defective delinquents'.

Although diagnosis and the admission of defectives to special schools and institutions was to be controlled by doctors, such legislation betrays the influence of contemporary social factors and indicates the importance of social control of mental defectives in this period. 'Idiots', 'imbeciles', and the 'feeble-minded' were defined primarily according to their social aptitude (i.e. by their inability to look after themselves) rather than on the basis of educational standards. In addition, the British 1913 Act authorised the segregation of defectives who were found to be guilty of a criminal offence, who were in a prison, asylum, or reformatory, who were habitual drunkards, or (in the case of women) were in receipt of poor relief when pregnant or had given birth to an illegitimate child.

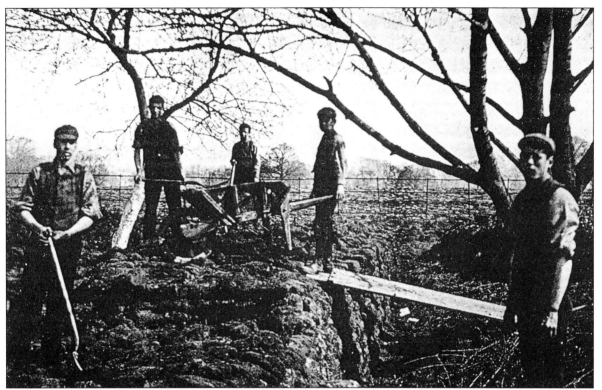

Group of feeble-minded boys working at Sandlebridge colony. Reproduced from Paget Lapage C. Feeble-Mindedness in Children of School-Age. *Manchester: Manchester University Press; 1911. Plate 1, frontispiece.*

Medical classifications and aetiology

For much of the nineteenth century, the words 'idiot' and 'mental defective' had been used as blanket terms, covering all grades of educational and social backwardness. At the turn of the twentieth century, though, more complex classifications of deficiency and more elaborate understandings of aetiology emerged.

In addition to classifying defectives according to the degree of their deficiency, doctors also did so according to its supposed cause, and arranged these individuals whenever possible into clinical types. By the 1910s, medical experts in the field of mental deficiency on both sides of the Atlantic agreed that most cases were primary, i.e. caused by the inheritance of a 'neuropathic taint'. In this context, it was hoped that the long-term segregation of mental defectives in colonies would reduce their opportunities to reproduce, thereby preventing racial decline. In only 10% of cases could the deficiency be attributed to some external agent, the most obvious example of which was syphilis. Here, the deficiency was associated with characteristic physical stigmata: a stunted body, keratitis, Hutchinson's teeth, scars, and a depressed nose.

Although there were also very few clear-cut clinical varieties of mental deficiency in this period, conditions such as cretinism (now referred to as congenital hypothyroidism), mongolism (now referred to as Down's syndrome or trisomy 21), and microcephaly were regularly presented in medical texts as exemplars of a perceived link between mental ability and physical form. It was the prevalence of such presumptions about the close association between mental and physical health that dictated the need for careful physical examination of all suspected defectives by medical experts.

Diagnosis of mental deficiency was to be made on a number of grounds. The presence of physical stigmata, particularly deformities of the cranium, was central (see opposite). In some cases, even the presence of a 'defective expression' or a characteristic gait was thought to betray the feeble mind. The educability and intelligence of a child, or the social aptitude of an adult, were also to be assessed by appropriate questioning and observation. Increasingly during the 1910s, doctors, teachers, and psychologists achieved this by employing some form of standard intelligence test, such as the Binet–Simon test or a modified version of it (Chapter 1, p. 27). In addition, since mental deficiency (and a whole range of related pathologies) was thought to be inherited, a family history of insanity, feeble-mindedness, alcoholism, or tuberculosis was often included as substantive or collaborative evidence of deficiency. Finally, diagnosis could be confirmed by reference to behaviour: criminal propensities, giving birth to illegitimate children, poverty, and disruptive behaviour in school could all contribute.

Treatment

In the 1910s, there were very few medical treatments available to cure, improve, or prevent mental deficiency. Thyroid extracts had been used successfully to treat cretinism since the late nineteenth century and were routinely employed in English mental deficiency institutions. Otherwise, there were no pharmaceutical agents directed solely at alleviating the mental and physical symptoms.

Some doctors forcefully advocated compulsory sterilisation, which they believed would serve to prevent mental defectives from reproducing, at the same time as preserving their liberty. Interest in sterilisation (a procedure sometimes referred to at this time as 'asexualisation') was particularly prominent in North America and in some parts of Europe, such as Scandinavia. Between 1905 and 1922, 18 American States passed laws permitting the sterilisation (by vasectomy or salpingectomy) of the insane, the mentally defective, or criminals in institutions. Although the implementation of these laws varied widely between States, this legislation resulted in the sterilisation of many thousands of people in the early decades of this century. In Britain, while many doctors and politicians continued to advocate the merits of compulsory sterilisation, legislation was consistently rejected as politically unacceptable.

In most countries, institutionalisation was regarded as the principal means of both protecting a mentally defective person from society and of safeguarding society against the manifold social ills thought to be caused by an expanding population of defectives. Institutional life reflected the special educational and medical needs of mental defectives, but also revealed contemporary anxieties about the importance of training, managing, and controlling them. Children in special schools and classes were to be given mainly manual instruction, rather than being taught reading and writing. Once they reached the school-leaving age and entered a colony for mental defectives, they would then be expected to work, e.g. in a laundry or on gardens and farms (see previous page). Productive occupation of this nature was thought to serve the dual purpose of generating income for the institution and of discouraging an otherwise degenerate and wasteful section of the population from becoming a further economic and moral burden on society.

Conclusion

Although the First World War delayed the implementation of much contemporary legislation, local and national authorities throughout the world increasingly established systems to coordinate the ascertainment and management of defectives both in institutions and in the community. In subsequent decades, increasing numbers of people identified as mentally defective were admitted to an expanding network of special schools and colonies. This process was legitimated by dominant medical views of deficiency as an inherited, pathological condition that posed substantial threats to individual and social health and welfare. Public and professional support for such institutions eventually crumbled under the combined weight of political, ideological, economic, and scientific objections. However, the implementation of these policies did create an opportunity for more elaborate scientific studies of mental deficiency, and set the agenda for its treatment in much of the twentieth century.

FURTHER READING

Shell-shock

Butler AG. Moral and mental disorders in the war of 1914–18. In: *Australian Army Medical Services in the War of 1914–1918*, Vol. III. Canberra: Government Printing Office; 1943.

Johnson W, Rows RG. Neurasthenia and war neuroses. In: *History of the Great War Based on Official Documents. Diseases of War*, Vol. 2. London: HMSO; 1923.

Lerner P. *Hysterical Men: War, Neurosis and German Mental Medicine, 1914–1926* (Forthcoming).

Medical Department of the United States Army in the World War, Vol XI. *Neuropsychiatry*. Washington, DC; 1929.

Merskey H. Shell-shock. In: Berrios GE, Freeman H, eds. *150 Years of British Psychiatry*, Vol. 1. London: Gaskell; 1991.

Myers CS. *Shell-Shock in France*. Cambridge: Cambridge University Press; 1940.

Report of the War Office Committee of Enquiry into 'Shell-Shock'. London: HMSO; 1922.

Roudebush MO. *A Battle of Nerves: Hysteria and its Treatment in France during World War*. PhD Thesis, University of California at Berkeley; 1995.

Shephard B. The early treatment of mental disorders: RG Rows and Maghull 1914–1918. In: Freeman H, Berrios GE, eds. *150 Years of British Psychiatry*, Vol. II. *The Aftermath*. London: Athlone; 1996.

Trillat E. *Histoire de l'Hysterie*. Paris: Seghers; 1986.

The emergence of psychoanalysis

Abraham K. *Selected Papers on Psychoanalysis*. New York: Brunner-Mazel; 1927.

Abraham N, Torok M. *The Wolfman's Magic Word*. Minneapolis: University of Minnesota Press; 1986.

Ferenczi S. *First Contributions to Psychoanalysis*. London: Maresfield; 1952.

Freud S. New introductory lectures on psychoanalysis. In: *Standard Edition of the Complete Psychological Works of Sigmund Freud*, Vol. 22. London: Hogarth; 1933.

Gay P. *Freud: A Life for Our Time*. New York: Norton; 1988.

Horney K. *The Neurotic Personality of Our Time*. New York: Norton; 1937.

Mahler MS. *The Memoirs of Margaret S Mahler*. New York: Free Press; 1988.

Reich W. *Sex-Pol: Essays 1919–1934*. New York: Random House; 1966.

Stanton M. *Sandor Ferenczi: Reconsidering Active Intervention*. Northvale, NJ: Aronson; 1990.

Stanton M. *Out of Order: Clinical Work and Unconscious Process*. London: Rebus Press; 1997.

Sigmund Freud

Borch-Jacobsen M. *The Freudian Subject*. London: Macmillan; 1989.

Forrester J. *Dispatches from the Freud Wars*. Cambridge Mass: Harvard University Press; 1997.

Gay P. *Freud: A Life For Our Time*. New York: Norton; 1988.

Jones E. *The Life and Work of Sigmund Freud*, 3 Vols. New York: Basic Books; 1953.

Roazen P. *Freud and His Followers*. Harmondsworth: Penguin Books; 1976.

Timms E, Segal N, eds. *Freud in Exile*. New Haven: Yale University Press; 1988.

Emil Kraepelin

Berrios GE, Hauser R. The early development of Kraepelin's ideas on classification: A conceptual history. *Psychological Medicine*. 1988; **18**:813–821.

Brink L, Smith EJ. Emil Kraepelin, psychiatrist and poet. *Journal of Nervous and Mental Diseases*. 1933; **77**:134–152; 274–282.

Engstrom EJ. Emil Kraepelin: Psychiatry and public affairs in Wilhelmine Germany. *History of Psychiatry*. 1991; **2**:111–132.

Engstrom EJ. Kraepelin. In: Berrios G, Porter R, eds. *A History of Clinical Psychiatry: The Origins and History of Psychiatric Disorders*. London: Athlone; 1995: 292–301.

Hoff P. *Emil Kraepelin und die Psychiatrie als klinische Wissenschaft*. Berlin: Springer; 1994.

Hoff P. Kraepelin. In: Berrios G, Porter R, eds. *A History of Clinical Psychiatry: The Origins and History of Psychiatric Disorders*. London: Athlone; 1995: 261–279.

Janzarik W. 100 Jahre Heidelberger Psychiatrie. *Heidelberger Jahresbuecher*. 1978; **22**:93–113.

Kraepelin E. *Memoirs*. Berlin: Springer; 1987.

Roelcke V. Biologizing social facts: An early 20th century debate on Kraepelin's concepts of culture, neurasthenia, and degeneration. *Culture, Medicine and Psychiatry*. 1997; **21**:383–403.

Shepherd M. Two faces of Emil Kraepelin. *British Journal of Psychiatry*. 1995; **167**:174–183.

Weber MM, Engstrom EJ. Kraepelin's 'diagnostic cards': the confluence of clinical research and preconceived categories. *History of Psychiatry*. 1997; **8**:375–385.

Eugen Bleuler

Asperger H. Autistic psychopathy in childhood. In: *Autism and Asperger Syndrome*. Cambridge: Cambridge University Press; 1991. (Translated and annotated by Frith U. from Die 'autistischen psychopathen' im Kindesalter. *Archiv für Psychiatrie und Nervenkrankheiten*. 1944; **117**:76–136.)

Berrios GE, Hauser R. The early development of Kraepelin's ideas on classification. A conceptual history. *Psychological Medicine*. 1988; **18**:813–821.

Bleuler E. *Dementia Praecox or the Group of Schizophrenias*. New York: International Universities Press; 1911. (Translated by Zinkin J. Dementia Praecox oder der Gruppe der Schizophrenien. In: Aschaffenburg, PG, ed. *Handbuch der Geisteskrankheiten*. Leipzig: Deutike; 1950.)

Kanner L. Autistic disturbances of affective contact. *Nervous Child*. 1943; **2**:217–250.

Kraepelin E. Dementia praecox. In: Cutting J, Shepherd M, eds. *The Clinical Roots of the Schizophrenia Concept*. Cambridge: Cambridge University Press; 1896:15–24. (Translated from Lehrbuch der Psychiatrie, 5th edition. Leipzig: Barth; 426–441.)

Mental retardation

Jackson M. Images of deviance: visual representations of mental defectives in early twentieth century medical texts. *British Journal for the History of Science*. 1995; **28**:319–337.

Jackson M. Institutional provision for the feeble-minded in Edwardian England: Sandlebridge and the scientific morality of permanent care. In: Wright D, Digby A, eds. *From Idiocy to Mental Deficiency: Historical Perspectives on People with Learning Disabilities*. London: Routledge; 1996: 161–183.

Kanner L. *A History of the Care and Study of the Mentally Retarded*. Illinois: Charles Thomas; 1964.

Noll S. *Feeble-Minded in Our Midst: Institutions for the Mentally Retarded in the South, 1900–1940*. Chapel Hill: University of North Carolina Press; 1995.

Reilly PR. *The Surgical Solution: A History of Involuntary Sterilization in the United States.* Baltimore: Johns Hopkins University Press; 1991.

Rose N. *The Psychological Complex: Psychology, Politics and Society in England, 1869–1939.* London: Routledge and Kegan Paul; 1985.

Simmons HG. Explaining social policy: the English Mental Deficiency Act of 1913. *Journal of Social History.* 1978; **11**:387–403.

Thomson M. 'Though ever the subject of psychological medicine': psychiatrists and the colony solution for mental defectives. In: Freeman H, Berrios GE, eds. *150 Years of British Psychiatry*, Vol. 2: *The Aftermath.* London: Athlone; 1996: 130–143.

Thomson M. *The Problem of Mental Deficiency: Eugenics, Democracy, and Social Policy in Britain, c.1870–1959.* Oxford: Clarendon Press; 1998.

Tredgold A. *Mental Deficiency (Amentia).* London: Baillière, Tindall and Cox; 1908.

Trent JW. *Inventing the Feeble Mind: A History of Mental Retardation in the United States.* Berkeley: University of California Press; 1994.

Trombley S. *The Right to Reproduce: A History of Coercive Sterilization.* London: Weidenfeld and Nicolson; 1988.

Wright D, Digby A, eds. *From Idiocy to Mental Deficiency: Historical Perspectives on People with Learning Disabilities.* London: Routledge; 1996.

1921–1930

Chapter 3
Evolution of Clinical Concepts

1921–1930 CHAPTER 3

Major world events

1921	Leow in Germany demonstrated a chemical basis for neurotransmission
1921	Einstein in Germany received the Nobel Prize for Physics
1922	A diabetic patient was treated with insulin for the first time
1925	Charlie Chaplin (USA) triumphed with *The Gold Rush*
1927	First transatlantic telephone call made
1927	First televised transmission by John Baird, Glasgow
1928	Alexander Fleming (Great Britain) discovered antibiotic properties of penicillin
1929	The Wall Street crash

Major events in psychiatry

1921	The Serbsky Central Research Institute of Forensic Medicine established in Moscow
1921	K Bonhoeffer founded the Department of Child Neuropsychiatry at the Charité Hospital, Berlin
1921	Ernst Kretschmer's book *Physique and Temperament* published in Germany
1921	Sweden established an Institute of Racial Biology
1921	Clérambault became director of the Special Infirmary of the Central Police Station, Paris
1922	Klaesi published results of deep-sleep treatment, which then became widely adopted
1922	The Psychoanalytic Institute founded in Berlin
1922	Henri Claude appointed Professor of Clinical Psychiatry, Paris
1923	The first group analysis started by Trigant Burrow, at Johns Hopkins Hospital, Baltimore
1923	Joseph Capgras, a psychiatrist at the Sainte-Anne Hospital, Paris, described 'the illusion of doubles', or *'l'illusion des 'sosies'*
1923	René Laforgue established a psychoanalytic service at the Sainte-Anne Hospital, Paris
1923	The Maudsley Hospital, London, was opened jointly by the London County Council and London University, headed by Edward Mapother
1923	William Alanson White's *Insanity and the Criminal Law* published in the USA
1924	The 'twin method' of genetic investigation developed independently by Curtis Merriman in the USA, and Hermann Siemans in Germany
1924	Hans Berger introduced electroencephalography in Germany
1926	Death of Emil Kraepelin
1926	*The Rolleston Report* published in Britain by the Interdepartmental Committee on Morphine and Heroin Addiction
1927	*Psychopathology*, by Bernard Hart, published in London
1927	Pneumoencephalography first applied to the study of schizophrenia by the German psychiatrists Jacobi and Winkler
1927	Julius Wagner-Jauregg awarded the Nobel prize for Medicine
1928	The General Medical Association for Psychotherapy founded in Germany
1929	Holland passed a law on psychopathy which acknowledged 'defective development or pathological disturbance' as accounting for some criminal actions
1930	Freud received the Goethe Award in Frankfurt
1930	The first child psychiatry clinic established in Baltimore, headed by Leo Kanner

THE 1920s: AN OVERVIEW

by Edward Shorter

The 1920s marked the beginning of a competition in psychiatry that was to stretch into the 1990s and beyond: the contest between psychopharmacology and psychotherapy. Although both are now seen as essential in the treatment of individual patients, at the theoretical level the doctrines are often in competition. This is a rivalry whose genesis goes back to the 1920s, though then the battle lines were much less clearly drawn. It was in those years that the great paradigms of psychiatric illness — the psychogenic and the neurogenic — came into direct conflict with each other. Their competition built up throughout the decade with the result that, by 1930, many doctors had two clearly articulated alternatives to choose between. From the 1930s to the 1960s, this competition tilted towards Freudian psychodynamics in North America, and from the 1970s to the 1990s, back again in favour of biological models supporting psychopharmacological approaches. The 1920s are thus crucial in the making of modern psychiatry.

The rise of psychotherapy

At the outset of the 1920s, both psychopharmacology and Freudian-style psychotherapeutics were just beginning to make a clinical impact. The first out-patient clinic for training psychoanalysts was founded in Berlin in 1920. Psychoanalytic notions began to infiltrate the educated public, and consequently in Central European cities, people would chat about their 'Minko's, short for '*Minderwertigkeitscomplex*', or inferiority complex. In Paris, Henri Claude, Professor of Clinical Psychiatry in the years 1922–1939, encouraged René Laforgue in 1923 to establish a psychoanalytic service at the Sainte-Anne mental hospital, where a generation of French analysts was trained. In 1926, Claude organised a series of lectures on psychoanalysis in his own department.

What accounts for the rapid gains of analysis in these years? At the level of the psychoneuroses, there was a theoretical vacuum. By the 1920s, the hysteria doctrines of the Paris neurologist Jean-Martin Charcot, which had dominated psychiatric thinking in the late nineteenth century, had collapsed. With Charcot's views about genetically predisposed hysterical 'constitutions' now discredited, the way was opened to non-biological interpretations, and Freud's doctrine of hysteria seemed plausible. (Initially, Freud had seen hysteria as the conversion of childhood trauma, but by the 1920s, this changed to the result of sexual repression.) So psychoanalysis barged through a door partly opened: much of the biological thinking of the nineteenth century had been dismantled.

But the onrush of psychoanalysis also had a social dimension. Until the First World War, psychiatry as a discipline had been concentrated almost entirely in mental hospitals, the treatment of neuroses in private practice being left to neurologists, physicians, and hydrotherapists. Yet by the 1920s, many psychiatrists were chafing at their imprisonment in the asylum, and wanted to open lucrative private practices. In a fictional dialogue that appeared in the *Annales Médico-Psychologiques*, the main French psychiatry journal, a wise old alienist says to a young practitioner, "In France, psychiatric practice is almost exclusively asylum medicine and allows complete scientific impartiality. The alienists have not given to Freud the enthusiastic reception that [Emil] Kraepelin got. But new winds are blowing. Since the War, the excess number of women, the distaste for arduous thought, the love of making money and of dangerous sport: all have guaranteed to sexual Freudianism a magnificent future, and the patients are shaping the doctors to suit". This deliciously cynical quote brings home the point that the spread of psychoanalysis required both sympathetic doctors and receptive patients: by the 1920s each, for its own reasons, was ready — at least in some major cities.

The rise of psychopharmacology

The 1920s also saw the rise of what would later be called psychopharmacology (Chapter 10, p. 352). One must distinguish between the brain-biological thinking of the nineteenth century — by the 1920s already very much in decline — and the empirical willingness to use new medication of proven value. The old brain-biology school was already on its way out by the 1920s. Aldous Huxley mocked it in a limerick:

> There was a young girl of East Anglia
> Whose loins were a tangle of ganglia
> Her mind was a webbing
> Of Freud and Krafft-Ebing
> And all other sorts of new fanglia.

The reference to Freud is whimsical, yet when Huxley pointed to the Viennese professor of psychiatry, Richard von Krafft-Ebing, and to loins as "a tangle of ganglia" presumably influencing the brain, he was aiming directly at the old psychiatry that attributed cerebral events to degenerate constitutions and peripheral irritations. The death in 1919, of Augusto Tamburini, professor of clinical psychiatry in Rome and editor of the *Rivista sperimentale di freniatria*, was a landmark of the decline of the old 'brain-mythology' approach to psychiatry, filled with speculation about cerebral 'excitement' as the cause of mental symptoms.

In the 1920s several new, non-theoretical approaches to treating biologically the major mental illnesses arose, coming from clinicians who accidentally chanced across ways of improving patients by medication. These innovations gave hope and excitement to a field that would, in the 1950s and after, be called 'psychopharmacology'.

Malarial-fever treatment

The first innovation occurred during the First World War: Julius Wagner-Jauregg, Professor of Psychiatry at the University of Vienna, discovered in 1917 a method of arresting the progress of neurosyphilis by infecting the patients with malaria, thus creating the 'malarial-fever treatment' (this chapter, p. 74). After years of experimenting with various infections as a means of raising patients' temperatures (the spirochaete that causes syphilis wilts in the presence of elevated temperatures in the central nervous system), Wagner-Jauregg discovered that giving patients malarial infection would keep the disease from progressing to its hitherto invariably fatal end — a progression accompanied by the full display of psychiatric symptoms. After the patients had experienced repeated attacks of fever, and by now often much improved mentally, they would then be cured of their malaria with quinine. It was an epochal discovery, the first virtual cure of a major cause of mental illness, and it won Wagner-Jauregg the Nobel Prize in 1927.

But the malarial-fever therapy was quite demanding to apply. Only certain strains of malaria worked, and they had to be maintained intact in a human reservoir so that sufferers could be inoculated. When, for example, in 1930 a centre for malaria therapy was created at the Hôpital Cochin in Paris, it was in response to complaints of provincial doctors that, when they sent patients to Paris to be treated with malaria, the strain would die out before anyone else locally could be treated. (It was also a highly sensitive matter, in conservative provincial France, for patients to let it be known that they were receiving malaria therapy. That could only mean that they had led a dissolute lifestyle.)

By 1930, the malarial-fever therapy had become the most successful single method in psychiatry, for it actually did cure at least some patients of their neurosyphilitic psychoses. Given that in some institutions up to half of all male patients had 'progressive paralysis', 'general paralysis', 'tabes dorsalis', 'general paralysis of the insane', or one of the other terms designating the symptoms of neurosyphilis, the fever cure represented a major landmark. Yet neurosyphilis was a special kind of psychiatric illness, because the cause was manifestly organic.

More difficult to treat, by contrast, were the 'functional' psychoses, such as schizophrenia and manic–depressive illness, called functional because the cause was unknown. The first promise of a cure for these devastating diseases came from a treatment now forgotten: deep-sleep therapy. The therapeutic agent was barbituric acid, introduced in 1903, the stem compound of the barbiturates.

Deep-sleep therapy

Yet the barbiturates did not represent the first sleep cure in psychiatry. The notion of relieving major psychiatric symptoms by inducing patients to sleep for weeks at a time — rousing them periodically to give them a few tablespoons full of milk or letting them go to the toilet — had surfaced in medicine some decades previously. But by the time of the First World War these earlier attempts, conducted with bromium, had been forgotten.

Then in 1915, Giuseppe Epifanio, a young psychiatrist at the university psychiatric hospital in Turin, used the barbiturates to put patients with major illnesses into prolonged slumber. His work, too, went virtually unnoticed, except perhaps by Max Cloetta, Professor of Pharmacology in Zurich, who in the early 1920s called to the attention of Jakob Klaesi, a staff member at the Burghölzli university psychiatric clinic, the possibility of using the barbiturates for prolonged, therapeutic sleep. Klaesi actually had little fundamental commitment to biological psychiatry, but wanted to use drug treatment as a way of making patients accessible to psychotherapy (where, he believed, the true cure would take place). He published his results in 1922 in a major journal in the world's then

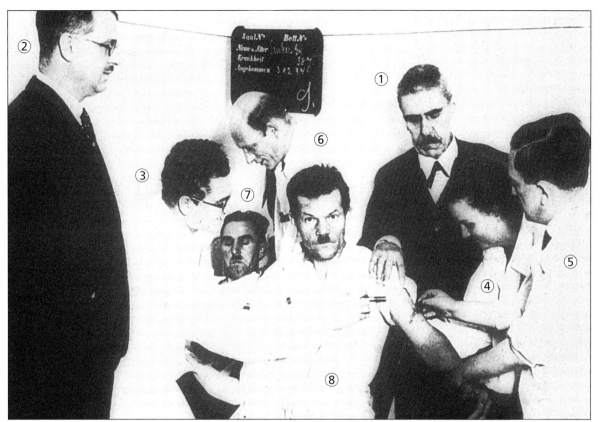

Wagner-Jauregg (1) and Otto Kauders (2) attending a malarial blood transfusion. Dr Th. Dussik (3) draws the blood; Dr Ch. Milz-Palisa (4) and Dr E. Horn (5) assist. Patient (8) is malarial blood donor; patient (7) receives malarial blood. Nurse Rieder (6) is in the background. Reproduced with permission from the Institut für Geschichte der Medizin der Universität Wien, Vienna.

most prestigious scientific language — German. Klaesi's deep-sleep cure became widely adopted. As Marcel Monnier and others showed, it was in fact quite successful in the treatment of schizophreniform illnesses (although it had something of a mortality rate, later reduced with other barbiturates). The therapy also required intensive nursing, which made it less suitable for the crowded public asylums. Yet so successful was sleep therapy that, in retrospect, it does appear — along with malaria therapy — to be the first true cure in the history of psychiatry and therewith an early building block in the history of psychopharmacology.

Twin studies and genetics

The 1920s also saw a third triumph in the development of scientific psychiatry: the advent of twin studies in understanding the genetics of psychiatric illness. Yet the baby in this case was birthmarked with racism, and the story is an ambiguous one. It begins in 1917, when Emil Kraepelin (Chapter 2, p. 49) established the German Psychiatric Research Institute (*Deutsche Forschungsanstalt für Psychiatrie*). The Institute's genesis was a somewhat lengthy one and only in 1928 did its new quarters in the '*Kraepelinstrasse*' open (Kraepelin himself died in 1926). By that time, the Institute had acquired an extraordinarily distinguished group of researchers in neuropathology, neurochemistry, clinical psychiatry, and genetics. It was in this latter area — led by the Swiss psychiatrist Ernst Rüdin — that the most significant progress was achieved. Twin studies carried out by Hans Luxenburger established that monozygotic twins had much higher concordance for schizophrenia than did dizygotic twins, which was a finding of major significance. Unhappily, both this genetics research and a proportion of the work of the whole Institute were tainted by the kind of racist thinking that later became the pseudoscientific basis of the Holocaust. For example, Julius Hallervorden, an early collaborator of the Institute (but not on staff), later became notorious for his research on the brains of patients killed in the Nazi euthanasia programme. Rüdin became one of the chief theorists of Nazi racialism, and even the intensely Catholic Luxenburger served the Nazi geneticists for a while. The whole story of what became, after the Second World War, the Max-Planck-Institute for Psychiatry had a kind of unlovely beginning in the German nationalism and racialism of the years following the First World War. Yet researchers at the Institute also laid the basis for modern psychiatric genetics, and during the 1920s, it was probably the single most distinguished institute for psychiatric research in the world.

Psychiatry in Europe

In the 1920s, Germany was almost certainly the epicentre of world psychiatry. In the psychiatry chairs of its 23 faculties of medicine there sat such major figures as Karl Bonhoeffer in Berlin, one of the founders of research in alcoholism (a kind of 'exogenic' reaction, as he put it). Hans Berger, discoverer in 1924 of electroencephalography, occupied the chair of psychiatry at Jena, while Karl Wilmanns, one of the founders of modern forensic psychiatry, had the chair at Heidelberg.

But the German-speaking lands embrace Austria and part of Switzerland as well. Here again, the 1920s saw university psychiatry dominated by figures of world renown. Wagner-Jauregg stepped down from the chair of psychiatry in Vienna in 1928, to be followed by Otto Pötzl (under whose aegis Manfred Sakel later tested insulin-coma therapy). Eugen Bleuler, who in 1908 coined the term 'schizophrenia', was head of psychiatry in Zurich until 1927 (Chapter 2, p. 52). In short, it was the German-speaking lands that, in the 1920s, consolidated their grip on world psychiatry — a grasp first acquired late in the nineteenth century. It is an astonishing comment on the unpredictability of human events that these scientific triumphs were so casually thrown away after 1933.

In France, the 1920s represented a fallow period. The basic French problem was the dominance of the entire university system by Paris. With good people at the centre, such predominance can focus and marshal the energies of the nation. With people of indifferent quality, this kind of centralisation is a recipe for stagnation, and Henri Claude, Clinical Professor of Mental Illness, did not rank among the discipline's most luminous figures. Yet alongside his school there were other lights in the Parisian firmament. Historically, the French have contributed to the study of psychosis particularly by isolating unusual delusional disorders. This tradition goes back to Esquirol's 'monomania' in the early nineteenth century, and includes the chronic nihilistic delusions that Jules Cotard described in 1880 and after (now known as 'Cotard's syndrome').

Yet in the 1920s, the French did make two major new contributions. It was in 1905 that Gaétan Gatian de Clérambault joined the Special Infirmary of the Central Police Station in Paris. Through this intake clinic for the Paris mental-hospital system passed all the mental pathology of the great city. And by 1921, the year he became director, Clérambault had seen enough individuals who were out of control in love, jealousy, and other passions to allow him to speak of 'the passionate delusions' ('*les délires passionnels*') as an independent category of illness. The only member of this category to survive has been what Clérambault called 'pure erotomania', the delusional sense that someone else is in love with you. Often called (incorrectly) 'Clérambault's syndrome', erotomania has come to occupy a prominent place in the description of the human condition, though it is no longer considered an independent illness entity.

Secondly, in 1923, Joseph Capgras, a psychiatrist at the Sainte-Anne Hospital, described 'the illusion of doubles', or '*l'illusion des 'sosies'*' (continuing the work that he and Paul Sérieux had begun in 1909 with their systematic discussion of chronic delusional disorders). The illusion of doubles meant that an apparently familiar person was in reality a double, or impostor. This became known as 'Capgras' syndrome', although it too has lost the independent status which Capgras wished for it. Thus, the French enriched the understanding of delusions with these curious eponymous conditions, which rank among the main historic monuments of their psychiatry in the 1920s.

In Britain, the profession of psychiatry was largely unaffected by these trends. Yet in London, the tension between psychoanalysis and biological psychiatry did play out in the rivalry between the psychoanalytically orientated Tavistock Clinic, founded by Hugh Crichton-Miller in 1920, and the Maudsley Hospital, opened in 1923 and headed by organicist Edward Mapother (who in 1936 became England's first professor of psychiatry). The Maudsley was modelled after Kraepelin's Department of Psychiatry (*Nervenklinik*) in the Nussbaumstrasse in Munich, and aspired similarly to cover both neuroscience and clinical psychiatry.

Yet the most significant representative of the psychological approach in the 1920s — the psychoanalyst Bernard Hart — was associated with neither institution. Hart was appointed Consultant in Psychological Medicine at University College Hospital in 1913. By the 1920s, his book *The Psychology of Insanity* (first published in 1912) had become the single most influential work in what was being called 'the new psychiatry', meaning the psychodynamic orientation. Hart's 1927 book *Psychopathology* attempted to put a psychoanalytic spin on the psychological interpretation of symptoms, an approach launched by Karl Jaspers before the Great War.

The Achilles heel of British psychiatry has always been its chronic shortage of money for research, in contrast to the State-endowed German psychiatric clinics. In the 1920s, British psychiatry registered few triumphs that depended on the expenditure of money, such as genetic surveys of the population. Where the British have excelled has been in their scepticism of scientific fads. One thinks of the dubiety with which Charcot's 'hysteria' was received in the UK, or the national scepticism towards the syndrome building that cluttered much of psychiatry elsewhere. [Similarly, today, the British are wary of such trendy new diagnoses in American psychiatry as attention deficit hyperactivity disorder (Chapter 7, p. 195).]

Psychiatry in America

So massive has been the development of American psychiatry since the Second World War that there is a tendency to forget that before the 1940s, it was very much a tail wagged by a large European dog. The centre of American psychiatry in the 1920s was the Henry Phipps Psychiatric Clinic at the Johns Hopkins University in Baltimore, directed by Swiss-born Adolf Meyer, who had become Professor of Psychiatry there in 1910, three years before the Phipps opened its doors. Because Meyer trained an entire cohort of American psychiatrists (as well as a small group of admirers from the UK), he has received a generally favourable press in the history of American psychiatry (Chapter 4, p. 103). In retrospect, however, Meyer probably did more to muddy the waters with his outlandish neologisms and his belief that every patient is so unique that general classification is arbitrary and probably undesirable. Meyer's influence on American psychiatry delayed for many years the adoption in the USA of the systematic, quantitative, comparative studies that became the norm in psychiatry elsewhere. When, after the Second World War, the USA came to dominate the psychiatric mainstream, it would be under the leadership, not of Hopkins but of such government agencies as Jonathan Cole's Psychopharmacology Service Center, part of the National Institute for Mental Health.

Conclusion

By the end of the 1920s, the concept of psychopharmacology — though it was not yet called that — was becoming established in psychiatry. Scientifically orientated psychiatrists — such as the staff of the Rockwinkel Sanatorium in Bremen — would be expected to have a working knowledge of fever-treatment drugs for schizophrenia. (It had been in 1920 that David Macht at Johns Hopkins used the word 'psychopharmacology' for the first time.) Interestingly, when in 1930 the Swiss held a conference on 'pharmacology and psychiatry' in Perreux (near Neuchâtel), one of the speakers was the young Ernst Rothlin, who later became research director of Sandoz in Basel and, in 1957, co-founder of the Collegium Internationale Neuro-Psycho-pharmacologicum — today the premier world body for exchanging findings in psychopharmacology. In terms of curiosity about drugs and the mind, the 1920s laid the base for the dramatic quickening that occurred in the 1930s in the form of insulin-coma and metrazol-convulsion therapy.

Similarly, psychoanalysis poised in the 1920s for its spring into clinical medicine. And the budding analysts clearly perceived themselves in rivalry with the budding organicists. In his 1926 essay 'On the Question of Lay Analysis', Freud wrote of the typical medical education, "[The aspiring analyst] has no use for the great bulk of information that the medical schools teach. Be it the knowledge of the tarsal bones, or the composition of hydrocarbons, or the course of the nerve fibres in the brain: everything that medicine teaches about bacillary causes of disease and their treatment, about serum reactions and tumour neogenesis: all to be sure most valuable, but all completely useless to the young analyst". All this biological knowledge was of no value whatever in the treatment of neurosis, said Freud; the analysts scorned pharmacological approaches in particular. (The prominent American psychoanalyst Jules Masserman later dismissed chlorpromazine as "a glorified sedative".)

Yet it must not be forgotten that many psychiatrists saw no tension between psychoanalysis and biological psychiatry: so desperate were psychiatrists to mitigate the suffering in the asylums that they were willing to grasp after anything that worked. Thus it was that in 1919, the Swiss novelist Friedrich Glauser was admitted as a patient for the first time to the Münsingen asylum. During the 1920s, Glauser was in and out of this institution on several occasions. He went on to have an important literary career, and in his 1936 novel *Matto Regiert* ("The Madman is in Charge"), the protagonist, a Swiss police inspector, investigates an apparent murder in the asylum. The inspector encounters the acting medical superintendent 'Dr Laduner'. Of interest is that Laduner simultaneously administers psychoanalysis to his private patients, and hydrotherapy to his public ones, seeing no contradiction between the two modes. Laduner was modelled on the psychiatrist Max Müller, who later became director of Münsingen and whom Glauser first met in 1925. Müller also saw no contradiction between the use of psychoanalysis in psychotherapy, and the introduction in the 1930s of the new physical methods of treatment such as insulin-coma, of which he was a major advocate.

In terms of psychiatric care, the 1920s are associated with the long period of stagnation in the life of the asylum, in which the patients vegetated in back wards. The scientific developments of the 1920s remained on the surface, scarcely affecting the quality of clinical care for the great masses. Yet it was in scientific terms that the 1920s saw important new departures, pointing the way for psychotherapy and psychopharmacology in the next half century.

THE CONTRIBUTION OF FRENCH PSYCHIATRY

by Pierre Pichot

From the beginning of the nineteenth century, Philippe Pinel and his followers had given the French school of psychiatry a leading position in Europe. The anatomo–clinical perspective had been introduced into France in 1821 with AL Bayle's description of general paralysis of the insane and its specific brain lesions. Although a pathogenic concept which met with great success until the First World War, having been proposed in 1857 with BA Morel's theory of degeneracy, the main contribution of the French school was in the description of the various forms of mental disorder. The faithfulness of the clinical approach had been demonstrated by Pinel's pupil, Esquirol. His *Treatise on Mental Disease*, published in 1838, opened a direction to be followed by French alienists of the subsequent generations, and also had a deep influence in other European countries.

At the beginning of the 1870s, German psychiatry progressively took the place until then occupied by the French school. One of its most symbolic expressions was the success, around 1900, of Kraepelin's nosological system (Chapter 2, p. 50). Its main feature was the classification of the psychotic states: manic–depressive psychosis, dementia praecox, and paranoia were the three new basic entities. Kraepelin's ideas were known early in France, where the concept of manic–depressive psychosis was readily accepted: Esquirol's pupil, JP Falret, had described it as far back as 1851 under the name of circular madness (*folie circulaire*) or bipolar disorder. But some aspects of dementia praecox, which associated the clinically very different manifestations of hebephrenia, catatonia, and paranoid psychosis in a single category because of their allegedly common evolution towards a final state of mental deterioration, were criticised in France. It was certainly possible to admit that the hebephrenic and catatonic forms belonged to a single disease with an evolution towards dementia — several decades before, Morel had described cases with relatively similar symptoms under the name *démence précose*. However, the inclusion of the great majority of the chronic delusional states into the paranoid form conflicted with prevalent French conceptions.

Nosology of the delusional states

The restriction of the criteria for dementia praecox — and later of schizophrenia — led to a specific contribution of French psychiatry: the creation, on psychopathological criteria, of an original classificatory system for the chronic delusional states. This was a group which included many cases considered in the other nosologies as belonging to the paranoid form of dementia praecox — and later of schizophrenia — as well as to Kraepelin's paranoia. Some elements of this system, such as Clérambault's erotomania syndrome, have been more or less accepted in other countries. Others have, at least temporarily, had their counterpart in the international classifications — the paraphrenia of ICD–9 was very similar to the French chronic hallucinatory psychosis — but on the whole, use of this system has been limited to France, which is still the case today.

Although established in its classic form between 1921 and 1930, the French system of delusional states incorporated various concepts already proposed during the preceding decade, and was slightly modified during the following one.

Serieux and Capgras: 'chronic interpretative delusional state'

In 1909, Serieux and Capgras had described the 'chronic interpretative delusional state' which "developed gradually in vulnerable individuals". These had five main diagnostic criteria: (a) the complexity and coherence of the delusions; (b) the absence of hallucinations or their manifest subordination to the delusional core; (c) unimpaired intelligence; (d) progressive extension of the delusional network; (e) incurability without significant mental and social deterioration. These criteria resembled Kraepelin's paranoia — Serieux had introduced his ideas into France — but they differed from it in two respects. On the one hand, the French criteria were more flexible: disorders best classified under this heading are diagnosed more frequently in France than is the *paranoia vera* of German authors. On the other hand, in accordance with the name given to the disorder, it was defined by a fundamental psychopathological mechanism of an intellectual nature. This was the interpretation of phenomena by "false reasoning, originating in the misinterpretation of correctly perceived fact or facts, to which logical but erroneous inferences lend misconstrued subjective meaning". Serieux and Capgras contrasted their new category with the 'vindictive delusional states' in which emotional factors were decisive and whose features were quite similar to those of Kraepelin's *Querulantenwahn*.

Ballet: 'chronic hallucinatory psychosis'

In 1911 and 1913, Gilbert Ballet described 'chronic hallucinatory psychosis'. Schematically, this delusional state was characterised by: (a) persistent and prominent hallucinatory activity; (b) delusional — most frequently persecutory, but also grandiose — ideas; (c) a clear sensorium, unimpaired speech, appropriate behaviour, and intact higher intellectual functions, contrasting sharply with the co-existing delusional and hallucinatory syndrome. In addition, a late onset — after the age of 40 — was the rule. This description was schematic, in so far as it did not mention the possibility of minimal deficits in the intellectual sphere and did not discuss a possible evolution towards a final deterioration. It aimed to separate a large group of patients from the paranoid form of dementia praecox — or of paranoid schizophrenia, described in the same year by Bleuler. In modern terms, these would be said to show positive symptoms — hallucinations and delusions — predominating massively over the negative ones. Like the concept of Serieux and Capgras, this category emphasised the role of a psychopathological mechanism for the definition of the entity: the hallucinations were the primary phenomena here, as the interpretations were in the interpretative delusions.

Dupré and Logre: 'chronic imaginative psychosis'

The importance of the psychopathological mechanism as the criterion for the delimitation of the various chronic delusional states was stressed by Dupré and Logre who, also in 1911, described 'chronic imaginative psychosis'. They contended that the 'imaginative psychosis' could be considered as valid a construct as the 'interpretative mechanism' or the 'hallucinatory mechanism'. Chronic imaginative psychosis seemed to them to "parallel chronic interpretative psychosis in its development, symptoms and course", but differed fundamentally in the origin of the delusional ideas. In their view, "the delusionally interpretative and delusionally imaginative individual are opposite in temperament and mental make-up". However, since chronic imaginative psychosis was far less frequent than the interpretative and hallucinatory forms, it initially attracted little attention.

It was between 1921 and 1930 that these clinical entities were incorporated definitively into the French nosological system, thanks to a comprehensive survey by Serieux and Capgras, published in 1926. At the same time, though, the concepts that were already established were submitted to revision, while other new ones were introduced.

Clérambault's studies

A central role was played in this process of revision by GG de Clérambault. Head of the small psychiatric department of the Paris central police station (the *Depot*), he had to examine subjects who were arrested by the police because of their abnormal behaviour and suspected to be mentally ill. These numbered about 2000 per annum; after observing them for 2 or 3 days, he would write a concise case history and send them eventually to a mental hospital. Through his informal weekly lectures, during which he submitted the patients to a clinical examination, and through his publications in an extremely precise but somewhat mannered style, he acquired considerable prestige. In recent years, he has been described as the 'last great French clinical psychiatrist', and his life and works have been the subject of several books. Clérambault's studies concentrated on the description and pathogenic interpretation of the symptoms of chronic hallucinatory psychosis, as well as the delimitation, within the group of the non-hallucinatory chronic delusional states, of the specific class of *psychoses passionnelles*.

Clérambault gave a minute description of the symptoms of chronic hallucinatory psychosis, isolating with great accuracy the various pathological phenomena such as thought insertion, thought broadcasting, and thought withdrawal (previously called 'pseudo-hallucinations' by Kandinsky). For these, he coined the term 'mental automatism', known today in France as 'Clérambault's syndrome'. He affirmed that this was the core manifestation of the disorder, and claimed that it was provoked directly by a biological functional impairment of the brain cortex.

our experience of our personal mother. The more autonomous the complex, the less conscious (and so more problematic) will be relationships that touch it off. The task is not to 'overcome' or 'outgrow' our complexes, because they are the very substance of our personal unconscious, but rather to relate to them more consciously in a continuing work of psychic integration.

In the development of his theory, Jung was able to draw on a wide education in both the natural sciences and the humanities. He had embarked on a medical training at the University of Basel without much enthusiasm, but knowing that as the son of a modest country pastor, he must get himself a livelihood. In a 'flash of illumination', however — or so he remembered it at the end of a long life — he saw when he first opened a textbook of psychiatry that this was the discipline in which his interests could flow together. "Here was the empirical field common to biological and spiritual facts, which I had everywhere sought and nowhere found. Here at last was the place where the collision of nature and spirit became a reality". So he threw up good prospects in the medical mainstream and in 1900, became an assistant at the Burghölzli mental hospital in Zurich, under Eugen Bleuler (Chapter 2, p. 52). Psychiatry, therefore, offered Jung the chance to reconcile two fundamental aspects of his own character. He also felt from the start that psy-

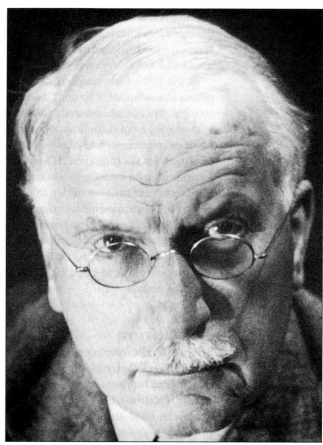

Carl Gustav Jung. Reproduced with permission from the Eranos Foundation, Ascona, Switzerland.

chiatric understanding must have to do with the subjective perceptions of the doctor as well as objective facts. It was this interaction of the objective and subjective worlds, this call to the 'whole of the personality' that drew him irresistibly, and continued to inform his understanding of psychic process.

The making of analytical psychology
1900–1909: Apprenticeship
During his nine years at the Burghölzli, Jung had little interest in welding symptoms into diagnostic categories. For him, the 'burning question' was 'What actually takes place inside the mentally ill?' In his search for answers, he now added the insights of contemporary psychology to those of the Romantic philosophers of the unconscious. His psychological masters were Bleuler himself, Pierre Janet, with whom Jung studied for a semester in Paris, Alfred Binet, and Theodore Flournoy. From Janet, he learned particularly about 'psychological automatism', dual personality, the *abaissement du niveau mental* and 'subconscious fixed ideas' — all of which would inform his own theory of *complexes*. Binet's influence can be discerned in Jung's work on *typology* (Chapter 1, p. 27). Flournoy's insistence on the importance of 'occult' and 'psychical' phenomena to understanding unconscious processes greatly influenced Jung's choice of doctoral dissertation, which examined a case of apparent 'mediumship'. Bleuler's influence was even more direct. His own concern to understand his patients and build a rapport with them set the tone of work at the Burghölzli. And early on, he encouraged Jung to acquaint himself and his colleagues with the work of Sigmund Freud.

The first recorded exchange of letters between these two progenitors of modern depth psychology, in 1906, was prelude to a relationship whose intensity of creativity was matched by the intensity of bitterness and pain with which it ended. In 1909, however, there was no sign of that final rift. By then, Jung was well-established in a large house of his own design by the lake at Kusnacht, married since 1903 to the wealthy Emma Rauschenbach, with whom he would have five children. He was professionally successful as second-in-command at the Burghölzli and lecturer at the University of Zurich. And just as he had abandoned his mainstream prospects in medicine when he opted for psychiatry, he now did exactly the same, by resigning from the Burghölzli and throwing in his lot with the controversial new discipline of psychoanalysis.

1900–1913: Psychoanalysis

It would be quite wrong to see Jung's *analytical psychology* as a distortion of or deviation from psychoanalysis. Although he was certainly influenced by Freud's thinking before they met and early in their relationship, he was continually developing his own distinctive understanding of the psychic process. The intensity of relationship between the two men was founded more on personal factors than professional ones: Jung needed a strong father figure as much as Freud needed an 'eldest son', and 'crown prince' who would carry his teaching beyond the largely Jewish circle in which it had begun. Their cooperation was close. They travelled and lectured together in the United States; Jung became the first president of the International Psychoanalytic Association and managing editor of the *Jahrbuch*, the first psychoanalytic periodical; he also gave a course of lectures on psychoanalysis at Zurich University. But the archetypal dynamics of father and son increasingly brought about anger and disappointment in both. In 1913, Jung resigned from the International Psychoanalytic Association and editorship of the *Jahrbuch*. He also resigned his post at Zurich University. Once more, he gave up what might seem good prospects of advancement, just as he had at university and the Burghölzli.

In 1912 and 1913, Jung published his two-part *Symbols of Transformation*. With this hugely sprawling amplification of the mythological themes behind and below a series of fantasies a young American woman had sent to Flournoy, he burst out of the psychoanalytic frame. The *libido* that Freud so insistently identified as sexual here expanded to become *psychic energy* itself, expressed by the universal symbols of mythology and transformed by the hero's descent into the deep unconscious and return to an enriched consciousness. The urgency of Jung's exploration of these themes not only signalled the inevitability of his break with Freud, but presaged his own 'confrontation with the unconscious' and the enrichment of his developing theory.

1913–1919: 'Confrontation with the Unconscious'

The description is Jung's own, of a period during which he worked to relate to and understand the personal and mythological meanings of the images that flooded through his dreams, visions, and fantasies. He recalled that he 'consciously submitted' himself to these products of the unconscious, though that suggests a greater control than he often felt. Yet it was out of the extraordinary and often terrifying experiences of these years that Jung felt his entire remaining life-work came. It was at this time that he deeply understood, through his own encounters with personified images of archetypal energies, that the human psyche is not only personal but collective as well. It was also at this time that he began to understand the working of the Self as the 'principle and archetype of orientation and meaning', in which psychic life is rooted and towards which its highest purposes seem to strive.

Jung's influence

Jung's thinking has gone wide and deep into the fabric of Western culture. Not everyone, for instance, could name his theories of *shadow projection* or *complexes*; but the notions that we all tend to condemn in others what we least like in ourselves, or that we are made up of different and often squabbling 'selves' are hardly strange. Yet between individual experience and academic interest, a gulf remains. It is only relatively recently that analytical psychology has been taught in universities; the only academic field that has yet engaged seriously with Jung's work has been religious studies, rather than psychology or his own discipline of psychiatry.

Many reasons could be suggested for this. Jung's studies in mythology, and particularly his fascination with alchemy in later years, have led many who lack both his intellectual curiosity and the depth of his learning to dismiss him as a 'mystic', or 'New Age guru'. They forget, perhaps, that Jung was a scientist as well as a philosopher. His theory of complexes, for instance, was founded on the objective findings of the word association test that he adapted from the work of Sir Francis Galton; today's psychological measurement of 'introversion' and 'extroversion' rests on *typology* first described by Jung in 1921.

The fact that Jung himself was an introvert has also played its part in his relative professional neglect. His insistence on the journey of individuation as psyche's goal hardly made for an interest in the founding of schools and institutes: "Thank God I'm not a Jungian!" was his reported reaction to such activities. Research indicates that those attracted to the 40 or so training institutes in analytical psychology which have nevertheless grown up in the last 50 years tend to be introverted themselves; so the extroverted work of making Jung's theories more widely known has tended to be relatively neglected. In addition, the early psychoanalytic insistence on medical training for its practitioners has given them a professional place which the more eclectically based analytical psychologists have never had. More profoundly, however, a psychology that takes its value from the inner world, as does Jung's, is both out of step with and challenging to a collective culture that values above all adaptation to the outer world. Jung himself insisted that the end of the individuation process was a conscious return to society and its responsibilities, rather than any 'individualistic' retreat from it. Nevertheless, his psychology is coloured by a deep mistrust of collective values and Freud's goal of enabling his patients 'to love and to work' may seem more immediately accessible. That does not make Jung 'elitist'. His insistence on a psychic foundation common to all human beings was informed by his work with a great variety of psychiatric patients, often poor, schizophrenic, or 'borderline' — a very different clientele from that of Freud's middle-class Vienna. But it does mean that people working in collective psychiatric settings may not feel immediate attraction for Jung's theories.

Yet his first 'burning question' — 'What actually takes place inside the mentally ill?' – remains vital. And crucially, the answer offered by his theories demands a second question: 'What is the purpose of this?' Freud's question is rather 'Why has it happened?' That certainly accords more with the pursuit of causal relationships which has characterised the mainstream of post-Enlightenment intellectual endeavour. But Jung's insistence that subjective experience and individual symptom have both meaning and purpose remains a challenge to psychiatric theory and practice.

The value of this challenge is beginning to be recognised, particularly as many 'Jungian analysts' now adopt a more eclectic theoretical position. Anthony Stevens draws on his own disciplines of psychiatry and analytical psychology to bring together Jung's archetypal theory, Bowlby's work on attachment, and the ethologists' *innate releasing mechanisms* to posit the *frustration of archetypal intent* as the root cause of psychological distress. This work has since been elaborated into an 'evolutionary psychiatry' which describes familiar psychiatric conditions in terms of archetypal adaptive responses. It offers an understanding of the essential question 'To what purpose?', as well as the necessary therapeutic optimism on which individual treatment can be based.

The complexities of Jung's character and thought have invited extravagant projections, both positive and, more recently, negative. Assessment of his contribution to the understanding of the human condition has sometimes been obscured by *ad hominem* argument about his relationships with women and the extent of his complicity with the German National Socialist government in its early years. The most extreme interpretations have been refuted, however, and Stevens has provided a useful introduction to the way in which the life informed the thought. Comprehensive assessment of both will have to wait until private material is made publicly available. Meanwhile, there is more than enough in the more than 20 volumes of Jung's published works to occupy students and scholars, as well as psychiatrists, for a long time ahead.

JULIUS WAGNER-JAUREGG (1857–1940)

by Magda Whitrow

Julius Wagner-Jauregg (1857–1940), the Austrian psychiatrist who was awarded the Nobel prize in 1927, is all but forgotten now, unlike his contemporary and fellow student Freud, who has become a household name all over the world. In his life-time, he received many other honours and was one of the best known psychiatrists, but his great achievements have either been superseded or become so much part of medical practice that they are no longer thought of in connection with his name.

Julius Wagner-Jauregg was born in 1857, a year junior to Freud, and died in 1940 a year after his famous contemporary. He did all his medical studies at the University of Vienna and apart from a short period at the University of Graz, spent most of his professional life at his original university and the two psychiatric clinics there. His preferred field was internal medicine, but having failed to obtain a post at either of the two clinics, he accepted a post of assistant at the First Psychiatric Clinic, which was part of the Asylum of Lower Austria in Vienna, under Max Leidesdorf. When Leidesdorf retired in 1889, Richard von Krafft-Ebing, Professor at Graz, was appointed his successor, and Wagner-Jauregg followed him as Director of the Psychiatric Clinic there. After Theodor Meynert's death in 1892, Krafft-Ebing moved to the Second Psychiatric Clinic, which was the more prestigious and which included a neurology clinic. Wagner-Jauregg succeeded him at the First Clinic and was appointed to a Chair of

Psychiatry at the University. When Krafft-Ebing died in 1902, Wagner-Jauregg moved to the Second Clinic, where he worked until his retirement in 1928.

Wagner-Jauregg's two great achievements were the development of malaria therapy for general paralysis of the insane (GPI), for which he was awarded the Nobel Prize, and his campaign to reduce the incidence of cretinism, which was then endemic in parts of Austria. Experiments on animals early in his career convinced him that removal of the thyroid produced all the symptoms of cretinism. On the strength of his investigations, Wagner-Jauregg followed the lead of some English physicians and began to treat patients with myxoedema and cretinous children with thyroid extracts or thyroid tablets, with spectacular success. Some years later, he began his campaign for the prophylaxis of goitre. As early as 1898, he had proposed a method for the prevention of goitre and cretinism by the addition of iodine to food, and he continued his campaign for the issue of iodised cooking salt until the end of his life.

Wagner-Jauregg's interest in fever therapy also dates back to his early days at the First Psychiatric Clinic. Soon after he began work there, a woman patient contracted an attack of erysipelas and subsequently recovered from a severe mental illness. Anxious to ascertain whether the relationship between psychoses and fever was causal or merely incidental, he began a search of the literature and observed the description of a number of patients who recovered from mental illness after a severe attack of fever. As a result of this research, he embarked in 1887 on a programme of generating fever as a therapy for psychoses. He inoculated several patients with a culture of streptococci originating from erysipelas, with negative results. After this disappointment, he temporarily abandoned his experiments and only resumed them when one of his colleagues brought from Berlin a few bottles of tuberculin. Wagner-Jauregg thought that this would provide him with a method for producing artificially the effect of bacterial infection, above all fever, without the dangers of a real infection. During the winter of 1890–1891, he treated a number of patients with favourable results, two of whom were quickly cured of their psychoses. Unfortunately, he felt obliged to discontinue these experiments because of alarming reports of the dangers of the therapeutic use of tuberculin. Nevertheless, when sufficient experience had been gained of safe dosages of tuberculin, he arranged for 33 patients to be treated, but there were few remissions. However, he realised that amongst those who benefited from tuberculin treatment, there were many more patients with dementia paralytica (or GPI) than those suffering from other forms of mental illness. Although there were a considerable number of complete remissions, they only lasted in a minority of cases; best results occurred when some feverish illness intervened. This circumstance suggested to Wagner-Jauregg that he should produce real infectious diseases in patients with dementia paralytica.

As early as 1887, Wagner-Jauregg had suggested the artificial production of tertian malaria. A chance event caused him to take up the idea again, and this led to the beginning of malaria therapy in 1917. A soldier had been admitted to hospital suffering from tertian malaria on his return from the Macedonian front, and the idea occurred to Wagner-Jauregg to inoculate GPI sufferers with the blood of this malaria patient. On 14 June 1917, he took blood from the vein of the soldier during an attack of fever and inoculated two paralytics with it. From the blood of these, three more patients were infected by subcutaneous injection and two more were injected with the blood of one of this group. Of the nine patients thus treated, six showed considerable improvement. The experiments were temporarily discontinued because of a setback, when a malignant type of malaria tropica was unfortunately used. They were resumed in September 1919 and then continued at the Vienna Psychiatric Clinic on a large scale without interruption. By 1925, the number treated exceeded 1000; generally, the success rate was about 30% full remission and 20% partial remission; until then, improvement had been virtually impossible. The therapy was used in many European countries as well as in the United States, until the discovery of penicillin made it redundant.

Julius Wagner-Jauregg. Reproduced with permission from the Institut für Geschichte der Medizin der Universität Wien, Vienna.

FURTHER READING

The 1920s: an overview

Berrios G, Freeman H, eds. *150 Years of British Psychiatry, 1841–1991*, Vol. 1. London: Gaskell; 1991.

Pichot P. *A Century of Psychiatry*. Paris: Dacosta; 1983.

Shorter E. *A History of Psychiatry from the Era of the Asylum to the Age of Prozac*. New York: Wiley; 1997.

The contribution of French psychiatry

Pichot P. The diagnosis and classification of mental disorders in the French-speaking countries: background, current views and comparison with other nomenclatures. *Psychological Medicine*. 1982; **12**:475–492.

Pichot P. *Un Siècle de Psychiatrie*, 2nd edn. Le Plessis-Robinson: Synthélabo; 1996.

Carl Gustav Jung

Ellenberger HF. Carl Gustav Jung and analytical psychology. In: Ellenberger HF. *The Discovery of the Unconscious: The History and Evolution of Dynamic Psychiatry*. New York: Basic Books; 1970: 657–748.

Jung CG. *Memories, Dreams, Reflections* (1963). London: Fontana Press; 1995.

Jung CG, von Franz M-L, Henderson JL, Jacobi J, Jaffé J. *Man and His Symbols* (1964). London: Penguin; 1990.

Stevens A. *On Jung*. London: Routledge; 1990.

Stevens A, Price J. *Evolutionary Psychiatry: A New Beginning*. London and New York: Routledge; 1996.

Storr A. *The Essential Jung: Selected Writings Introduced by Anthony Storr*. London: Fontana Press; 1998.

Julius Wagner-Jauregg

Whitrow M. *Julius Wagner-Jauregg (1857–1940)*. London: Smith–Gordon; 1993.

1931–1940

The Development of Physical Treatment

1931–1940 CHAPTER 4

Major world events

1933	Hitler appointed Chancellor of Germany
1934	Vitamin C synthesised by Hirst and Haworth in Great Britain
1936	Margaret Mitchell published *Gone with the Wind* in the USA
1937	Production of the first Walt Disney cartoon in Hollywood
1939	Second World War broke out
1940	Graham Greene published *The Power and the Glory* in London

Major events in psychiatry

1931	Karl Jaspers published *The Intellectual Situation of our Time* in Germany
1931	Ernst Rüdin appointed chairman of the Institute of Psychiatry in Munich
1931	Donald W Winnicott published *Clinical Notes on Disorders of Childhood* in London
1932	Melanie Klein published *The Psychoanalysis of Children* in London
1933	Insulin coma treatment for schizophrenia introduced by Manfred Sakel in Berlin
1933	East London Child Guidance Clinic, the first in England, opened under the direction of Dr Emmanuel Miller
1933	The Maudsley Hospital in London opened a children's department under Mildred Creak
1934	Ernst Rüdin appointed President of the German Association for Neurology and Psychiatry
1934	First use of chemical convulsive therapy by Meduna in Budapest
1934	Moritz Tramer founded the *Zeitschrift für Kinderpsychiatrie (Journal of Child Psychiatry)*, which later became *Acta Paedopsychiatria*, in Switzerland
1935	The first use in English of the term 'child psychiatry' occurred when Leo Kanner published his textbook under that name
1935	Publication of Anna Freud's book *Das Ich und die Abwehrmechanismen* (The Ego and the Mechanisms of Defence) in Vienna
1935	Egas Moniz and Almeida Lima first carried out a 'prefrontal leucotomy' in Lisbon
1936	Edward Mapother became England's first Professor of Psychiatry in London
1938	First use of electroconvulsive therapy by Ugo Cerletti and Luigi Bini in Rome
1939	Hitler's written authorisation for the killing of psychiatric patients on 1 September, the first day of the Second World War
1939	Bargue Hubert and Norwood East jointly published a *Report of the Psychological Treatment of Crime* in England
1939	Sigmund Freud died on 23 September, having finished his last great work *Moses and Monotheism*
1940	Foundation of the *Deutsche Gesellschaft für Kinderpsychiatrie und Heilpädagogik* (German Society for Child Psychiatry and Curative Education)

FOCAL INFECTION

by Andrew Scull

The notion that some or even all forms of mental disorder were the product of focal infection attracted a number of prominent adherents on both sides of the Atlantic during the first three decades of the twentieth century. Though it never became professional orthodoxy, the idea that psychoses might be caused by the presence, in a variety of organs, of chronic untreated reservoirs of infection, at times enjoyed a considerable vogue, particularly in the 1920s and 1930s. In a pre-antibiotic era, the adoption of such a perspective on psychiatric disorders was associated with attempts to stimulate the immune system via the production of 'vaccines' and — more commonly still — by the employment of a variety of surgical interventions, most commonly directed at the teeth, tonsils, and sinuses, but in other instances involving the excision of the colon, spleen, stomach, and uterus. Such operations provoked increasing controversy, and by the 1940s, most psychiatrists were highly sceptical of the focal sepsis hypothesis. Though the theory still attracted a handful of die-hard enthusiasts into the early 1950s, in essence it had lost its scientific credibility before the advent of the modern psychopharmacological era.

During the last third of the nineteenth century, there had been a number of speculations about the toxic origins of mental illness. Henry Maudsley (1835–1918), for example, asserted that "There is no want of evidence that organic morbid poisons bred in the organism or in the blood itself may act in the most baneful manner upon the supreme nervous centres. The earliest and mildest mental effect by which a perverted state of the blood declares itself is not in the production of positive delusion or incoherence of thought, but in a modification of mental tone. The further effect is to engender a chronic delusion of some kind. A third effect of its more acute action is to produce more or less active delirium and general incoherence of thought".

By the turn of the century, these ideas were increasingly couched in the terminology of the new bacteriological medicine. Such well-known British surgeons as William Arbuthnot Lane (1904) and William Hunter (1929) were warning of the perils of "intestinal stasis" — particularly its likely effects on mental stability — and were urging their colleagues to respond by developing a "surgical bacteriology". Psychiatrists soon followed suit. The Scottish alienist, Lewis Bruce, advocated careful attention to the problem of focal sepsis as early as 1906 and Henry Upson, the superintendent of the Cleveland State Hospital in Ohio, had written articles in 1907 and 1909 on the relation of tooth decay to focal infection and thence to insanity.

The growing appeal of the hypothesis that the psychoses had an infectious aetiology obviously owed much to the general advance of bacteriological models of disease. Within general medicine and surgery, though the initial claims of Pasteur, Koch, and Lister had often been greeted with scepticism and even ridicule, powerful gains in both aetiological understanding and therapeutic efficacy had rapidly followed the elaboration of the "germ theory" of disease. Here too, however, a number of chronic, debilitating disorders remained frustratingly recalcitrant in the face of every attempt to unravel their secrets. And here too, a number of leading medical figures on both sides of the Atlantic turned to the notion of focal sepsis for an explanation, Billings suggested that such chronic diseases as arthritis, nephritis, and degenerative disorders of the arteries "might be caused by bacteria disseminated through the lymph or blood-streams from a hidden primary focus of infection". He was dean of the University of Chicago Medical School, and sometime President of both the American Medical Association and the American Association of Physicians. Other prominent American physicians who embraced focal infection included Osler's successor at Johns Hopkins, Llewellys F Barker, William Thayer (also of Hopkins), and Edward Rosenow and Charles Mayo of the famed Mayo Clinic in Minnesota. British adherents, besides Lane and Hunter, included Sir William Wilcox, Chalmers Johnson, and Sir Berkeley Moynihan, sometime President of the Royal College of Surgeons.

Focal sepsis as cause of mental disorder

Seen in its historical context, therefore, the psychiatric flirtation with the doctrine of focal sepsis was neither eccentric nor extreme. Moreover, amongst alientists desperate for some therapeutic purchase on the problem of chronic mental disorder, the plausibility of the hypothesis that infection played a primary role in the genesis of psychiatric disorders soon received a dramatic boost with the documentation of the long-suspected syphilitic origin of general paresis. Victims of GPI formed a very sizeable fraction of mental hospital admissions in the early twentieth century. It thus should come as no surprise that once Noguchi and Moore in 1913 had definitively confirmed that it was the syphilitic spirochaete which produced the brain lesions which in turn caused paresis, many in the psychiatric profession hoped that the pathology of GPI would provide a paradigmatic model of the origins of mental disorder. This was a harbinger of what harnessing the new laboratory science would bring to the understanding and treatment of mental disorders.

Psychiatrists like Bruce and Upson had suggested that focal sepsis was one of a number of factors that could produce mental illness. Within a decade, however, leading proponents of the doctrine of focal infection were increasingly stressing a monocausal account of all serious mental disorders, rejecting both hereditarian and psychodynamic explanations of mental illness. In the words of Henry Cotton (1923), the superintendent of the Trenton State Hospital in New Jersey,

> "The most constant [cause], and, from the standpoint of treatment, the most important one, is the intra-cerebral, biochemical cellular disturbance arising from circulating toxins originating from chronic foci of infection…. Instead of considering the psychosis as a disease entity, it should be considered a symptom, and often a terminal symptom, of a long-continued chronic sepsis or masked infection, the accumulating toxaemia of which acts directly or indirectly on the brain cells".

Following seven years of laboratory investigation and increasingly radical therapeutic intervention, he and those who followed his lead had been led to reject the very idea of distinguishing amongst different types of mental disorder:

> "as a result of our work, I do not believe there is any fundamental difference in the functional psychoses. The more we study our cases, we are forced to conclude that distinct disease entities in the functional group… do not exist. The aetiological factors are the same… [in] the whole so-called functional group, such as manic–depressive insanity, dementia praecox, paranoid conditions, the psychoneuroses, etc.".

Attempts to eliminate focal infection

Independently, Thomas Chivers Graves, who was superintendent of the Hollymoor and Rubery Mill Mental Hospitals from 1920, and of all the mental hospitals in the Birmingham area from 1926 onwards, had reached very similar conclusions. The two men forcefully argued for the elimination of focal sepsis both in print and in person, both addressing the Medico-Psychological Association on the topic in 1923 and again in 1927. Graves targeted the teeth, tonsils, and sinuses for particularly close scrutiny, coupling surgical intervention with sinus irrigation, injections of colloidal sulphur, and the administration of autogenous vaccines. By 1930, continuous colonic irrigation was added to the therapeutic mix. Cotton intervened still more aggressively. To routine tonsillectomies and wholesale extraction of teeth, he added an extensive programme of abdominal surgery, excising the stomach, gall bladder, spleen, uterus, and especially colon, in an attempt to detoxify his patients. Both men brought an array of outside consultants into the hithero closed world of the mental hospital to assist with tracking down and eliminating sepsis. Their hospitals routinely employed both X-rays, and serological and bacteriological analyses in a period where such diagnostic tests were only beginning to be employed in general medicine.

Graves and Cotton won a considerable number of converts to their approach, though most of those endorsing their claims about focal sepsis seem to have treated it as one of a number of factors producing psychosis, rather than its primary cause. Even sceptics, after all, were hard put to assert that physical ailments could safely be left untreated, and there was no shortage, particularly amongst working-class patients, of troublesome chronic infections in evident need of treatment. The proceedings of the joint annual meeting of the British Medical Association and the Royal Medico-Psychological Association in 1927 document widespread support for focal infection theory amongst the British medical, surgical, and psychiatric elite, and a substantial number of medical superintendents adopted Graves' techniques. Cotton, too, could point to endorsements of his approach from a number of his fellow psychiatrists in the United States.

Diminishing enthusiasm

Perhaps because of the very extravagance of Cotton's therapeutic claims, however (he claimed cure rates approaching 80% when focal infection was eliminated), his work almost immediately attracted criticism. Private objections to his 'monomania' on the subject of focal sepsis were particularly harsh, though curiously and significantly, neither Cotton's willingness to operate without the consent of his patients nor his publicly reported mortality rates of over 36% in his abdominal surgery attracted unfavourable comment. A series of papers emanating from the New York State Psychiatric Institute, however, claimed that Cotton's methods for discovering infection were arbitrary, scientifically unreliable, and even worthless, and that the therapeutic effects of treating sepsis were minimal or non-existent. These findings appear to have sharply diminished North American interest in focal sepsis as a cause of mental disorder, though Cotton continued to proselytise in its behalf until his death in 1933. The mental hospital he had headed, Trenton State Hospital, professed its adherence to the doctrine even into the mid-1950s.

In Britain, the focal sepsis hypothesis died a more lingering death. Graves continued to head all the mental hospitals in the Birmingham region until the formation of the National Health Service, and used his position as the longest-serving president in the RMPA's history (1940–1944) to argue strenuously for the centrality of focal infection in the genesis of psychosis. With the advent of a spectrum of new somatic therapies from the mid 1930s, however — treatments Graves fiercely rejected as useless — most of his psychiatric colleagues displayed diminishing enthusiasm for claims about the aetiological significance of focal sepsis. And in the aftermath of the psychopharmacological revolution in the 1950s, the whole episode became nothing more than a historical curiosity.

ENVIRONMENTAL INFLUENCES ON CHILD PSYCHIATRY

by Melvin Lewis, David Musto, Linda Mayes, & Katharina Buhl

An important antecedent to the specialty of child psychiatry was the social recognition of childhood as a special phase of life with its own developmental stages, starting with the neonate and eventually extending through adolescence. Until the early eighteenth century, the dividing line between childhood and adulthood was when the young person assumed responsibilities in the adult world. However, this simple division was subsequently challenged by the introduction of formal education for a greater proportion of children. At the same time, an appreciation of childhood as psychologically distinct from adulthood was found in many countries, perhaps related in part to the ideals of the French Revolution and the new humanism that was now part of Western culture. Also about this time, defects observable from birth, such as deafness and blindness, further focused attention on children's development.

Eventually, mental retardation (or 'learning difficulties') was separated from the emotional difficulties that many children experienced. The prevailing economic and political environment also became more receptive to an enlightened approach to the care of the mentally retarded child, as well as being concerned with emotional disorders in children who appeared otherwise normal.

As early as 1899, the term 'child psychiatry' (in French) was used as a subtitle in Manheimer's monograph *Les Troubles Mentaux de L'Enfance*. However, the Swiss Moritz Tramer (1882–1963) was probably the first to define the parameters of child psychiatry in terms of diagnosis, treatment, and prognosis within the discipline of medicine, in 1933. In 1934, Tramer founded the *Zeitschrift für Kinderpsychiatrie* (Journal of Child Psychiatry), which later became *Acta Paedopsychiatria*. The first use in English of the term child psychiatry occurred when Leo Kanner published his textbook under that name in the USA in 1935.

Psychopathology of childhood
The causes of childhood behaviour problems were generally (but not universally) ascribed to both the biological constitution of the child and to the immediate environment — the nature versus nurture debate. Specific views on childhood psychopathology in the decade 1931 to 1940 included: genetic defects, prenatal damage and congenital abnormalities, post-natal brain damage, the effects of maternal deprivation, neglect and abuse, severe parental dysfunction, and unconscious conflicts.

The most prominent symptom that attracted the attention of early investigators was misbehaviour (juvenile delinquency). Why did children, mostly boys, behave violently, or steal, or be unable to stay in school? Why did girls become promiscuous? To help answer such questions, the first Juvenile Psychopathic Clinic was established in 1909 in Chicago, USA (the same year that Freud published *Little Hans* in Vienna) under the direction of a neurologist, William Healy. Healy applied the early concepts of psychoanalysis to child psychiatric treatment. He subsequently developed a tripartite model — of child psychiatrist, child psychologist, and psychiatric social worker — for the ambulatory care of children in child guidance clinics, which were supported by the Commonwealth Fund. Other countries, including England (which received Commonwealth Funding from America) and Sweden quickly followed. The East London Child Guidance Clinic, the first in England, was opened in 1933 under the direction of Dr Emmanuel Miller. Guidance for the parents was an important component of the treatment, and this model of mental health care subsequently became a mainstay of child psychiatric treatment in those three countries and some others. Since delinquency and related problems were then thought to be at least in part a result of a bad environment, it was hoped that early intervention through these clinics and the use of psychotherapy would essentially change a 'bad child' into a normal one.

The use of medication in the treatment of children also began in the 1930s, when Charles Bradley opened a neuropsychiatric unit and was the first to use amphetamine for brain-damaged and hyperactive children. Generally available treatments throughout the 1930s included guidance for parents, sympathetic handling of the child based on an understanding of needs at each stage of development, more accurate diagnosis, and improved knowledge of the aetiology of early psychiatric disorders. Psychotherapy based on psychoanalysis was used to help the child resolve inner conflicts, together with multi-disciplinary treatment approaches. Still to come was the alliance of child psychiatry with other related fields, including the neurosciences, child development research, paediatrics, and developmental and social psychopathology.

Describing the environmental influences on the development of services for child and adolescent psychiatry in Britain, Wardle cited first the influence of trans-Atlantic exchanges, particularly in regard to the idea of the child guidance clinic, which was strongly supported by Sir Cyril Burt, the most influential psychologist of that period. Psychiatric services for children thrived best when the prevailing political and social environment was "tolerant, [and] loving, sought good qualities to augment... and succeeded in balancing structure and control with flexibility and freedom to grow".

Theories of child development

Several complex theories of child development began to emerge in the 1930–1940 decade. One was a simple maturational point of view, in which a species-specific, genetically determined, more or less continuous unfolding of various skills could be observed at different ages. Arnold Gesell was perhaps the quintessential maturationalist. In the 1930s, working at what was then the Yale Child Development Clinic, he focused on four aspects of behaviour: motor, language, adaptive, and personal–social, using the then new technology of cinematography for scientific research.

At the same time, more complex developmental–structural types of theory emerged. These postulated a genetically determined capacity for the development of a fixed sequence of thoughts, feelings, and behaviour that both act upon and are influenced by the environment. Two major examples are Freud's psychoanalytic and Piaget's cognitive–developmental theories, while another is Bowlby's concept of attachment. The clinical implication of the developmental–structural theories of stages was that some kind of internal reorganisation within the child is required for development to proceed. Such reorganisations included resolution of intrapsychic conflict through psychotherapy, modification of maladaptive family homeostasis through guidance and family therapy, or acquisition of new cognitive schemata through education and experience.

A third category — of reactive theories — eschewed the developmental approach and relied instead on principles of reaction. Starting with Locke's (1632–1704) idea of the child's mind as a *tabula rasa* that is then influenced and shaped by the environment, the category of reactive theories included stimulus–response, classic and operant conditioning, and the learning theories elaborated by Watson, Skinner, Bandura, and others (Chapter 6, p. 175). The clinical implication of these was that the child's symptoms were to be regarded as learned, and that re-learning or environmental change would lead to the disappearance of the symptoms. Of these three types of theory, developmental–structural stage theories rapidly assumed dominance in child psychiatry in the 1930s.

Freud's psychoanalytic theory

Freud initially focused on developmental stages of sexual development during childhood ('oral', 'anal', 'phallic-oedipal', 'latency', and 'adolescence'). A developmental structural theory ('id', 'ego', and 'superego') was then conceived, along with a psychodynamic view of conscious, preconscious, and unconscious aspects of inner conflicts. Theories of mechanisms of defence and transference were also developed by Freud.

A major expansion of psychoanalytic theories and treatments in child analysis occurred during the 1930s: Melanie Klein published *The Psychoanalysis of Children* in 1932 and Anna Freud's book *The Ego and the Mechanisms of Defence* appeared in 1936. Hermine Hug-Hellmuth in Vienna had been the first child analyst to use some form of play in therapy with a child in 1919, but Melanie Klein in Berlin in 1920 was the first to conceptualise the developmental theory and uses of play in the psychoanalytic treatment for this age-group.

Meanwhile, differences in viewpoints about psychoanalytic theory and practice between Klein and Anna Freud became prominent and at times acrimonious. Klein, who had moved to England in 1926, was probably most influential there and was regarded as a pioneer in object relations theory, while Anna Freud's teachings and views generally prevailed in the United States.

Donald W Winnicott (1896–1971) was an Englishman, dedicated to children but not dogmatic, and astonishingly original in his observations. He was a non-conformist, a kind of rebel, and described as at times quite 'clown-like'; he flourished in the environment of a country that then seemed to cherish the eccentric in its midst. Quite unafraid to state where he thought Sigmund Freud, Melanie Klein, and Anna Freud were wrong, he also appreciated where they were right. He was also not afraid to be alone in his theoretical position and clinical practice. Having completed his medical studies at St Bartholomew's Hospital, London, he made the transition from paediatrics to psychoanalysis, became a consultant at Paddington Green Children's Hospital in 1923, and held that post for 40 years. Winnicott's early publications include a paper in 1931 on anxiety and a book *Clinical Notes on Disorders of Childhood* in the same year. In 1935, he published a paper on the manic defence, followed by other contributions. In his account, the mother initially provides a "holding environment", and through "good-enough mothering", enables the child to begin to develop the "capacity to be alone" and to become aware of his or her own self. Subsequently, the child would also become aware of the relationship between that self and the self of others. Winnicott then described the development of "transitional phenomena" and the "transitional object" — a corner of a favourite blanket or a cuddlesome toy — which he thought represented for the child a step in the transition from the self to the "not-me". He believed that this intermediate realm of transitional phenomena, i.e. between the child's inner fantasies and the external reality, continued to be present in the inner life of an adult who might experience an "ineffable moment", e.g. while listening to a particular moment in music, seeing and being affected by a work of art, or having a religious experience.

Winnicott also developed the technique of the "squiggle game" in which, through exchanges of spontaneous squiggles and drawings between clinician and child, there might emerge a theme that reveals to both of them some insight into the child's inner life. Winnicott, who had a unique capacity to communicate with young children, added to child psychiatry important insights into their inner life.

Psychoanalysis, which was eagerly received in America, soon dominated the fields of general psychiatry and child psychiatry, these reaching their zenith in the 1950s. David Levy in New York was the first American child psychoanalyst. However, at that time, child psychiatrists who were not analysts, such as Leo Kanner at Johns Hopkins University, viewed Freudian theory at best as without scientific foundation and at worst as perhaps potentially dangerous. In the 1970s, however, research in the neurosciences began to blossom and soon overtook psychoanalysis as the dominant foundation for American child psychiatry. This came about in part through the use of standardised research diagnostic criteria, more sophisticated statistical methods, neuroimaging techniques, and an explosion of knowledge in such sciences as genetics, psychopharmacology, brain function, and neurophysiology. There was also accumulating clinical experience in the use of psychotropic medication.

Piaget's cognitive–developmental theory

In the 1920s, Jean Piaget at Geneva began to develop a cognitive–developmental theory of an unvarying sequence of stages, using the concept of the growth of schemata through the twin mechanisms of assimilation and accommodation. This concept had four major stages: sensori-motor (0–2), pre-operational (2–7), concrete operations (7–11), and abstract operations (11+). These ideas and observations became widely used in the education of the school-age child and in understanding the child's developing concepts of one's own body and illnesses.

Bowlby's attachment theory

John Bowlby was supervised in his child analytic training by Melanie Klein; he initially worked at the Maudsley Hospital and then at the Islington Child Guidance Clinic in London. He soon became aware of the mother's contribution to the development of her infant, and in this particular respect, differed from Klein's views concerning the child's earliest relationship with the mother. Klein had focused almost entirely on the child's perceptions and fantasies, paying virtually no attention to the actual mother. Bowlby, however, who was an independent thinker, began to develop further his interest in the impact of the early maternal environment on the infant's relationship to the mother. He was especially concerned with the possibility of a mother's negative attitude toward her infant, which would give rise to a "broken mother–child relationship" during the first three years. These broken relationships included major separation of the mother from the child, leading to emotional withdrawal and possibly the symptom of stealing during adolescence. This latter syndrome of "affectionless thieves" became an important part of the foundation for his later major contributions — the formulation of attachment theory and descriptions of attachment behaviour.

With the later help of others such as Mary Ainsworth and Mary Main, Bowlby went on to describe four types of attachment: secure, anxious-avoidant, anxious-resistant, and disorganised. Each of these had stages in a developmental pathway. Some of his work was built on earlier ethological studies by Konrad Lorenz in Germany.

New syndromes

A discovery of new syndromes also occurred at this time, particularly in America and England. Alfred Tredgold introduced the term 'minimal brain damage' in 1908, Kahn

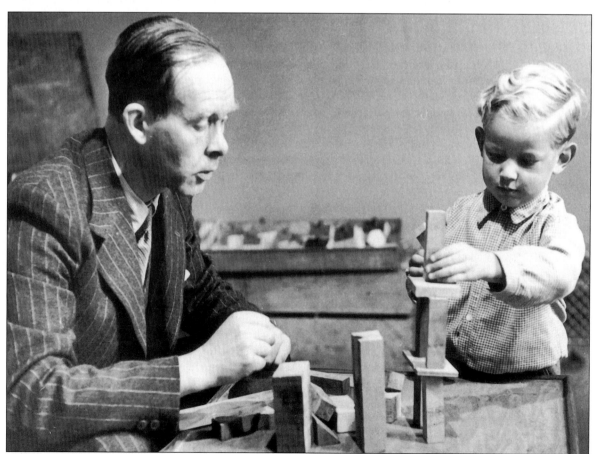

Child psychiatrist, Dr John Bowlby (1907–1990), playing with wooden building blocks on a board, in a therapy session with Richard (c.1950). Reproduced with permission from the Wellcome Institute Library, London.

and Cohen in 1934 described similar children who had 'organic driveness', Lewin described restlessness in children. All of these linked such abnormal behaviour with brain damage. The condition is now called 'attention deficit hyperactivity disorder' (DSM–IV) and is presently perhaps the most commonly made diagnosis in child psychiatry in America. Similar lines of developments in psychopathology occurred in other diagnoses, e.g. anorexia nervosa and bulimia. In 1943, Kanner made his original description of autism.

Organisational developments

Academic divisions of child psychiatry began to develop, particularly in the USA, in the 1930s. The first 'pediatric psychiatry clinic' was established in 1930 in Baltimore, headed by Leo Kanner. In 1933, The Maudsley Hospital in London opened a children's department under Mildred Creak, and research in child psychiatry began to increase.

Although similar overall early developments took place in many countries, there were also important differences as a result of differences in the relationship between the specialty and the particular environment in which it emerged. The phenomenon can perhaps best be illustrated by two strikingly different environments — Sweden and Germany — during the years 1930–1940.

Sweden

Amongst the many complex forces influencing the environment in which child psychiatry emerged in Sweden were: (a) the political–social climate, (b) the strength of the Karolinska Institute in Stockholm, and (c) an enlightened corps of paediatricians.

The political leaders moving Sweden toward a democratic Welfare State were energetic people with many ideas. From 1932 to the 1970s, Sweden enjoyed a stable democratic government that not only actively promoted social democracy and neutrality, but also aimed to create an ideal living environment for all its citizens, particularly for its children. Its parliament passed a Child Social Welfare Act specifically to develop programmes supporting the social needs of children, and highly successful child guidance clinics were started in Stockholm. Beginning in 1934, Torsten Ramer was the pioneer director of these clinics, which thrived in the context of Sweden's supportive humanist approach to the care of mentally ill children throughout the 1930s. At the same time, interested in making Swedes stronger and 'less defective', the government used enforced sterilisation to bring about selective breeding, as did Denmark, Estonia, Finland, Germany, Norway, and Switzerland. Sweden had established an Institute of Racial Biology in 1921, and this policy remained in the official record as late as 1976.

In 1845, the Karolinska Institute in Stockholm created the world's first university chair in paediatrics. Subsequently, the major encouragement for the emergence of child psychiatry in Sweden came from that specialty. Isaak Jundell, Professor of Paediatrics at the Karolinska Institute from 1914 to 1932, founded *Acta Pediatrica Scandinavia* and encouraged the publication of child psychiatry papers. He had advocated a new discipline of child psychiatry as early as 1915 in a publication called *Broken Minds*. He also funded his own child psychiatric out-patient department at Nortull's Children Hospital in Stockholm as early as 1918. Swedish paediatrics essentially provided a safe nurturing harbour for child and adolescent psychiatry until the first chair in that subject could be founded in 1958; Sven Ahnsjo was the first professor.

Germany

In Germany, a very different set of environmental circumstances greatly influenced the form of child psychiatry in general, and psychodynamic child psychotherapy in particular, during the decade 1930–1940. Prior to this period, there had been several important pioneer texts on mental illness in children. For example, H Emminghaus (often regarded in the German literature as the father of child psychiatry) published a textbook *Die Psychischen Störungen des Kindersalters* (Psychic Disturbances in Childhood) which included the contributions from both adult psychiatry and paediatrics, in 1887.

In 1921, K Bonhoeffer founded the Department of Child Neuropsychiatry at the Charité Hospital in Berlin, developing research on psychopathology in childhood and adolescence. Psychoanalysis had been rapidly developing in both Austria and Germany from at least 1909. Then came National Socialism and the appointment of Hitler as Chancellor in 1933. From its beginning, the Eugenics movement and Social Darwinism began to take an ominous form in Germany. Initially, as in neighbouring countries, forced sterilisation was used to prevent the birth of 'undesirable' children. Then in 1939, the Knauer family asked Hitler for permission to have their handicapped child killed. Hitler referred the case to his personal physician, Karl Brandt, who saw the child, and recommended that the child be killed. Hitler than empowered Brandt and Bouhler to kill not only that child but any similar ones. This marked the beginning of the escalation of the 'action' to kill both mentally ill and physically disabled children under the guise of 'treatment'. The methods of killing included barbiturates, morphine, and death by slow starvation. Some children also died during 'research'. More than 5000 children, including 'juvenile delinquents', were killed through this escalating action, parents being required to pay the cost of the 'treatment'. Furthermore, as the result of generalised anti-semitism in Germany, normal children who happened to be Jewish also began to be killed.

Amongst German doctors who were involved in this 'action' that involved the killing of children were Werner Catel, Professor of Psychiatry at Leipzig, Professor Hans Heinze at Görden (near Brandenberg), and Ernst Wentzler, a paediatric psychiatrist in Berlin. However, reponsibility for the final decision and actual killing of such children was difficult to determine; it was diffused through numerous agencies and committees, who also used vague medical terms to disguise the brutal killing that was actually carried out. The violent terror of Krystallnacht on 10 November 1938 became a defining moment for all Germans who were Jews to make desperate attempts to leave the country. Included amongst those who frantically attempted to emigrate to other countries were child psychoanalysts, who were doubly at risk: besides being Jewish, they practised the psychoanalytic treatment developed by Freud, a Jew. These circumstances resulted in a virtual migration in the 1930s within the field of child psychoanalysis from Germany and Austria (this chapter, p. 92).

In 1939, the *Deutsche Gesellschaft für Psychiatrie* formed a committee for child psychiatry, which was followed in 1940 by the foundation of the *Deutsche Gesellschaft für Kinderpsychiatrie und Heilpadagogik* (German Society for Child Psychiatry and Curative Education). Schröder, who was the first president of this society, held ideas that were similar to those used by the National Socialists, but the war interrupted the activities of the society, and publication of the organisation's journal was stopped.

Slowly following the Second World War, the first attempts at reconstituting a society for child and adolescent psychiatry were made at Göttingen in 1948. However, it was only later that child psychiatrists in Germany begin to confront issues such as the national shame which resulted from the events that had taken place under National Socialism, particularly the behaviour of German doctors.

Meanwhile, a group of European child psychiatrists had met in 1935 for the initial discussions of what was to become the Association for Child and Adolescent Psychiatry and Allied Professions. Helmuth Remschmidt is the current president.

Postscript

Environmental influences on the development of child and adolescent psychiatry are presumably continuously at work. The recent social–political forces that led to the growth of managed care in the United States, with its consequences for the mental health care of children, child psychiatry research, and child psychiatry training, are clearly most important. As we approach the next century, the development of child and adolescent psychiatry will no doubt continue to be affected by environmental changes. Service delivery systems, patient care, research, training, and administrative leadership are all likely to show the effects of this influence.

GERMAN PSYCHIATRY

by Uwe Henrik Peters

The period 1931–1940 was the most anomalous one, both in German history and in German psychiatry. On the political level, in 1931 the Weimar Republic with its vivid intellectual and cultural life was still in existence. German psychiatry was then at the height of its worldwide influence; a racist tendency did exist, but was of almost no significance. In 1940, by contrast, Nazi Germany had reached the peak of its power and the country had lost 600 of its best psychiatrists by emigration. Nazi psychiatry and its *führer*, the Swiss psychiatrist Ernst Rüdin, were all-influential. The killing of — eventually — 300,000 psychiatric patients had started.

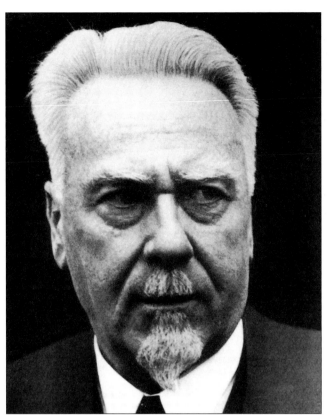

Professor Dr Ernst Rüdin. From 'People and Race', an illustrated journal for the German people (1944). Reproduced with permission from the LWV archive, photo collection.

Classical psychiatry

German classical psychiatry had three principal characteristics: its positivistic philosophy, the establishment of an accepted psychiatric nosology, and the encouragement of phenomenology. The latter involved careful observation of patients' clinical presentations — particularly symptom profiles — while minimising inferences about aetiology.

As a theory of mental illness, classical psychiatry continued to be acknowledged in Germany in this decade, though the different academic centres of gravity within the country had quite separate emphases. With the eighth edition of his textbook, Kraepelin had, to use Kurt Schneider's metaphor, rammed the foundations of an accepted psychiatric nosology into the ground (Chapter 2, p. 50). This was true, though, only for the categories of 'general psychiatry', 'dementia praecox', and 'manic– depressive insanity'. In the textbook, their descriptions were enlarged so that 'dementia praecox' eventually occupied 584 printed pages, but only small sections of Kraepelin's writings have been translated into other languages. The first volume of the eighth edition, containing 'general psychiatry' together with the all-important phenomenon of *'Zerfahrenheit'* (inaccurately rendered in English as 'incoherence'), has never been read by non-German speakers. Kraepelin's school of psychiatry stopped where he left it, when he died unexpectedly in 1926, but remained accepted in Nazi Germany. Though many former students remained, as well as the first psychiatric institute in the world, there was no real psychiatric successor to him. Johannes Lange (1891–1938), who took over the chair in Breslau (now Wrocslav, Poland) in 1930, was the editor of a ninth edition, but it had no real influence. In other writings, Lange had hailed the sterilisation laws of 1933, and thus accepted Nazi ideology.

In 1911, Eugen Bleuler had published his account of schizophrenia, which constituted the first volume of the first psychiatric handbook in the world (Chapter 2, p. 52). The editor was Gustav Aschaffenburg, Kraepelin's first student, and the style was more accessible than that of many other works. The new term 'schizophrenia' was taken from the Romantic idea of a split personality, but Bleuler also made use of association and psychoanalytic theories, as well as presenting a grouping and weighting of symptoms, which had been neglected by Kraepelin. In the period 1931–1940, Bleuler's book remained a standard work and was to be found in every institutional library.

Starting in 1911, under the leadership of the psychiatrist and philosopher Karl Jaspers together with Karl Wilmanns, a third centre of classical psychiatry had developed at Heidelberg. This school was represented by two main books. The first was *General Psychiatry* by Jaspers. At the beginning of the decade, Jaspers had published new philosophical writings, *The Intellectual Situation of our Time* (1931) and three volumes of *Philosophy* (1932). In 1937, he was forbidden to teach or publish any longer because his wife was Jewish. During the subsequent years, however, he again turned to psychiatry and wrote the fourth edition of *General Psychopathology*, which was completed in 1942. It was published in 1948 and has remained in print ever since; it is this fourth edition which has been translated into other languages. The English-language version was produced by Hamilton and Hoenig in 1963. Secondly, *Schizophrenia*, edited by Karl Wilmanns (1873–1945), came out at the end of 1932. Though a very important book in its own time, it was without later resonance and has never been translated, because the Heidelberg school was destroyed within the very first weeks of Nazi rule. Wilmanns himself was under arrest for a couple of weeks, because he had called Hitler a hysteric, and lost his chair through his wife being a 'three-quarters Jew'.

The Heidelberg school of psychopathology had been critical of Kraepelin, as well as of Bleuler. Its strong point was the working out of psychopathological 'phenomena', i.e. signs of mental illness that are 'carved' so clearly as to make them recognisable even to those clinicians who had never come across them before. The metaphor was taken from the description of the microscopic picture of a cell by histologists. Out of the contributors to this book on schizophrenia, Willy Mayer-Gross, emigrated to England, while Gabriel Steiner and Alfred Strauss went to the USA. Wilmanns survived the Nazi period in Germany, first in a monastery and later in a private apartment.

Psychoanalysis and psychotherapy

By the end of the 1920s, psychoanalysis was widely accepted in Germany. There had been a psychoanalytic institute in Berlin since 1922, which was even older than the one in Vienna. In Frankfurt, another institute which, amongst others, included Erich Fromm, was founded in 1929. In 1930, Freud received the Goethe Award in Frankfurt, the only such recognition he was ever given. In the decade of the 1930s, important psychoanalytic writings, which defined the discourse up to the end of the 1950s, were published in German for the first time. Amongst these were Anna Freud's book *Das Ich und die Abwehrmechanismen* (The Ego and the Mechanisms of Defence) (1935) and Heinz Hartmann's *Ich-Psychologie und Anpassungsproblem* (Ego Psychology and the Problem of Adaptation) (1939). However, between 1933 and 1939, psychoanalysis in Germany was virtually extinguished. Freud emigrated to Britain, where he died just after the Second World War had begun. Only a handful of psychoanalysts, such as Richard Nepalleck and August Aichhorn, stayed. For psychoanalysis as a whole, which had been forced by the Nazis to leave central Europe, the time of its great influence only began towards the end of the 1940s.

At least 100 years before Freud, a more general psychotherapy had existed, as Ellenberger described in his *Discovery of the Unconscious*. These were a variety of theories and therapeutic techniques, which centred on the doctor's psyche as the main therapeutic agent. In the 1920s, this form of psychotherapy had also grown more influential and was even stronger than psychoanalysis. From 1926, there were annual meetings which were organised by Wladimir Eliasberg. The General Medical Association for Psychotherapy was founded in 1928 and published its own journal. This association was open to psychotherapists of all orientations, and many psychoanalysts were amongst its members. Its officers included Robert Sommer, Ernst Simmel, Johannes Heinrich Schultz, Wladimir Eliasberg, Kurt Goldstein, Arthur Kronfeld, and Ernst Kretschmer — all renowned psychotherapists. But Hans Prinzhorn, Carl Gustav Jung, Paul Schilder, Erich Stern, and Alfred Adler were also members. The annual congress of the Association for 1933 was scheduled and completely prepared for 6–8 April in Vienna. Charlotte Bühler, Anna Freud, Heinz Hartmann, and many others were among the expected speakers, while several thousand psychotherapists had promised to participate. However, because of Nazi pressure, Ernst Kretschmer, then president of the Association, had to cancel the congress on 27 March 1933 and then resigned from the presidency.

Rather surprisingly, CG Jung accepted the vacant presidency, but the Nazis declared this not to be enough. Therefore, a new National Psychotherapeutic Association was founded, the president of which was to be Matthias Heinrich Göring (1879–1945), a cousin of Hermann Göring. This remained the only national association of what was now called the International Federation of Psychotherapy, chaired by Jung. Göring wrote that members of the Association should make Hitler's *Mein Kampf* the basis of all psychotherapy. In 1935, 1938, and 1940 the Association organised congresses and in 1936, Göring founded the *Deutsche Institut für psychologische Forschung und Psychotherapie* in Berlin. This 'Göring Institute' had no important influence, however. Göring died during the Russian siege of Berlin at the end of the war, in circumstances which are not known.

Bonhoeffer's psychiatric school

One of the weaknesses of Kraepelin's textbook had been the lack of an acceptable systematisation of organic psychiatric disturbances, although in the eighth edition, the whole second volume was devoted to this topic. On the other hand, starting in 1908–1909, Karl Bonhoeffer (1868–1948) had described a system of acute brain syndromes, which are now known as Bonhoeffer's forms of exogenous reactions. This concept then became generally accepted in Germany. It proposed that a great variety of disorders which can cause psychic disturbances correspond to only a handful of psychopathological syndromes. Each one of these syndromes, therefore, could be caused by many changes in the body — Bonhoeffer's Rule of Non-Specificity. His theories, however, have only been published in journals and special monographs. Until 1938, Bonhoeffer was the uncontested head of Germany's greatest school of psychiatry, in Berlin. Among his many students were: Lothar Kalinowsky (later USA), Franz Josef Kallmann (later USA), Georg Stertz, Erwin Strauss (later USA), Jörg Zutt, and Erich Sternberg (later Soviet Union). In 1938, Bonhoeffer reached retiring age, and was followed by the Austrian Nazi psychiatrist Max de Crinis. In April 1945, a few weeks before the end of the war, Bonhoeffer had the misfortune to see two of his sons (Dietrich and Klaus), two of his sons-in-law (Hans von Dohnanyi and Rüdiger Schleicher), and his cousin Paul von Hase hanged or shot by the Nazis because of their resistance to Hitler. Later, Dietrich Bonhoeffer in particular became the symbol of this resistance; to make a living for his grandchildren, he started working as a psychiatrist again. By contrast, de Crinis committed suicide on 1 May 1945, one day before the capitulation of Berlin.

Nazi psychiatry

Nazi psychiatry was not different in all respects from classical psychiatry. A shared belief between them was that endogenous psychoses were somatic, with mainly genetic causes, and they also shared a therapeutic nihilism. Nazi psychiatry was further characterised by fundamental racism. A very illuminative example of this is the life of Ernst Rüdin. As an editor of the racist *Archives for Racial and Social Biology*, Rüdin had constantly proposed a "merciless extinction" of patients with dementia praecox and alcoholism, as well as criminal offenders. This was before his involvement in psychiatry, but after he had started as an assistant to Kraepelin, he appeared to have proved the genetic determination of dementia praecox. He subsequently took over the psychiatric chair at Basel, and in 1931, in succession to Kraepelin, was appointed chairman of the Institute of Psychiatry in Munich. In 1933, he became full professor of psychiatry there and in 1934, President of the German Association for Neurology and Psychiatry. All of these offices were held by him until 1945.

In July 1933, a few months after their rise to power, the Nazis launched a 'Law for the Prevention of Offspring with Hereditary Diseases', or 'Sterilization Law'. Rüdin became the principal commentator on this legislation, and every German doctor was required to buy his book about it. The killing of psychiatric patients had been planned since at least 1935, but action was postponed until Hitler's written authorisation for it on 1 September 1939, the first day of the Second World War. The text of this authorisation was that only "patients who, on the basis of human judgement, are considered incurable, can be granted mercy death after a discerning diagnosis". This assumed, however, that an application had been made for the euthanasia to be carried out. The intellectual centre of the holocaust of psychiatric patients was therefore the Munich Psychiatric Institute. Kurt Schneider had in fact been director of the clinical department since 1931, and his role has not yet been studied thoroughly, but other psychiatrists were actually responsible. Some of these were Nazis like Carl Schneider, the follower of Karl Wilmanns in Heidelberg in 1933–1945. Others were well known in the German psychiatric world; they included Friedrich Panse, Kurt Pohlisch, Friedrich Mauz, Werner Villinger, and Berthold Kihn. However, this enormous killing action could not have been put into effect without at least the passive assistance of many psychiatrists. The facts are well known, but we still need an answer to the question — what theoretical or other ideas made so many psychiatrists who were not Nazis break their Hippocratic oath?

The so-called 'Euthanasia' decree from Adolf Hitler, 1 September 1939. The translation is as follows: "Reichsleiter Bouhler and Dr med Brandt are responsibly instructed to extend the authority of certain named doctors to grant euthanasia to, as far as one can judge, incurably ill patients, under the most critical assessment of the patients' condition". Reproduced with permission from the Bundesarchiv, Berlin. Photograph courtesy of the LWV archive, photo collection.

The smaller centres

In addition to the better known centres of psychiatry at German universities, there were smaller places where teaching and research went on, some of them with more than a local reputation.

Kraepelin's student Johannes Lange, who had taken the chair at Breslau in 1930, died unexpectedly in 1938. Mainly because of the presence of the great neurologist Ottfried Förster, the University of Breslau had a very good psychiatric reputation. But Lange's successor was the Nazi psychiatrist, Werner Villinger, who was able to play an important role in child psychiatry after the war, in spite of this. At Danzig (now Gdansk), which was a Free State from 1920 to 1939, a new chair of psychiatry was inaugurated in 1934. The first professor was Franz Kauffmann. During the winter of 1944–1945, most of the population left the city, but he remained with his patients and is understood to have died in June 1945.

In Frankfurt, Karl Kleist (1879–1960) was the most eminent leader in psychiatry, holding the chair from 1920 to 1950. Deeply influenced by the years during which he had worked with Carl Wernicke, he continued Wernicke's work in neurology and psychiatry, much of it based on the study of traumatic brain injuries. Kleist was a pioneer both of descriptive psychopathology and of a comprehensive neuropathology. To this school, we owe mainly the concept of schizo-affective psychoses or disorders, and their work is currently continued in the International Wernicke–Kleist–Leonhard Society, which first met in 1989. Kleist was succeeded in 1936 by Karl Leonhard (1904–1988) as head of the academic department at the University Psychiatric Hospital. Leonhard developed a complex classificatory system of the endogenous psychoses, based on clinical, genetic, and follow-up studies. This was the forerunner of a current classifications of psychoses.

At Frankfurt, there was a second institute of international standing, founded and directed between 1917 and 1930 by Kurt Goldstein (1878–1965), The Research Institute for the Sequelae of Brain Damage. In 1930, Goldstein became chairman of the Neurological Department of Moabit (Berlin), but in 1933, he was first arrested for a few weeks and then allowed to emigrate to Holland, where he waited a year before receiving permission to go to the USA. During this time, he was supported by the Rockefeller Foundation. Goldstein was a determined person and during this year was able to write his magnum opus, *Der Aufbau des Organismus*. The German original was published in The Hague in 1934, but the English translation *The Organism: A Holistic Approach to Biology*, which appeared in 1939, became the better known. Although Goldstein was mainly recognised as a neurologist in Germany, in the USA, he was considered primarily a gestalt psychologist.

Also in Frankfurt, Freud's famous patient Bertha Pappenheim ('Anna O', 1859–1936) had lived and worked since 1906. She was the head of a large institute for unmarried mothers, prostitutes, and delinquent women. She had also published many books, mainly on Jewish history. Being strongly against the idea of emigration from Germany, she remained and was interrogated by the Gestapo, but died a natural death soon after, in 1936.

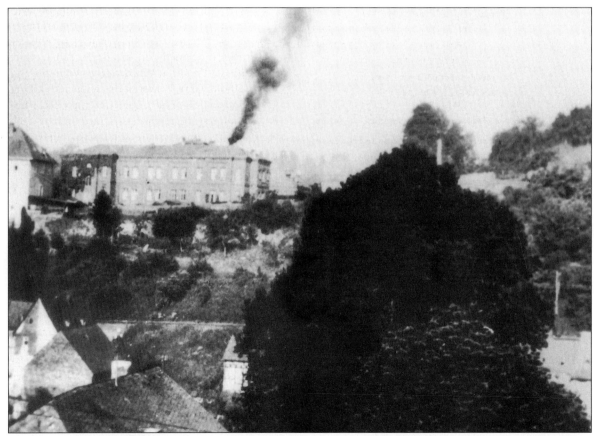

The Euthanasia Institute, Hadamar. This photograph was secretly taken in 1941. Reproduced with permission from the LWV archive, photo collection.

In the old university city of Göttingen, Gottfried Ewald took over the psychiatric chair in 1934. He was one of the few German psychiatrists who actively resisted the killing programme of the Nazis, although even he allowed his patients to be taken away for that purpose. He was able to publish a new textbook of psychiatry in 1944, but the chapters about sterilisation were cut out and their content is unknown.

In Jena, Hans Berger (1873–1941) held the chair of psychiatry until 1938, having spent practically his whole academic life there. It was in this seclusion that he invented and elaborated the electroencephalogram (EEG), almost all the basic papers about this being published between 1930 and 1940. Psychiatrist emigrants brought this new method to Britain and the USA, but Berger had the pain of seeing a Nazi psychiatrist become his successor in 1938. Berthold Kihn (1895–1964) had published 'scientific' papers on such subjects as "The elimination of the inferior from society"; beginning in 1940, he sent some hundred patients to their death every week.

At Kiel, the university had a high reputation related to its long history that was connected with the kingdom of Denmark. There, Georg Stertz had occupied the chair of psychiatry since 1926. He was known for his research on the midbrain, and papers published in 1929, 1931, and 1933 described what was then known as the 'Stertz midbrain syndrome'. The key symptom was a particular lack of initiative, described as 'midbrain dementia' because the sequel was an apparent lack of intelligence and memory. Stertz was married to the daughter of Alois Alzheimer, who's wife had been Jewish. Therefore in 1937, the Nazis demanded that he divorce her or lose his chair; he chose the latter. Since his well-known colleagues Edmund Christian and Kurt Kolle had supported him, they too were forced to give up their academic careers. It was only in 1947, when he was called to the chair at Munich, that he was able to continue his scientific work. At Kiel, his successor was Hans Gerhard Creutzfeldt, who had described Creutzfeldt–Jakob disease. Creutzfeldt was interrogated by the Gestapo a number of times because he had criticised Nazism in his lecture courses.

In Cologne, Gustav Aschaffenburg (1866–1944) had to give up the chair of psychiatry in 1934 because he was Jewish. He was mainly known as an outstanding forensic psychiatrist, yet was actually close to the Nazis in some of his ideas. It was surprising that in 1939, after the beginning of the war, he was officially permitted to accept an invitation to go as research professor to Washington, and that he continued to receive his German pension there until 1942. His successor in Cologne, however, was the disreputable de Crinis, who remained until 1938 and then went to Berlin. Among Aschaffenburg's outstanding students in Cologne was Eduard(o) Krapf, who emigrated to Buenos Aires in 1933, immediately after his inauguration lecture. In 1956, he became the Director of the WHO Mental Health Division in Geneva. Another student was Kurt Schneider, who after 20 years of work in Cologne, went to the Psychiatric Institute in Munich in 1931. Most of Schneider's original writings were done in Cologne, but were revised many times in later editions.

At Marburg, Ernst Kretschmer (1888–1964) held the chair of psychiatry from 1926 to 1946. His book *Physique and Temperament*, was first published in 1921, and went through 24 editions. It was translated into many languages and was the model for other constitutional typologies, such as that of WH Sheldon in the USA. The continuing commercial success of the book can be attributed to Kretschmer's ability to give very impressive descriptions of different kinds of character. However, Kurt Schneider, while praising the book's "unsurpassed intuitive clearness", felt that it would apply only to a few varieties of personality. In Germany, Kretschmer was even better known as being the describer of the "sensitive ideas of reference" (*Der Sensitive Bezieungswahn*), having published a book with that title for the first time in 1918. Kretschmer was also the intellectual founder of a school of psychotherapy that was independent of psychoanalysis, but not anti-psychoanalytic. Even during the Nazi period, schizophrenic patients received psychoanalytically orientated treatment from Theodore Winkler in his department.

The German University of Prague (*Karlsuniversität*), founded by Emperor Charles IV in 1348, was the oldest in the Empire. A chair of psychiatry was established in 1886, held by Arnold Pick (of Pick's disease), Otto Pötzl, and — since 1929 — by Eduard Gamper. Gamper was well known for his report of a case of arhinenzephalia, which became known as 'Gamper's midbrain child'. This child almost completely lacked activities of the cerebral cortex. Gamper was also the first to describe the anatomical changes in the mamillary bodies in Korsakoff's syndrome. In 1938, Gamper was killed in a traffic accident, together with his wife. His best-known student, with whom he had published many papers between 1932 and 1938, was Adalbert (Vojtech) Kral (1903–1988). After the death of Gamper, Kral had to give up his academic career and in 1942 was sent to the *Ghetto Theresienstadt*, where he was one of the very few survivors. He was, however, forced by the Russian commander to stay there until August 1945, because of an outbreak of epidemic encephalitis, which he later described. When he was finally freed, he tried to return to his university, but in the meantime it had been closed by the Czech Government. In 1948, Kral was able to go to Canada, where he continued to work as a psychiatrist. The successor of Gamper had been Kurt Albrecht, a disciple of Bonhoeffer, but he was murdered in Prague in May 1945.

At the University of Tübingen, Robert Gaupp (1870–1953) had held the chair of psychiatry since 1906; he retired in 1936. Gaupp was mainly known for his extensive studies of the mass murderer, Ernst Wagner. This case was considered to be the purest prototype of 'paranoia', and was known in German psychiatry as 'paranoia Gaupp'. In 1938, Gaupp published a follow-up after 37 years of observation of Wagner, who had died in the same year. The ironic title, in the circumstances of the time, was 'About a paranoic mass murderer'. Gaupp was followed by the insignificant Nazi psychiatrist Hermann Hoffmann (1891–1944); his main contribution to psychiatry had been an article in 1934 entitled, 'The psychiatrist and the New Time', which welcomed Hitler.

The psychiatric chair of Würzburg was incorporated in a very special way into the service of Nazi psychiatry. Martin Reichardt (1874–1966), who had held this chair since 1925, retired in 1939 and was succeeded by his assistant, Werner Heyde. Heyde became a member of the SS and ended as a captain in the 'Death's Head' units and psychiatric expert for the Gestapo. It was only the influence of his close personal friend Theodor Eicke, SS commander of the Dachau camp, murderer of Ernst Röhm, and finally chief inspector of all concentration camps, that promoted his career. In 1939–1941, Heyde was medical supervisor of the 'euthanasia programme'. After the war, he was arrested, but escaped. Under the name of Dr Sawade, he worked in several professional roles and finally for nine years as a psychiatric expert. It was only in 1959 that his identity was discovered by Hans Gerhard Creutzfeldt. Heyde committed suicide in prison in 1961. His follower as medical supervisor for the killing of patients was Paul Nitsche, medical director of the oldest psychiatric asylum, Sonnenstein. After the war, Nitsche was executed in the Soviet zone.

The emigration of German psychiatrists

Most of the psychiatrist emigrants continued to feel deeply involved in German psychiatry and German culture in general, but understandably, often with very ambivalent feelings. Although the main stream of emigration was to the USA and Britain, the exodus involved a great variety of countries.

The reason for emigration in general, though not exclusively, was that these psychiatrists were Jewish; there were two phases: 1933 and 1938. The emigration of psychoanalysts was almost total, but due to the founding of many new psychoanalytic institutes in other countries, the movement preserved a cohesion even after geographical dispersal. This did not hold true for other psychotherapists, however, let alone for other groups of psychiatrists.

In general, the emigrants had been thrown out of their accustomed professional life, had to adapt to a new language, and often had difficulty making a living. Yet a high degree of creativity emerged from them again in the 1950s and 1960s. In fact, there was never a time, either before or after, during which so much was published about German psychiatry and general culture, in languages other than German.

Theory and practice of schizophrenia

When the emigration movement began, Kraepelin's theory of dementia praecox was well known in many countries. In the USA, though, it had been seen with the critical eye of Adolf Meyer, who had introduced the concept there after visiting Kraepelin in 1896. Meyer added a cultural–psychodynamic theory, which resulted in an extension of the diagnosis of schizophrenia (this chapter, p. 103). The Heidelberg school of phenomenology, though, was less known in the USA and because of its completely different philosophy, was not well understood. In the *Interpretation of Schizophrenia*, Silvano Arieti referred to the 'Von Domarus Principle'. Elmar von Domarus, who worked at Heidleberg, had published papers about disturbances of thinking in schizophrenics, and had described 'paralogic identification'. His paper, 'The specific laws of logic in schizophrenia' provided Arieti with the nucleus of his theory of 'paleological thought'. This theory was replaced, however, by the double-bind model of Gregory Bateson. Bateson also stressed the role which Frieda Fromm-Reichmann had played in the development of his thinking. After her emigration in 1933, she spent one year in Palestine and finally arrived in the USA in 1935, then still the wife of Erich Fromm. During her years at Chestnut Lodge private hospital, she cooperated closely with Harry Stack Sullivan. It was during this time that she coined the term 'schizophrenogenic mother' — which was so much abused later by the anti-psychiatry movement.

Another once very well known researcher on schizophrenia with a classical–psycho-dynamic orientation was Arthur Kronfeld (1886–1941). In 1935, he emigrated to Russia, after receiving a very good offer from the Gamuschkin Neuropsychiatric Research Institute in Moscow. However, except for some repetition in Russian of his previous studies in Germany, he was unable to develop his work. When German troops came close to Moscow, he committed suicide, together with his wife. Kronfeld had no influence, however, on the later Moscow school of 'sluggish schizophrenia'. This also holds true for Bonhoeffer's former assistant, Erich Sternberg (1903–1980), who also emigrated to Moscow. Kronfeld and Sternberg at first published a number of papers together, but in 1938 Sternberg disappeared into Stalin's Gulag in Siberia, from which he returned 16 years later. He was then able to start a new psychiatric career as a close associate of Snesznewski at the Moscow Institute of Psychiatry (Chapter 8, p. 276). He published many papers in Russian about schizophrenia in the elderly, and became the founder of Russian gerontopsychiatry.

One of the great researchers in schizophrenia in Heidelberg had been Willy Mayer-Gross (1889–1961), but after his emigration to Britain, he did not continue his work in this field of schizophrenia. It was only in the textbook *Clinical Psychiatry*, which he published with Slater and Roth as late as 1954, that he made use of his earlier studies and knowledge. This book was the leading textbook of psychiatry in the English-speaking world for at least a decade.

Leopold Bellak (born 1916) emigrated to the USA in 1938. There, he collected the literature on schizophrenia in several languages and produced successive reviews of the subject. Friedrich Karl (Frederick C) Redlich (born 1910), who also emigrated to the USA in 1938, became known as the founder of a theory of social class levels and their relation to schizophrenia. Heinz Edgar Lehmann emigrated to Canada from Berlin in 1937. His schizophrenia chapters in the first two editions of the *Comprehensive Textbook of Psychiatry*, edited by Freedman, Kaplan, and Sadock, are among the best clinical–classical descriptions of the disorder. It was Lehmann who introduced the neuroleptic treatment of schizophrenia to the American continent, after reading about it in a French psychiatric journal in 1953.

Conclusion

The 1930s were a time of extreme contrast and change for German psychiatry. At the beginning of the decade, classical psychiatry, psychoanalysis, and general psychotherapy were at their highest level of creativity and influence. During the next 10 years, important books were published, German psychiatrists invented the EEG, and they also developed the first shock treatment (this chapter, p. 96).

On the other hand, the 1930s were also the time of the most important emigration movement in the history of psychiatry. At the end of the decade, psychoanalysis was extinguished and Nazi ideology was dominant. This had as a sequel first the sterilisation and then the murder of hundreds of thousands of psychiatric patients.

MENTAL HEALTH NURSING

by Peter Nolan

Mental health nurses currently exist as a discrete professional group in only about nine countries worldwide. The origins of the profession can be traced to antiquity, but more recently within the mediaeval monastic system. There, specially chosen monks devoted their time to caring for people who, because of their state of mind, were unable to continue their lives unassisted. Perhaps the most famous of the religious orders dedicated to the care of the mentally anguished was that founded by St John of God in Portugal. The first hospital in England for mental patients, St Mary of Bethlehem, opened in London in 1247, and the first continental European hospital of that kind was built in Valencia in Spain in 1409. With the Reformation and the dissolution of the monasteries, mental health care in England was taken over by privately run institutions and local parishes. In the eighteenth century, France made a critical contribution to humanising the care of the mentally ill with the work of Philippe Pinel and his chief nurse, Jean Pussin, at the Bicêtre asylum.

During the eighteenth and early nineteenth centuries, those entrusted with the care of the mentally ill in England were called 'keepers', to indicate their custodial role. Even in nineteenth-century asylums, the most important role of the keeper was to control the inmates. Female attendants, however, were generally referred to as 'nurses' and by the beginning of the twentieth century, 'nurse' had become a term applied to both male and female carers.

The United States was very much to the fore in the training of asylum nurses, with the McLean Psychiatric Asylum in Waverly, Massachusetts mounting a formal training course in 1880 under the direction of its Matron, Linda Richards. Ten years later, the first national training scheme for asylum nurses started in Britain and this was soon emulated by many countries of the Empire. Those who successfully completed their training were awarded the MPA (Medico-Psychological Association) qualification and were entitled to put these letters after their name, to distinguish them from unqualified staff. In the 1920s, a second national training course for mental nurses was started in Britain under the aegis of the General Nursing Council. This led to the RMN (Registered Mental Nurse) qualification, which eventually replaced the MPA scheme when the National Health Service began in 1948. Until then, the RMPA (as it had been since 1926) held twice-yearly examinations for nurses; it also produced the most widely used psychiatric textbook for nurses in the United Kingdom.

A worldwide perspective

The images we have of mental nurses and the descriptions of what they did in the 1930s are, unfortunately, based on limited historical sources. For most of the twentieth century, mental nursing has transmitted its values and practices from one generation to the next by means of an oral tradition, with little in writing to support it. The most that can be gained from the predominantly British and American sources that are available from that time is an overview of the profession as it was in the inter-war years, when it was shaped by the culture of the mental hospitals in which it was so deeply embedded. Both in Europe and North America, the 1930s saw the mental hospitals in their most developed phase; many were functioning as complete, self-contained societies — busy, purposeful, and largely autonomous because of their often physical isolation. The description provided by the son of a physician superintendent who grew up at that time in the Wiltshire County Asylum in England suggests a highly ordered community, much akin to an English boarding school, in which everyone had their allotted tasks and where deviations from the daily routine were poorly tolerated. The work of mental nurses was primarily to supervise patients and ensure that as many as possible were productively employed on the farms, in the gardens, in the workshops, in domestic duties, and on the wards. Effective supervision was always difficult, though, due to inadequate staff, increasing numbers of patients, and ward accommodation which was often overcrowded.

There is a persistent myth that mental nursing at this time was characterised by practitioners who were poorly educated, servile, and lacking in initiative. Apathy and demoralisation may, of course, characterise members of any professional group, but it is incorrect to imply that mental nurses in the 1930s generally had low professional standards. In many British mental hospitals, staff and patients engaged in a varied social life that paralleled and sometimes exceeded that available in the outside community. Nurses and patients knew each other well; many had grown up together in the same or adjacent areas and attended the same schools. In the hospital, they worked and played together, so that strong and enduring friendships were often forged.

At the same time as this vigorous interaction between nurses and patients was manifest in mental hospitals, the profession was developing new theories which attempted to analyse the experience of mental illness and what might constitute effective care. Throughout the nineteenth century, attempts had been made to replace a custodial approach to mental illness (as exemplified in the first institutions) by a 'moral management' approach, as developed in the Retreat at York, Pinel's work in Paris, and the American reforms inspired by Dorothea Dix. From this developed the person-centred approach of the twentieth century which emphasised the importance of the activities of daily living — a good diet, exercise, social involvement, and family care — as well as the benefits of specific therapies such as massage, hydrotherapy, and later electroconvulsive therapy. For mental nurses to be able to make the transition from control to compassion and deliver a new kind of care, the issue of what kind of training and education they required was crucial. This was to remain near the top of the professional agenda for mental health nurses until the present day.

In considering the extent to which mental nursing has been successful in transforming itself during the twentieth century, the influence of seminal figures in the early part of the century, such as Sigmund Freud, Adolf Meyer, and Clifford Beers needs to be acknowledged. Freud's ideas about the links between personality and behaviour began to be absorbed into mainstream psychiatry during the 1930s (Chapter 2, p. 47). Adolf Meyer, a Swiss psychiatrist, became Director in 1913 of the purpose-built psychiatric clinic at the Johns Hopkins University Hospital in Baltimore (this chapter, p. 103). Firmly rejecting any dualistic philosophy which separated mind and body, he insisted that the aetiology of mental disorders involved both brain dysfunction and exposure to a hostile environment. He devoted himself to improving the care of patients, and his commitment to nursing facilitated the writing of the first psychiatric nursing textbook in 1920 by Harriet Bailey, who worked alongside him. This book became a standard text in English for nurses for the next 20 years.

Clifford Beers (1876–1943), a distinguished American businessman, wrote a highly influential account of his own experience of being mentally ill in *A Mind that Found Itself*. Beers described the poor care he had received in mental hospitals and analysed its effects on patients with psychiatric problems. Almost single-handedly, he helped to bring about a change for the better in public consciousness towards the mentally ill. The mental hygiene movement which was born out of his book was influential in its turn in the rise of preventive psychiatry and the growth of child guidance clinics across the USA and then Europe (this chapter, p. 85).

The work of such influential thinkers helped psychiatry to move out from the mental hospitals and to begin to deal with the mental health needs of a far wider population than simply of those patients within institutions. Thus it was that during the 1930s, some psychiatrists began to interest themselves in the workplace and in treating the widespread depression that was associated with chronic unemployment during the worldwide economic slump. In attempting to understand how individuals relate to their work, to other workers, and to their bosses, mental health care became increasingly active along the boundaries between the individual and society. This broader, more worldly perspective enabled the formulation of a relatively new idea — that to seek to influence people's relationships may help them cope with the effects of mental illness.

In Europe and especially in Sweden, the 1930s saw a wide-scale effort to recruit female general nurses into psychiatric hospitals. Both ideology and self-interest on the part of medicine led it to attempt to reinforce the view that psychiatric conditions were akin to physical illnesses, and therefore best treated by doctors assisted by nurses. Doctors also wanted to counter the threat posed by male psychiatric nurses, whose power was increasingly being felt as a result of well-organised trade union activity. Some doctors, such as Herman Simon who worked at Guterloh in Germany, were strongly opposed to recruiting female nurses on to wards for male patients. Simon felt that work

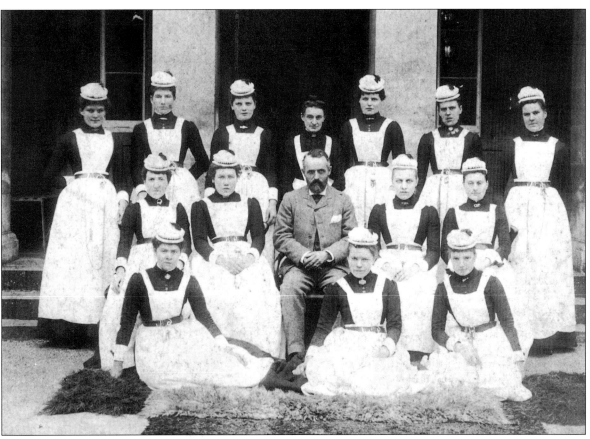

A group of female nurses at the Wiltshire County Asylum (later known as Roundway Hospital, Devizes, UK), in the early 1920s, who had been successful in their RMPA exams.

was the best therapeutic activity in which patients could engage, and that this should be supervised by male nurses who would accompany patients to the workshops, the farms, and gardens. By the end of the 1930s, Holland and most Scandinavian countries had adopted Simon's ideas and were providing various forms of occupational and industrial therapy. Doctors prescribed a specific number of hours of work for each patient, on the very simple premise that "if you have something to do, there is less time for preoccupation with yourself".

In the United Kingdom also, there was support for the critical role played by nurses in creating a therapeutic environment for patients. While Glasgow Royal Asylum provided a wide range of treatments in the 1930s, including light therapy, prolonged narcosis, insulin coma, leucotomy, and ECT, the nurses were in fact seen as the mainstay of the hospital. The hospital was complimented in a British textbook in 1936 on the quality of the nursing care it provided, and held up as a model for psychiatric services elsewhere.

In the 1930s, in some countries at least, nurses were ready to respond to a rapidly changing world, and consequently the care of psychiatric patients was evolving alongside the more widely publicised and celebrated developments in medical treatment.

ORIGINS OF CONVULSIVE THERAPY

by Max Fink

At the beginning of the twentieth century, no effective treatment for the major mental illnesses — dementia praecox (schizophrenia), manic–depressive insanity, or dementia paralytica (neurosyphilis) — was known. Hospital superintendents encouraged experimental treatments; many such experiments, previously untested, were risky and had high mortality rates. Consent was not sought, but was assumed, as the patients were wards of the State and the desperate nature of the illnesses warranted desperate cures.

Neurosyphilis was as widespread and as feared a disease, as HIV and AIDS are today. Large doses of arsenic and mercury were the principal treatments, but were only occasionally successful. In the third stage of a chronic inflammation, neurosyphilis mimics the symptoms of paranoia, depression, mania, and dementia. In this form, it does not elicit fever, and the idea developed that if fever could be induced, the disease might be extinguished. In 1917, Professor Wagner-Jauregg of the University of Vienna reported that three patients had recovered, three were much improved, and three remained unchanged as the result of the artificial induction of malarial fever. None died. Despite its modest results, the treatment was widely adopted and widely hailed (Chapter 3, pp. 64,74).

Chemical convulsive therapy

This success engendered a theory of antagonism of diseases: that it was possible to treat a mental disease by introducing another disorder. A clue to such an antagonism was found in reports that patients with dementia praecox who developed epileptic seizures, perhaps after a head injury or encephalitis, were occasionally relieved of their mental symptoms. Some doctors, believing there was a biological antagonism between dementia praecox and epilepsy, sought unsuccessfully to halt intractable epilepsy with transfusions of the blood of psychotic patients.

In the early 1930s, Ladislas Meduna, a physician trained in neurology and neuropathology, was studying the concentration of brain glia cells in human postmortem specimens at the Hungarian Psychiatric Research Institute in Budapest. He found fewer than the normal number of glia in the brains of those who had had dementia praecox, and an excess in those who had had epilepsy. Meduna inferred that the relief of the symptoms of dementia praecox in the patients who had developed epileptic seizures must have resulted from the increase in the number of glia, and he sought ways to induce seizures safely in patients. In 1933, he settled on the intramuscular injection of camphor-in-oil to produce a grand mal convulsion. It did not incapacitate or kill experimental animals.

Most psychiatrists believed that dementia praecox was an inherited genetic disorder and therefore irremediable. The idea that it might be treatable was academic heresy. Fearing criticism at the institute, Meduna moved his research activities to a state hospital for the long-term mentally ill, at Lipotmezö outside Budapest.

Amongst his patients was a 33-year-old man who had been psychotic, mute, and negativistic for four years, often requiring nasogastric tube feeding. Since all other measures had failed, on 23 January, 1934, Meduna injected camphor-in-oil into an arm muscle and, "after 45 minutes of anxious and fearful waiting, the patient suddenly had a classical epileptic attack that lasted 60 seconds". According to Meduna, the patient recovered from the seizure without harm.

Following the model of malarial treatment for neurosyphilis, Meduna repeated the camphor injections at three- to four-day intervals, and "two days after the fifth injection, on February 10 in the morning, for the first time in four years, [the patient] got out of his bed, began to talk, requested breakfast, dressed himself without help, was interested in everything around him, and asked about his disease and how long he had been in the hospital. When we told him he spent four years at the hospital, he did not believe it". After three additional seizures, the patient's symptoms were relieved and he returned home; he was well when Meduna left Europe in 1939.

Each of five other patients treated with injections of camphor also improved. Reports that pentylenetetrazol (Metrazol) safely induced seizures in animals led Meduna to try this compound in place of camphor, and because the seizures were immediate and predictable, Metrazol quickly became the principal agent for treatment. During the next two years, Meduna treated 110 patients, and in 1937 reported the remission of mental illness in 53 (50%). Amongst those with illnesses of under four years, the remission rate was even higher. Since seizures elicited by Metrazol and by camphor were both effective, this suggested that the therapy was inherent in the seizure, not in the mode of induction, a conclusion that led directly to seizures elicited by electricity. In 1939, Meduna sought asylum in the United States; he worked in Chicago until his death, in 1964.

Electroconvulsive therapy

The induction of a safe seizure by either Metrazol or camphor was difficult. Immediately after the injection, the patient experienced terror as the heart raced, breathing became difficult, and consciousness was lost. On awakening, headache and back pain were severe, and fractures were common. Many patients refused treatment.

An alternative method was therefore sought. As electric currents had been used in experimental epilepsy, electrical induction was studied in animal experiments, and a method was designed by a research team headed by Ugo Cerletti and Luigi Bini in Rome. In April 1938, a 39-year-old man suffering from a manic–psychotic episode was admit-

Thymatron device. Modern devices modify the energy to square wave currents. The controls measure skull resistance and deliver specific energies. Seizure durations and characteristics are monitored by EEG, EMG, and ECG. The EEG is analysed quantitatively to determine whether a treatment is effective. Photo courtesy of Dantec Electronics Ltd, Bristol.

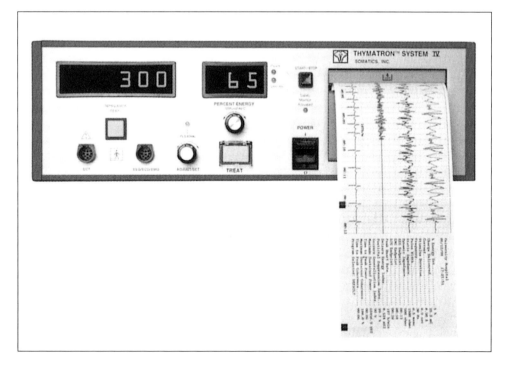

ted to the University Hospital. He had experienced a similar episode a few years earlier, at which time he had responded well to Metrazol convulsive therapy. The initial application of electric current was subconvulsive, but a second induction at a higher energy setting, immediately induced a grand mal seizure. Seizures were repeated on alternate days over the next three weeks, following the same design as had been used for Metrazol seizures. The patient recovered.

Interest in Metrazol convulsive treatments had already galvanized psychiatric practice. By 1940, at least 3000 cases had been treated in the United States, and more than 2000 in Europe. The greater ease of use with ECT and the immediate loss of consciousness without initial terror encouraged its quick replacement of Metrazol treatment.

At the time when the convulsive therapies were devised, the profession learned of two other methods that were said to relieve schizophrenia: insulin coma, introduced by Manfred Sakel in Vienna in 1933, and leucotomy, developed by Egas Moniz in Lisbon in 1935. All three forms of treatment were intimately related in the minds of both the public and the profession, and many assumed that the treatments were equivalent in efficacy and in mode of action.

Insulin coma treatment

Manfred Sakel, after graduating from the University of Vienna in 1925, managed a clinic for the treatment of opiate dependence in Berlin. The discovery of insulin to treat diabetes led him to apply it in cases of opiate withdrawal. Insulin improved appetite, increased weight, and decreased the craving for opiates. The dosages of insulin, however, were imprecise, and often a patient's blood sugar dropped so low that he suffered stupor or coma. But even after such accidental experiences, restless and agitated patients became tranquil, tractable, and more amenable to treatment.

Sakel returned to Wagner-Jauregg's (Chapter 3, p. 74) clinic in Vienna in 1933 and was assigned to care for patients with schizophrenia. Impressed by the beliefs of eugenicists that schizophrenia resulted from the malignant influence of abnormal but less robust brain cells, Sakel sought to destroy the weaker cells by the stress of hypoglycaemia. He induced repeated comas with large doses of insulin in severely agitated patients. The number of the comas and their duration were increased until the patient had one a day for from two to four weeks. After he had treated 50 patients, Sakel optimistically reported full remission in 70% and a social remission in another 18% of his patients.

His report was met with disbelief in Vienna, but others sought to replicate his work. In May 1937, the insulin treatment of schizophrenia was described by 46 reports at a meeting of the Swiss Psychiatric Society; most were favourable, although no experimental assessments had been done. As with malarial fever therapy, the results were relatively poor — improvement rates varied from 20 to 50% and there were death rates of 1 to 5%. Nevertheless, insulin coma units were quickly developed at leading mental hospitals throughout the world.

The introduction of chlorpromazine in 1953 provided an alternative treatment for psychosis, and three random assignment studies were done to compare insulin coma and chlorpromazine. No specific benefit was found for insulin over the comparison treatment. A devastating review by in *The Lancet* by Bourne —'The Insulin Myth' — showed that the optimism engendered by insulin coma was unfounded. In 1958, Ackner *et al.* reported a controlled comparison of comas induced by insulin and barbiturates respectively, which showed no significant difference between the two. By 1960, insulin coma treatment facilities in most countries had been shut down.

Leucotomy

The leucotomy era is yet another example of reckless enthusiasm accorded a dramatic procedure alleged to be helpful in treating the mentally ill (Chapter 6, p. 159). Metrazol seizures, insulin coma, ECT, and leucotomy were only four of many such treatments introduced in the first half of this century. The long list of poorly tested, risky, and unsound therapies includes sleep deprivation, continuous sleep, light therapy, acetylcholine infusions, nitrous oxide, ether and carbon dioxide inhalations, histamine injections, megavitamin and rare metal diets, atropine and scopolamine coma, haemodialysis, LSD, methamphetamine, megimide, hypothermia, photoshock, regressive electroshock, subcoma insulin, cerebral pneumotherapy, high-dose reserpine, and acupuncture. Each was introduced without adequate experimental evaluation. The same casual attitudes encouraged the uncritical use of the many unproven forms of psychotherapy.

PIERRE JANET (1859–1947)

by Paul Brown

Janet's death in 1947 went virtually unnoticed; it occurred some eight years after the death of Freud, and coincided with a newspaper strike in Paris. However, just over two decades later, Ellenberger's publication, *The Discovery of the Unconscious* (1970), augured a rebirth of interest in Janet's oeuvre.

Two hypotheses have been advanced to explain the initial abandonment of Janet's ideas: he discouraged the establishment of a psychological school, and he was eclipsed by Freud. A more likely explanation is that his comprehensive biopsychosocial approach to psychiatric disorder was before its time. Janet's models of neurosis, encompassing hysteria and 'psychasthenia', represented the apotheosis of nearly three centuries of evolution of psychiatric nosology.

Janet's conceptualisation was misrepresented by Freud and his followers as essentially biological and reflecting constitutional vulnerability. While acknowledging the biogenetic contribution to mental illness, Janet never regarded it as more than one of a range of biopsychosocial factors contributing to the essential mechanism: a complex failure in psychological synthesis. To understand this failure, he proposed a psycho-economic model encompassing a hierarchy of integrated biopsychosocial functions.

Biographical résumé

Most of Janet's active professional life spanned the half-century between 1885 and 1935. Prior to this, he was a philosophy professor in Le Havre, also engaging in experimental and clinical studies of dissociation. The results of his researches were reported to Charcot. They formed the basis of his doctoral dissertation, published as *L'automatisme psychologique* in 1889.

Janet was invited by Charcot to head the psychological laboratory at the Salpêtrière. He was awarded his MD in 1893, the year of Charcot's death. Although Janet maintained his prodigious output of studies on the neuroses, collaborating with Charcot's successor at the Salpêtrière, Raymond, he found himself increasingly marginalised. Babinski emphasised the roles of suggestion and malingering, while Déjerine found hypnosis — a technique advocated by Janet — morally reprehensible. In 1910, Janet left the Salpêtrière; he had already obtained the Chair of Experimental Psychology at the prestigious College de France, and held this post from 1902 to 1934. Janet's studies became known internationally, particularly through the Harvard Lectures in 1906, and those given at The Lowell Institute in 1919.

During the 1920s and 1930s, Janet pursued his clinical research, as well as publishing prolifically, teaching, and carrying on a private practice. In the twilight years, Janet maintained active participation in mainstream psychiatry through attendance at his pupil Jean Delay's seminars. The latter incorporated Janet's ideas into his hierarchical classification of psychotropic drug treatment (Chapter 6, p. 152).

Clinical and conceptual constellations

Three clinical and conceptual constellations pervade Janet's oeuvre: (a) trauma and dissociation, (b) psychopathology and mental economic hierarchy, and (c) treatment integration. Post-traumatic hysteria rather than post-traumatic psychasthenia was his paradigmatic post-traumatic category, but since the economic model encompasses post-traumatic dissociation, it will therefore be described first.

Originally, Janet had proposed two levels of personality functioning — automatic and synthetic. Later (1903), he expanded these into a five-level economic hierarchy, which provided

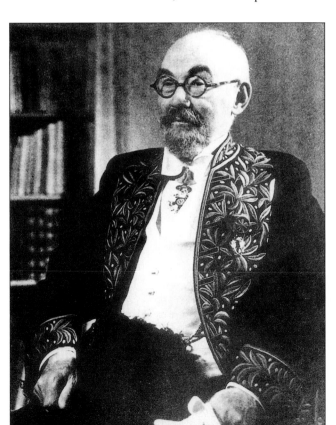

Pierre Janet. Photo courtesy of the Société Pierre Janet, Paris, France.

an over-arching model of personality functioning, neurosis, and mental illness in general. Janet sought to explain this hierarchy of reality functioning by using an economic metaphor, which invoked two hypothetical constructs — psychological force and psychological tension. The latter can be compared with Freud's concept of ego strength. The hierarchy of reality functioning may also be seen as an economic hierarchy. Following trauma (and in mental illness in general), there is a lowering of organisational and adaptive capacities or psychological tension, reflected in reduced mental synthesis and clinically in 'psychological misery'.

Janet compared and contrasted hysteria and psychasthenia in *Les Néuroses* (1909): in hysteria, lowering of mental activity is manifested in diminished consciousness and dissociation. Hysterical phenomena originate outside central consciousness. In psychasthenia there is a heightened albeit primitive consciousness, accompanied by conscious attempts at repression. Psychasthenic phenomena occur in collaboration with the total personality, and are manifested in anxiety, agitation, and obsessive–compulsive symptoms.

Hysteria, stress and traumatic stress

For Janet, hysteria was the quintessential paradigm for exploration of disorders of behaviour and consciousness, dissociation theory, and the impact of psychological trauma. These concepts were summarised in his magnum opus, *Les Médications Psychologiques* (1919), translated as *Psychological Healing* (1925).

Consciousness consists of a central active state, in free contact with inactive sub-conscious states at the periphery. In the dissociated state, there is narrowing of the field; subconscious ideas, emotions, and memories are pathologically split off from the main focus of attention. They do not contribute to the individual's central sense of self.

Although Janet dichotomised hysteria into core symptoms (stigmata) and contingent phenomena (accidents), both were seen to be founded on stress-induced dissociation: mild-to-moderate stress in the first case, and traumatic stress in the second. The causes of hysteria (and mental illness in general) extend to include severe physical illness and constitutional factors. Stigmata encompass somatoform (mostly conversion) symptoms, e.g. anaesthesias, paralyses, and contractures. Loss of skills range from impaired standing and walking, to loss of complex functions. There is also suspension of critical functions associated with suggestibility, and impairment of volition, or abulia. Ultimately, Janet regarded post-traumatic states as disorders of 'realisation', in which the patient is fixated at the point of traumatisation.

Three stages were described in the natural history of post-traumatic hysteria. The acute stage is characterised by massive emotional arousal, with failure to assimilate the primary experience of trauma. A dissociative phase ensues, with narrowing of consciousness; traumatic memories are dissociated as subconscious fixed ideas. Reactivation of traumatic phenomena gives the disorder its essentially bi-phasic character in which acute transient re-experiencing of the trauma alternates with amnesia, phobias, and other avoidance phenomena. In the final stage, there is increasing failure of psychological assimilation, extending beyond memory to the gamut of cognitive, psychophysiological, and somato-sensory functions.

Post-traumatic hysteria represents a global failure of mental integration, subsuming a specific failure to integrate traumatic memory. Essentially, this is a disorder of the biographical function, or memory-processing. There are important differences between experiential traumatic memories and ordinary reconstructive memories. Traumatic memories are highly resistant to deliberate modification — by auto-suggestion or by therapist-induced suggestion, e.g. Janet's therapeutic substitution technique. Thus, traces of the traumatic memory linger as subconscious fixed ideas that cannot be 'liquidated' until they have been translated into a personal narrative.

Primary fixed ideas range from partial experiences of traumatic memories, in which a single subconscious fixed idea forms the basis of partial intrusion as flashbacks or distressing physical sensations, to the complete encapsulation of traumatic experiences, e.g. fugue states. Secondary fixed ideas are derived from primary fixed ideas by a process of generalisation. Further traumatic stress leads to the superimposition of further accidental phenomena, with stratification of fixed ideas. Reactivation is then of more complex intermingled phenomena in hysterical 'attacks', or somnambulistic 'crises'.

Later, Janet considered traumatic memories and their corresponding fixed ideas to be subject to post-event modification. Even though the traumatic memories can be reproduced, they are not exact reflections of the original events. This theoretical work is of great interest in relation to the more recent concept of post-traumatic stress disorder (Chapter 8, p. 248).

Multiple personality disorder

The most complex forms of post-traumatic hysteria were said to comprise multiple personality disorder, in which successive traumata are encapsulated and stratified as separate personalities. Each has its own life history, but this cannot be recalled coherently. Although Janet acknowledged the contribution of psychological trauma and the pathogenicity of traumatic memories, he initially emphasised the role of acute emotions and emotional exhaustion.

In one of these cases (Marie), hysterical dissociation was linked with psychological trauma, although the emotional rather than cognitive disorder was then still seen as primary. This patient experienced symptoms for two days after each menstrual period, which included a sensation of coldness rising up to her waist. Janet traced this symptom to her menarche, when she had attempted to staunch the flow of blood by immersion in an ice-tub. Subsequently, two antecedent traumata were uncovered: seeing an old woman fall down some stairs and die, and even earlier than this, sleeping with a child who suffered from disfiguring facial impetigo. However, the substantiality of multiple personality disorder as a clinical entity has now become very controversial (Chapter 10, p. 334).

Treatment approaches

Janet called his treatment approach 'psychological analysis'. He fostered therapeutic rapport, while also applying specific treatment techniques, notably hypnosis. Over the course of time, he gradually moved towards methods of therapeutic integration.

In building rapport, Janet first used directive approaches. More severe cases of hysteria were complicated by the development of a pathological rapport. This was characterised by an increased tendency to dissociate, accompanied by dependency on treatment, with a craving for hypnosis and psychological guidance. At first, Janet did not acknowledge suggestion, either in the formation of hysterical symptoms or in shaping therapeutic responses. Later, however, he began to understand the contribution of both direct and, more importantly, indirect suggestion.

Discussing the sub-conscious transmission to the patient of the clinician's ideas, Janet outlined three sequential stages of hypnotic influence: fatigue, therapeutic influence proper, and a state of idealised dependency on the therapist. These were said to be common to all the neuroses, but attempts to direct and influence patients frequently met with resistance. The therapist should therefore seek to foster relative patient autonomy in the therapeutic alliance, reflected in what he called the 'act of adoption'. Pathological dependency is minimised by progressive reduction of direction in treatment, by enhancing awareness, and by regulation of the degree of therapeutic contact.

Instead of focusing on internal determinism and unconscious psychosexual factors as Freud did, Janet emphasised external attachments and the influence of expectation, in particular suggestion. He acknowledged the possible aetiological contribution of so-far unidentified cerebral cellular changes to therapeutic influence, but felt that psychological factors contribute no less than organic ones.

Janet dichotomised treatment into methods of economic augmentation, aimed at psychological growth, and methods for conserving the mental economy, aimed at psychological restitution. The former centred on hypnotic approaches, which transform the patient through suggestion. The latter, which aim at "reducing the work of the mind and at promoting the storage of its energies", include rest, isolation, and diminution of the impact of stress, particularly traumatic stress.

These methods were systematically incorporated into a three-stage treatment of post-traumatic hysteria. The inaugural stage was aimed at stabilisation of the patient, general reduction of symptoms, and preparation for integration of traumatic memories. It consisted mostly of rest (including hospitalisation), simplification of the lifestyle, and establishing the therapeutic relationship. Hypnosis was also used to produce relaxation, relieve symptoms, and alleviate potentially life-threatening conditions.

Secondly, integration or 'synthesis' of traumatic memories was the key to resolution of post-traumatic stress; he called this process 'liquidation'. Its essence was to facilitate recounting, reconstruction, and controlled re-experiencing of the trauma. Hypnotic liquidation was the most direct approach to uncovering and modification of traumatic memories. Two indirect techniques were also developed: substitution of positive for negative images, and conceptual re-framing. These were applied when symptom-orientated hypnotic approaches were considered too superficial, and liquidation too traumatising.

The final stage pursued the goals of personality integration and rehabilitation. Further clinical issues which had to be dealt with included prevention of relapse, and management of residual symptoms. Treatment included education, stimulating graduated activity, and emotional guidance. Drug treatment was not avoided, although its limitations were acknowledged.

Janet was well aware that psychotherapy was still at a pre-scientific stage, and that it was less specific than drug treatment in medicine generally. However, his work demonstrated that psychological analysis, as he practised it, was efficacious in many cases.

Janet and Freud

Dynamic psychiatry was conceived at the Salpêtrière Hospital in Paris, just over 100 years ago. In 1892, Janet made the revolutionary proposal that in hysteria, it was the *idea* representing the organ or its function which was lost to consciousness. In 1893, following seminal publications by Janet in the previous year, Freud was able to begin developing his own positive characterisation of hysteria. He incorporated Janet's thesis and developed his post-traumatic ideational model to cover all hysterical symptoms. At first he acknowledged his debt to Janet, but 30 years later, denied that psychoanalysis was based on that research.

Janet presented his first major critique of Freud and psychoanalysis at the Seventeenth International Congress of Medicine, in London in 1913, and subsequently published this in the *Journal of Abnormal Psychology* (1914/15). These articles drew a critical response from Ernest Jones in a later issue of the same Journal on behalf of psychoanalysts.

Janet's most comprehensive critique of Freud, however, is to be found in his *Psychological Healing* (1919/1925). His methodological criticism concerned Freud's approach to data collection, and included the unreliability of free association as well as the limits of interpretation of the proposed unconscious processes. Janet also noted Freud's tendency to select evidence to support his theories linking trauma to repressed sexual wishes, even to the point of subordinating current trauma to what was claimed to be fantasised childhood sexual abuse.

Janet next criticised Freud's aetiological approach, describing repression as an independent, conscious process, which could be partly invoked as an explanation for dissociation. Finally, he questioned Freud's "unrestricted (sexual) generalization", making linguistic and logical objections, and drawing attention to the ubiquity of sexual issues and themes. Thus, Janet differentiated non-sexual from sexual emotions and memories in patients.

Janetian and equivalent Freudian concepts	
Janet	**Freud**
• Unconscious, repressed complexes (theoretically inferred)	• Subconscious, dissociated, fixed ideas (represented in observable phenomena)
• Transference	• Rapport, somnambulistic influence, and the need for direction
• Free association	• Automatic talking
• Psychoanalysis	• Psychological analysis
• Abreaction with equilibration through the discharge of affect	• Therapeutic synthesis and integration on the one hand, and treatment by emotional 'discharge' on the other
• Working through	• Dissociation as a therapeutic process
• The reality principle	• Function of reality
• Ego and ego strength or weakness	• The self and levels of psychological tension and degrees of psychological synthesis
• Complementary series	• Constitutional stigmata with incidental or 'accidental' traumatic stress factors
	• Abreaction

Janet emphasised multi-factorial causation, asserting that we must not interpret symptoms historically, unless clinical observation makes such an interpretation indispensable, and we should never indulge in risky hypotheses. Ellenberger saw the influence of Janet on Freud as a controversial problem, which has never been objectively studied. At first, Freud's methods and concepts were modelled on those of Janet, but their paths diverged. Janet adopted a biopsychosocial, health-orientated model, based on personal growth. It included external factors such as objective trauma, and social factors such as therapeutic suggestion. Janet and Freud both continued to focus on intra-psychic processes, but Janet emphasised the interaction of exogenous and psychosocial factors within the biogenetic matrix. This compared with Freud's more endogenous psychological and physiological approach. Janet's writing extended to 23 books, 18 chapters, and 159 papers. Clearly, his oeuvre would richly repay further study.

ADOLF MEYER (1866–1950)

by Michael Gelder & Hugh Freeman

Adolf Meyer was born in November 1866 in Niederwenigen near Zurich, where his father was a minister. He studied medicine at the University of Zurich, one of his teachers being August Forel. He qualified in medicine in 1890, and won a travelling scholarship which enabled him to go first to Paris, where he attended lectures by Déjerine and Charcot, and then to Edinburgh and London. At the National Hospital for Neurology, he observed the work of Hughlings Jackson, Horsley, Ferrier, and Gowers. On his return to Switzerland, Meyer undertook research in neuropathology as a preliminary to clinical training. He then decided to set off for America, thinking that the career opportunities would be better there than in Switzerland.

On arrival, he wrote to the University of Chicago, enquiring about work in neuropathology; an appointment was offered him, but it was to be unpaid. Nevertheless, Meyer accepted it, and also worked as a general practitioner to earn enough to live on. Although disappointed by several rebuffs, he eventually obtained a post, again unpaid, as attending physician to the Neurology Department of the College of Physicians and Surgeons. Here, he was able to teach medical students, see patients, and meet local neurologists.

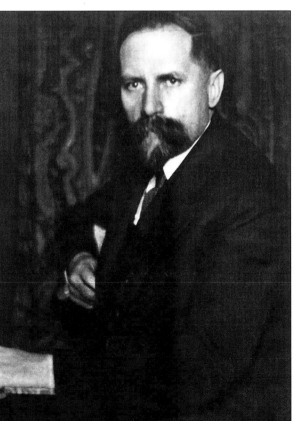

Meyer (1866–1950), a Swiss-born American clinical psychiatrist professor who specialised in the area of psychobiology. © Corbis.

However, this was not a happy time for Meyer. Not only did he have difficulty in obtaining satisfactory paid work, but he was also receiving worrying news about his mother. Eventually, the family persuaded Frau Meyer to see Forel, who diagnosed melancholia and arranged for her admission to the Burghölzli Hospital in Zurich.

In May 1893, Meyer had an unexpected offer. The Illinois Eastern Asylum was looking for a pathologist: at the age of 26, he went to work in his first psychiatric hospital. This was in Kankakee, 60 miles south of Chicago, and contained 3000 patients. Although appointed as a pathologist, Meyer was not impressed by what he saw of the clinical services of the hospital, and wrote a report to the governor of the state of Illinois suggesting reforms. It proposed that: "The ideal asylum or hospital for the insane should furnish the patients most of the advantages of home.… The attendants should be nurses not supervisors, they should live like patients, eat the same food… and share the recreations and amusements with the patients with as little bossing as possible. Everything that suggests detention in prison must be strictly avoided".

Meyer seems to have been as unimpressed by the quality of the hospital staff as he was in the care they provided, believing that, "more than any other physician the alienist must have a broad education". He tried to remedy matters by teaching them neuroanatomy, neuropathology, neurology, and features of the psychoses. Meyer based these lectures both on the teaching he had received from Forel and from his reading of the fourth edition of Kraepelin's textbook. But as he continued to work with psychiatric problems, he became increasingly dissatisfied with the emphasis Kraepelin and other authors of the time placed on heredity as a cause of mental illness. He began to think instead about environmental influences.

The year 1895 was a better one for Meyer: he was becoming known both locally and — after presenting his ideas at the annual meeting of the American Medico-Psychological Association — to a wider audience. Moreover, he was offered a new and more important post. This was as pathologist to the Worcester Lunatic Asylum in Massachusetts, with the possibility of a link with the nearby Clark University. In addition to the pathology work, Meyer was given responsibility for the training of the psychiatrists. To prepare for this, he was given leave to study in Europe, where he visited Kraepelin in Munich and Lombroso in Italy. Although impressed by their work, he continued to question the emphasis they laid on heredity and neuropathology as sources for the understanding of psychiatric disorders.

In 1901, at the surprisingly young age of 35, he was chosen to represent Clark University at the 450th anniversary celebrations of the University of Glasgow. In the following year, his growing reputation led to the offer of the post of Director of the New York State Pathological Institute. The purpose of this organisation was to improve the standards of medical work in New York State institutions, and Meyer threw himself into his new task with great enthusiasm. His experience at Worcester convinced him that to raise standards, clinical practice would have to improve.

Although Meyer understood the value of Kraepelin's system of diagnosis, he campaigned against what he saw as the unthinking use by others of these categories. His influence in New York grew steadily. He was appointed Professor of Psychotherapy at Cornell University Medical College, organised the first out-patient clinic in the city, and published many papers. One, on schizophrenia, was delivered in 1906 before the annual meeting of the British Medical Association, held in Toronto. The subject was dementia praecox: "Every individual is capable of reacting to a wide variety of situations by a limited number of reaction types... In psychiatry the facts occur in very complex combinations, and therefore one-word diagnosis is almost sure to fall short of what it ought to do". Meyer's emphasis on clinical standards led him to propose a change of name for the Pathological Institute, which became the New York State Psychiatric Institute.

In 1908, he received an offer from Johns Hopkins University Medical School in Baltimore, where a new psychiatric clinic was being established with an endowment from Henry Phipps, a wealthy financier. However, the clinic did not open until five years later, in April 1913. Meyer now had a position of great influence. He demanded high standards of clinical work from his staff and was active in teaching medical students, while at the same time continuing pathological work of his own. The reputation of the clinic grew, and many young psychiatrists went there to improve their training.

Meyer remained in charge of the Phipps Clinic until his retirement at the age of 74. During these years, he achieved much and received many honours, but his ideas did not develop in important ways after the first years in Baltimore.

Meyer's ideas

Psychobiology

Meyer used the term 'psychobiology' to indicate an approach to psychiatry that attended to the whole person and considered a wide range of factors in the aetiology of mental disorder. When he began to advocate this approach, most psychiatrists regarded psychoses as disorders with a predetermined and generally unfavourable course; in considering aetiology, they concentrated attention on hereditary factors, and for treatment they advocated custodial care.

Psychobiology was set up in opposition to these ideas. The mind/brain problem was rejected as insoluble, the two being regarded as equally essential aspects of the individual. Each person was seen as mainly a product of social forces and other life experiences, heredity being relatively less important. The psychiatrist had to understand his patients as individuals by studying their biographies. Psychiatric disorders were considered reactions of the person to cumulative events in his life, each person having a limited number of ways of reacting. Although Meyer was interested in Freud's work — and was an honorary member of the New York Psychoanalytic Society — he considered that the psychoanalytic approach embodied an excessive use of theory.

Psychobiology required a detailed assessment of patients' life experiences, which could be assisted by the drawing up of a 'life chart'. This had columns for life problems and for periods of psychiatric disorder, each of which was shown against the year that it began and ended.

Classification: the 'ergasias'

Meyer's view of psychiatric disorders as particular kinds of reaction to circumstances led him to propose a new system of classification. Although basically simple, the scheme was made unnecessarily difficult to understand by the terms chosen to denote each type of reaction. However, with the substitution of the words 'reaction type' for Meyer's term 'ergasia', the scheme was to become incorporated in an important British textbook and to influence the first edition of the American Psychiatric Association's classification scheme (DSM–I).

Treatment

Meyer taught that treatment began with the first interviews with patients, in which their assets and strengths were assessed, as well as their illnesses and handicaps. The aim was to help each patient find out for themselves, not to impose a conclusion. Then, patients were helped to build on their strengths, overcome their handicaps, and adapt better to their circumstances. As well as these psychological components, treatment included measures to improve sleep and nutrition, as well as a regular routine of living. Problems were dealt with at a conscious level, beginning with the most immediate and accessible, and avoiding speculation about unconscious processes.

Meyer stressed the need for 'habit training', by which he meant guidance, re-education, and other measures to help patients deal better with the stresses in their lives. Nurses were involved fully, and visits to the home were made by social workers; he also valued and encouraged the work of occupational therapists. At a time when physical treatments had little beneficial effect and when the diagnosis of schizophrenia often led to therapeutic nihilism, Meyer's therapeutic confidence was important.

Meyer was one of the pioneers of the reform of American psychiatric hospitals. His interest in social factors in mental illness led him to a concern for the care of patients after they left the hospital, and for prevention. In the early days of his clinical career, his wife helped him by visiting the families of his patients, becoming in effect the first psychiatric social worker. After initial caution, he supported the American "mental hygiene" movement started by Clifford Beers.

Teaching and training

Meyer believed that medical students should not learn just about mental disorders, but should also understand personality and its development. In 1914, he introduced the first course on psychology for medical students at Johns Hopkins Medical School. So far as postgraduate training was concerned, he believed that it should emphasise the detailed study of individual patients. When President of the American Psychiatric Association in 1928, he made a strong plea for the specialist certification of psychiatrists, and referred approvingly to the diplomas in psychological medicine which already existed in Britain. Psychoanalysis was to be part of it, but as "an incident in a broader training to be limited to specially talented clinicians and well chosen patients".

Influences on British psychiatry

Meyer's influence on the teaching and practice of clinical psychiatry was arguably greater in Britain than in America. The importance of his 'psychobiology' was seen as a trend of thought that paved the way for the acceptance of psychodynamic concepts and the movement towards community mental health. Meyer never mastered a clear style of writing in English, and the volumes of his collected papers remain largely unread. However, his influence was carried to Britain by psychiatrists who worked with him, of whom the two most influential were Sir David Henderson and Sir Aubrey Lewis.

In 1915, Henderson returned to Glasgow from Baltimore to work in the Royal Mental Hospital and at the University. At that time, none of the current British textbooks of psychiatry set out the kind of clinical approach that Henderson had learnt from Meyer, and he decided to join with another of Meyer's pupils, RD Gillespie, to produce a new one. This appeared in 1927, and was dedicated to Adolf Meyer. Unlike other current textbooks, the chapter on methods of examination emphasised history-taking as much as the examination of the mental state. It contained many illustrative case histories, constructed on psychobiological lines, to illustrate the importance of understanding the patient as a unique individual. Aetiology was presented in psychobiological terms, emphasising the interplay of causes. A second edition appeared in 1930, and further versions until the late 1970s, more than 50 years after its first appearance.

Sir Aubrey Lewis introduced Meyer's ideas to Britain in a different way, relating it to other approaches. He respected Meyer's wide general knowledge of literature and philosophy, and his scholarly approach to psychiatry. He was also strongly impressed by Meyer's personal and professional integrity.

Three aspects of Meyer's thought were particularly influential in Lewis' teaching and practice. These were: Meyer's clinical method; the psychobiological approach with its emphasis on multiple causes and on the study of each patient as a unique individual; and the idea of a research centre in which clinicians could work closely with basic scientists. It was the expansion of British psychiatric training after the Second World War and Lewis' appointment to the Chair of Psychiatry at London University in 1945 that enabled him to exert great influence. His trainee psychiatrists learnt a clinical method which emphasised extensive history-taking, leading first to a diagnosis and then to an understanding of the individual patient. Life charts were used to show relationships between social or psychological changes, and episodes of mental disorders.

Meyer's influence was also seen in Lewis' plan for the Institute of Psychiatry attached to the Maudsley Hospital. Just as the staff of the Phipps Clinic included basic scientists such as Horsley Gantt and Kurt Richter, so Lewis introduced departments of psychology and physiology, as well as more traditional neuropathology. Although Meyer was influenced by Swiss thinkers and by American psychologists and philosophers such as James, Peirce, and Dewey, the ideas of British writers on biology and medicine were also very important to him.

These included three ideas of TH Huxley: "his definition of science as organised common sense; second his presentation of the theories of Darwin and the critical philosophy of Hume… and third, his extreme version of parallelism which made mind a mere epiphenonomenon". Meyer also praised "Hughlings Jackson's capacity for observation; his use of the principles of evolution and dissolution rather than of a narrower concept of structure and function, and his caution in the use of psychological terms and concepts".

During the post-war years, however, a wave of enthusiasm for psychoanalysis swept through American medical schools, and Meyer's less spectacular ideas became neglected. In Britain, though, psychoanalysis never achieved the same influence. As the tide of psychoanalysis in America receded, it was soon replaced by another enthusiasm — 'biological psychiatry', a name which suggests a relationship with psychobiology but which is in reality very different from Meyer's notion of reaction types. The biological approach is also associated with a system of diagnosis that relies more on the patient's present state than on the evolution of personal problems, while treatment relates more closely to the diagnosis than to the unique features of the individual.

In Britain, with its more conservative approach, the ideas of biological psychiatry were absorbed into previous teaching and practice. Nevertheless, there are continuing pressures to return to an approach to psychiatry which focuses on the illness at the expense of the ill person, and in which the doctor thinks that the investigative work is done when a diagnosis has been made. Meyer warned against the doctor who has no use for the actual study of cases, beyond the search for a few diagnostic signs, and who asks "What is the use of any special study of the case if the diagnosis is already made?".

Acknowledgements

This contribution has been modified from Gelder MG. Adolf Meyer. In: Berrios GE, Freeman H, eds. 150 Years of British Psychiatry, *Vol. 1. London: Gaskell; 1991.*

ANNA FREUD & MELANIE KLEIN

by Meira Likierman

In the early 1920s, the psychoanalytic method developed by Sigmund Freud for the treatment of neurotic patients began to be adapted to therapeutic work with children. This pioneering endeavour was carried out by two strong-minded women, Freud's daughter Anna and the slightly older, Vienna-born Melanie Klein. The method developed through their efforts led to the establishment of a new profession — child psychoanalysis — followed by that of psychoanalytic child psychotherapy. This is now a well-established method of treating children, both in the UK and other countries. In addition, there has been a worldwide dissemination of psychoanalytic knowledge in the field of child mental health.

Anna Freud and Melanie Klein had much in common. Their similar cultural background, interest in psychoanalysis, and dedication to child mental health should have naturally brought them into some form of professional association. Both women also had to contend with issues that emerged from belonging to a minority group twice over — ethnic and professional. Though the difficulties that psychoanalysis initially encountered are well documented, along with the challenges faced by some of its women members, the ethnic dimension of the problem is perhaps less familiar. The lives of Anna Freud and Melanie Klein followed a pattern that owed much to a shared female Jewish identity, in a particular historical context. Yet paradoxically, they were not particularly conscious of the significance of this background; if anything, they lived as what Isaac Deutscher labelled "non-Jewish Jews". They belonged to a well-known genre of Jewish thinker who was concerned with universal issues and addressed the whole of society, rather than just the Jewish community. Such thinkers also included radical women who since the late nineteenth century had been taking up struggles for causes outside Jewish society. Such women tended to experience painful, confrontational struggles, because they could not easily gain acceptance, either in the Jewish community or beyond.

While Anna Freud and Melanie Klein did not think of themselves as rebels or radicals, they none the less poured their considerable energies into a universal cause — revolutionising the understanding of infancy and childhood through psychoanalytic knowledge. Far from joining forces, though, the two could agree on very little and in fact became lifelong professional antagonists.

In this way, the technique of child analysis developed through disputes and conflict, leading finally to an open confrontation described as the 'controversial discussions'. These took place between 1941 and 1945 in London, to which both Melanie Klein and Anna Freud had by this time emigrated, and were debated within the British Psycho-Analytical Society. By this time, both women had achieved a great deal in their own right. On the basis of their observations and work with children, they had made significant contributions to psychoanalytic theory. Their insights had immediate relevance to psychoanalysis in general, in as much as they were derived directly from data that held clues to the earliest and most formative experiences in life. It was for this reason that, by the time they confronted each other in 1941, they did so not specifically as child psychoanalysts, but as representatives of two opposing streams within the British psychoanalytical establishment. However, no consensus on key issues could be reached, either by the two women or by the Society itself.

Melanie Klein believed that the infant is born with a readiness for social interactions and is immediately capable of forming 'object relations', even though these are rudimentary and incomplete. But it does respond to maternal nurturing, and becomes attached to a part of the mother that carries immediate significance for it — her feeding breast. The latter represents not only food, but, by virtue of offering also comfort and pleasure, acquires the significance of 'good'. However, the infant can also be deprived of the maternal breast, can then react with frustrated aggression, and experience it as 'bad'. The concept of 'object' originated in Freud's drive theory. According to this, primary motivational forces, or 'drives', propel human needs and urges to seek need-fulfilling objects. In infancy such an object might be the mother's feeding breast, but later in life, needs are fulfilled in much more complex ways, and the individual is driven to seek valued others or 'love objects'. Klein felt that this developmental progression was far from simple, even in its origin. She suggested that the infant has inevitable emotional responses to its earliest need-fulfilling objects, and soon establishes with them primitive 'object relationships' of attachment or aggression.

To Anna Freud, such advanced differentiating abilities in the infant were hardly credible. This proposal also threatened her father's model of development, according to which the infant is initially sheltered in a foetus-like 'primary narcissism'. Freud had envisaged the young infant as noticing very little of the outside world, since its existence was governed by the pleasure principle and its primitive mind drifted into dream-like, hallucinatory states that hindered the full apprehension of worldly frustrations. Only gradually does the infantile mind accommodate the 'reality principle', and only then are object relations tenable. Such a difference of opinion might seem insufficient to have caused a fundamental rift between the two women, but Melanie Klein proceeded to hypothesise a rudimentary psychical activity that exists from birth and that she termed 'phantasy'. It is early phantasy, she felt, that both gives form to infantile instinctual life and also represents worldly events internally. Gradually, it enables clearer cognitive capacities to emerge in the infant.

Klein envisaged that the content of early phantasy was complex, and suggested that it could be used by the infant for defensive purposes. On this basis, overwhelming disturbance and anxiety in the infant could trigger phantasies that reinforce a primitive mental mechanism of 'splitting'. (By 'splitting' Klein was referring to a mechanism underpinning dissociation processes, employed by the psyche to distance feelings from thoughts, and so reduce the impact of painful experiences. In this thinking, she was relying on Eugen Bleuler's view of dissociation processes in his 1924 '*Textbook of Psychiatry*', where he noted the typical schizophrenic state of 'defects in affectivity'.) Klein felt that this helped to explain the mechanisms at work in adult psychiatric conditions, including schizophrenia, manic–depression, and obsessional disorders. According to this view, all the important mental ingredients of adult psychotic illness are genetically present in early psychic life, and are only gradually rendered harmless through healthy development. This model indicated a radically different approach to analytic interpretations from the one favoured by Anna Freud. She continued to attribute complex processes and pathologies only to much later stages of development. Between them, though, Anna Freud and Melanie Klein articulated different but crucial issues, and it is the contributions of both that add up to a rounded definition of child mental health needs. Perhaps the different angles that they each brought to bear on the subject emerged from their almost opposite personalities and lifestyles.

Anna Freud, who never married, devoted her life single-mindedly to the cause of psychoanalysis, and later also to the care of her ailing father. She was by nature traditional and orderly, and so inclined to follow in her father's footsteps. His influence on her thinking was increased by the fact that she had also been his analytical patient for a period. Initially, her main efforts were devoted to adapting her father's existing psychoanalytical method as faithfully as possible. Yet the continuity that she sought with his thinking did not merely reflect an uncritical devotion to him. She actually favoured an approach that tended to being more 'scientific', in the sense that she attempted to study existing models, proceed logically in applying these, and systematically collect data to verify their value.

In such tasks, her orderliness and industry were obvious assets, and these virtues appear to have been a feature of the Freud household more generally. Like her father, Anna spent a good deal of time writing, corresponding, and systematically ordering her documents and reports. Her mother, equally well organised, seems to have derived confidence not only from an efficient household, but also from a belief that integrity and correctness reigned in the rest of society. Two telling incidents highlight these inclinations, particularly as they put both Anna and the Freud household to a severe test. They occurred in March 1938 in Vienna, on a day when the Nazis invaded the Freud apartment. They were later recalled by Freud's son Martin (all the following quotations are from the biography of Anna Freud by Young-Bruehl, 1988):

> "The first was the view I had from the window of Anna being driven off in an open car escort-
> ed by four heavily armed SS men. Her situation was perilous; but far from showing fear, or even much interest, she sat in the car as a woman might sit in a taxi on her way to enjoy a shopping expedition".

This self-possessed, courageous behaviour fits in well with Martin's second memory from the same day:

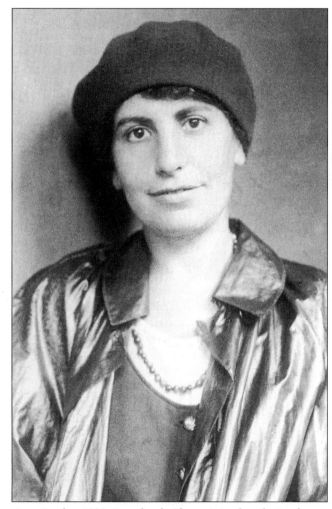

> "The second scene... is of mother, highly indignant with an SS man who, on his way through a passage, paused at a large cupboard, pulled open its doors and began roughly dragging out her piles of beautifully laundered linen, all efficiently arranged in the way dear to her housewifely heart, each package held together by coloured ribbons.... Without showing the slightest fear, mother joined the fellow and told him precisely what she thought of his shocking behaviour in a lady's house".

Years later, at the child analysis clinic that Anna Freud founded in Hampstead, London she was to leave all her documents divided and tied with string in the same careful fashion that her own mother had kept linen:

> "At the end of each year, all the papers for the year were punched with two holes in their left margins and tied up with a string into six-inch-thick book-like parcels... there were exactly five parcels for each year. The system never varied".

Indeed, this exactitude characterised Anna Freud's handling of her literary estate, which:

> "resembled an archaeological site, keyed precisely to the day-by-day, year-by-year living of her life. She filed away every piece of paper that came her

Anna Freud, c. 1932. Reproduced with permission from the Freud Museum, London.

way at 20 Maresfield Gardens from the end of the Second World War to 1982, and she kept carbon copies of every typewritten communication that left the house".

An orderly approach extended also to her clear written style as well as to the mode of training and research that she favoured. Within her Clinic, she developed a comprehensive indexing system which was taught to all the staff and used for the collection of an impressive archive of data. She also designed a profiling system that allowed the development of a consistent, detailed approach to the diagnosis of children.

By comparison with this, Melanie Klein's life appears turbulent and unconventional. Rather unusually for the period, Klein divorced her husband early, and later had a stormy battle with her daughter, when the latter grew up and also became a psychoanalyst. Tragically, she also lost her son when he had a climbing accident. Over the years, she appeared to many to be fanatical in her total absorption in her work, while being hopeless about household details. Her biographer, Phyllis Grosskurth, describes how her housekeeper arrived home one afternoon to find the kitchen smeared from end to end with a red substance. Fearing that her employer had injured herself, she rushed into Mrs Klein's bedroom, only to find to her calmly reading in bed. It appeared that she had spilled a jar of beetroot.

This impatience with mundane tasks was consistent with a personality that was passionate, spontaneous, and imaginative, but at times capable also of taking an uncompromising stance. Her early liveliness and flamboyance were noted by a devotee and fellow trainee, who was instrumental in encouraging her efforts. Having embarked on her psychoanalytic training in Berlin, Alix Strachey was in analysis with Karl Abraham, who was also analysing Melanie Klein at the time.

Alix Stachey's enthusiasm, though, was tinged with some ambivalence. Writing to her husband James, who translated Sigmund Freud's writings into English, she concluded that: "She's a dotty woman. But there's no doubt whatever that her mind is stored with things of thrilling interest. And she's a nice character". Melanie Klein's mind was felt by others to be highly original but anarchic, and Ernest Jones suggested that it was "neither scientific nor orderly". Indeed, the approach that characterised her work could be described as more artistic than scientific, proceeding through intuition and emotion, exploring the depths of primitive phantasy life and favouring evocative description as a main explanatory tool. In line with this, Melanie Klein developed no systematic indexing or recording methods. She left behind only a handful of papers that expound her basic concepts, and these are intricate, dense, and repetitious. Yet each of her papers contains highly original contributions, with a scope that covers everything from the earliest mental experiences to mechanisms that underlie major psychiatric afflictions. The fundamental differences between the personalities and lives of Melanie Klein and Anna Freud had implications for the theoretical heritage which they have left.

It is perhaps not surprising that Anna Freud, who approached the profession conventionally, began with the logical first step of training as a teacher and gaining experience with children. This left a lasting mark on her future work, which could never be confined entirely to a private consulting room. She continued to cultivate community-based work, extending her expertise to children who were deprived, orphaned, handicapped, poor, delinquent and, for one reason of another, a concern of the State.

During the war years, with the help of a grant from the American Foster Parents Plan for War Children, she opened the Hampstead War Nursery. Children were sent to her by the emergency accommodation authorities, by hospitals from poor parts of London, and by psychiatric social workers from the rest centres for victims of bombing. The Nursery offered places to children from bombed homes, to those who

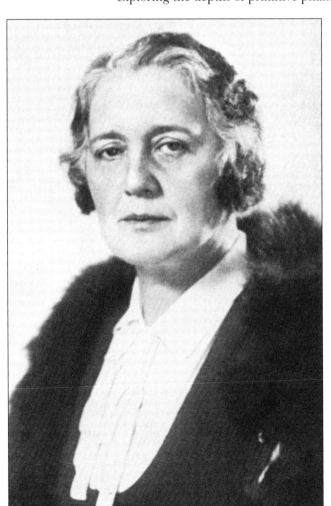

Melanie Klein, c. 1935. Reproduced with permission from Sigmund Freud Copyrights, Colchester.

had spent their nights on noisy underground platforms and developed sleep difficulties, to children who had been sent back from evacuation after failing to settle down, to those whose fathers had joined the armed services and whose mothers were at work, and other similar cases. Anna Freud not only organised expert care for those children, but trained the staff to observe and record all the important psychological details that emerged. This project typifies her vision of the ideal child mental health provision: it combined a humane public service with a rigorous scientific research programme.

Melanie Klein's initial approach to the profession equally left its mark on her long-term work, but it differed considerably from Anna Freud's. Klein was neither trained herself to work with children nor followed any other conventional career path. Around 1914, she sought psychoanalysis for her own difficulties, and while engaged in this, began also to observe her own children and discuss them with her first analyst, Sandor Ferenczi. Having tried out some rudimentary analytical work with her son, she wrote this up and presented it to the Hungarian Psychoanalytical Society, as a prelude to joining it. From then on, her work was focused on the private treatment of children in her own consulting room.

Anna Freud's first observations of children had been professional and slightly more distanced. Klein's personal involvement in the first observations of children led to a closer and most detailed look at their inner lives. Her observations were domestic, intimate, and close to the source. In the privacy of her own consulting room, she was able to respond naturally and intuitively to the children she saw, and so develop the crucially important psychoanalytic play technique. Yet while Anna Freud continued to underscore the importance of work with children who are a concern of the State and a responsibility for society as a whole, it was paradoxically the work of Melanie Klein that put on the agenda for the first time the right of the child to a separate analytic consideration.

Unlike Anna Freud, Klein felt free to challenge accepted psychoanalytic views. Unencumbered by dogmas, she boldly asserted a much earlier onset of human relations that had hitherto been imagined. Her observations of infants convinced her that they were capable of a rudimentary recognition of their mothers from the very beginning of life. In her view, this ability to relate to separate others developed rapidly, with the result that even within the first year of life, the infant could come to a fuller recognition of the mother and other significant adults. This in turn implied that even the young child patient was able to relate to the analyst as a separate adult who was understood to be outside the family circle. Therefore, like the adult patient, such a child could form a transference towards its analyst, transferring its typical patterns of relating to the arena of the analytic session.

Anna Freud objected to this notion. While agreeing that "The child indeed enters into the liveliest relations with the analyst", she still concluded that it did not form a transference neurosis. In her view, "The child is not, like the adult, ready to produce a new edition of its love-relationships, because, as one might say, the old edition is not yet exhausted". This, she reflected, is due to the fact that:

> "(The child's) original objects, the parents, are still real and present love-objects, not only
> in phantasy as with the adult neurotic; between them and the child exist all the relations of
> everyday life, and all its gratifications and disappointments still in reality depend on them.
> The analyst enters this situation as a new person… but there is no necessity for the child to
> exchange the parents for him, since compared with them he has not the advantages which
> the adult finds when he can exchange his phantasy-objects for a real person" (from *The Psycho-
> Analytical Treatment of Children*, 1946).

As far as Melanie Klein was concerned, an 'old edition' of love-relationships already existed for the child, and this was the archaic, rudimentary one of earliest infancy. This version had already been internalised and integrated into the child's view of reality, colouring its relationships with all the adults in its life, including the parents. The child's perception of ordinary parental behaviour was therefore tinged with primitive elements that exaggerated its different facets. Thus, parental affection seemed more ideal to the young child than it was in reality and by the same token, parental disapproval could be heard by the child as more persecutory and threatening than it actually was.

Klein held that the young infant gradually creates primitive mental representations of both the good and bad aspects of its first relationship with the mother. These representations — or internal objects — were already integrated into the ego of the young child. They were revived in the analytic relationship, endowing the child analyst with either malevolent or ideal qualities.

However, Klein also had another reason for believing that the child could form a transference to its analyst. Her observations convinced her that the infant's circle of significant adults expands in the first place through transference-like processes. Even from the time of weaning, when the infant realises the limitations of its first relationship with the mother, it begins to explore other possibilities by reaching towards the father and later, other family members. Yet each new relationship also symbolises the first one in life, since the infant brings to it expectations arising from its previous experiences.

These beliefs were more than just a question of theoretical outlook. Her views also fitted into something broader — her ambition to establish a complete equality between child and adult analysis. Through developing later than adult analysis, child analysis was in danger of seeming like a derivative of a more pure discipline, and hence as of a lesser scientific and clinical value. By underscoring that the child was able to form a transference that was no different from an adult's, Klein took the first step towards asserting an equal clinical status for this work with children.

Not only was a transference relationship possible, she suggested, but the obstacles traditionally imagined to be inherent in child analysis were surmountable. The child analyst need no longer worry that the child was unable to offer free associations in its sessions. Play provided the solution, for it was the equivalent of adult free association, making the child's deep unconscious available to the analyst. The phantasy elements revealed through play came from the same primitive source as adult dream material, and so they also comprised a "royal road to the unconscious", as Sigmund Freud had described dreams.

Anna Freud was uneasy about this. The adult, she argued, engaged with free associations voluntarily, while stopping other activities and lying down on the analytic couch. The child, however, could not easily separate meaningful play from its general activities in the consulting room. How was one to ascertain which of its activities was a symbolic expression? Furthermore, in the child's play, a

> "car collision may be reproducing some happening in the street; and the child who runs towards a lady visitor and opens her handbag is not necessarily, as Mrs Klein maintains, thereby symbolically expressing its curiosity as to whether its mother's womb conceals another little brother or sister, but may be connecting some experience of the previous day when someone brought it a little present in a similar receptacle".

Anna Freud thus underscored the child's continuous engagement with its changing external environment, and not only with its unconscious life. Unlike dreaming, play can express not only symbolic unconscious material, but also the impact of real events. So she could accept that often, young children do not narrate external events coherently. Indeed, they may prefer to express the impact of these through play, by repeating elements of what they had actually observed, rather than by symbolising them.

Logical though this thinking was, it failed to impress Melanie Klein. One reason for this may well have stemmed from the broader problems that were emerging about the status of child analysis. Klein seems to have intuitively grasped the antipathy that was in store from the international psychoanalytic establishment for child analysis. To forestall this, she opposed potential objections from a theoretical, rather than from a professional standpoint, arguing that play had the fully revealing status of free association. Since she objected to the child–analytic session being used for any purpose other than pure analysis, educative measures, for instance, had no room in her technique. As with the adult, the child–analytic session was set aside entirely for the exploration and interpretation of the child's unconscious life.

Klein's claim of equality for child analysis on these theoretical grounds perhaps showed a pragmatic approach to psychoanalytical politics. When, years later, Anna Freud fought the same battle, she was to discover that her decision to do so on purely professional grounds was to end in failure. During the 1960s and 1970s, she had a demoralising struggle to win a full professional standing for the child analysts trained under her. She felt, quite reasonably, that since psychoanalysis was so concerned with childhood experiences, direct work with and observation of children would be of crucial scientific value to it. Yet in spite of her efforts, the status of child analysts was left just as it had always been, and the situation has remained unchanged since then. Nowadays, a training in child psychotherapy does not lead to any form of affiliation with the British Psycho-Analytical Society. In the UK, however, child psychotherapists, unlike psychoanalysts, are recognised as specialists by the Department of Health.

Ironically, through her initial reluctance to grant full theoretical status to the child's transference, Anna Freud might have inadvertently reinforced the prejudice of the psychoanalytical establishment against child analysis. For her part, Melanie Klein lost international support because of her refusal to express her findings in a way that took into account more than the influence of primitive reality on the individual child.

Perhaps in this respect the failure of the two women to collaborate represents a loss that was both scientific and professional. Melanie Klein felt unable to emphasise areas of the child–patient's experience that were other than the internal, free association material that formed the core of adult psychoanalysis. Her technique ultimately suffered from a lack of emphasis on external factors that are normally of far greater significance in children's lives. As Anna Freud had logically pointed out, children continue to depend on their environment, and this has to be taken into account when trying to ascertain their analytic needs. For her part, Anna Freud did not find a way of dealing with the very early onset of object relations and their most archaic expression in the child's later mental life.

While Anna Freud would merely regard the child from an adult stance, and hence describe it as, for example, undergoing a particular 'phase' of development, it was Melanie Klein who first offered insights into what the child's subjective world view might be like. She underscored how the beliefs of the older child are not the products of rationality alone, but derive their essence from the operation of malign or nurturing internal objects, now integrated into the child's world view. These determine whether the older child has an internal unconscious scenario which predisposes it to feel disliked and persecuted, or one which predisposes it to approach others with confidence. Without awareness that subjective phantasy patterns operate continually in the child, and that internal objects, now parts of the child's own psyche, continue to 'treat' it in characteristic depriving or nurturing ways, progress in the psychotherapeutic treatment of children is limited.

None the less, the heritage left by both women is substantial, and further research saw succeeding generations of Kleinians and Freudians move into less extreme positions. Child analysts have been able not only to apply the findings of both pioneers, but also, on the basis of these findings, to extend the scope of child analytic work. It now covers the full spectrum of psychological difficulties encountered in contemporary society. It is used for conditions as varied as autism, developmental failure, sexual or physical abuse, trauma, bereavement, serious physical illness, delinquency, and eating disorders. Through the efforts of both Anna Freud and Melanie Klein, it is now possible to have a psychoanalytic mental health service for children that addresses their needs at different levels, whether for intensive individual therapy or for a more facilitating environment. Intensive therapy is obviously a scarce resource, especially in public health services. However, its timely use needs to be weighed up against the cost of later mental illness, youth offending, teenage pregnancy, drug abuse, and other such much more costly outcomes. As well as this, the principles of psychoanalytic work with children are now regularly used to inform a range of interventions of different kinds, such as brief parent–infant psychotherapy, and adolescent and student counselling.

Acknowledgements

This contribution has been modified from Likierman M. The debate between Anna Freud and Melanie Klein: a historical survey. *Journal of Child Psychotherapy. 1995;* **21***:313–325.*

FURTHER READING

Focal infection

Andrews J, Briggs A, Porter R, Tucker P, Waddington K. *The History of Bethlem*. London: Routledge; 1997: 682–683.

Billings F. *Focal Infection*. New York: Appleton: 1916.

Bruce L. *Studies in Clinical Psychiatry*. London: Macmillan; 1906: 5, 6, 8–10, 37–38, 227.

Bynum WF. *Science and the Practice of Medicine in the Nineteenth Century*. Cambridge: Cambridge University Press; 1994.

Cotton HA. The relation of oral infection to mental disease. *Journal of Mental Research*. 1919; **1**:273.

Cotton HA. The relation of chronic sepsis to the so-called functional psychoses. *Journal of Mental Science*. 1923; **69**:434–465.

Cotton HA. The relationship of chronic sepsis to the so-called functional mental disorders. *Journal of Mental Science*. 1923; **69**:433–445.

Graves TC, Turner, DE. A method of continuous colonic irrigation. *Journal of Mental Science*. 1930; **76**:306–317.

Grob G. *The Inner World of American Psychiatry 1890–1940: Selected Correspondence*. New Brunswick, NJ: Rutgers University Press; 1985: 108–123.

Hobbs AT. A survey of American and Canadian psychiatric opinion as to focal infections (or chronic sepsis) as a cause of mental disorder. *Journal of Mental Science*. 1924; **70**:542–553.

Hobbs AT. Diphasic vascular variation in the treatment of mental inefficiency arising from a common somatic cause. *Journal of Mental Science*. 1940; **86**:751–766.

Hobbs AT. Symposium on ear, nose, and throat disease in mental disorder. *Journal of Mental Science*. 1941; **87**:477–528.

Howell J. *Technology in the Hospital: Transforming Patient Care in the Early Twentieth Century*. Baltimore: Johns Hopkins University Press; 1995.

Hunter W. Oral sepsis as a cause of disease. *British Medical Journal*. 1990; ii:215–216. (See also idem, Chronic sepsis as a cause of mental disorder. *Journal of Mental Science*. 1927; **73**:549–563; and The relation of focal infection to mental diseases. *Journal of Mental Science*. 1929; **75**:464–466.)

Keen WW, White JW. *Standard American Textbook*. Philadelphia, PA: Saunders; 1892.

Kopeloff N. Is the stomach a focus of infection. *American Journal of the Medical Sciences* (2nd series). 1923; **165**:120–129.

Kopeloff N, Cheyney CO. Studies in focal infection: its presence and elimination in the functional psychoses. *American Journal of Psychiatry*. 1922; **2**:139–156.

Lane WA. *The Operative Treatment of Chronic Constipation*. London: Nisbet; 1904.

Maudsley H. The physiology and pathology of mind quoted in TC Graves, 'The relation of chronic sepsis to so-called functional mental disorder'. *Journal of Mental Science*. 1923; **59**:465.

Noguchi H, Moore JW. A demonstration of treponema pallidum in the brain in cases of general paralysis. *Journal of Experimental Medicine*. 1913; **17**:232–238.

Scull A. Focal sepsis and psychosis. In: Freeman H, Berrios GE, eds. *150 Years of British Psychiatry*, Vol. 2. London: Athlone; 1996: 529.

Shaw A. Physical treatment for mental disorders: a summary of expert commentary upon Dr Cotton's work at Trenton. *Review of Reviews*. 1922; **66**:625–636.

Upson HS. Nervous disorders due to the teeth. *Cleveland Medical Journal*. 1907; **6**:458–459. (Idem, Dementia praecox caused by dental infection. *Monthly Cyclopedia and Medical Bulletin*. 1909: 648–651; and Serious mental disturbances caused by painless dental lesions. *American Quarterly of Roentgenology*, 1910; **11**:223–243.)

Environmental influences on child psychiatry

Bowlby J. *Forty-Four Juvenile Thieves: Their Characters and Home Life*. London: Ballière, Tindall and Cox; 1946.

Bowlby J. *Attachment and Loss* (3 vols). London: Hogarth Press; 1969–1977.

Cunningham H. Histories of childhood. *American Historical Review*; 1998.

Gesell A, Thompson H. *The Psychology of Early Growth*. New York: Macmillan; 1938.

Goldhagen DJ. *Hitler's Willing Executioners. Ordinary Germans and the Holocaust*. New York: Alfred A Knopf, Inc; 1996.

Grosskuth P. *Melanie Klein: Her World and Her Work*. New York: Alfred A Knopf, Inc; 1986.

Kanner L. *Child Psychiatry*. Spring, IL: Charles C Thomas; 1935.

Klein M. The early development of conscience in the child. In: *Psychoanalysis-Analysis Today*. New York; 1933.

Klein M. The *Psycho-Analysis of Children* (1932). London: Hogarth Press; 1960.

Klemperer V. *I Will Bear Witness: A Diary of the Nazi Years, 1933–1941* (trans. by M Chambers). New York: Random House; 1998.

Lewis M, Vitulano L. A historical perspective on views of childhood psychopathology. In: Last C G, Hersen M, eds. *Handbook of Child Psychiatric Diagnosis*. New York: Wiley; 1989: 3–11.

Lifton RJ. *The Nazi Doctors*. New York: Basic Books; 1986.

Parry-Jones WL. History of child and adolescent psychiatry. In: Rutter M, Taylor E, Hersov L, eds. *Child and Adolescent Psychiatry*, 3rd edn. London: Blackwell; 1994.

Piaget J. *The Language and Thought of the Child*. London: Routledge and Kegan Paul; 1926.

Rydelius P-A. History of Swedish child and adolescent psychiatry. *Acta Paediatrica*. 1995; **84**:703–704.

Viner R. Melanie Klein and Anna Freud: the discourse of the early dispute. *Journal of the History of Behavioural Sciences*. 1996; **32**:4–15.

White House Conference on Child Health and Protection. Psychology and Psychiatry in Pediatrics: The Problem. Report on the Sub-Committee on Psychology and Psychiatry. New York: Century; 1932.

Winnicott D. *A Note on Normality and Anxiety in Clinical Disorders of Childhood*. London: Heinemann; 1931.

Winnicott D. *The Maturational Processes and the Facilitating Environment*. London: The Hogarth Press; 1965.

German psychiatry

Jaspers K. The phenomenological approach in psychiatry. *British Journal of Psychiatry*. 1968; 114:1313–1323.

Kalinowsky LB. In: Ponztatz LJ, ed. *Psychiatrie in Selbstdarstellungen*. Bern: Hans Huber; 1979.

Peters UH. Die Heidelberger phönomenologishe Schule und die psychiatrische emigration. In: Bühler KE, Weiß H, eds. *Kommunikation und Perspektivität*. Wurzburg: Koningshausen & Neumann; 1985.

Mental health nursing

Arton M. The development of psychiatric nurse education in England and Wales. *Nursing Times*. 1981; **3**:124–127.

Beers CW. *A Mind that Found Itself*. New York: Doubleday, Doran and Company, Inc; 1937.

Berrios GE. *The History of Mental Symptoms*. Cambridge: Cambridge University Press; 1996.

Digby A. *Madness, Morality and Medicine – A Study of the York Retreat*. Cambridge: Cambridge University Press; 1985.

Freeman H, Berrios GE, eds. *150 Years of British Psychiatry*, Vol. 2: *The Aftermath*. London: Athlone; 1996.

Gordon C. Psychiatry as a problem for democracy. In: Miller P, Rose N, eds. *The Power of Psychiatry*. London: Polity Press; 1986.

Hunter R. The rise and fall of mental nursing. *Lancet*. 1956; **1**:98–99.

Kneisl CR, Wilson HS. Historical perspective. In: Wilson HS, Kneisl CR, eds. *Psychiatric Nursing*, 3rd edn. California: Addison-Wesley Publishing Company, Health Science Division; 1988.

Leech J. *The Lunatic Years – Growing up in the Wilts County Mental Hospital*. Trowbridge: Shires Press; 1992.

Nolan P. *A History of Mental Health Nursing*. London: Chapman Hall; 1993.

Scott DH, Masterton JF, Hainsworth M, Mayne WS. *Modern Mental Nursing*. London: The Caxton Publishing Company Ltd; 1936.

Origins of convulsive therapy

Fink M. *Convulsive Therapy: Theory and Practice*. New York: Raven Press; 1979: 303.

Fink M. Meduna and the origins of convulsive therapy. *American Journal of Psychiatry*. 1984; **141**:1034–1041.

Marti-Ibanez F, Sackler AM, Sackler MD, Sackler RR. *The Great Physiodynamic Therapies in Psychiatry: An Historical Reappraisal*. New York: Hoeber-Harper; 1956.

Meduna L. Versuche über die biologische Beeinflussung des Ablaufes der Schizophrenie: Camphor und Cardiozolkrampfe. *Zeitdchrift für die Gesamte Neurologie und Psychiatrie*. 1935; **152**:235–262.

Meduna L. *Die Konvulsionstherapie der Schizophrenie*. Halle: Karl Marhold; 1937.

Meduna L. Autobiography. *Convulsive Therapy*. 1985; **1**:43–57; 121–138.

Pierre Janet

Brown P. Pierre Janet: alienist reintegrated. *Current Opinion in Psychiatry*. 1991; **4**:389–395.

Brown P. Janet and Freud: Revealing the roots of dynamic psychiatry. *Australian and New Zealand Journal of Psychiatry*. 1996; **30**:480–491.

Brown P, Van der Hart O. Memories of Sexual Abuse: Janet's Critique of Freud, a balanced approach. *Psychological Reports*. 1998; **82**:1027–1043.

Ellenberger HF. Pierre Janet. In: *The Discovery of the Unconscious: The History and Evolution of Dynamic Psychiatry*. New York: Basic Books; 1970.

Janet P. *The Mental State of Hystericals*. New York: Putmans; 1901. (Reprint: Janet P. *The Major Symptoms of Hysteria* (1907), 2nd edn. New York: Macmillan; 1929 and New York: Hafner; 1965.)

Janet P. *Psychological Healing*. New York: Macmillan; 1925. (Reprint: New York: Arno; 1976.)

Pitman R. Pierre Janet on obsessive compulsive disorder (1903): review and commentary. *Archives of General Psychiatry*. 1987; **44**:226–232.

Van der Hart O, Friedman B. A Readers Guide to Pierre Janet on dissociation: a neglected intellectual heritage. *Dissociation*. 1989; **2**:3–16.

Van der Kolk BA, Van der Hart O. Pierre Janet and the breakdown of adaptation in psychological trauma. *American Journal of Psychiatry*. 1989; **146**:1530–1540.

Adolf Meyer

Betz BJ. Adolf Meyer: youth and young manhood 1866–1896: part II. *American Journal of Social Psychiatry*. 1981*a*; **1**:34–40.

Betz BJ. Adolf Meyer: youth and young manhood 1866–1896: part III. *American Journal of Social Psychiatry*. 1981*b*; **1**:32–40.

Frank JD. *Adolf Meyer in Retrospect*. Unpublished manuscript; 1980.

Gelder MG. Adolf Meyer. In: Berrios GE, Freeman H, eds. *150 Years of British Psychiatry*, Vol. 1. London: Gaskell; 1991.

Grob GN. Adolf Meyer on American psychiatry in 1895. *American Journal of Psychiatry*. 1963; **119**:1135–1142.

Henderson DK. Adolf Meyer: a tribute from abroad. *American Journal of Psychiatry*. 1966; **123**:322–324.

Henderson DK, Gillespie RD. *Textbook of Psychiatry*, 1st edn. London: Oxford University Press; 1927.

Lewis AJ. The study of defect (the Adolf Meyer Lecture). *American Journal of Psychiatry*. 1960; **117**:289–304.

Lidz T. Adolf Meyer and the development of American psychiatry. *American Journal of Psychiatry*. 1966; **123**:320–332.

Meyer A. *Report to the Governor of Illinois 1895*. (Reprinted: Lief A. In: *The Commonsense Psychiatry of Dr Adolf Meyer*. New York: McGraw-Hill; 1948: 53–60.)

Anna Freud & Melanie Klein

Ellenberger H. *The Discovery of the Unconscious* (1970). London: Fontana; 1994.

Freud A. *The Psycho-Analytical Treatment of Children*. London: Inigo; 1946.

Freud A. *Infants Without Families (1939–1945)*. London: Hogarth Press; 1974.

Gay P. *Freud: A Life for Our Time*. London: Dent; 1988.

Grosskurth P. *Melanie Klein*. London: Hodder and Stoughton; 1986.

King P, Steiner R, eds. *The Freud–Klein Controversies 1941–1945*. London: Tavistock Routledge; 1991.

Klein M. Eine Kinderentwicklung. *Imago*; 1921.

Klein M. The psychogenesis of manic–depressive states. In: *Love, Guilt and Reparation* (1935). London: Hogarth Press; 1975.

Roazen P. *Freud and his Followers*. New York: Knopf; 1975.

Shepherd N. *A Price Below Rubies: Jewish Women as Rebels and Radicals*. London: Weidenfeld and Nicolson; 1993.

Young-Bruehl E. *Anna Freud*. London: Macmillan; 1988.

1941–1950

Chapter 5
The Impact of World Events

1941–1950 CHAPTER 5

Major world events
1944 Avery, McCarty and McLeod in the USA identified the role of DNA
1945 Birth of the United Nations Organization
1947 Indian Independence
1948 State of Israel established
1950 First television programmes in colour in the USA

Major events in psychiatry
1942 Walter Freeman and James Watts published *Psychosurgery*
1944 Publication of *An Introduction to Physical Methods of Treatment in Psychiatry*, by Eliot Slater and William Sargant
1946 Walter Freeman introduced transorbital leucotomy, using an ice pick, inserted from below
1946 Aubrey Lewis appointed Professor of Psychiatry in the University of London, and united the old Bethlem Royal Hospital with the newer Maudsley, creating the Institute of Psychiatry
1946 The National Mental Health Act passed by Congress in America
1947 Pierre Janet died
1947 Maxwell Jones opened the Henderson Hospital, London
1948 Foulkes' *Introduction to Group Analytic Psychotherapy* published in London
1948 The *International Classification of Diseases* (ICD) first published by WHO
1948 Publication of the fourth edition of *General Psychopathology* by Karl Jaspers in Germany
1948 Jacobsen and Hald in Denmark discovered the value of disulphiram ('Antabuse')
1948 Inauguration of the National Health Service in Great Britain
1949 *The Biology of Mental Defect* by Lionel Penrose published in London
1950 First World Congress of Psychiatry held in Paris
1950 A Mental Hygiene Act passed in Japan

1941–1950

by John Crammer

Medicine has been defined by an English philosopher as no more than "the name of a somewhat arbitrary consortium of more or less loosely connected inquiries and techniques". This is certainly true of the medical specialty which since about 1920 has been called 'Psychiatry' in English. Psychiatry has no grand common theories, or even an internationally agreed practice. It is a mixture of knowledge from several distinct sources about: (a) people with abnormal behaviour and feelings who are socially disabled or anti-social and may need to be restrained (e.g. psychotics, often confined in asylums since about 1800); (b) people suffering from unpleasant feelings, often with bodily symptoms like those of known physical illness ('neurotics'), frequently treated by general physicians since the seventeenth century or later by neurologists; (c) ideas and practices derived from both experimental and dynamic psychology since about 1870; (d) relevant discoveries in biological sciences and physical instrumentation (brain anatomy and physiology, virology, biochemistry; radiology) which were increasingly applied through the twentieth century, particularly after 1950.

What distinguishes psychiatric illness from the rest of medicine is that its diagnosis and treatment always involve special forms of interview and conversation with the patient, that the symptoms are often long-lasting, or if acute, liable to return at intervals through life, and that it impairs the social being of the sufferer. That being involves the ability to form harmonious relationships with other human beings, in the family, in sexual and social life, and at work. The term 'mental illness' tends to be applied to psychosis; 'psychiatric' (or psychological) illness is generally a much wider term, implying the existence of psychological symptoms (anxiety, depression, etc.), without assuming anything about their origin in either a mental or somatic disturbance. The ultimate causes of such illness may not be known, but the brain's functioning is always involved in some way.

Cultural differences in psychiatry

However the content of psychiatry may vary, from time to time and place to place, it always remains a part of European–North American or 'Western' medicine. But alongside it there may be other organised ways of coping with mental disturbance (Chapter 10, p. 338). In Brazil, for instance, there are many more religious centres (Umbanda, or Kardecismo) than there are psychiatric out-patient departments. Chinese medicine as late as 1940 made no division between mental and somatic illness, ascribing disease to imbalance of non-material entities such as 'wind', 'air', or 'heat'; care was a family matter, except for a tiny provision of asylums, mostly by Christian missionaries. But after the communist triumph and unification in 1949, Western medicine was rapidly introduced, albeit in an organisation peculiar to itself because of the vast size of the country with 80% of the population scattered in far rural communities and in great poverty. This was a discipline shaped by communist ideology, by people's continued reliance on belief in the somatic basis of all illness, and by the coherence of the family, with Chinese traditional medicine continuing alongside it.

Although Japan began to adopt German medicine after 1869, mental illness was regarded as incurable, impossible to understand, dangerous, and shameful to families. Sufferers were secluded at home or in distant private institutions, and had no legal rights. A Mental Hygiene Act (1950) marked the beginning of only a very slow change towards more modern care of the mentally ill.

The need to restrain the antisocial person and to control the cost to the community of psychiatric illness leads governments to intervene both administratively and legally with these disorders, and usually to provide institutions and personnel for that purpose. The patient may have a personal explanation of his/her experienced disability, while the community may take a different view (fear, repugnance, condemnation, amusement). This can be a spiritual, moral, magical, or medical explanation of the changed behaviour, which may or may not be shared by society. The doctor has to use medical knowledge and understanding to satisfy these legal and community expectations, as well as helping the patient. Thus, the practice of psychiatry is at the mercy of public passions and political directives, as well as being modified in each country by the national culture and history.

When the war came in 1939, different countries suffered in different ways. In some there was extensive destruction of homes and hospitals, or diversion of medical services away from civilian care. Large numbers of particular populations (in German concentration camps, Japanese prisoner of war camps, but also in mental hospitals and similar institutions) suffered from extreme malnutrition or starvation. This resulted in many deaths, as well as a degree of organic dementia amongst survivors later. Even in England, there had been numerous deaths amongst mental hospital patients during the First World War, though not in 1939–45.

One remarkable piece of scientific research was carried out in the appalling conditions of Japanese prison camps. De Wardener and Lennox recorded 52 typical cases of Wernicke's encephalopathy in prisoners at Changi, Singapore, most of whom also showed typical neurotic, cardiac, or oedematous signs of beri-beri. It was thus confirmed that thiamine deficiency was alone responsible for the encephalopathy, and the link was forged between the cerebral and systemic manifestations of that nutritional depletion. In almost all these cases, the encephalopathy appeared when some other factor, such as epidemic dysentery, had intensified the vitamin deficiency. These records had to be made in secret and were buried just before the end of the war, but retrieved while they were still legible.

After 1945, with the British empire in decline and the victorious USA's cultural influence spreading globally — aided by Hollywood films, and fast air travel — medicine (including psychiatry) became internationally more uniform. The World Health Organization (1946) and its mental health branch sponsored the accurate translation of technical terms into many languages, using them to describe syndromes which psychiatrists from different cultures could agree on and use in diagnosis. The major pharmaceutical companies promoted international use of their products, and a plethora of congresses began, starting with the first World Congress of Psychiatry (Paris, 1950). This was mainly concerned with the researches of the wartime decade, particularly in Scandinavia, Switzerland, France, Britain, and the USA.

In its first third, the twentieth century showed rather slow and patchy evolution in psychiatry. But the Second World War speeded up some of the social changes and technological developments that had begun earlier. In many countries, war caused a forced reorganisation of daily life, an urgency to counter the psychological stresses of new and abnormal experiences, and an opportunity in the ensuing peace to rebuild from the ruined landscape in a new way.

After 1945, Eastern European countries became communist, under Soviet influence in psychiatric services as in other matters, while Japan was occupied by the USA. Before this, Germany had had two important influences on the development of psychiatry. From 1933, the Nazi Government had pursued a policy of sterilising the mentally handicapped and chronically ill, which was later converted into systematic killing of these groups. There was also a policy to exterminate the Jews, but a proportion of them, including some psychiatrists and psychoanalysts, were able to escape, mainly to Britain and the USA, where they were to exert a great influence (Chapter 4, p. 86).

The spread of academic psychiatry

For at least three-quarters of a century before 1933, Germany had been a world leader in science. Since Griesinger in 1865 became the world's first professor of psychiatry (at Berlin), there had been teaching departments at German university medical schools, with special hospital and clinic facilities, while medical students were obliged to study the subject and pass an examination in it. There were public asylums, private psychiatric institutions, research laboratories (some concentrating on brain anatomy), and special institutes, notably at Munich, where study of the inheritance of mental illnesses became internationally known. In contrast, Britain had no university teaching departments for the subject, except at Edinburgh, and from 1923 at the new Maudsley Hospital (London). Mental illness was a postgraduate study — with optional self-teaching and an optional diploma examination — and standards of learning and practice were generally low. Drs Mott and Maudsley had worked for many years to persuade London University to establish with the London County Council a research and teaching hospital like the one at Munich. The Maudsley Hospital was the eventual result — with 250 beds and some laboratories. In the USA, academic psychiatry had begun to develop in the earlier years of the century, and psychiatric units were established in a number of general teaching hospitals by the 1930s. Paris and Vienna were also centres of psychiatric teaching, but few other European cities had anything comparable.

The eugenics movement

The eugenics movement was active in Britain, the USA, and some European countries in the first half of the twentieth century, with the idea that people with inheritable diseases should be discouraged from mating, or should even undergo sterilisation. With a disease like

Huntington's chorea, rare but clearly due to a dominant gene, it seemed possible to eliminate it altogether in this way. But little was known about the inheritance of mental retardation (now called 'severe learning difficulty'), and even less about that of schizophrenia, so it was not possible to identify who should theoretically be persuaded to refrain from reproduction. In Germany, however, there had been great concern that inheritable defects were on the increase, and that the future health of the German nation was being challenged (Chapter 4, p. 86). Discussions from at least 1920 amongst some geneticists, psychiatrists, and lawyers were based on 'Social Darwinism' (the survival of the fittest, or elimination of the unfit) and on the idea of "permission for the extinction of worthless life". In that view, people with mental retardation or incurable chronic psychosis were deemed 'mentally dead', and should therefore have their lives terminated by 'euthanasia'.

Sterilisation and starvation

When the Nazis came to power in 1933, they legalised a campaign of compulsory sterilisation, initially of children of severe alcoholic or mixed black and German parentage, and those with congenital mental retardation, epilepsy, etc. (Chapter 4, p. 86). Up to 1939, about 350,000 individuals are thought to have been sterilised. At first, state hospitals had to send a report on each case for decision to act taken by an 'expert' panel of four; the police had reported to the panels about 10% of the cases. However, some institutions ended children's lives by starvation plus barbiturates, their relatives simply being told they had died. About 5000 (up to age 17) were finished off in this way. Once the war started, instruction was given secretly (without any law or ministerial decree) to start killing supposedly incurable patients, sexual deviants, psychopaths, gypsies who were asocial and "good for nothing", severe epileptics, and alcoholics. Belief in the inheritable nature of all these conditions far outran the slender genetic information that was available, but there was felt to be a need to preserve the (mythical) racial purity of the Germans, so as to keep the nation from evil. The Jews, of course, were believed to have a malign anti-German influence too, and for most of them the Holocaust was to be the answer (Chapter 4, p. 86).

Trials of carbon monoxide poisoning were started in Brandenburg Hospital (near Berlin), and extended to other sites. By September 1941, over 70,000 mental patients in Germany had been killed. Meanwhile, in the wake of the invasion of Poland, 4400 'incurables' in institutions there were simply shot by a special army unit. Starvation was deliberately practised at a number of Bavarian institutions.

The killing policy provoked some protest by clergy, as well as unease amongst relatives of the dead and those civilians who knew something of the scale of what was going on. As a result, the official policy was stopped after 1941. 'Wild' killing still continued, however: by 1945, it was estimated only 15% of the German mental hospital population still survived. In occupied France, the mental in-patient population of about 115,000 was halved. However, at St Alban, near Vichy, the asylum doctors, seeing how food supplies were being denied their patients, discharged numbers of them into the care of neighbouring villages, where they were able to survive with the help of the Resistance. In Japan, 30,000 mental hospital patients are believed to have died from starvation, but to what extent this was the result of a deliberate policy remains uncertain.

The German concentration camps

German concentration camps were notably stressful environments, both physically and mentally. They contained an immense number of prisoners of all ages, from young children to the old, crammed together in a small space without privacy, quiet, warmth, food, toilet provision, or any activity except work, and a liability to constant physical assault. They were

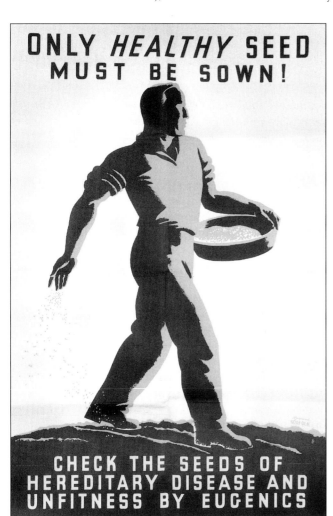

Poster: "Only healthy seeds must be sown!" by Haywood, Norfolk, n.d. (c. 1935?). Reproduced with permission from the Galton Institute. Photo courtesy of the Wellcome Institute Library, London.

separated from friends and relations in a constantly changing mass, as groups of those who were sick, or could not work, or broke any rules were moved away to their deaths, and their places taken by newcomers. Chronic humiliation, destruction of self-identity, impossibility of any relief or release except illness and death (or execution), with continual uncertainty from day to day, were all part of the trap in which the individual was held. Kral (1951) gives some details about Theresienstadt in northern Bohemia. It held at least 30,000 people at any one time, and from November 1941 to 1945, almost 140,000 passed through it: 33,500 died there, over 86,500 were sent east for killing, and only 19,300 survived. The young did best, while the elderly became apathetic and liable to collapse. Yet apart from the psychoses of malnutrition (Korsakov, pellagra), there was no evidence of an increase in schizophrenic breakdown or severe depressive illness as a result of camp conditions, and pre-existing neurotic states appeared to clear up. Being a prisoner was a horrible experience, and produced some personality change, but did not appear to be a cause of recognised psychotic or neurotic breakdown. Nor did survivors after release develop such illness (unless they had been liable to it already in pre-camp life), though they showed depressive reactions and a degree of social withdrawal in some cases. Of course, the difficulties of studying such a diverse and selected population, albeit large in number, make firm conclusions impossible. Nevertheless, the evidence is suggestive that this kind of general stress is not significant in precipitating psychiatric breakdown — at least in the short term.

During the war, some German psychiatrists were uneasy and tried to avoid knowing about the Camps, others were willing practitioners, and some attempted to carry out research, e.g. preparing 500 brains of mentally retarded and epileptic patients for detailed study, after the patients had been examined physiologically and psychologically before death. Concentration camp inmates also served as 'experimental animals'. Killing in places like Auschwitz became highly organised by 1943, with special gas chambers using cyanide, and crematoria which could dispose of 4756 bodies per day. Xenophobia, anti-Semitism, disgust at human deformity, and the fear of possible consequences of appearing disloyal to official policy, combined with a belief in the German 'mission', allowed doctors to take part in this irrational eugenic programme. However, the research was abortive, there was no evidence that the incidence of most diseases was altered, and some Jews survived, including a number of eminent scientists who helped the Allied war effort. Eugenics obtained a very bad name from then on.

Emigration of leading psychoanalysts

The official anti-Semitism had allowed about 600 Jews out of a total of 3000 German psychiatrists to emigrate before 1939. Some of these were leading psychoanalysts: many went to the United States, and much fewer to Britain, where the Rockefeller Foundation helped several to join the Maudsley Hospital. Those in Britain included, Mayer-Gross from Heidelberg, Alfred Meyer (neuropathologist) from Bonn, Guttmann, Hoffer, Last, Stengel, and Bierer from Vienna, Freudenberg (who had been Sakel's assistant) and Glatt from Berlin, and Foulkes (Fuchs) from Frankfurt. This gave a great boost to the teaching of psychiatry, which had been so backward in Britain. Stengel became a notable professor at Sheffield, Bierer started the day hospital and social clubs, Freudenberg brought the technique of insulin coma therapy, Kalinowsky brought ECT (though he went on to the USA), and Foulkes largely invented group therapy (this chapter, p. 141). The analysts who went to the USA — including Alexander, Fenichel, Fromm-Reichman, and Horney — were also influential, but in a much wider way. It was largely a case of "psychoanalysis in one country at this time", though small groups also became established in South America.

Psychoanalysis had been offered as: (a) a coherent practical method of psychological treatment, and (b) a theory of how the human mind worked — known as psychodynamics. These two contributions were largely distinct. The theory could be studied as a part of psychology, even if the treatment in the clinic did not work; and *per contra*, what the analyst did with a patient in an interview might be different or more complex than the theory supposed.

With his emphasis on repeated long interviews, on the patient's childhood history, on the importance of sexual drive and expression, on the revelation of hidden motives, and on awareness of patient–therapist emotional interactions, Freud made fundamental advances in the study and practice of psychotherapy. However, when he ran into some shocked opposition from the medical profession, he responded as if he were the leader of a religious faith by insisting that all his procedures and hypotheses were correct and must be followed exactly. Disciples were welcome, but if they began to disagree, they were regarded as heretics, to be condemned and expelled. Freud's ideas were often based on single cases, mostly arising in the cultural setting of nineteenth-century Vienna, and he

Psychoanalysts in various countries

	1931	1954
Austria	57	12*
Belgium	–	11
France	32	46
Germany	50	15*
Italy	–	22
Netherlands	21	60
Switzerland	28	44
Israel	–	22
Britain	54	147
USA	69+29+= 98	2754
Hungary	22	–
Argentina	–	49
Brazil	–	36
Spain	0	0
India	26	Not known

- **1931**: *International Journal of Psychoanalysis* 1931; **12**: 527–538. Number of analysts and associates registered with national societies in the International Psychoanalytical Association. (Not all in active practice; two societies listed in USA, but care taken to count an individual only once when the name appears twice.)
- **1954:** Nigel Walker. *A Short History of Psychotherapy in Theory and Practice*. London: Routledge and Kegan Paul; 1957; 152: note 19.

* Note decrease from 1931, at least partly due to emigration after 1933.
+ Twenty-nine in New York Society, additional to 69 names in American Society.
Nine out of 12 societies had less than 50 members in 1954.

did not support his generalisations by study of additional cases, e.g. from foreign cultures, or by enquiring what the effect of time on *untreated* neurosis might be. If a patient changed during analysis, this was assumed to be due to the treatment, and (it was claimed) thereby proved the correctness of the interpretations.

Freud's dominance of his group up to his death in 1939 fostered both the persistence of his doctrines and the slow spread internationally of Freudian psychoanalysis. At the same time, hypnotism and suggestion, and the ventilation of feelings by talking and abreaction, as well as interpretation of dreams had begun to be offered by Janet, Jung, Adler, and a few others. During the First World War, the experience of 'shell-shock' and its sometimes successful treatment by short-term psychotherapy (in which classical Freudian psychoanalysis had no part) encouraged the expansion of psychotherapy in Britain (Chapter 2, p. 33).

Psychoanalysis in America

In the USA in the 1920s and 1930s, training institutes for psychoanalysis were established in New York, Chicago, San Francisco, and elsewhere. The new schools of social work also taught psychodynamic theory. In the late 1930s, refugees from Europe, amongst a diversity of medical practitioners of all backgrounds, swelled the modest number of analysts in private practice. The American public was more welcoming of Germanic doctors than the British had been, and the Press enthused about the new psychology, which amongst other things, seemed to authorise greater sexual freedom. There were good opportunities in the larger cities for private practice, and the psychoanalytic societies fought to establish their right to control it and to claim it for those whom the institutes had chosen and trained. In this, there was frequent consultation with Freud and his daughter, Anna, in Vienna for approval. Up to 1938, some Americans went to Vienna every year for personal training analysis; when Nazi Germany took over in Austria, 12 out of the 23 candidates in training there were American citizens.

Yet at the time America went to war, in December 1941, analysts were still a small minority of the psychiatric profession; neurologists and mental hospital doctors still provided most psychiatric treatment. When the US army found itself unprepared to cope with psychiatric casualties, the few psychoanalysts enrolled in its medical branch seemed the only

vidual's capacity or avoids hostility. Or it may be possible to educate the family or co-workers to provide a different emotional environment.

Britain at war needed productive work from everyone, and a Medical Research Council (MRC) study of 3000 workers with sickness absence (10% of the workforce in 13 factories) revealed that more than a quarter of them were absent from work for neurotic symptoms, often aggravated by disturbed domestic relationships. Studies of Royal Air Force aircrew and of soldiers in units overseas showed similarly that breakdown occurred quite often in those already predisposed to neurosis in civilian life. Since very limited education and low IQ were also vulnerability factors, the US Army found it helpful to screen all new recruits with intelligence tests, and to reject those who scored low. At Mill Hill Emergency Hospital (London) under Sir Aubrey Lewis, soldiers with neurotic breakdowns were treated, but also given short courses in engineering or clerical work to improve their employment opportunities, as well as a personality assessment. As a considerable number of them returned to military duty, Lewis persuaded the War Office to take psychiatrists' and tutors' reports on each man into account in deciding his posting, with resultant better outcome.

Seemingly independently of Mill Hill and of the therapeutic community, at Northfield Military Hospital, Joshua Bierer, a refugee analyst from Vienna who was working at a mental hospital in Essex, began treating hospital patients along group lines. He set up social clubs, which they could then run themselves to provide support and encouragement, both in and out of hospital. Later, in London, he opened the first day hospital in Britain, which patients living at home could attend regularly; the name 'day hospital' had been originated by Ewen Cameron of Montreal, about the same time.

Post-war British social psychiatry led in many directions: the *International Journal of Social Psychiatry* (Bierer), the Institute for Group Analysis in London (Foulkes), and the Henderson Hospital (Maxwell Jones) with its influence in the USA, Sweden, and elsewhere. Also, the MRC Unit for Occupational Adaptation under Lewis examined the conditions under which people of very limited intelligence (IQ 20–50) or suffering from the impairments of chronic schizophrenia could undertake regular work. It found that many could be interested and motivated, provided the tempo of instruction was slow enough, and the work supervised in an encouraging way. This work was important in leading later to the establishment of industrial therapy units in mental hospitals, and the rehabilitation of long-stay in-patients and their discharge into the community, with the possibility there of employment in sheltered workshops. It was recognised that work could be therapeutic through contacts with fellow workers, the provision of a supportive routine, and the improvement of self-esteem by the development of a skill. Later, it emerged that schiz-

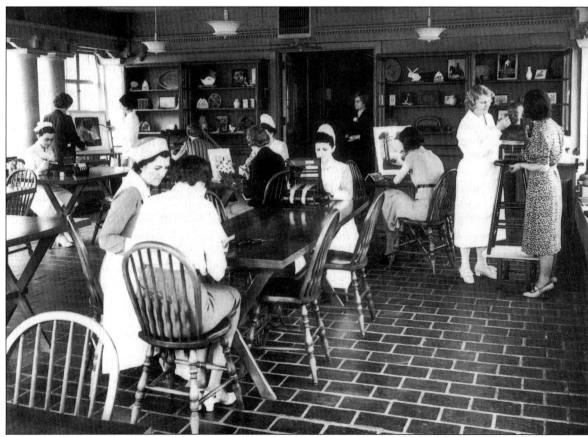

Occupational Therapy Department, Phipps Psychiatric Clinic (c. 1939). Reproduced with permission from the Chesney Medical Archives, Johns Hopkins Medical Institutions.

ophrenic patients discharged home after a prolonged hospital stay might do better living with strangers, or in a hostel, than with their relations, since family criticism and relationships proved disturbing. Further work showed that this 'expressed emotion' of family members might be therapeutically modified (Chapter 9, p. 311).

This British interest in social psychiatry reflected a general cultural–political belief that the community had a responsibility to its members: to provide free education and medical care, financial help for the unemployed and the disabled, decent housing, and pensions for the old — a Welfare State. For a long time, people had been meeting through organisations such as the Workers' Education Association, or to hear cultural or political ideas broadcast on BBC radio. With the war came the establishment of the Army Bureau of Current Affairs, which organised meetings in all units to debate war aims, the future of welfare, and other morale-boosting subjects. After peace and a general election which resulted in a Labour government, there was a widespread public faith that nationalisation of major industries on behalf of the nation would solve financial problems and benefit workers. The new National Health Service (1948) was another expression of the same group feeling, and it was in this setting that British social psychiatry developed. As a result, over the next 30 years or so, the focus of medical activity was to shift from the mental hospital to crisis intervention in the community, and then to community care for the mentally ill. The decade 1940–50 showed great changes in Britain in these aspects of psychiatric practice, leading to new specialisms, innovative services, research, and public education. Some of these developments had international influence.

Social psychiatry in other countries

The differences between countries have primarily been in: (a) the provision for compulsory hospital admission, and the laws and procedures for achieving this; (b) the extent to which people who do not need compulsion should be treated, in or out of hospital; (c) the focus of psychiatry — on neurotic, psychotic, or other types of disorders; and (d) payment of the doctor by salary or fee for service.

In other countries, similar examples of social psychiatry appeared as independent local initiatives. In the late 1930s, Professor A Querido had organised a successful service for the Amsterdam municipality, in which teams including social workers assessed the mentally ill at home or at an out-patient centre, to forestall admission to mental hospital and offer early treatment. This in turn had been based on an earlier private initiative in Frankfurt. In post-war Paris, there was another development — in the 13th arrondissement — to pro-

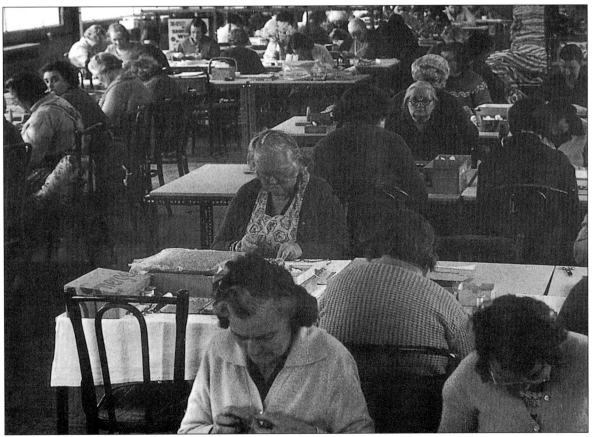

Patients busy at work making 'bows' for ladies underwear at Severall's Hospital near Colchester, UK (c. early 1960s). Reproduced with permission from the North East Essex Mental Health NHS Trust.

vide a range of community-based services (Chapter 7, p. 213). But neither in Germany nor France could the existing administration and finance of mental health services allow the widespread development of community-based services. In both countries, individual private practice and state mental hospital treatment remained quite separate. German practice was financed by a multitude of distinct insurance schemes, while hospital services were divided between university centres and State hospitals. From Paris, the central government controlled the mental hospitals and preferred its money to be spent in that way. From the late 1950s, the USA was to discharge very many chronic psychotic patients from immense state hospitals (559,000 in-patients shrank to 107,000 by 1988), but the community mental health centres set up at the same time preferred to treat the 'worried well' rather than care for the mentally disabled. Social psychiatry depends on modes of organisation, adequate funding, supervision, teamwork with non-medical professionals, public concern, and forensic facilities as well as physical and psychiatric care. What suits one country in respect of these complexities does not appeal to another.

Psychiatry in Britain as a public service

In every population there are mentally ill people; a minority of them are suicidal, homicidal, or socially disruptive. Some simply tolerate their disturbance or disability, others seek help from religion or folk medicine, while yet others come to doctors or nurses. They may then be treated by a general practitioner, or by a medical specialist (perhaps a neurologist or neuropsychiatrist). This may be at home, in a private clinic if the family can afford it, or in a public mental hospital if they cannot. The actual practice of psychiatry depends greatly on what the State offers and controls, as well as on people's expectations and wealth. Unless the State pays for medical care, numbers of the sick population must remain untreated, while a larger group will receive only minimal help — far less than current medical knowledge can offer.

In 1939, Britain's hospitals were going bankrupt. Both the charitable infirmaries and the teaching hospitals, which were independently governed and maintained by donations, as well as the public general and mental hospitals run by elected councillors, were mostly in physical decay, lacking equipment and staff. To treat the expected civilian casualties of war, as well as the military wounded, all hospitals were united in an Emergency Medical Service. A National Blood Transfusion Service and a Public Health Laboratory Service were also created, paid for by the national Treasury. The success of this wartime nationalisation encouraged a similar hospital plan as part of the post-war National Health Service. For psychiatry, the vital change was that the mental hospitals were to be regarded henceforth as on a par with general hospitals, all equally eligible for money, equipment, and staff, under a common administration. Under the previous system, the biggest concern of local management bodies was to keep down costs, which had to be met through local taxes. Then, mental illness tended to come last in a competition for funds. There were too few doctors for the hospital work, and they were paid less than other doctors, mostly received no specialist training, and had to operate in an atmosphere generally of custodial stagnation.

Under the NHS, however, the money all came from national taxation, via the Ministry of Health to Regional Hospital Boards. Each Board had an executive (architects, engineers, doctors, and nurses) which had professional understanding of hospitals and was less parochial than the previous administration had been.

All hospitals now had a similar hierarchy of medical staff, regarded as in training under senior specialists, who were salaried but also able to undertake private practice. The mental hospitals shared in this structure and became eligible for larger staffs, while the need for training — in psychiatry as much as in other specialties — was now officially recognised. New out-patient clinics, day hospitals, and other extramural facilities such as hostels began to be established. Later, new sub-specialties (old age, childhood, drug dependence, liaison, etc.) would be developed. Occupational therapists, radiographers, laboratory technicians, psychologists, and social workers were appointed to the services. There was an injection of enthusiasm and innovation: research and experiment began; long-stay patients were reviewed; many were rehabilitated and some discharged; doors were unlocked; it was possible for patients to come and go without legal formality.

But the greatest change was in professional training. The medical schools began to improve the teaching of psychiatry to undergraduates and the universities to offer courses to postgraduates, while a body was established (the Royal College of Psychiatrists) to hold specialist examinations which would guarantee the expertise of new specialists. Psychiatric nurses also shared in this process, to some extent (Chapter 7, p. 208).

The British psychiatric hospital service was thus given an immense boost from the late 1940s, but where the plan largely failed was over care outside hospital. Responsibility then passed to the family doctor and to local government social services, both lacking in specialised knowledge of psychiatric problems. This split in responsibility for longer-term patients also existed in many other countries (e.g. France, Germany, USA), where private practice operated extensively.

American psychiatry

The Second World War has been seen as a watershed in American psychiatry and mental health policy. From that experience, it was generally concluded that psychiatric disorders were a more serious problem than had hithero been recognised, that environmental stress contributed to mental maladjustment, and that early, non-institutional treatment could produce favourable outcomes. Whilst these new views were a useful influence in many ways, they involved an assumption about the relationship between minor and major psychiatric disorders which was not scientifically founded and which would lead to a fairly disastrous pursuit of the goal of 'primary prevention' in the 1960s and 1970s.

The leading historian of American psychiatry, Gerald Grob, has emphasised that whereas in 1941 this discipline had only marginal status in either civilian or military life, by 1945, it appeared to be on the threshold of a new era. However, the speciality that emerged anew in the late 1940s was not one based primarily in public mental hospitals, but was rather trained in a psychodynamic and psychoanalytic ideology, dealing mainly with non-psychotic disorders in private practice.

In 1946, the National Mental Health Act was passed by Congress, providing federal funds for psychiatric research, the training of mental health personnel, and grants to states to help establish clinics and demonstration studies. None of this money, though, was to be directed towards State mental hospitals. A National Institute of Mental Health was established under Robert Felix, who continued to direct it until 1964; his emphasis was on mental health as a part of biomedical science — a portrayal which was effective in obtaining steadily increasing financial support. Both through its intramural research and its grants to scientists and clinicians throughout the country, the NIMH was to be the driving force in American psychiatric research over the next few decades.

From the beginning, the NIMH encouraged States to develop alternatives to their mental hospitals, arguing that early identification of disorders and their treatment in the community would minimise the need for in-patient admission. This view was very attractive to the States, since it seemed to promise an end to the endless growth of mental

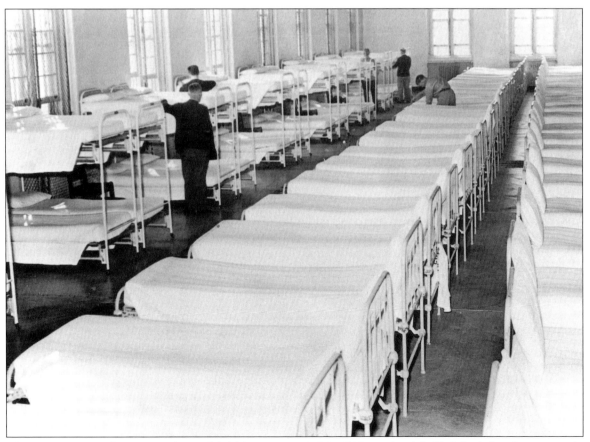

The increased number of patients at Byberry (Philadelphia State Hospital) in 1941 necessitated double-decker beds and a centre row in one of the men's dormitories. Reproduced with permission from the Philadelphia Bulletin, Urban Archives, Temple University, Philadelphia, Pennsylvania.

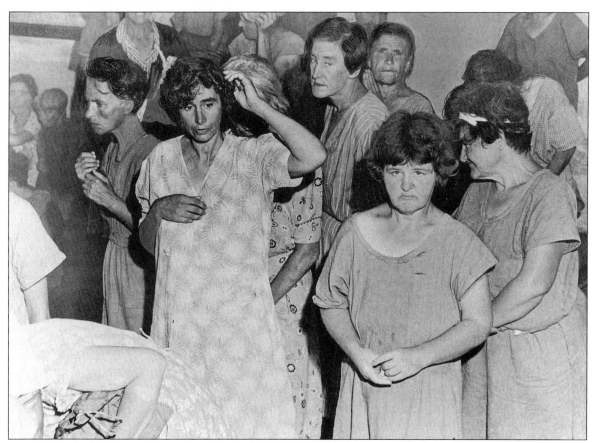

With no place to sit except on the floor, female patients wander aimlessly in an overcrowded ward at Byberry (Philadelphia State Hospital) in 1946. Reproduced with permission from the Philadelphia Bulletin, Urban Archives, Temple University, Philadelphia, Pennsylvania.

hospital populations, which was a heavy financial burden, notwithstanding the generally poor standards of care and accommodation in those institutions. The rapid expansion in numbers of non-medical health professionals, which began in this period, also tended to move the emphasis towards extramural services, since relatively few of these new practitioners went to work in the older mental hospitals.

The optimistic view that NIMH (and particularly Felix) promoted — that medical scientific research could reveal the causes of psychiatric disorder and develop effective treatment for it — was never seriously challenged. As consumers, more and more Americans were now seeking help with mental health problems, and had the resources to pay for this intervention from the growing number of professionals. In this situation, the role of mental hospitals tended to be overlooked, even though their in-patient populations continued to grow.

If any attention was given to the State hospitals, it was usually of an unfavourable kind. In the mid-1940s, revelations of appalling conditions appeared in a number of films, newspaper and magazine articles, and even novels. The most notable of these exposés was the *Shame of the States* by Albert Deutsch, which pointed out that not a single public institution met all the minimum standards laid down by the American Psychiatric Association. Amongst films, *The Snake Pit* attracted the most attention, but the temporary concern which was aroused by these portrayals had little long-term effect in improving mental hospital conditions. One of the biggest problems for many of these institutions was their size. In 1950, the Georgia State Sanatorium had 10,000 beds, and even larger numbers would be found during the next decade. For their part, psychiatrists mostly "voted with their feet", by settling in private practice, particularly in more favoured areas. A few — notably Fritz Freyhan — pointed out that it was misleading to equate effective treatment with individual psychotherapy, and that the emphasis on 'prevention' had no scientifically valid basis. But these were voices crying in the wilderness. In several States, there was public and political concern about their mental hospital systems; surveys were undertaken and discussion took place between State Governors, but the practical results were few. Psychiatric nursing declined in significance at this time, although its numbers slightly increased, and there was no agreed training for attendants who carried out most of the actual care of patients.

Whilst psychodynamic theory then seemed to be all-conquering — in psychiatry, psychology, and social work — the somatic treatments that had been developed in the 1930s were also being widely used, but mainly in the mental hospitals. Leucotomy in particular was being most widely practised in the late 1940s (Chapter 6, p. 159). But the gener-

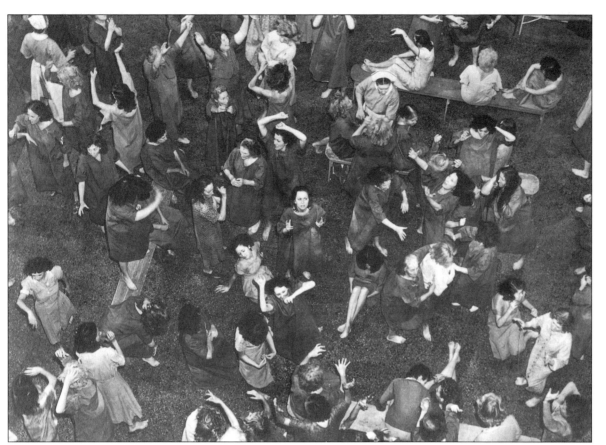

A scene taken from the 20th Century–Fox production of "The Snake Pit". Reproduced with permission from The Museum of Modern Art, Film Stills Archive.

al rejection by psychoanalysts of the somatic approach tended to widen divisions between those psychiatrists who were still practising in institutions and the majority now focusing on individual psychotherapy. The scene was set for more fundamental changes, which would gradually emerge over the next 15 years.

An era of physical treatment

Rather suddenly in the 1930s, a number of new physical therapies had appeared, and the decade 1941–1950 saw their further exploration and the clearer definition of their use. They were empirical in origin, but supported by clinical observation, and were taken up enthusiastically because schizophrenia and melancholia had seemed such unchanging disorders that to see patients improving at all was exciting and encouraging.

Insulin

In the early 1920s, pancreatic extracts had been used in Canada to treat diabetics, and eventually the active principle, crystalline insulin, had been isolated and studied. Sakel, a young Austrian doctor working in a private Berlin clinic, was withdrawing addicts from morphine, which can cause restlessness, abdominal cramps, sweating, and vascular effects. He found that insulin injections brought relief from these symptoms, and speculated that the same treatment might also tranquillise schizophrenics. He then persuaded the Professor of Psychiatry at Vienna to let him try it on patients who were regarded as hopeless cases. To everyone's surprise and initial disbelief, the first 50 cases yielded 35 who "remitted" and went home, with a further nine showing some "social improvement". Though the results in a further series of cases were less impressive, some improvement nearly always took place, and the therapy began to spread to asylums in Austria, Germany, and Switzerland, and then further afield. However, it required considerable investment in skilled nursing, a special ward, and much time. An increasing injection of insulin was given day after day, until a dose produced coma about three hours later. The patient was allowed about 20 minutes in coma and then revived with intravenous glucose, followed by oral glucose; this routine was followed for 6–10 weeks, with breaks every sixth or seventh day. It was a dangerous procedure: some patients had epileptic fits, others had a prolonged coma and were only revived with difficulty, while a few died. Patients put on a lot of weight and some became mentally much improved (Chapter 4, p. 96).

The British Board of Control (of mental hospitals) sent Dr Isabel Wilson to Vienna, and she made an official report of her experiences there, which was generally favourable. The technique was also brought to Britain at a private hospital in London by Sakel's assistant, Rudolf Freudenberg, while Willy Mayer-Gross, an international authority on schizophrenia and a refugee from Heidelberg, introduced it to the Maudsley Hospital. Similarly, Pullar-Strecker brought insulin coma to Edinburgh, under Professor Sir David Henderson. Sakel himself emigrated to New York, where psychoanalysts tried to prevent publication of the method and Sakel from practising. Different centres disagreed about how effective it was, as appeared in discussions at the 1950 World Congress in Paris. There was much inconclusive biochemical study, particularly trying to make it less dangerous. It was clear that epileptic fits could be avoided, but that much depended on skill in dosing to achieve a safe level of coma, which was variable according to the individual. It was generally agreed that a significant depth and duration of coma were needed for successful treatment.

But with the coming of the neuroleptic drugs, which were much safer and easier to use, and with the publication in 1958 of a controlled trial of insulin coma compared with barbiturate coma, which showed no difference in therapeutic outcome between the two groups, insulin therapy died away. This did not prove that insulin was ineffective, merely that it did not do better than barbiturates used in the same way. Previously, some had thought that continuous narcosis with barbiturates relieved schizophrenic symptoms, though this was not scientifically established.

During the Second World War, William Sargant had used insulin in safer doses to tranquillise soldiers with anxiety and depression following battle experience: the men put on weight and their symptoms were often relieved. Eliot Slater, who wrote a textbook of physical treatments with Sargant in 1944, asked why insulin coma cases had generated such enthusiasm if it did nothing for acute schizophrenia. Was it a *folie à cent* amongst psychiatrists? This was before controlled trials compared drugs against each other or against placebo. The published clinical series of insulin coma cases were weak in three areas: diagnosis, prognosis, and assessment of benefit. Centres differed in their selection of patients, and some included as 'schizophrenic' cases whom others would have regarded as manic–depressive, etc. Although insulin coma is not now a practical therapy, there may still be a case for looking at insulin as a psychotropic drug, e.g. in decreasing anxiety.

Cure by epileptic fit

It was an old asylum observation that a patient might improve mentally for a certain time after a spontaneous epileptic fit. Meduna, a Hungarian neuropathologist, examined the brains of patients with either epilepsy or schizophrenia who had died suddenly. He thought that the morbid anatomy was different in the two groups, and wondered whether epilepsy and schizophrenia might be antagonistic to each other. He therefore gave schizophrenic patients epileptic fits, first by injections of camphor, and later with Metrazol (Cardiazol), trying to find a drug with a reliable effect. The fits seemed beneficial to the mental state, though the patients found the initial feelings after injection very unpleasant.

Cerletti in Rome had learned how to create epileptic fits in dogs, to test the value of drugs in preventing convulsions. To be safe, an electric shock as stimulus of the fit had to be given only to the head. With Bini and others, he found that even one fit would remove schizophrenic symptoms for a time. However, a short series of electrically induced fits — two or three times a week — was particularly effective in abolishing human melancholia, though the muscular contractions of the fit could be so violent as to break bones. In 1940, Bennett in the USA introduced curare, which would paralyse the musculature briefly during treatment; the absence of contractions did not alter the therapy, which depended on the nervous discharge in the brain. Later, better muscle-relaxing drugs (such as succinyl choline) were found.

The technique spread to Britain and the USA, carried by Kalinowsky, a refugee from Berlin who had spent time in Rome and Paris. It was accepted in Britain and quickly became a widely used and beneficial technique. But in the USA, as mentioned above, it was greeted with disfavour by the psychoanalysts. Sargant reported that in the first half of 1955 at St Elizabeth's Hospital, Washington, DC, electroconvulsive therapy (ECT) had been used only on 12 out of 7500 patients. In this same period, 20–30 patients a week were receiving it at the Maudsley Hospital, London (Chapter 4, p. 96).

Throughout the 1940s, ECT was a subject for clinical and biochemical study. It was also the target of an emotional hate by people who wanted to think of the human mind as spiritual, above the material world. In spite of such adverse propaganda, ECT is now used in most places round the world, though a wide range of antidepressant drugs has much reduced the need for it.

Treatment of epilepsy

Epilepsy used to be an important problem amongst asylum in-patients, but the development of effective medication changed that. In the twentieth century, phenobarbitone (1912) was for long the only anti-epileptic drug apart from bromides, which had troublesome side-effects. However, in 1938, Merritt and Putnam made an electrical apparatus for producing convulsions in cats, which have a stable threshold for the stimulation of a major fit. They then examined about 50 drugs for their ability to raise the seizure threshold and prevent convulsions. This confirmed the value of phenobarbitone over that of other barbiturates, and revealed the great effectiveness of diphenylhydantoin (phenytoin). This drug had no sedative action, but did have some effect on temporal lobe epilepsy, encouraging further research to find other drugs with value for different types of epilepsy — tridione (trimethyl oxazolidine dione) (1945), phenurone (phenyl acetyl urea) (1949), and mysoline (1952). This marked the beginning of intensive research by pharmaceutical companies for new drugs affecting mental functioning.

The electroencephalograph (EEG), developed in Germany by Berger in the 1930s, revealed various characteristic electrical changes in the brain. These occurred in waking, sleeping, delirium, some dementias, psychoses, and psychopathies, as well as in a variety of clinical patterns of epilepsy. This work was being developed particularly in the 1941–1950 decade. It was also a period when surgery for temporal lobe epilepsy, in particular by Penfield in Canada, was providing new information, as well as successful treatment where there was a focal scar or benign tumour from which the epileptic discharge started.

Leucotomy

For many years, clinical experience had shown that damage to the frontal lobes of the brain caused a personality change in injured people, with the disappearance of tension, anxiety, and temper tantrums and their replacement by a cheerful happy-go-lucky disinhibited state. Chimpanzees in the laboratory reacted similarly. This induced Egas Moniz, a Portuguese neurologist (whose real name was de Abreu Frêire), to ask a surgical colleague to resect part of the frontal lobes in 20 chronic asylum patients (1936): seven were 'cured', seven improved, and six showed no change. Freeman, an American neurologist, with Watts, a surgeon, followed this up with enthusiasm, and published a very influential book in 1942: *Psychosurgery: Intelligence, Emotion, and Social Behaviour Following Prefrontal Lobotomy for Mental Disorders*. It was followed more cautiously in Britain, with papers in the *Lancet* in 1941 and 1943, and a psychiatric conference on the procedure in London, in March 1943 (Chapter 6, p. 159).

In 1946 Freeman introduced transorbital leucotomy, using an ice pick which he inserted from below. Others developed special cutting instruments, or modified cuts, attempting more anatomically precise and limited operations. In Britain, the subjects were mostly mental hospital in-patients who were severely affected by their psychosis, and therefore suffering badly, or proving very difficult management problems because of violence. Freeman, on the other hand, toured the USA and seems to have accepted patients with a wide diagnostic range from their own homes.

Leucotomy was a mutilating operation, which could not be reversed. It came to be restricted to very disturbed schizophrenic patients, severe obsessionals, and melancholics who responded poorly to ECT. Time showed that it could have undesirable side-effects, behavioural as well as physical. On the other hand, before the arrival of chlorpromazine it offered a proportion of patients relief and benefit, which could not be obtained otherwise. By 1954, the British Ministry of Health estimated that there had been 12,000 such operations in the UK. Grob states that by 1951, there had been 18,600 in the USA: one-third of patients were said to have shown good results, one-third were judged somewhat better, and the rest were unchanged or worse. With the coming of the psychotropic drugs, leucotomy rather quickly ceased to be used on any significant scale, though it still exists in a much modified form today.

Abreactions

The intravenous use of barbiturate or methylamphetamine may make the mute speak, the stuporose become active and feed themselves, and the inhibited talk more freely and display emotion. Working with soldiers who had anxiety and hysterical symptoms at the Sutton Emergency Hospital near London, Sargant found that with these intravenous drugs, patients would remember stressful experiences, or at least fantasies of them. They would then become extremely emotional and eventually fatigued and quiet, after which they were often symptom-free. The material described might be of diagnostic value (e.g. reveal schizophrenic thought disorder) or might sometimes reflect the therapist's expectations, rather than the individual's own preoccupations. Sargant thought that the therapeutic value lay in the degree of emotion that was expressed, and he had been impressed by the excitatory abreaction which occurred when ether was used instead of barbiturate (as discovered by Harold Palmer). He felt that what happened in psychoanalysis or hypnosis was basically the same as with a drug, depending on the therapist's ability to achieve emotional relief.

The combination of drug and psychological handling, again with suggestibility as a possible factor, was seen also in the treatment of chronic alcoholism by inducing vomiting with emetine or apomorphine, whenever alcohol was taken (aversion therapy). This was a Russian development, theoretically based on Pavlovian conditioning. An early report of this was by Voegtlin in 1940 (Chapter 6, p. 173). In the same field, Jacobsen and Hald in Denmark discovered in 1948 the value of disulphiram (Antabuse) in discouraging the detoxicated drinker from again taking ethanol. Methadone, synthesised in Germany in the 1940s, later became important in the management of the narcotic addict.

In this first phase of testing the new physical treatments, two basic questions had to be resolved. The first was that of diagnosis — how to select patients with similar symptoms and syndromes, representing some common pathology, whatever the range of quantitative differences. The second was how to measure the effects of the treatment, bearing in mind the many changing influences of environment (diet, activity, relationships, etc.) which might simultaneously be acting on the patient. Ways had to be found of reducing reliance on the subjective impressions of the doctor, both in diagnosis and in assessment of the therapeutic outcome. The introduction of physical and biochemical laboratory measurements, as well as of rating scales and planned comparisons and statistical analyses, was about to begin.

A basis in biological research

Because no physical basis had so far been discovered for schizophrenia, some people said that therefore there could be none, and that it was a gross error to waste time and money in searching for one.

This ignored medical history. Epilepsy, general paralysis of the insane, and Alzheimer's disease accounted for a considerable number of patients in asylums before 1920. But thanks to successful research, these illnesses had either been partially conquered or transferred to more appropriate non-psychiatric care. More importantly, such a negative view ignored the particular difficulties of research into mental illness. Although there was quite extensive biochemical research in the 1931–1950 period — partly metabolic, partly endocrinological — it seemed at the time to lead nowhere in most cases. Yet it did enlarge understanding of how to avoid mistakes and helped towards the successes of later years.

Much study of the chemistry of urine yielded contradictory or unrepeatable results, which were often due to unappreciated difficulties in psychiatric diagnosis (e.g. schizophrenia as a label could not guarantee a single pathology, and was applied differently in different clinics). In other cases, the inconsistencies were due to patients' unanticipated quirks of behaviour (e.g. licking boot polish, smoking). Many attempts to display an effect of the endocrines (thyroid, adrenal cortex, sex hormones) on mental state foundered on the lack of sufficient sensitivity of the chemical analyses then available. Biochemistry itself had to develop new techniques of measurement involving radioactive labelling, fluorescence, or purification by chromatography before progress was possible.

As an example, the treatment of diabetics with insulin was adjusted by testing the patient's urine for glucose. Urine from healthy people or from diabetics receiving enough insulin did not give the same result, but some seriously depressed patients had urine which appeared to produce the positive diabetic test. Henri Ey was amongst those interested (see below). But was the positive urine test in depression due to glucose, other sugars, uric acid, or an unknown substance ('x')?

A new enzyme, glucose oxidase, which specifically destroyed glucose, had no effect on a positive urine test. Paper chromatography, a recently discovered technique for analysing urine, suggested that 'x' was a mixture of things. The explanation came from the serial collections of urine from the same severely depressed patients. During a phase of depression, they drank very little, became dehydrated, and produced scanty, very concentrated urine; it was only this which gave a test positive for 'x'. If their fluid intake was maintained, the test remained negative throughout.

Studies of mental hospital patients, comparing their urine with that from nurses in the same hospital who were eating the same food, showed differences that were not due to mental illness as such. They were eventually traced to the fact that the patients drank more coffee than the staff, or took less vitamin C. To get meaningful results from research, a patient had to be strictly controlled for diet and observed at all times. The work of Gjessing in Norway (1925–1950) was a demonstration of this, and led to therapeutic success in a rare condition.

In his mental hospital, there were a few cases of periodic catatonia, regarded as a variety of schizophrenia. In one form, a man who was averagely active and talkative suddenly passed into a mute state, standing like a statue for long periods. This might go on for several weeks and then suddenly remit; after more weeks, it would recur — and then spontaneously remit again. Gjessing put such patients in isolation, with special nursing control, and fed them on the same amount of the same milk diet, day after day. Every day, all urine and faeces were collected for chemical analysis, while detailed records were kept of behaviour, clinical phenomena (temperature, pulse, body weight, blood pressure, etc.), and mental state. Normally, the amount of nitrogen excreted daily equalled the amount in the fixed daily diet. Gjessing found that during stupor, more nitrogen was excreted than swallowed, but that during remission, after achieving a level balance, nitrogen began to be retained, to a peak at the onset of the next stupor. Thus, nitrogen was being rhythmically retained and expelled, in step with mental change. Perhaps some nitrogenous toxin was being intermittently formed, causing the stupor, but if nitrogen retention could be prevented, no stupor might appear. He knew that thyroxine caused catabolism and excess nitrogen excretion, so although his patients had no evidence of any thyroid disturbance, he started giving them thyroxine. *Mirabile dictu*, the patient's periodic catatonia vanished, and stayed away as long as the thyroxine was continued. This was confirmed by others; but unfortunately, it was only in the rare catatonia, and not in any other psychotic state, that thyroxine was effective. Unfortunately too, with only the biochemical knowledge of 50 years ago, Gjessing could not discover what precisely thyroxine was doing in his patients. Then chlorpromazine arrived, successfully treated periodic catatonia, and the world lost interest in his work.

Also in Norway, in 1934, Fölling discovered an abnormality — phenylpyruvic acid in the urine of two mentally retarded children: the condition was named phenylketonuria. Three years later, Penrose in England showed that this was a genetically determined (recessive) condition — an inability to metabolise the phenylalanine which was the component of a normal protein diet. Other work in the 1940s, e.g. by Jarvis in the USA, demonstrated that this biochemical anomaly could be created in rats, and that it was a failure to convert phenylalanine to tyrosine. At first, the anomaly was supposed to be simply coincident with and not causative of mental retardation. But when special diets lacking phenylalanine were fed through childhood to babies with liability to phenylketonuria, their intelligence developed normally.

The psychopharmacology that began in 1952 arose from earlier dynamic neurochemistry. About 1942, Hoffmann in Switzerland discovered a hallucinogen, lysergic acid diethylamide (LSD-25), while working on alkaloids extracted from ergot. About 1945, serotonin (5-hydroxytryptamine) was discovered in certain areas of the brain, and was shown to be involved in some way in nervous activity. It proved to be affected both by LSD-25, the hallucinogen, and by reserpine — a newly isolated plant derivative which had antipsychotic potency. This was the start of a whole new approach to mental illness — one in which animal experiment could play a useful part, and was to yield great therapeutic benefit. The research laboratories of (chiefly) Swiss and American pharmaceutical companies, together with the teams of S Kety and BB Brodie at the newly founded National Institute of Mental Health in Washington, DC, began to uncover the metabolism and effects of chemical neurotransmitters. Alongside these developments, a new form of psychotherapy — behaviour therapy — was also to arise from animal experimentation which had led to the description of Pavlovian conditioned reflexes and Skinnerian operant conditioning (Chapter 6, p. 173).

But the decade's greatest contribution lay in human genetics, because this made clear the great extent, as well as the limitations of the physical contribution to mental health. Penrose, by a vast study of the mentally retarded and their families, separated conditions due to gene defects from those resulting from other causes. In 1945, Kallman, a German refugee in New York State, identified 691 schizophrenic patients with a traceable co-twin — some fraternal and some identical (monozygotic). In the latter case, nearly 86% of both twins were psychotic, whereas in the fraternal ones, only 14.7% were both affected. Slater in London, in a comparable series, found similar results. Earlier, Rosanoff in Los Angeles had also found the importance of inheritance in the incidence of both schizophrenia and manic–depressive disorder. However, since about a quarter of identical twins presented with only *one* of the pair mentally abnormal, non-genetic factors must also be at work. Inheritance might strongly predispose, but the actual situation determined the result.

Mental illnesses pose complex problems of causation, not least because individual psychological states present great variations, which conceal any common underlying pathology. We cannot connect thought and feeling to micro-physiological change, but progress can come — on the clinical side by study of very large numbers of patients, and on the pathological–therapeutic side, by isolating questions which can be examined by animal experimentation and bioscience. Experimental observations on human beings are always bound to be ethically limited. They are always also bedevilled by the difficulties of diagnosis, and by the dynamic nature of illness.

Practices and diagnoses: work of the decade

The last half century has seen astonishingly rapid changes in treatment, in the organisation of mental health services, and in molecular biology and neuroscience.

But in 1940, psychiatry still meant chiefly public mental hospital psychiatry, treating people with schizophrenia, manic–depressive psychosis, epilepsy, organic dementia (including GPI), or mental retardation. Sometimes, such people also had some physical disability (deafness, blindness, a neurological disorder, etc.). These patients were mostly admitted under compulsion by a legal process (varying from country to country), and they tended to stay in for a long time. In the hospital, there might be as little as one doctor per 500 patients, and one attendant per 15 patients, to cover the 24 hours. The patients were locked in, mostly with nothing to do. Amphetamine for depression, barbiturates and morphine plus hyoscine by injection for heavy sedation, and chloral or paraldehyde for sleep at night, represented the total of available drug treatment.

However, certain special treatments were occasionally in use. Immersion in hot baths calmed the excited (usually manic) patient, but needed experienced nursing, and the calming effect was usually only short-lasting. In Europe, spa treatment (including hydrotherapy) was in vogue for the well-to-do, with uncertain results.

Continuous narcosis or sleep, which again needed careful nursing supervision, could be produced by repeated doses of hypnotics, on a regular schedule. The patient lay in bed in a quiet, warm, dark room and was undisturbed, asleep for 20 hours out of 24 every day, for anything up to three weeks. He was briefly wakened three or four times per day for excretion, consumption of fluids and food, and a further dose of barbiturate to keep the sleep going. As time went on, the patient might reach the point of continuing to sleep without further medication. However, the risks of fever, bronchopneumonia, cardiovascular collapse, and a certain unpredictability of effects meant that extreme nursing vigilance was needed. The method could produce good results in disturbed patients with severe anxiety attacks, agitated melancholia, or excited schizophrenia — in the days before ECT and psychotropic drugs.

Neurosyphilitic GPI could be stopped by infecting the patient with tertian malaria, and allowing about eight rigors before eliminating the malaria with quinine (Chapter 3, p. 64). This treatment needed a centre where malaria-carrying mosquitoes were bred to infect the patients. There was still a minority belief in focal sepsis as a cause of mental illness, and mass tonsillectomy, colonic lavage, etc. were practised at certain hospitals to remove infection (Chapter 4, p. 79).

Apart from their mental illnesses, asylum patients were prone to tuberculosis, malnutrition, and gastrointestinal infections, all of which could lead to death. The conditions of overcrowding, dirt, inadequate sanitary provision, and poor food in many mental hospitals predisposed to this situation. Tuberculous patients there often could not be isolated, put into the fresh air, or given extra food — all part of the recognised treatment of pulmonary TB before the arrival of antibiotic drugs. Facilities for chest X-rays, sputum examination, and blood sedimentation rate measurement might also be lacking.

While lack of food seemed to encourage active tuberculosis, a restricted institutional diet might also lead to cases of scurvy or pellagra. Even the timing of meals could be wrong. For financial economy, the last food of the asylum day might be a light meal at 4.30pm. Patients were sent to bed early, and were often restless and disturbed through the night, unless given paraldehyde regularly. It was eventually discovered that if they were given a bigger meal at 6.30pm, most would sleep without the need for drugs. Doctors pointed out that many psychotics were under-weight and that feeding them better should be a good general treatment, but the asylum management, anxious to save money, was usually disinclined to agree.

Even in 1945, this was the asylum doctor's work — largely physical medicine and administrative management (a sort of public health), though the new physical treatments meant more clinical concern. Nursing, too, was becoming more demanding, both of medical knowledge and of befriending skill. The mental nurse or attendant had in the past been regarded as a domestic servant or handyman, recruited with difficulty from the pool of the unskilled or unemployed. They had to learn to deal with epileptics having a fit at night, and to help patients to eat. They had to turn bedridden patients frequently to avoid bedsores, supervise regular excretion by the incontinent, render first aid for fractures, and treat cuts from fights or accidents. They received some training on the spot, but were not State-registered nurses who had trained in a general hospital, though this was beginning to undergo some change (Chapter 7, p. 208).

Historians, sociologists, and others have frequently misunderstood the asylum, and judged it by the scandals of the worst managed. It may have been called a hospital, but no-one involved in it thought of it as a place of cure, because it was clear that few cures took place. It was rather a situation of refuge, physical care, and symptom-relief. It aimed to protect disabled people who were poorly treated outside, to protect society from the attacks of the aggressive few, and to allow the spontaneous recovery that would occur in perhaps 30% of newly admitted patients within a few months. The character of its regime depended in part on its finance and in part on staff morale, particularly a vigilance for the abuses which can creep into any human institution. The asylum doctor often had a lower social status than other doctors or those people who took the financial decisions, and usually had no say in who was sent to his institution, which could be a legal decision, made by outsiders. There were whole areas of psychiatric disorder with which he was not concerned. But by 1950, changes were on the way in some countries.

The neuroses, personality disorders, drug dependencies, and questions of mental capacity to make a will or recognise right from wrong, were work for the family doctor, the general hospital physician, or neurologist. Very occasionally, a private psychiatric specialist or psychotherapist was involved. Hypochondriasis, anorexia nervosa, anxiety expressed through somatic symptoms, and hysterical conversions were cases which might have gone into a general hospital ward or, in some European countries, to a spa. By and large, results were no better there than in the asylums: some symptomatic relief, and spontaneous lessening of severity could be expected in time, but in these settings, the doctor could give more time to these individuals. In addition, a spa offered a quiet routine away from the stress of work and family life, a regulated diet, and hydrotherapy, without the stigma of 'mental illness'.

In the British system, even before the NHS, the family doctor was the controller of access by the patient to any more specialised doctor. In most other countries, on the other hand, a patient who could afford it could go directly to the specialist of his or her own choice, and the specialist was often both neurologist and psychiatrist. At this time, there was no special consideration of old age psychiatry, and very few special investigations (blood, X-ray, etc.) were available. Child psychiatry in the full sense was only just coming into being (Chapter 4, p. 81). Adolescents were not regarded as a distinct problem, drug dependence was not recognised except on a very minute scale, and much alcoholism was missed. There were initiatives in self-help by patients and lay workers: Alcoholics Anonymous came to Britain in 1947, and the Samaritans (available to listen on the telephone to those troubled and possibly suicidal) started there in 1953. Attempted suicide, like sexual abuse of children, was both less common and less a matter of great concern than it became decades later.

Diagnoses were needed as a short-hand way of stating the future course and outcome of the patient's symptom-complex, and indicating the current requirements of care, which might include placement in hospital. Involutional depression was then seen as a separate type of illness, while neurosis was classified as neurasthenia, anxiety-state, or hysteria. In English-language psychiatry, Meyerian psychobiology was the prevailing basis, with a diagnosis of reaction-type (schizophrenic, manic–depressive, etc.) rather than illness. Some practitioners believed that neurosis was constitutional, others that it arose from early psychic traumas. Most believed in the Kraepelinian division of the psychoses, but a few maintained that all were manifestations of different stages in one illness. There was a tendency to assume that a name such as 'paranoid schizophrenia' meant a specific illness with specific pathology — not a type of reaction (as 'epilepsy' represents grand and petit mal, Jacksonian, etc., caused by drugs, trauma, electric shock, etc.). Clear organic illness (e.g. endocrine disorder, deafness, hepatolenticular degeneration, pernicious anaemia) was less recognised than it is today as a basis for mental disorder. This was the starting point from which more fundamental changes were to take place in psychiatry in the 1950s.

HENRI EY (1900–1977)

by John Crammer

Born of a medical family in Banyuls dels Aspres near Perpignan in Catalan France, Henri Ey gained his medical education in post-First World War Paris and wrote his MD thesis on "Glycaemia in Mental Disorders". He combined literary, artistic, and philosophical interests with great energy for organisation and teaching. He became a leading influence in French psychiatry in the period 1935–1970, and particularly in the decade from 1940, when he began to direct and build up the mental hospital at Bonneval near Chartres. There, he organised a series of conferences which brought together clinicians, philosophers, and historians to discuss the relationships between neurology and psychiatry, the unconscious, the psychogenesis of neuroses and psychoses, heredity, and other theories. Their proceedings were later published as stimulating books. He organised the first World Congress of Psychiatry, held in Paris in 1950, which reviewed and re-launched psychiatry after the interruption of the war. He was also an influential adviser to the French Government on the reorganisation of mental health services.

His contribution to psychological medicine was that of a clinician–philosopher. He reported a detailed examination of the different kinds and settings of hallucinations and degrees of consciousness. He developed a theory (organo-dynamism) of the whole brain–mind which would explain the working of both normal mental processes and breakdowns in psychosis. For him, there was no sense in trying to discern distinct mental illnesses, to diagnose collections of symptoms as implying different psychoses, or to make exogenous/endogenous or organic/functional distinctions. Following the British neurologist Hughlings Jackson (1834–1911), he accepted the brain as an organ which had evolved in stages, in which new levels of inhibitory activity were successively imposed on older levels of excitation. Psychosis was therefore a movement of regression towards a more primitive archaic mental functioning, when the higher inhibition was partly lost. But some of the resulting pathological behaviour was due not simply to release, but to compensatory responses by unaffected parts of the brain. All clinical types were said to arise from variations in the same mechanism: he was a believer in monopsychosis (unitary psychosis, *einheits psychose*). The reality of consciousness was central to his thinking, but he was as opposed to the crude mentalism of Freudian ideas as to the naïvety of equating depressive illness with monoamine transmitter failure. His work is out of fashion at present, but it would be a valuable corrective and stimulant to psychiatric thought, if it was available in English translation.

SIR AUBREY LEWIS (1900–1975)

by John Crammer

Nineteen hundred and forty-six was a key year in the history of British psychiatry, both at home and in its influence abroad. This was when AJ Lewis was elected Professor of Psychiatry in the University of London, in succession to E Mapother (first professor 1936–39), and proceeded to unite the old Bethlem Royal Hospital with the newer Maudsley, and so create the Institute of Psychiatry, making a 500-bed teaching centre. It was the first and for long the only academic teaching and research unit in England, and was to become a powerful influence in upgrading the training and practice of psychiatry throughout Britain. It was also an important support internationally to the work of the World Heath Organization, and an attractive centre for the education of many foreign doctors. Many of his pupils became professors and directors at home and abroad.

He had a clear vision of what both psychiatric education and service organisation ought to be. His teaching demanded precise use of words and clarity of underlying concepts in describing the detailed personal, family, and illness histories of each patient. These were to avoid psychodynamic speculations, and record the patient's own words wherever possible, as in the psychobiology of Adolf Meyer (Chapter 4, p. 103). At the Maudsley, there was a three-year course for trainee psychiatrists, rotating through various departments (children, old age, emergency clinic, etc.) with regular case conferences and seminars, and a requirement to present a thesis based on a piece of research. For the Institute, he drew in men of ability and largely left them to make their own research programmes. These were in endocrinology, biochemistry, neuropathology, pharmacology, but first and foremost in psychology, where HJ Eysenck developed psychometric tests of personality, promoted behaviour therapy, and trained generations of clinical psychologists.

Lewis' own research was primarily in the field of industrial health. In 1947, he became director of the MRC Occupational Psychiatric Research Unit, renamed (1952) the Unit for Research in Occupational Adaptation. This was concerned with the mental and emotional characteristics of industrial workers, how the mentally handicapped or chronic psychotic might be encouraged to do productive work, and how the psychiatric interview might reliably define a personality. Some of the findings were of great practical importance to later rehabilitation and discharge programmes, in showing how people with low IQ (20–50) or chronic schizophrenia, could be managed outside hospital. It was shown that they could be interested in work, and could concentrate and learn skills, if given time and suitable supervision.

Lewis was born, an only child, in Adelaide (Australia), his father a Jewish watchmaker who had emigrated from London 10 years before. At the Christian Brothers (Catholic) College and later at the Adelaide Medical School, he was a notable student, graduating in 1923. After junior posts at his hospital and some physical and psychological research on Australian aborigines, he went in 1927 as a Rockefeller Travelling Fellow to McFie Campbell in Boston, Adolf Meyer in Baltimore, then to Germany (Beringer at Heidelberg, Bonhoeffer at Berlin), and finally to Sir Gordon Holmes at Queen Square (London).

The Maudsley Hospital, a new acute psychiatric hospital, opened (1923) jointly by London County Council and London University primarily to teach the staffs of the London mental hospitals, was struggling to become a clinical research centre. Lewis arrived there in 1929, became clinical director in 1936, and when war came in 1939, led half the hospital to Mill Hill, where he brought in Maxwell Jones and HJ Eysenck. After the war, he directed research in social psychiatry at the Maudsley, and showed great administrative talents in creating a large research programme at the Institute of Psychiatry. For Britain, he was the outstanding academic psychiatrist of the century.

ELIOT SLATER (1904–1983)

by John Crammer

Slater was associated with the Maudsley Hospital (London) from 1931, and in addition a consultant in psychological medicine at the National Hospital for Neurology (Queen Square) 1946–64 and director of the MRC Unit for Psychiatric Genetics (1959–1969). He was primarily a clinical scientist who gained an international reputation in psychiatric genetics.

His beginnings had been very unpromising. His parents were in India and he was sent to an English boarding school and then to Cambridge University, at both of which he did poorly, and was unhappy, being attracted to literature but having to study medicine. He was convinced he would never make a scientist. At St George's Hospital, he remained uninterested until a chance experience of neurology, with its logical analysis of symptoms and signs in relation to pathology, caught his interest. However, he was not accepted for a neurological job, and became a provincial mental hospital doctor, where there was little to do. He began appealing to the Maudsley Hospital for help, and was finally taken on there in 1931.

The staff there were friendly and stimulating. Mayer-Gross taught him the phenomenological approach in diagnosis, he went for special teaching in statistics to RA Fisher, Aubrey Lewis suggested genetics might be his research field, and the Rockefeller Foundation financed him to spend 1934–35 in Germany, chiefly at Munich, which was then a world centre for psychiatric genetics. He interviewed manic–depressive patients and their families. On return to England, he began interviewing pairs of twins in the London area; where one was diagnosed as suffering from manic–depressive disorder, schizophrenia, neurosis, or psychopathy, he investigated what illness, if any, the co-twin shared. He was able to continue this work right through the war, in addition to his ordinary duties, at Sutton Emergency Hospital, on the south-west fringe of London.

Delayed by the war, the analysis was only published in 1953, but showed clearly that where one twin had schizophrenia, the other was likely to have the same disorder, though not necessarily

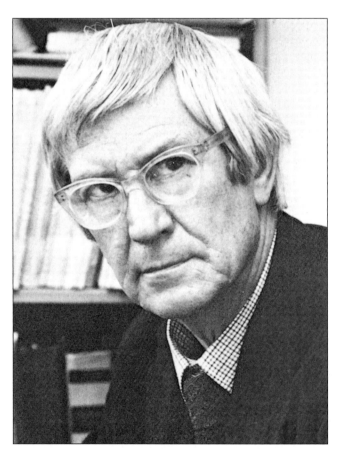

Eliot Slater. Photo courtesy of The Royal College of Psychiatrists, London.

of the same severity and duration. On the other hand, in about a quarter of the identical cases and in the majority of fraternal twins, there was no concordance. In other words, genetic identity was a strong predisposition to psychotic breakdown, but other (environmental?) factors also played a part. A similar result was obtained for manic–depression, but in neurosis, there was little concordance, even in identical pairs. Rosanoff in California, and Kallman in New York made similar studies, with similar findings. However, his wartime study of 2000 soldiers admitted for neurotic breakdown while on active service showed that while Army stress provoked breakdown, a majority of the men in fact had shown a variety of previous maladaption in childhood, civilian employment, and marriage, suggesting that they were constitutionally vulnerable in a non-specific way — a possibly polygenic effect.

In a different field, he published important work on the schizophrenia-like psychoses of epilepsy (1963). Arising from his wartime experience at Sutton Emergency Hospital, he published in 1944 with William Sargant *An Introduction to Physical Methods of Treatment in Psychiatry* — one of the first books to describe the practical use of insulin, ECT, leucotomy, and drug and abreactive therapy in hospital practice. Ten years later, with Mayer-Gross and Roth, he produced what became the standard English textbook in the field, *Clinical Psychiatry* (1954). He revived and re-created the *British Journal of Psychiatry* in 1961–72, and with Cowie published *Delinquency in Girls* (1968), and *The Genetics of Mental Disorders* (1971). In retirement, he published poetry, had an exhibition of his paintings, and gained a PhD from Cambridge for Shakespearean studies.

LIONEL PENROSE (1898–1972)

by John Crammer

The Biology of Mental Defect (1949) was a book which shone a searchlight of new information on a neglected subject (mental retardation, or now learning disability), where ignorance had encouraged widespread fears of national intellectual degeneration and racial decay. Just at a time when, in Germany, compulsory sterilisation and 'mercy' killing of defectives on a large scale were proceeding, partly out of eugenic panic, Penrose was engaged on "A clinical and genetic study of 1280 cases of mental defect" (1930–1938), published in about 30 papers and then in his book. He studied over 100 disorders which are productive of severe mental defect, and showed that while some defects were pathological and genetically determined (Down's syndrome; phenylketonuria), many others were part of the normal variation of human qualities. These individuals were simply at the lowest end of the population curve — a polygenic subcultural group. In this group of defectives, their parents were predominantly of normal or high intelligence, and their children (if any) could well be of higher intelligence again. There was no good evidence of national decline in successive generations, but some suggestion that polygenic variation produced a healthier stock. Sterilisation of this group, therefore, could not affect the national incidence of mental defect. In the pathological group also, the genetic determination differed in different disorders, and sterilisation might well be ineffective in preventing their perpetuation.

This major work had involved examining not only 1280 patients in the Royal Eastern Counties Institution at Colchester, but also their 2560 parents and 6629 siblings. It had necessitated the development of new intelligence tests which were non-verbal, so as to avoid any effect of the patient's lack of reading and education. The study of mental retardation became Penrose's life work. How did he come to it?

His parents were strict Quakers, who had brought him up with a religion which emphasised pacifism and lack of ostentation. He went to the same school and Cambridge college as Eliot Slater, where he read Mathematics and Moral Sciences and came under the influence of WHR Rivers, the most noted British dynamic psychotherapist of his day.

Penrose became interested in mental illness, visited Fulbourn, the Cambridge mental hospital, and in 1922 went to Vienna, and had a short analysis by Freud himself. He returned to London to study medicine at St Thomas's Hospital, qualifying in 1928, and proceeding to MD in 1930. This was with a thesis on a long-term study of a single schizophrenic patient whom he saw while working at Cardiff City mental hospital.

From there he went to Colchester, where he remained till 1945, except for the six years of war, when he conducted a large survey of in-patient psychotics and their relatives in the mental hospitals of Ontario. He became Professor of Human Genetics at University College, London until 1965, directing the Galton Laboratory there and editing scientific journals. Penrose's work resulted in significant advances in the scientific study of mental retardation.

AUTISM AND ASPERGER'S SYNDROME

by Lorna Wing

Leo Kanner, in the USA, and Hans Asperger, in Austria, are both best known for describing and naming, in the early 1940s, a group of children who had in common a pattern of strange behaviour. The two groups differed in many ways, but both authors used the term 'autistic' to capture the essential quality of aloneness and lack of social sense in the children they observed.

Although Kanner and Asperger were the first to recognise the existence of groups of children with social impairment as the common characteristic, the history of autistic disorders stretches far back into the mists of time. Some versions of the myths of 'changeling children' sound remarkably like children with autism. In factual history, scattered examples of individuals, who, with hindsight, seem to have had autistic disorders, can be found. The most famous of these is Victor, the boy found living wild in the woods of south central France, who was described in reports written at the beginning of the nineteenth century by the physician, JMG Itard. There was no suggestion that such children could be grouped together until, in the UK, Dr James Haslam, in 1806, and the psychiatrist, Henry Maudsley, in 1867, wrote accounts of children they described as 'insane', some of whom can now be identified as probably autistic.

In the first half of the twentieth century, various workers tried to define sub-groups amongst these children. In 1943, Leo Kanner in the USA wrote his classic description of young children who were, from birth or very early in life: (a) socially aloof and indifferent; (b) were mute or had echolalia and idiosyncratic speech; (c) were intensely resistant to change in their own repetitive routines; and (d) who had isolated skills in visuo-spatial or rote memory tasks, against a background of general delay in learning. He thought that they were of potentially normal intelligence, and coined the name "early infantile autism" for this syndrome.

One year later, in 1944, Asperger in Vienna published his first paper on older children and adolescents who: (a) were naïve, inappropriate, and egocentric in social interaction; (b) had good grammar and vocabulary but repetitive speech with poor intonation and poor body language; (c) were absorbed in their circumscribed interests; and (d) usually had poor motor coordination. They were of borderline, normal, or superior intelligence, but often had specific learning difficulties. He referred to this syndrome as "autistic psychopathy".

Amongst those in the field in the early years, Kanner and Asperger are the only ones whose names have become well known throughout the world. Kanner was the first to have his work widely recognised. Asperger achieved this status in the English-language literature much later, though his work had been known in mainland Europe. It was not until the 1980s that interest in Asperger's work began to grow in the UK, following some publications discussing his ideas.

Kanner originally thought that his syndrome was genetic in origin. However, in 1949, influenced by views prevailing in the USA at the time, he wrote that the cause was emotional, not physical, due to abnormal child rearing by cold, over-intellectual parents who were of high social class. He also suggested that infantile autism was the earliest form of schizophrenia. Asperger always considered that the syndrome he described was due to abnormality of aspects of brain development that were very probably genetic in origin. He believed that it was not schizophrenia or any form of psychosis.

Scientific methods of investigation into autism

The 1960s saw the introduction of scientific methods of investigation into the field. Victor Lotter carried out the first epidemiological study of autism in the former English county of Middlesex, and found the prevalence of Kanner's syndrome to be nearly 5 in 10,000. Michael Rutter and his colleagues in London observed that many of the children had mild or severe mental retardation and that the long-term prognosis was closely related to their level of intelligence. Other workers have found no objective evidence that the parents caused their children to be autistic. Most of the studies that examined the parents' occupations found that they came from all walks of life. In a series of studies published in 1971, Israel Kolvin and his colleagues in Newcastle and Oxford compared autism and childhood schizophrenia, and found many differences between them. For example: (a) those with childhood schizophrenia had hallucinations and delusions as in adult schizo-

Alexander Wolf in New York — became passionately interested in this form of therapy, and powerful advocates of it. Foulkes, however, had more confidence than Wolf in using an unstructured group situation. Sensitive to the unconscious life of groups and identifying common themes, he began to elaborate the theoretical structure of group analysis. Wolf, more cautious and more traditionally psychoanalytic, believed that the concept of group dynamics was anti-therapeutic: he relied more on the analysis of the individual transferences to the group therapist, as well as those between members. Also in New York, Samuel Slavson developed 'activity group therapy' for adolescents. A powerful advocate and administrator, he founded both the American Group Psychotherapy Association, and the *International Journal of Group Psychotherapy*, and became the acknowledged leader of this form of treatment in North America. Jacob Moreno, an Austrian psychiatrist fascinated by the theatre, devised a method for patients to act out their conflicts in a group setting; he believed that releasing blocked spontaneity and creativity had healing powers. Under the direction of the trained psychodramatist, a group member (protagonist) brought to life significant events in his own life, with other group members acting as characters from that life. One important psychodramatic technique was role-reversal, where the protagonist changes place with the person he is facing — a process in which I become you: you become me. Thereby, the first person is enabled to see herself through the eyes of the other. Another technique was 'doubling', where one person standing behind the protagonist speaks out thoughts and feelings that the protagonist is not aware of, thereby deepening that person's self-awareness. Moreno emigrated to the United States, where he created an influential school of psychotherapy, started the journal *Sociometry*, and with Slavson was a founder of the International Association of Group Psychotherapy. Moreno was a far-seeing, charismatic leader whose major written work is characteristically entitled *Who Shall Survive?*. His sociometric method charts the vectors of attraction and repulsion between the members of the group and has become a useful clinical and research tool. However, Moreno and Slavson — the leaders of their respective empires — were in conflict: Slavson espoused and advocated psychoanalysis, which Moreno repudiated.

Freud's group psychology

After the First World War, Freud has turned his attention to group psychology, publishing *Group Psychology and the Analysis of the Ego* in 1921. Drawing on the influential work of the French theorist le Bon, who wrote on the effect of crowd behaviour particularly during the French Revolution, Freud showed how the relationship of the group to its leader resulted in mutual identification between the members. They share the leader as their own beloved and feared master, which lays the ground both for identification and for group cohesion. Groups require both a central figure, so that they can establish themselves as a group, and enemies to help define the difference between groups.

The war years — 1939–1945

The war years opened up the study of both small and large group dynamics, since psychiatrists, psychoanalysts, social scientists, and psychologists were drawn into military service in Britain, America, and some other countries. Armies are very large groups. Huge numbers of soldiers have to be allocated to appropriate duties, so that they can become useful members of units; battle casualties have to be treated, and rehabilitated where possible, while large numbers of men who show the potential to be effective leaders have to be selected and trained. In the United Kingdom, this became imperative after the fall of France, when the defeated British Expeditionary Force had to be greatly enlarged to form an efficient war machine. Brigadier JR Rees, Director of the Tavistock Clinic in the 1930s, had been put in charge of army psychiatry and called in his Tavistock Clinic colleagues to form an 'invisible college', which was responsible for both personnel selection and treatment. Military psychiatry had to become functional, not custodial in the way that the current mental hospitals were. Psychiatrists and psychotherapists collaborated in the War Office Selection Boards for potential officers (Bion and JD Sutherland), the conversion of a hospital into a therapeutic community (Foulkes, Bion, H Bridger, TF Main), and the rehabilitation of returned prisoners of war. Thus the concept of the 'therapeutic community' was born out of military psychiatry, since the term was coined by Main to describe the organisation of a psychiatric hospital which was now designed to facilitate treatment (Chapter 6, p. 155). This work was at Northfield Military Hospital in Birmingham. The hospital was seen as a whole functioning institution, with its activities systematically scrutinised to understand their effects on the process of rehabilitation. During this time, Maxwell Jones had moved from physiological investigations of 'effort syndrome' to an appreciation of the

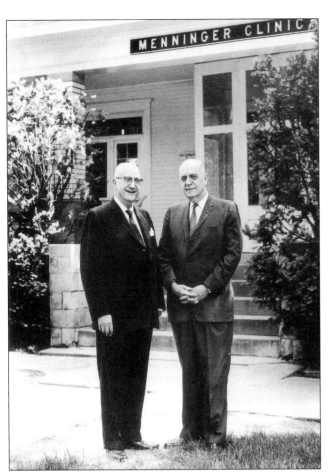

Karl A Menninger (left) and William C Menninger (right), 1960. Reproduced with permission from The Menninger Foundation Archives.

power of group discussions to reveal and release group tensions and conflicts.

The work at Northfield was in two phases: Northfield 'Experiment One' was limited to six weeks, when the psychoanalysts Bion and John Rickman converted a conventional ward for neurotic soldiers to a situation where large and small group discussions were going on all the time. The disruption of the rest of the hospital caused by this experiment led to these doctors being removed, but from 1943 onwards, Foulkes, Main, Bridger, and others restructured the whole hospital to form a 'therapeutic community'. The impact of this experience on American military psychiatry was radical. Generals Karl and William Menninger, powerful officers in American psychiatry and directors of the Menninger Clinic in Topeka, Kansas, who visited this hospital, were so impressed that orders were given that American army psychiatrists should begin to practise group psychotherapy. Special training began for this purpose. The 1946 issue of the *Bulletin of the Menninger Clinic* contained papers on the subject, which have become classics. These were WR Bion on 'The Leaderless Group Project', Harold Bridger on 'The Northfield Experiment', SH Foulkes on 'Principles and Practice of Group Therapy', and TF Main on 'The Hospital as a Therapeutic Institution'. In this way, the experience gained in wartime by British psychodynamic psychiatry was made available worldwide. It was followed in 1948, by Foulkes' *Introduction to Group Analytic Psychotherapy*, which outlined the theory and practice of his technique, and became an influential work.

In the post-war years, Bion, Sutherland, and H Ezriel dominated the scene of group psychotherapy at the Tavistock Clinic, London. Much influenced by the theories of Melanie Klein, Bion wrote *Experiences in Groups*, in which he postulated that the Work Group represented the more rational attempts of the group's members to use the situation as one in which to work on their personal problems. However, those problems which arose through membership of the group were opposed by the underlying Basic Assumptions. These are primitive regressed states of mind — compromises between impulses and defences — which represent the unconscious disowned mental life of the group members, pooled together to form three types of mentalities. He postulated that the group is driven: (a) to seek a dependent relationship with the therapist, which involves giving up their own autonomy and work capacities, or (b) to adopt fight-and-flight to counter the dominance of the leader, or else (c) to engage in 'pairing', waiting for some pair to create together the wherewithal for the group's salvation. Erziel elaborated Bion's ideas into a system which, as Malan's follow-up study of groups held at the Tavistock demonstrated, did not yield good results. At the Maudsley Hospital, Foulkes taught generations of psychiatrists a form of group psychotherapy which was less systematic, but more adaptive to the needs of individuals. It has proved clinically effective and influential in both the United Kingdom and Continental Europe. In the United States, the work of Wolf and Schwartz was the most influential throughout this decade.

Therapy of the group, in the group, by the group

An overall view of mainstream approaches to group psychotherapy can be gained by classifying in the following way:

Psychoanalysis in the group

This is the method of Wolf and Schwartz, where the emphasis is on the group leader's work with each individual member, predominantly through the recurrent behaviour patterns that emerge in transference to both the leader and to the 'sibling' members of the group. Family dynamics are then played out again, and can be corrected.

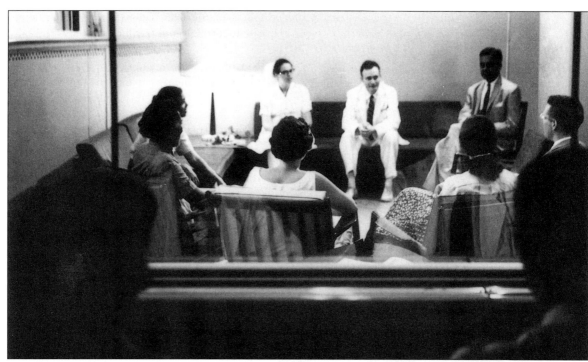

Group therapy session at Phipps Psychiatric Clinic, Johns Hopkins Medical Institutions (c. 1965). Reproduced with permission from the Chesney Medical Archives, Johns Hopkins Medical Institutions.

Psychoanalysis of the group

This is the approach originated by Bion and Erziel at the Tavistock Clinic: the therapist's interventions are not directed to individual members of the group, who play their unconscious parts in combined attitudes towards the group therapist and to the other group members. The interpretation and theorisation is on primitive, regressive compromises between impulses and defences.

Psychoanalysis by the group

In Foulkes group analytic technique, the therapist weans the members from excessive and inappropriate dependency towards becoming their own therapists — both to themselves and to the other group members. Foulkes's emphasis was on facilitating communication and helping the members to learn to deal with the basic issues of social life through self-understanding and the understanding of others.

After his war service, TF Main became Director of the Cassel Hospital, London, which developed into an internationally known centre for the application of group psychotherapy in a psychoanalytic setting. However, at the Henderson Hospital, Maxwell Jones eschewed psychoanalytic ideas for those derived from social psychology. The Cassel retained individual psychotherapy, whereas the Henderson relied totally on group methods. The research of Rappaport in the 1960s on the therapeutic activities of the Henderson Hospital showed that democratisation, permissiveness, reality confrontation, and communalism — the sense of participating in a set of close relationships — were the working principles.

Army psychiatrists returned from the war and, imbued with a new spirit of dynamic psychiatry, initiated therapeutic community-style practices in many psychiatric institutions in the UK, USA, and some other countries in Europe. This movement retained its vigour for some 20 years, but gradually declined in the face of institutional resistance, funding difficulties, the dominance of individual psychotherapy over group methods, and finally advances in psychopharmacology and the biological treatments. But the lessons of the effects of institutionalisation had been learned. Russell Barton's *Institutional Neurosis* (1959) was influential in drawing attention to the administrative abuses which psychiatric patients had been enduring for decades. 'Administrative psychiatry' — a recognition that psychologically informed administration was an essential part of a hospital psychiatrist's training — was formulated by DH Clark at Cambridge and became widely recognised in Britain, North America, and Japan.

Training

In the United Kingdom, the principal centres for training in the NHS were the Tavistock Clinic and the Maudsley Hospital. Informal training began under SH Foulkes and developed into the Institute of Group Analysis. In the USA, many centres opened treatment programmes, and Moreno's psychodramatic method was widely taught and practised. Bion's ideas were closely studied at Herbert Thelen's Laboratory at the University of Chicago, though this work did not begin until the 1950s.

Group psychotherapy in Europe

Following the Second World War, the most considerable developments have been in:

(a) Scandinavia — where group analytic psychotherapy on the Foulkesian model has been widely taught.

(b) Germany — as well as the Foulkesian method, an indigenous German technique, the Gottingen method, was developed by Heigl and Heigl-Evers. This is a form of analytically orientated group therapy which takes note of unconscious processes in the group, but carefully monitors the level of regression to ensure that individual members are not overwhelmed. The patient is helped to name and distinguish feelings and to recognise the nature of their inner worlds.

(c) France — a form of psychoanalytic psychodrama was developed which involved the use of several therapists to play out aspects of an individual patient's inner world. Naturally, this is a complex and expensive procedure. French approaches have been outlined by Anzieu, Kaes, and Rouchy.

(d) Italy — There are many group training institutions in Italy. Some follow the model of Bion, and others that of Foulkes. This work is well represented in Claudio Neri's monograph *Group*.

Conclusion

In the decades of the 1920s and 1930s several developments led towards an enlargement of the therapeutic situation from dyadic to group. Conventional psychiatrists, Freudian analysts, and Adlerians all contributed to this process. Social psychological research under Lewin had shown that group processes could be studied scientifically, and attention was drawn to group psychology — a field previously neglected. Isolated projects in small-group psychotherapy in the 1930s became in the 1940s urgent situations for therapy under wartime conditions. Mental hospital psychiatry and psychodynamic psychotherapy then came into a fruitful collaboration, giving birth to the concept of the therapeutic community. Systems of group therapy were elaborated by Bion and Foulkes in the United Kingdom, and by Wolf, Schwartz, and Slavson in the United States, where Moreno also established his psychodramatic method. Group psychotherapists nowadays continue to draw on the experiences and publications of this decade; those theories have remained dominant for over 40 years and still retain considerable influence.

FURTHER READING

1941–1950

Bennett DH, Freeman HL, eds. *Community Psychiatry*. London: Churchill Livingstone; 1991.

Ellenberger H. *The Discovery of the Unconscious: The History and Evolution of Dynamic Psychiatry*. New York: Basic Books; 1970.

Fenichel O. *The Psychoanalytic Theory of Neurosis*. New York: WW Norton; 1945.

Gjessing RA. *Contribution to the Somatology of Periodic Catatonia*. Gjessing LR, Jenner FA, eds. Oxford: Pergamon Press; 1976.

Grob GN. *From Asylum to Community*. Princeton: Princeton University Press; 1991.

Hale NG Jr. *The Rise and Crisis of Psychoanalysis in the United States*. New York: Oxford University Press; 1995.

Hoskins RG. *The Biology of Schizophrenia*. London: Chapman & Hall; 1946.

Müller-Hill B. *Murderous Science* (trans. GR Fraser). Oxford: Oxford University Press; 1988.

Penfield W, Erickson TC. *Epilepsy and Cerebral Localisation*. London: Ballière Tindall Cox; 1941.

Penrose LS. *The Biology of Mental Defect*. London: Sidgwick and Jackson; 1949.

Shorter E. *A History of Psychiatry*. Chichester: Wiley; 1997.

Henri Ey

Ey H. *Etudes Psychiatriques*, Vols 1–5. Paris: Desclée de Brouwer; 1954.

Ey H. Hughlings Jackson's principles and the organo-dynamic concept of psychiatry. *American Journal of Psychiatry*. 1962; **118**:673–682.

Sir Aubrey Lewis

Lewis AJ. *The State of Psychiatry: Essays and Addresses*. London: Routledge; 1967.

Shepherd M. A representative psychiatrist: the career, contributions and legacies of Sir A. Lewis. *Psychological Medicine*. 1986; monograph 10.

Eliot Slater

Shepherd M, Davies DL, eds. *Studies in Psychiatry*. London: Oxford University Press; 1968.

Shields J, Gottesman II, eds. *Man, Mind and Heredity: Selected Papers of Eliot Slater on Psychiatry and Genetics*. Baltimore: Johns Hopkins; 1971.

Lionel Penrose

Penrose LS. Contribution of mental deficiency research to psychiatry — the 40th Maudsley Lecture. *British Journal of Psychiatry*. 1966; **112**:747.

Watt DC. Lionel Penrose and eugenics, parts one and two. *Notes and Records of the Royal Society of London*. 1998; **52**:137–151, 339–354.

Autism and Asperger's syndrome

Attwood T. *Asperger's Syndrome: A Guide for Parents and Professionals*. London: Jessica Kingsley; 1998.

Frith U. *Autism: Explaining the Enigma*. Oxford: Blackwell; 1989.

Frith U, ed. *Autism and Asperger Syndrome*. Cambridge: Cambridge University Press; 1991. (Includes a translation by U Frith of Asperger's 1944 paper, pp. 37–92.)

Gerland G. *A Real Person*. London: Souvenir Press; 1997. (An autobiography by a woman with Asperger's syndrome.)

Gillberg C. The Emmanuel Miller Memorial Lecture 1991. Autism and autistic-like conditions: subclasses among disorders of empathy. *Journal of Child Psychology & Psychiatry*. 1992; **33**:813–842.

Howlin P. Prognosis in autism: Do specialist treatments affect outcome? *European Child and Adolscent Psychiatry*. 1997; **6**:55–72.

Howlin P. *Autism: Preparing for Adulthood*. London: Routledge; 1997.

Jordan R, Powell S. *Understanding and Teaching Children with Autism*. Chichester: Wiley; 1995.

Kanner L. *Childhood Psychosis: Initial Studies and New Insights*. New York: Winston/Wiley; 1973. (Includes Kanner's 1944 paper, pp. 1–43.)

Wing L. Asperger's syndrome: A clinical account. *Psychological Medicine* 1981; **11**:115–129.

Wing L. *The Autistic Spectrum: A Guide for Parents and Professionals*. London: Constable; 1996.

Wolff S. *Loners: The Life Path of Unusual Children*. London: Routledge; 1995.

Group psychotherapy

The International Library of Group Analysis (Editor, Malcolm Pines) has published a number of important books with Jessica Kingsley Publishers, London.

Alonso A, Swiller HL. *Group Therapy in Clinical Practice*. Washington, DC: American Psychiatric Press; 1993.

Aveline M, Dryden W. *Group Therapy in Britain*. Milton Keynes: Open University Press; 1988.

Bion WR. *'Experiences in Groups' and Other Papers*. London: Tavistock; 1961.

Foulkes SH. *Introduction to Group Analytic Psychotherapy*. London: Heinemann; 1948. (Reprinted: London: Karnac Books; 1983.)

Foulkes SH, Lewis E. Group analysis: studies in the treatment of group psychotherapy along psycho-analytical lines. *British Journal of Medical Psychology*. 1994; **20**:175–184.

Kaplan HI, Saddock BJ. *Comprehensive Group Psychotherapy*, 3rd edn. Baltimore: Williams and Wilkins; 1993.

Main TF. The hospital as a therapeutic institution. *Bulletin Menninger Clinic*. 1966; **70**:1946.

Malan D. A follow-up study of group psychotherapy. *Archives of General Psychiatry*. 1976; **33**:1303.

Marsh LC. Group therapy and the psychiatric clinic. *Journal of Nervous and Mental Disease*. 1935; **82**:281–293.

Moreno JL. *Who Shall Survive? Foundation of Sociometry, Group Psychotherapy and Psychodrama*. Washington, DC: Nervous and Mental Disease Publishing Co; 1953.

Rutan JS, Stone WN. *Psychodynamic Group Psychotherapy*. New York: Macmillan; 1984.

Wender L. Group psychotherapy: a study of its application. *Psychiatric Quarterly*. 1940; **14**:708–718.

Wolf A. The psychoanalysis of groups 1. *American Journal of Psychotherapy*. 1949; **3**:525–558.

Wolf A. The psychoanalysis of groups 2. *American Journal of Psychotherapy*. 1950; **3**:16–50.

1951–1960

1951–1960 CHAPTER 6

Major world events

1953 Kruschev became First Secretary of the Soviet Communist Party
1953 Inaugural Boeing 707 flight (USA)
1957 European Economic Community established
1957 The Soviets launched Sputnik I into space, followed by the first living creature, a dog called Laika
1960 Creation of OPEC, 'The Organisation of Petroleum Exporting Countries'

Major events in psychiatry

1952 Max Lurie and Harry Salzer in Cincinnati discovered that isoniazid could be used as an antidepressant
1952 The *Diagnostic and Statistical Manual* (DSM–I) introduced by the American Psychiatric Association
1952 A critical evaluation of psychoanalytic therapy — *The Effects of Psychotherapy* published by Hans J Eysenck in London
1952 Delay and Deniker described a psychological disturbance treated with chlorpromazine
1954 Nathan Kline in New York reported that rauwolfia serpentina exerted a therapeutic effect on both anxiety and obsessive–compulsive symptoms
1954 Delay and Deniker, Noce in the USA, and Steck in Switzerland, reported that reserpine had a favourable effect on mania
1954 Mayer-Gross, Slater, and Roth produced the standard English textbook on *Clinical Psychiatry*
1954 The first community psychiatric nurse post established in Britain
1954 Led by Paumelle, a group of psychiatrists created a sector-based service in the 13th arrondissement of Paris
1955 The first benzodiazepine, chlordiazepoxide, synthesised
1955 Delay and Deniker proposed that drugs such as chlorpromazine and reserpine should be grouped under the heading of 'neuroleptics'
1956 The Narcotic Control Act passed in the USA
1956 Arvid Carlsson and Nils Ake Hillarp in Sweden discovered the catecholamine depleting effect of reserpine
1957 Imipramine introduced clinically in Switzerland as an antidepressant
1957 The characteristics of neuroleptics described by Delay and Deniker, who proposed a classification of psychotropic substances
1957 Royal Commission on the Law Relating to Mental Illness and Mental Deficiency published a report leading to the English Mental Health Act of 1959
1958 Carlsson *et al.* discovered dopamine in brain tissues and identified it as a neurotransmitter
1958 Janssen developed haloperidol, the first butyrophenone neuroleptic
1959 Publication of Russell Barton's *Institutional Neurosis* in England drew attention to the adverse effects of institutional regimes
1960 RD Laing's book *The Divided Self* published in London

EUROPEAN PSYCHIATRY

by Peter Berner

There is little doubt that the most important achievement of European psychiatry in the 1950s was the creation of new therapies. In the field of somatic treatments, the introduction of neuroleptics in 1952, of imipramine in 1956, and of inhibitors of monoamine oxidase in 1958 initiated important changes in strategy which became decisive during the following decades. Insulin coma and Metrazol shock treatment were gradually abandoned, while electroconvulsive therapy (ECT) (Chapter 4, p. 96) became increasingly restricted to severe depressive states, and leucotomy to those untreatable by any other means (this chapter, p. 159).

The application of these new drugs meant that physical restraint was no longer necessary; open-door psychiatric services could be set up in general hospitals, and sufferers who previously would have been sent to mental hospitals could now be treated as out-patients. In the general field of psychotherapy, behaviour therapy was developed after 1950 on the basis of learning theories. Unlike traditional dynamic psychotherapy, this method did not aim to raise awareness of underlying motives or conflicts but, focusing solely on the current problems, tried to remove the patient's actual symptoms or disturbed behaviour. In succeeding years, this strategy has found more and more application both in the out-patient and in-patient treatment of various psychiatric disorders, whatever their nosological basis (this chapter, p. 166).

Alongside these new therapeutic methods, but stimulated further by them, European psychiatry in the 1950s was characterised above all by the development of concepts which called in question the validity of classifications that had up till then served as accepted guidelines. During this period, previous attempts at classification were redefined in both France and Germany, in the form of very precise models.

The new German concepts

In Germany, three different concepts were developed: both Conrad and Janzarik suggested models for the genesis of psychoses deriving from the 'structural' psychology that had been developed at the turn of the century by Dilthey. William Dilthey (1833–1911) was a German philosopher who elaborated the viewpoint that the whole is 'more than the sum of its parts', in the same way that a melody is more than the sum of its notes. In this perspective, 'structure' means the manner in which the parts are arranged and combined; it gives unity to the whole and validity to the parts. Piecemeal analysis of the parts of experience, as carried out by experimental psychology, cannot provide an understanding of the whole. In this view structural psychology aimed to understand the wholeness of experience in which affect, drive, feelings, behaviour, and the way the individual understands the self in the world are combined. Leonhard, on the other hand, did not refer to the concept of structure, but applied himself particularly to the subdivision of psychoses into distinct entities according to their symptomatological and evolutionary features.

Conrad's morpho-analytical approach

It had first been proposed by Jaspers — and then clarified in respect of symptomatology by Kurt Schneider — that psychotic phenomena are characterised by their incomprehensibility. This view had exerted enormous influence in the psychiatry of German-speaking countries, but when Klaus Conrad developed his model, attempts were being made to refute it. Jaspers claimed that no phenomena which had a primary somatic origin could be understood through empathy. This led him to create a distinction between phenomena which were only quantitatively abnormal and those which were qualitatively abnormal. However, this viewpoint was particularly disputed by psychotherapists, whose fundamental approach involved considerations based on existential and phenomenological philosophy. They increasingly distanced themselves from an interpretation of psychopathological phenomena along the lines of Freud's theory of libido; instead, their attention was mainly focused on the relationship of a subject with the surrounding environment. From this arose an increasing tendency to concentrate less on understanding existing symptoms, but rather to consider them only as the expression of a modified 'being in the world', not fundamentally different from that of the normal person. It was assumed that this existential change differed from normality only in intensity and length of time involved. This new view of psychopathology was a return to the concept — introduced by structural psychology and further developed by Gestalt psychology — that any perceptual experience is a structured configuration in which the whole is more than the sum of its parts.

In this context, Conrad assumed that this configuration structuring is impeded in psychotic disorders and that this modifies the relationship between the subject and his environment. In his book on *Early Schizophrenia*, published in 1958, he emphasised that three phases can be distinguished during this process: the first is initiated by an increase in affective tension — of emotional background activity — which attributes increased importance to the aspects of the object or person which are perceived. This reduces the applicability of the 'epicritical' reference system that normally allows the subject to evaluate his relationship with the world realistically. The resulting impression is that something strange or unusual is happening. During the next stage, the epicritical reference system is gradually replaced by a 'protopathic' system, which is phylogenetically and ontogenetically older: the subject has the feeling of gaining special insight into his experiences and of being the centre of attention. He can then no longer take 'the view of Copernicus', i.e. admit that everything does not revolve around him. In the third phase, the fields of experience and cognitive links are destructured. Similar developments in symptomatology had been observed by Conrad in symptomatic psychoses of somatic origin. This led him to the conclusion that there are no harmful influences which produce specific symptoms; they only cause a functional change which results in the modification of performance. In organic psychoses, however, these influences can attain a degree of influence in consciousness which is not seen in schizophrenics. Conrad attributed this to a severe destructuring of the field of experience, preventing the subject from 'finding himself'. But what differentiated organic psychoses even more clearly, in his view, was that the psychotic stage in schizophrenics was followed by a loss of energy potential which caused residual deficit states to become established. In this 'loss of potential', he identified the specific modification of cerebral functioning which occurs in schizophrenics. Therefore, he believed that fundamental neurobiological and neuropsychological research should concentrate on the exact onset of this disturbance.

Conrad's efforts to obtain some kind of synthesis between phenomenological psychopathology and medicine as a natural science made him one of the most influential people in German-speaking psychiatry in the 1950s. After a post as director of the neuropsychiatric clinic in Homburg, he was appointed in 1958 to be director of the newly opened university neuropsychiatric clinic in Göttingen, which was at the time the most modern in Germany. In the same year, he was asked to advise on the reopening of the Institute of Psychiatric Research in Munich, and was expected to take up a position there, but his premature death prevented that appointment from taking place.

Conrad and Janzarik referred to the notion of 'structure' in different ways: Conrad described how the actual field of experience was structured during the successive phases of emerging psychoses, and called this "morpho-analysis". On the other hand, Janzarik reduced the term to a relatively stable personal hierarchical organisation of inborn recognition patterns and acquired mental representations. These determined how the subject experienced changes of feeling and drive.

Janzarik's 'structural-dynamic coherency model'

Conrad referred to the notion of structure mainly in relation to the configuration of perceptual experiences, whereas Werner Janzarik used this term with reference to the hierarchical organisation of the content of the mind. In his concept of 'structural-dynamic coherency', he designated as 'dynamics' a fundamental realm embracing affectivity and drive, in contrast to the 'psychic structure' which contains inborn recognition patterns and acquired representations. The inborn recognition patterns and parts of the psychic structure were described as 'dynamically invested', i.e. connected with positive, negative, or ambivalent feelings. These dynamically loaded parts of the structure were called 'values', but dynamics were not completely tied to structural elements. It was proposed that everybody has a certain amount of 'free floating dynamics' available, but subject to alteration. When these modifications reach the extent of morbidity, they correspond either to 'dynamic depletion', which is seen clinically as affective blunting, or to 'dynamic derailment'.

Janzarik defined three types of such derailment: dynamic 'expansion', as in mania; 'restriction', as in depression; and 'instability', which is characterised by rapid 'swings' between the first two states. Normally, inborn recognition patterns and personal values are continuously kept in the background by neutral representations. These form a hierarchy of reaction tendencies, based on learned experience, and permit a critical, realistic evaluation of the environment, which was described as the 'representative perception modus'. This reality-testing may, however, be distorted by the exaggerated influence of personal values, which is provoked by the derailment of the free-floating dynamics. This process sets in motion the 'impressive recognition modus', which is normally repressed.

Stable derailment actualises values corresponding to their mood tinge which can no longer be counterbalanced by a critical estimation of the real situation. In states of dynamic instability, rapid changes in different parts of the structure provoke a profound disturbance of reality-testing, which initiates the emergence of psychotic phenomena.

Janzarik held the view that the different types of endogenous psychoses are not separate disease entities, but rather result from a common predisposition to dynamic instability and may be triggered by somatic or psychosocial stress. The different forms of this 'unitary psychosis' are then determined by two pathoplastic conditions — the strength of the cognitive structure and the habitual dynamic level — which correspond to the familiar notions of 'character' and 'temperament'. Strong cognitive structures were thought to channel the resulting instability into stable derailment, whereas weak structures would allow the instability to become manifest as psychotic deterioration. The outcome may then take one of a number of forms: (a) If the normal dynamic level is high and the structure strong, the dynamic derailment is transformed — under the impact of the actual life situation — either into a depressive or a manic mood state. Very strong and rigid structures, accompanied by a low habitual dynamic level, transform the instability into depressive derailment. (b) On the other hand, weak structures fail to repress the instability and as a result, experiences of strangeness, mood-incongruent delusions, and hallucinations will appear. If structures are very weak, they collapse under the impact of the dynamic instability, which leads to a disorganisation of thought and behaviour. This may take one of two forms: (i) In subjects whose dynamic level is not abnormally low, the clinical picture then corresponds to positive schizophrenia. (ii) But if very weak structures are combined with a low habitual dynamic level, psychotic phenomena are not strongly evoked, whereas the dynamic deficiency and withdrawal reactions dominate the clinical picture. This latter constellation is thought to be the basis of negative schizophrenia. (c) In the presence of a somewhat stronger structure and a high habitual dynamic level, disorganisation of thought and behaviour does not occur. The initial delusional atmosphere then evolves into more structured, organised delusions, accompanied by more typical manic and depressive mood swings, without affective blunting. This situation corresponds to the schizoaffective type of the unitary psychosis. (d) The 'dynamic depletion' observed in schizophrenics is explained by a pre-existing low habitual dynamic level coming to the fore. In psychoses which can be attributed to an organic cause, Janzarik assumed that the clinical picture is triggered by a dynamic instability, caused by a somatic cerebral obstruction.

In 1959, Janzarik had first published his model, when he was still a university lecturer at Mainz. It became widely used in German psychiatry and was decisive in his being appointed director of the Heidelberg University Psychiatric Clinic in 1973.

Leonhard's classification

In 1957, Karl Leonhard published a classification which was based on the nosological approaches of Kleist. Contrary to the usual dichotomy into which endogenous psychoses had been split since the time of Kraepelin, he subdivided them into a large number of distinct entities. However, Leonhard replaced the cerebral-localising theories of Wernicke and Kleist by the hypothesis that the diversity of endogenous psychoses rests on different genetic predispositions. He therefore distinguished, firstly, between the 'pure form' (unipolar) and 'multi-form' (bipolar) psychoses, and secondly, in the schizophrenic group, between 'typical' (progressively deteriorating) and 'atypical' (characterised by recurrent episodes) forms. Each of these categories was subdivided into several sub-groups, according to their symptomatology and evolution. Leonhard was appointed professor in psychiatry and neurology at the Medical Academy of Erfurt in 1955 and director of the neurological university clinic at the Charité Hospital, Berlin in 1957. His opposition to dimensional approaches to the endogenous psychoses has stimulated discussion right up to the present day, both on the pros and cons of unitary psychosis as well as on the validity of definitions of schizophrenia and manic–depressive psychosis which had been suggested by the traditional European nosologies.

The French contribution

Ey's organodynamism

From the early 1930s, Henri Ey started to apply Hughlings Jackson's neurological principles in the field of psychiatry. Then, during the 1950s, the development of his 'organodynamic' concept made a deep impact on psychiatric thought in France. It was widely disseminated in the psychiatric manual published by Ey, Bernard, and Brisset in 1960. His model took as its starting-point Jackson's idea that the central nervous system constitutes an onto- and phylogenetic hierarchy of nerve centres arranged in layers, with the higher situated ones controlling (i.e. inhibiting) those of lower layers. In applying this approach to psychiatric problems, Ey assumed that mental illness has an organic origin which both suppresses the function at the affected level — producing negative symptoms — and releases functions which were until then under control — resulting in positive symptoms. In this context, psychoses and neuroses were no longer considered as entities, but as syndromes whose form is determined by the level at which disintegration causing regression to a lower level takes place. Ey attributed acute psychoses to a destructuring of the actual field of conscience by distinguishing three degrees: minor (mania or depression), average (brief delusional and schizophrenic-type disorders), and severe (confusional psychoses). Chronic disorders, on the other hand, were considered to result from a destructuring of the personality in which the degree of severity could also be defined: minor (pathological personalities and neuroses); average (chronic psychotic psychoses and schizophrenia); and severe (dementia). Ey's thinking incorporated the concepts of Janet and some of Freud's, but refuted the hypothesis of a psycho- or sociogenesis of mental disorders. His 'neo-Jacksonian' model has much in common with that of Conrad, with whom he had an intense and extremely cordial exchange of views. From 1948 onwards, Ey organised a number of symposia at the psychiatric hospital in Bonneval, where he had been medical director since 1933. In his position as editor-in-chief of *Evolution Psychiatrique*, he also contributed to lively discussions between the various currents of psychiatry in the 1950s (Chapter 5, p. 135).

Contributions by Delay *et al.*

Jean Delay had been professor at the Psychiatric Clinic of Saint Anne Hospital, Paris since 1946. In his book *Les déreglements de l'humeur* of 1947, he had proposed a distinction between two types of psycho-affective disturbance: 'hypothymic', considered to be the basis of schizophrenic hebephrenia, and 'hyperthymic'. In the latter, he identified a point of distress reached in depression and a point of euphoria reached in manic phases. This particular concept was prominent in discussions during the 1950s on the pathogenetic role of psycho-affective derailment. But Delay influenced the evolution of psychiatry even more strongly during this period by systematically pursuing his view of mental illness as a two-sided problem — to be explored in future by both biological and psychological methods.

In applying the first of these approaches, Delay undertook significant pharmacotherapeutic research with Pierre Deniker (this chapter, p. 179), in addition to studies of the experimental psychoses caused by hallucinogenic drugs. This research provided the impetus for the beginning of psychopharmacology, and led him to devise the term 'neuroleptic'. Central to this work was the use of psychometric tests at the onset of psychiatric disorders; it was described in a seminal work — *Méthodes Psychométriques en Clinique* — with P Pichot and J Perse in 1959. Delay's research on psychometric methods for in-patients had been strongly influenced by Pichot, who had worked on the appropriate use and validity of psychological tests since the 1940s. The results of these were published extensively in the 1950s, both in scientific journals and particularly in the book, *Les Tests Mentaux*, in 1954. The clarity with which Pichot analysed and grouped these tests according to their method and field of application played a major part in the effective integration of such techniques into current psychiatric research and practice.

Synthetic approaches

During the 1950s, European psychiatry made increased efforts both to harmonise the various schools of thought which had formed during the preceding decades and to integrate their new concepts. This was followed by the more effective application of multidimensional approaches to psychiatric problems, which subsequently also affected the treatment of patients.

Contributions from European countries participating in this development in the early stages varied according to the ideas in vogue at the time. In Germany, psychoanalysis had very little impact during this period; it was found only as part of a multidimensional concept, as envisaged by the Tübingen school. On the other hand, philosophical, phenomenological, and existential approaches played an important role — as they did in Spain and the Netherlands. In France, however, philosophical approaches held very little influence, while the psychoanalytic vogue, which sometimes attempted to find links with existentialism, only took hold to any significant extent towards the end of the decade. In Switzerland, both psychoanalytical hypotheses and existential approaches were widely influential, and both these points of view also held sway in Austria, though not in British or Scandinavian psychiatry. After emigrating to England in 1933, Willy Mayer-Gross was responsible for disseminating German nosological and psychopathological concepts in that country when he published his manual *Clinical Psychiatry* with Eliot Slater and Sir Martin Roth in 1954 (Chapter 00, p. xx). These German approaches also served as guidelines in Scandinavia, but were modified there by the importance attributed to distinguishing between psychogenic and endogenous psychoses and to the separation of schizophrenia from schizophreniform psychoses.

Confrontation of concepts

Two important efforts were made in the 1950s to obtain a convergence of the different current concepts: the organisation of the second World Congress of Psychiatry and the planning of a comprehensive account of contemporary psychiatry.

The second World Congress, held in 1957, was the only one to focus on a single topic: schizophrenia. This was not only due to it being held in Zurich, the city where Bleuler, the creator of the term 'schizophrenia' had worked. The main reason lies in the fact that this illness lent itself particularly to highlighting the differences between the various European approaches. These confrontations enabled the proponents of different schools to get to know one another, and significantly encouraged later exchanges of views.

The publication of a work on contemporary psychiatry arose from the fact that the standard German manual of psychiatry by Bumke had been out of print since 1936. In 1956, HW Gruhle, R Jung, W Mayer-Gross, and M Müller determined to fill this gap by planning a work which covered the international evolution of psychiatry during the previous decades. The section on clinical psychiatry — *Psychiatrie der Gegenwart, Vol. II* — appeared in 1960, followed by the other four volumes. Most of the authors contributing to this work, which attempted to summarise current psychiatric research in a number of countries, were Europeans who had played an active part in advancing these concepts. It therefore became a very important landmark in the process of understanding both the divergence and convergence between the various European experts.

Multidimensional approaches

Interest in interactions between somatic and environmental factors in the genesis of mental illness had already been shown earlier in the century, particularly by Eugen Bleuler and Ernst Kretschmer. They were both profoundly influenced by Freud's ideas, while maintaining a certain distance from his more dogmatic convictions. Bleuler had integrated psychoanalysis into his concept of schizophrenia, which he considered to have an organic basis, by attributing the formation of secondary symptoms to the coming into play of defence mechanisms. This viewpoint encouraged his followers, and especially his son Manfred, to pursue both biological and psychodynamic approaches simultaneously. The most striking achievement of this strategy concerned the elucidation of interactions between endocrine-based and psychological processes. Manfred Bleuler described these comprehensively in 1954 in his book on endocrinological psychiatry. It mainly highlighted the way that emotional and impulsive disturbances, triggered by an endocrine-based dysfunction of primarily organic origin, could be interpreted according to the psychological structure of each patient. Whilst acknowledging that the hypothesis of a psychogenesis of endocrine-based illness still required further investigation, Manfred Bleuler emphasised that endocrine-based features could reveal a liability to neurotic sequelae (Chapter 10, p. 347).

Earlier, Kretschmer had argued for the necessity of a 'multidimensional diagnosis' in psychiatric thinking. At the same time, in each individual case, treatment should take into consideration the particular biological, psychological, and social conditions that had been involved in the development of that patient's disorder. During the 1950s, this view spread from Germany to other countries, particularly Scandinavia, where the role of constitutional factors was also included. In England, where Sir Aubrey Lewis had stressed the importance of basing research on rigorous methodology, Mayer-Gross, Slater, and Roth put the case for a multidimensional diagnosis which would rest on definitions and measurements resulting from precise investigations, rather than on psychoanalytical hypotheses. This viewpoint strongly encouraged the evaluation of tests, the construction of rating scales, and the undertaking of epidemiological studies in that country.

In Austria at this time, the multidimensional perspective became the guiding force in psychiatry under the aegis of Hans Hoff, who occupied the chair of neuropsychiatry in Vienna from 1950 to 1969. Knowledge of depth psychology had awakened his interest in the question of how psychoses whose genetic basis he did not doubt could be influenced by other factors. Depth psychology is a generic term (coined in 1910 by Bleuler) for all psychotherapeutic trends which emanated from Freud's original concept. Thus, it embraced psychoanalysis, Adler's 'individual psychology' (Chapter 2, p. 42), and Jung's 'analytical psychology' (Chapter 3, p. 71).

Through an exchange of ideas with Manfred Bleuler and Ernst Kretschmer, Hoff therefore developed his multifactorial conception of 'endogenous' psychoses. In distinguishing between predisposing and triggering factors, he assumed that differing genetic predispositions to schizophrenia or manic–depressive disorder increased the risk of these psychoses occurring and determined their specific symptoms. But it was particularly emphasised that additional somatic factors, such as constitutional features, inherited illnesses, or drugs, as well as psycho-social influences, not only play a pathoplastic or triggering role, but can also become predisposing conditions. This viewpoint, which was first presented in his book, *Lehrbuch der Psychiatrie*, in 1957, contained the beginnings of concepts which would be seen later in vulnerability models.

Modifications to treatment

During the 1950s, changes in the treatment of psychiatric illness became increasingly important in Europe. The need for reform of this kind had already been demonstrated by both British and French psychiatrists who, on the basis of their experience in prisoner of war camps, had noted that the detrimental effects of such imprisonment were similar to the alienation often occurring in the asylum. This approach obtained solid support from social psychiatry which, through the results of epidemiological research, demonstrated the pathogenetic role of certain social and family structures. Towards the middle of the century, this began to stand out as a separate discipline. Its development was strongly encouraged by research which had focused on both cultural anthropology and group dynamics. In addition, the influence of the American mental health movement in Europe encouraged the influence of psychoanalytic concepts in socio-psychiatric discussions towards the end of the 1950s.

Institutional reform

While reform of the psychiatric services in Britain was mainly determined by the concept of the 'therapeutic community', in France also there was a move towards improved communication between staff and patient. Out of this came a movement for psychiatric carers to be more sensitive psychotherapeutically; team meetings with therapeutic aims were introduced, using group techniques such as that of Moreno (Chapter 5, p. 142). But these attempts, which involved trusting psychotherapeutic functions to nurses, were decried by many French psychiatrists. This was not only because they feared losing part of their power, but also because of their opposition to the psychoanalytic hypotheses which were often the inspiration for this type of approach. In the early 1950s, French resistance to Freudian theory was principally maintained by psychiatrists with quasi-Marxist views, who considered psychoanalysis to be "an instrument of the domination of capitalism". Though this anti-psychoanalytic position weakened with the political changes which followed Stalin's death in 1953, it was still a major influence as late as 1958.

In 1945, a syndicate of psychiatric hospital doctors, which had formed in France at the end of the war, presented some guiding principles on the reassessment of psychiatric treatment, stressing the unity of prophylaxis, prevention, treatment, and after-care. They underlined the fact that this unity could only be accomplished by the same care team, responsible for a defined territory. The psychiatrists at the heart of this reform were known as the 'Sèvres Group', whose leading lights included Bonnafé, Daumezon, and Le Guillant. Their name came from the fact that they organised two debates on these matters in an educational training centre in Sèvres. The first of these debates in 1958 was devoted to the role of staff and psychotherapy in psychiatric treatment; the second in 1959 to the conceptualisation of sectors. The 'Sèvres Group' were particularly concerned with the reform of psychiatric institutions, a process which remained largely centred on sociotherapy. This aimed at a resumption of normal relations between the patient and his environment, as well as the integration of varied psychotherapeutic techniques within 'institutional psychiatry'. A more strictly psychoanalytic direction would take hold only from the 1960s.

Sectorisation

The attempts of the 1950s to restructure institutional psychiatry by centring it mainly around social therapy highlighted the need to apply this equally to the out-patient field, by putting in place dispensaries in the patients' residential area. Encouraged by Paumelle, a group of doctors decided in 1954 to implement this concept by creating this type of sector-based service in the 13th arrondissement of Paris. This institution worked initially without a hospital by setting up in the premises of a traditional tuberculosis-prevention clinic, where with social security funding, it installed dispensaries centred around the "Association of mental health and struggle against alcoholism", created in 1958. This structure was completed in 1959 by the opening of a therapeutic workshop and the acquisition of land on which to build a hospital.

Implementation of the '13th arrondissement of Paris sector' resulted in an important change in the treatment of mental patients in France. This enterprise aimed to avoid or reduce hospitalisation to a minimum, but also to ensure that if it was necessary, it would take place in the patient's residential area. To this end, a series of facilities were opened in that locality: a mental health dispensary or consulting centre, a day hospital, an after-care home offering the patient meals and accommodation during the period of rehabilitation, and sheltered housing. This combination of out- and in-patient care in a defined geographical area served by teams of carers was recommended by the government in 1960 for all public mental health services, but would only become a reality 10 years later.

Repercussions

In much of Europe, the momentum deriving from these new visions for treatment led to a series of reforms. Aiming first to modify the legal conditions of psychiatric care, these focused on a reduction of in-patient admissions, but then inclined more and more towards the systematic organisation of out-patient services. Sectorisation was an important influence in these developments. In 1953, WHO set up an Expert Committee on Mental Health which encouraged the establishment of similar professional bodies in several countries. While these were concerned with implementing overall national plans, many independent initiatives were also being taken to create new services outside the psychiatric hospital. These proposals were often designed for the treatment or rehabilitation of specific groups of patients, such as alcoholics, drug addicts, criminals with mental illness, or schizophrenics undergoing rehabilitation. Implementation of most of the reforms and treatment projects set up in Europe during the 1950s began to take place only towards the end of this decade. In subsequent years, though, further progress was considerably helped by advances in pharmacotherapy and by the acceptance of multidimensional approaches to mental illness.

THERAPEUTIC COMMUNITIES

by David Millard

The use of therapeutic community techniques developed strongly during the 1950s, but for the origins of the movement, we have to look back over the preceding few years. A tendency exists to refer loosely to any form of residential regime which is broadly benign in its intentions and operation as a 'therapeutic community'. But the term is properly confined to a quite specific set of ideas and practices which developed from the work of a handful of British psychiatrists during the Second World War and the immediate post-war period. There were related developments in the United States, but the therapeutic community as it now exists in many parts of the world is essentially a British invention.

Its history is partly a matter of individuals and partly of the psychiatric institutions with which they were associated. Amongst the originators, the names of two British psychiatrists are pre-eminent. The first was Maxwell Jones (1907–1990), who in 1947 opened the Henderson Hospital — now an independent unit, but at that time a department in a traditional mental hospital in South London. He remained as its Director until 1959, later becoming Medical Superintendent of Dingleton, a psychiatric hospital in Scotland. The other was Thomas Main (1911–1990), Medical Director of the Cassel Hospital, London from 1946 to 1976. The pathways taken in these two centres towards an elaborated and largely agreed set of principles followed parallel, though somewhat separate lines.

Mill Hill to the Henderson

Having worked in Edinburgh and, more briefly, the United States, Maxwell Jones joined the staff of the Maudsley Hospital in 1938. His research interests then were in psychosomatic disorder — particularly in the physiological correlates of neurosis. With the outbreak of war, the Maudsley was evacuated and a section of the hospital was relocated in the buildings of a boarding school at Mill Hill in North London. Jones (almost universally known as 'Max') was placed in charge of a special unit of 100 beds for service personnel suffering from Da Costa's (or Effort) syndrome. Together with the cardiologist, Paul Wood, a number of papers were published in the early 1940s on biochemical indicators associated with the syndrome of left-sided chest pain, breathlessness, giddiness, etc. From the psychiatric perspective, there were attempts to treat these cardiac neuroses with individual psychotherapy — but with difficulty under the conditions of a large case load and a small staff. Hence, as Jones wrote in 1942 in his earliest paper in the field of social therapy, "It was decided to try a form of group therapy... The treatment was tried on a group of 50 patients, the remaining 50 being given individual psychotherapy".

This was the first manifestation of what has been called the 'proto-therapeutic community'. For the remainder of his career, Jones became a social therapist — or, as he liked to style himself, — an 'agent of social change'. At Mill Hill, the regime quickly came to include a meeting three times weekly of the whole community of patients and staff, which was educational in style. Beginning with a talk lasting 20 to 30 minutes, there followed time for 'open discussion'. The intention was that patients should begin to understand something of the nature of the psychosomatic mechanisms underlying their own illnesses. The other major emphasis was on group responsibility. Under the prevailing military conditions, this was seen as closely linked with morale and as involving some sacrifice of individual interests in favour of the larger group, the war effort, and a patriotic responsibility to the nation.

Two changes gradually evolved: firstly, by 1944, only about one-third of the patients had Effort syndrome, the remainder having anxiety states or depression and being, in Jones's words "the more chronically constitutionally endowed".

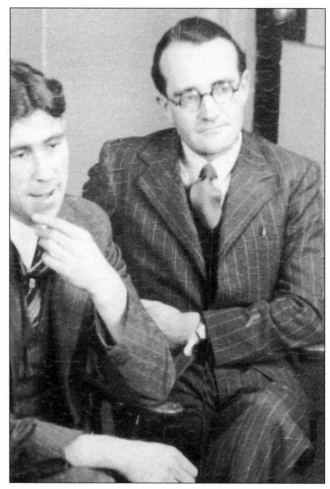

Maxwell Jones (right). Reproduced with permission from The Henderson Hospital, The St Helier NHS Trust.

Secondly, although educational techniques continued to be used, an increasingly reliance was placed on the potential of the group itself. As he later recalled:

> "It was all tremendously exciting as patients and staff were working together in furthering treatment with the patients themselves being a valuable resource for teaching... they listened with open ears to their peers. We were there as resource people and didn't say too much because there was always a nucleus of patients who understood their clinical state, as they learned what we had learned about the lack of homeostasis in relation to their exercise physiology".

Thus was born the use in psychiatry of the large group, although the Mill Hill regime also included the use of small groups. Moreover, Jones developed the idea that within the boundary of the unit, treatment was a continuous process operating throughout the working day and over every aspect of the life of the patient. Finally, he recognised that a more open style of communication inevitably resulted in changes in the power structure of the unit, with some flattening of the hierarchical relationship between doctors, nurses and other staff, and the patients.

All these are notions central to the therapeutic community ideology. They were transferred by Jones in 1946 to his next job as psychiatrist in charge of a 300-bed unit in a military hospital designed to assist in the rehabilitation of the most disabled amongst prisoners of war returning from Europe. Here, the work was expanded to include an important community dimension: facilitating the placement of patients in civilian work. So successful was this that the Ministry of Health was persuaded to establish at Belmont Hospital in Surrey an experimental Industrial Neurosis Unit. This was to deal with the rehabilitation of unemployed civilian casualties of society, rather than of war. In 1959, just as Jones was leaving, this unit was renamed the Henderson Hospital. By this time, the major features of the therapeutic community were well established. The figure opposite shows the main structural features of the Henderson model.

Contemporary therapeutic community theory still adheres to the principles established in the 1950s. The community meeting is a locus of the administrative discussion (itself therapeutic in intention), which is essential to a (at least partially) self-governing organisation. It is also the setting of more direct 'large group' therapy. Community meetings should be regularly associated with a staff group, whose function is to gain understanding of the material discussed by the community as a whole. Other groups comprise directly

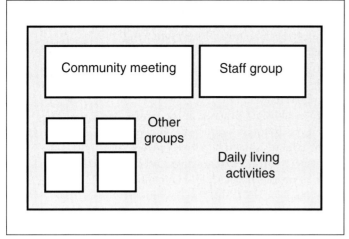

Therapeutic community structure. Adapted from Millard and Oakley, 1994, with permission from Routledge Publishers.

therapeutic groups, the exact nature of which varies between communities, but usually includes verbal (psychotherapeutic), creative (art or drama therapy), and work-related (community planning or maintenance) methods. The black lines in the figure above represent the boundaries. Members' observance or breach of these in their physical, temporal, personal, or symbolic aspects often constitutes the material for the community's discussion. The background of daily living activities (shaded in the figure) — i.e. the remainder of the available space/time — is also vitally important. It is central to the theory of therapeutic communities that no action-based programme is successful unless the gains (however small) made by patients are brought to some form of conscious recognition and verbal expression; while no verbal approach is complete unless the gains are tested and reinforced in action.

The close of the 1950s was marked by the publication of a major study of the Henderson which has become something of a classic in the therapeutic community literature, the Rapoports' *Community as Doctor* (1960). Here four principles that have since gained wide acceptance were defined: *permissiveness, communalism, democratisation,* and *reality confrontation.* Therapeutic communities act essentially on the meaningfulness of behaviour. Being socially relatively unstructured, they encourage members to act in accordance with their internalised rules of behaviour. Typically, they will then replicate in the community the difficulties which brought them there (*permissiveness*). All events in the community are regarded, in principle, as shared property (*communalism*) and are subject to observation and comment by other members (*democratisation*). Where these need to be modified (*reality confrontation*), the community will suggest how this should happen and will support the processes of change in the individual.

Northfield to the Cassel

Independently of Jones's work, developments occurred at a mental hospital in Birmingham which in 1942 had become the Northfield Military Hospital and included a rehabilitation unit for servicemen with neurosis. Under the Army Psychiatric Services, which were considerably influenced by personalities associated with the Tavistock Clinic, this was the site of what subsequently became known as the two 'Northfield Experiments'. The first was in 1943 and the second, for about 18 months, in 1944–46. Amongst the most influential figures involved here were the psychoanalysts Wilfred Bion, John Rickman, Harold Bridger, and SH Foulkes (who later founded group analysis) and the psychiatrist TF ('Tom') Main, who trained as a psychoanalyst after the war. The work of the second Northfield Experiment was written up in 1946 in the *Bulletin of the Menninger Clinic* where Main first introduced the use of the term *therapeutic community.*

"A Therapeutic Community

The Northfield Experiment is an attempt to use a hospital not as an organisation run by doctors in the interests of their own technical efficiency, but as a community with the aim of full participation of all its members in its daily life and the central aim of the resocialisation of the neurotic individual for a life in organised society".

The subsequent work of Main and his colleagues at the Cassel Hospital, throughout the 1950s and beyond, built on this experience.

The first, short-lived Northfield Experiment took place in the Rehabilitation Wing, where Bion was the commanding officer. It had developed serious problems of "slackness, indiscipline and aggressive untidiness". He tackled this by giving the soldiers opportunities to realise that the solutions were largely in their own hands. Bion gave the appearance of relinquishing responsibility for solving the problems brought to him — thus forcing the men to fall back on their own resources. He instituted a regime of a few simple regulations, including the requirement that all men were to belong to one or more activity groups and that they could create a new one if nothing suitable existed. A 30-minute parade would be held each day "for making announcements and conducting other business". He thereby set up in practice a system of small and large groups with some potential for patients to reflect upon their own behaviour, and perhaps come to understand it better.

This first experiment fell foul of the hospital authorities and was abruptly concluded, but the second took better care to involve the wider environment (in this case, the total hospital community and its administration). It therefore became possible, even in a military hospital, to sustain an unconventional regime in which there was a conscious modification of power relationships between staff and patients in favour of a more egalitarian, self-directed approach to treatment. The group programme, and a wide range of patient-organised activities, continued to be the principal substrate for therapy.

When Main went to the Cassel Hospital, it had an established practice in the psycho-dynamic treatment of the neuroses extending back to its foundation in 1919. However, he had brought from Northfield an insistence that the patients should be actively involved in the planning and organising of the daily life of the hospital and that tensions and conflicts, both in the whole hospital community and in its various parts, should be continuously studied. Without abandoning individual psychoanalytic work, this involved the use of daily community meetings, a variety of small groups, and staff groups — the whole contributing to what Main came to call a "culture of enquiry".

Three specific emphases developed at the Cassel during the 1950s. The first was the great emphasis placed upon staff groups. While these had been an inevitable part of every therapeutic community regime, they came to particular prominence here. This was both as a source of support in a particularly demanding form of work, and also as the forum for examining staff disagreements which (as became increasingly clear) are a potent contributor to patients' malfunctioning in therapeutic settings. Secondly, and linked to this, the changes in staff relationships led to the development of the concept of *psycho-social nursing*. Supported by senior nurses at the Cassel, and later more widely, this became an influential strand in the evolution of modern concepts of the role of the psychiatric nurse. It was now seen as being therapeutic, rather than custodial or simply caring. Thirdly, a particular patient of Main was unable to accept admission to the Cassel because she had a young child, and this led to the development of what was probably the first mother and baby in-patient facility. It also led to a strong emphasis on working with families — a further example of formative influence from the Cassel upon a mode of psychiatric practice which became widely adopted as the century progressed.

The wider context

All these developments had points of contact with the wider world of psychiatry. The 1950s saw what some (consciously employing a nineteenth-century concept) called the new 'moral treatment': that process of liberalising the mainly custodial regimes which had grown up in the large mental hospitals. This was a social movement within psychiatry, reflecting profound changes in the wider society, which preceded but was much assisted by the arrival of new psychotropic drugs. It included strategies such as reducing the size of institutions and their individual wards, open-door policies, encouraging easier contact with the wider community, modern occupational therapies, and the promotion of therapeutic attitudes within the multi-disciplinary staff team. It was recorded in publications such as Greenblatt *et al.*'s *From Custodial to Therapeutic Patient Care in Mental Hospitals* (1955) or Russell Barton's *Institutional Neurosis* (1959). Therapeutic communities were part (but no means the whole) of this trend. A significant number of British mental hospitals introduced replications of such regimes. Denis Martin in *Adventure in Psychiatry* (1962) described this process in one near London, while David Clark in *Social Therapy in Psychiatry* (1974) recorded similar work in Cambridge which had begun in 1953. Later, Clark was to make the important distinction between the *therapeutic community proper* — as at the Henderson — and the *therapeutic community approach*. The latter meant partial implementations of the concept in other psychiatric settings. Even today, those units which continue to hold a periodic ward or community meeting represent a persistent and often unacknowledged legacy of the therapeutic community movement.

The second contextual reference is international. During the 1950s, therapeutic communities were established sporadically in many countries. An example was a unit in Sydney, Australia which opened in 1959 and was described in the monograph *Fraser House: Theory, Practice and Evaluation of a Therapeutic Community* (1969) by Clark and Yeomans. But the main developments outside Britain were in the USA, where there was a rather different point of departure. From the 1930s, there had been an interest there in a psychoanalytic approach to work in psychiatric hospitals, but in the 1950s, this was joined by a wave of academic interest in such institutions by social scientists. The Cassel maintained links with a similar institution in the USA, Chestnut Lodge, where research by a sociologist and psychiatrist team, Stanton and Schwartz, was published in *The Mental Hospital* (1954). This included the first description of a virtual axiom of residential therapy theory — the causal relationship between covert staff disagreement and disturbed patient behaviour.

A number of major sociological studies of psychiatric hospitals appeared at about this time, the culmination of which was, perhaps, John and Elaine Cummings' *Ego and Milieu* (1962) and a somewhat more popular account, Ervine Goffman's *Asylums* (1961). Visits across the Atlantic in both directions were made by senior psychiatrists — as early as 1946 Karl Meninger wrote of British psychiatry: "One of the things that impressed us most was the skilful use the principles of group psychology and group dependency in therapeutic programs of various types". By 1966, Alan Kraft was able to contribute a confident chapter on 'The Therapeutic Community' to Volume 3 of the *American Handbook of Psychiatry*. Maxwell Jones himself moved to the USA in 1959, worked for three years in Oregon, and then returned to spend seven years in Scotland, before finally settling once again in North America.

Jones's own work remained within psychiatric and penal institutions, while 'democratic' therapeutic communities continued a significant presence within the conventional provision. However, the later growth of therapeutic communities in the USA was predominantly in the field of substance abuse, and is associated with institutions such as Synanon (of which Yablonsky published an account as early as 1965), Daytop Village, and Phoenix House in New York. These so-called concept houses, became known in subsequent decades as 'new' therapeutic communities; in contrast to the 'old' model of Maxwell Jones. They shared only partly in the old ideology. They were frequently set up and staffed by ex-addicts. Although they, like their predecessors, rejected the automatic assumption that most therapeutic potential resided in the formally qualified staff, unlike the earlier communities, they were often rather illiberal in their regimes and authoritarian in their social structures. Therapeutic communities of this type also flourished for a time in parts of Europe; although elsewhere, notably Holland and in Scandinavia, institutions based on the older model continued to be the norm. Efforts to reconcile the two models have had only limited success, and it seems possible that historians of the new millennium will find the principles and practices first established in the 1940s and 1950s to have an enduring place in the repertoire of mental health provision.

PSYCHOSURGERY

by George Fenton

The relationship between the frontal lobes and the mind was first highlighted by the dramatic story of Phineus Gage, a 25-year-old construction foreman employed by a railway in Vermont, USA. He was preparing a hole for blasting powder when an explosion occurred. This drove a long, steel rod through his left cheek, up through the frontal lobes and exiting from the skull near the sagittal suture. The young man was taken by ox cart to a local hotel, where he was attended by a small-town doctor named John M Harlow. To everyone's surprise, Gage survived. Though his physical recovery was complete, his personality changed dramatically following the frontal lobe trauma. Previously a stable, energetic, organised, and reliable worker, he became disinhibited, unreliable, foul-mouthed, euphoric, lacking in judgement, irritable, and tactless. He lacked initiative, had little ability to plan ahead, and was prone to act on impulse. Harlow cared for him until his death, and described his story in a letter to the *New England Journal of Medicine* in December 1848. The case of Phineus Gage was later referred to as the 'American crow bar case'.

Analyses of the cases of large numbers of soldiers with brain injuries suffered during the First World War in Germany showed that the changes in behaviour in many of those with frontal lobe damage were consistent with some of the behaviour that Phineus Gage had displayed.

Releasing demons

Trepanation — making a hole in the skull — began 4–5000 years ago, both in Europe and Northern Africa. It was aimed to release demons, and to relieve melancholia, unbearable pain, and a range of other disorders. The practice spread to the Americas, Asia, New Guinea, Melanesia, Tahiti, and New Zealand and the technique was particularly refined in Peru and Bolivia. In modern times, the first recorded neurosurgery for mental disorder was carried out in Switzerland by Burckhardt *et al.* in 1891. Based on data from early studies of cerebral localisation, areas of cerebral cortex were removed from the post-central, temporal, and frontal regions in six patients, who were described as aggressive and demented. The outcome in three was described as successful, partially successful in two, and the remaining patient died. Puusepp, a neurosurgeon in St Petersburg, acting on Burckhardt's report, operated on three patients with manic–depressive psychosis in 1910, resecting fibres between the parietal and frontal lobes. The results were not promising, though he did not publish the findings until 1937.

Becky, the neurotic chimpanzee

Further impetus for neurosurgery for mental disorder came from the work of Carlyle Jacobson and John Fulton on the frontal lobes of monkeys and chimpanzees at Yale in the early and mid-1930s. Following excision of both right and left anterior frontal association areas, there was no loss of ability to perform visual or auditory discrimination tasks or to recall the spatial orientation of objects, provided the tests involved immediate recall. However, the animals were unable to perform such tasks if a delay of more than a few seconds was introduced between the stimulus and the response. This phenomenon is the now classic delayed-response deficit, which has been shown to be specific for bilateral anterior frontal excisions in primates. The animals' behaviour changed in other important ways. They generally became more placid and lethargic, losing their characteristic inquisitive initiative, with bouts of aimless hyperactivity. They were easily distracted from a task, failing to maintain an attention-set for a given problem. They had great difficulty in adapting to changes in the directions of an already learned task, tending to perseverate. Relatively complicated goal-directed behaviour was no longer possible. These changes in behaviour after bilateral frontal lobectomy were very similar to those described by David Ferrier of Edinburgh in his classic book, *The Functions of the Brain*, published in 1878.

Changes in the behaviour of Jacobsen and Fulton's chimpanzees were particularly striking. Becky displayed a 'neurotic' behaviour problem during baseline testing. In delayed-response tests, she would become impatient, had temper tantrums, and threw herself on the floor, urinating, defaecating, and screaming. After a rest, it was difficult to get her to come back to the test situation. Following operation, however, her behaviour was dramatically different. She seemed pleased to participate in the delayed-response paradigm,

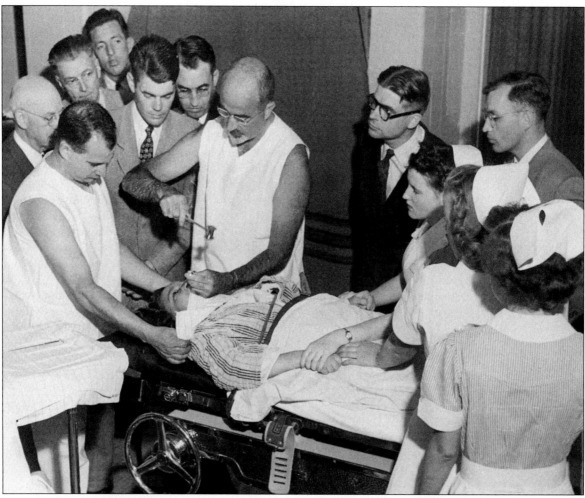

Dr Walter Freeman demonstrates his new surgical technique in an operation called 'transorbital lobotomy' at Western State Hospital (c. 1949). © Corbis/Bettmann.

even though she made many errors, of which she seemed unaware. She showed none of the pre-operative 'neurotic' behaviour. Indeed, Jacobsen commented that she seemed to have joined the 'happiness cult'. In contrast, the second chimpanzee, Lucie, responded in an entirely different way. She performed well on the delayed-response tasks prior to operation, and seemed to enjoy the process. Afterwards, she made many errors and had frequent temper tantrums over delays in food reward that were a consequence of the errors.

The Portuguese dimension

Jacobsen presented data from the experiments with Becky and Lucie at a symposium on frontal lobe function, chaired by Fulton, during the Second World Congress of Neurology, held in London in July 1935. Attending the congress was a former Portuguese Foreign Minister and current professor of neurology in Lisbon, who had distinguished himself by developing cerebral arteriography for the X-ray investigation of brain tumours and other lesions. Moniz (opposite) had an exhibit of his angiography work at the Congress. Next to it was one on ventriculography presented by Walter Freeman, neuropathologist and neurologist from Washington, DC. The two men met for the first time, and both attended the frontal lobe symposium. Both showed particular interest in Jacobsen's paper and in the effect of frontal lobe surgery on Becky's pre-operative 'neurotic' behaviour. Fulton, chairing the session, recalls Moniz getting to his feet after Jacobsen's paper and asking whether frontal lobe removal prevented the development of experimental neurosis in animals. If it eliminated frustrational behaviour, would it not be feasible to relieve anxiety states in humans by surgical means? Fulton was taken aback, thinking it a difficult and dangerous operation to carry out in humans.

Moniz was deterred neither by the potential surgical difficulties nor the fact that Lucie responded quite differently to frontal lobe ablation. On returning to Lisbon after the Congress, he and a young colleague, Almeida Lima, began immediately to develop a technique for psychosurgery. Their first approach was to make burr holes in the skull over the lateral surface of both frontal lobes under local anaesthesia. A long syringe needle was inserted into the white matter of the centrum ovale and absolute alcohol was injected at various sites, so as to make lesions in the frontothalamic pathways in the right and left frontal lobes. The first four patients — two with chronic depression and two with paranoid schizophrenia — were operated on in Lisbon on 12 November 1935. Within the next year, 20 operations had been completed, first using alcohol injections and later a leucotome — an instrument that made 4–6 core lesions in the white matter of each frontal lobe.

The results were presented in March 1936 to the Academy of Medicine in Paris, being published in *Le Bulletin de l'Académie de Médecine*. A monograph published by Masson followed shortly afterwards. Seven patients were considered 'cured', seven significantly improved, and six unchanged. Though considered of minor significance at the time, about half the patients displayed apathy, akinesia, retarded movements or inertia, and loss of initiative — phenomena later recognised as features of the frontal lobe syndrome.

During the autumn of 1936, a further 18 operations were carried out by Lima and Moniz and reported in the *American Journal of Psychiatry*. Moniz gave the name 'prefrontal leucotomy' to his procedure, and later coined the term 'psychosurgery'. Subsequently, he had difficulty recruiting patients because of the hostility of the local psychiatric establishment, but was awarded the Nobel prize for Medicine in 1949.

One Flew Over the Cuckoo's Nest

Several Italian groups, including that of AM Fiamberti from Varese and Dr Emilio Rizzatti, Director of the Racconiga Asylum near Turin, then became active in this field of treatment. Rizzatti's team had performed over 100 leucotomies by 1937. Indeed, the technique became widely adopted such that by 1940, at least 500 operations had been performed in many different countries, including Italy, France, Romania, Brazil, and the USA.

Walter Freeman reviewed Moniz's early work enthusiastically for the *Archives of Neurology and Psychiatry*. He was joined by James Watts, a neurosurgeon in Washington, to form the Department of Neurology and Neurosurgery at George Washington University. After the publication of Moniz's 1936 monograph, they obtained several leucotomes from Paris and performed their first leucotomy in September 1936, following Moniz's procedure, on a patient with agitated depression. Freeman and Watts soon modified Moniz's operation to divide the white matter tracts to and from the frontal lobes more completely. They used a lateral approach by making burr holes at a point behind the canthus of the eye and above the zygoma on each side. Through an avascular area of cortex, blind incisions were made to within a centimetre of the cortical rim, aimed at dividing white matter in the coronal plane. Freeman and Watts performed around 600 such closed operations, the technique being known as their 'standard prefrontal lobotomy'. Perhaps their most famous patient was Rosemary Kennedy, John F Kennedy's sister, who was operated on for depression in 1943, with a disastrous outcome. The Kennedys, however, maintained that she was mentally retarded, presumably to protect the family from the stigma of mental illness. (Paradoxically, this strategy greatly benefited mental retardation research and services, which attracted generous funding during the Kennedy years.)

Next, Freeman revised the technique of Fiamberti to develop transorbital leucotomy. This involved inserting an ice pick-like tool under the eyelids, through the roof of the orbit on each side, angled deep into the frontal lobe, and swept from side to side to sever the frontothalamic tracts. Anaesthesia was provided by two electroconvulsive treatments given in quick succession. This simple approach appealed to mental hospital psychiatrists, but horrified neurosurgeons because it was not carried out under the sterile conditions of the operating theatre and was performed by people who had no sur-

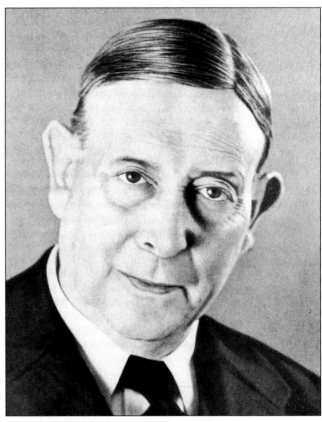

Egas Moniz. Photo courtesy of The Royal College of Psychiatrists, London.

gical training. Freeman promoted prefrontal lobotomy enthusiastically, in both medical circles and in the media. Despite serious reservations by some and vigorous opposition by others, the procedure caught on in American medical practice and by 1950, lobotomies were being carried out at the rate of around 5000 a year.

However, despite its apparent popularity at first, the practice of leucotomy has always aroused controversy and criticism. Ethical concerns focused on the use of a surgical procedure that deliberately damages the brain for its therapeutic effect, the problems of informed consent, and the potential for the operation to be misused to control awkward or socially disapproved behaviour in the absence of pathology. Scientific concerns came from doubts about case selection and the evidence for efficacy, since the published diagnostic and outcome data tended to be 'soft'.

Leucotomy comes to Britain

William Sargant, later to become head of the Department of Psychiatry at St Thomas' Hospital, London, spent a year (1938–39) at Harvard as a Rockefeller Scholar. There, he had met Freeman and examined some of the latter's patients who had been treated by prefrontal lobotomy. On his return to England, he was unable to obtain neurosurgical facilities at Belmont Hospital, outside London, where he then worked, but wrote to Professor Golla, suggesting that the latter should introduce leucotomy in Bristol.

The first operations in Britain were performed in 1940, and reported in the *Lancet* in 1941, accompanied by a cautious but encouraging editorial. EL Hutton, of the Burden Neurological Institute, Bristol, carried out a literature review of 330 patients operated on around the world. The mortality rate was then 2.4%. Of these, 43% were considered recovered, 23% improved, and the rest unchanged, the best outcome being when the predominant clinical features were chronic depression or anxiety. Long-term undesirable sequelae were considered rare, though Freeman's report on his first 54 cases commented that about half showed emotional flattening, diminished spontaneity, and lack of drive, while almost one-fifth displayed talkativeness, facetiousness, and euphoria. Restlessness, aggressiveness, perseveration, and indecent behaviour occurred in a few. In the same paper, eight new cases were reported— two of chronic depression, five of schizophrenics, and one man with intractable hypochondriasis — operated on by Wilfred Willway at the Bristol Royal Infirmary. Golla, the distinguished neuropsychiatrist of the Institute, had provided valuable guidance. Of these eight patients, the one with severe hypochondriasis died of myocardial ischaemia within

24 hours, one depressive patient and two schizophrenics showed marked improvement, the other depressed patient showed some improvement, while the remaining three schizophrenic patients were unchanged. Grey Walter, later to receive worldwide recognition for his neurophysiological research, did EEG studies on the seven surviving patients and demonstrated prominent delta wave discharges, often involving the whole of the cerebral cortex, which were reminiscent of the changes following head injury. However, this delta activity progressively decreased in amount, eventually becoming limited to the frontal areas.

In the same issue of the *Lancet* in 1941, JS McGregor, a psychiatrist, and JR Crumbie, a visiting surgeon at Warlingham Park Hospital, Surrey, reported results in four patients; one melancholic, two schizophrenic, and one suffering from 'delusional insanity' (probably schizophrenia). One died of bronchopneumonia on the eleventh post-operative day. The melancholic and one schizophrenic patient were greatly improved, while the other schizophrenics showed slight improvement only. The Bristol group continued to be active, Hutton reporting the outcome of 50 cases, in the *Lancet* in 1943. In nearby Gloucester, Dr Fleming, Medical Superintendent of Barnwood House, teamed up with Wylie McKissock, a neurosurgeon who was later to perform over 1400 leucotomies, and develop the rostral leucotomy — a more limited operation. They described a series of 15 cases, mainly suffering from intractible melancholia; seven made a complete recovery, as did the single obsessional case, and there were no deaths.

These early studies provided the stimulus for the widespread use of prefrontal leucotomy throughout Britain, other European countries, and elsewhere in the world. The Board of Control, which regulated psychiatric institutions in England and Wales, started an enquiry into psychosurgery by questionnaire, and collected data on 1000 cases who had had operations between 1945 and 1947. Of these, 60% suffered from schizophrenia and 25% had intractible depressive disorder. The operative mortality rate was 2.7%, the major cause of death being cerebral haemorrhage; 35% were discharged from hospital as recovered or improved, and a further 32 were improved but unable to leave hospital. The condition of 25% remained unchanged, and in 1% the mental state after operation was worse; the patients with depressive disorder were twice as likely to do well as the schizophrenics. Post-operatively, 2.1% had recurrent fits, but these were invariably mild and easy to control.

Analysis of the effect of the operation on individual clinical features found that mood-related symptoms, suicidal ideation, and obsessional phenomena responded best, while delusions and hallucinations were least affected. However, the questionnaire did not contain enough detail to permit meaningful observations on change in personality. The Board of Control concluded that prefrontal leucotomy was a relatively simple operation to perform, and that it produced significant improvements in patients with severe mental illness who had failed to respond to other treatments. Many became well enough to leave hospital, which would otherwise have been unlikely. Of the 57% who remained in hospital, about half were more placid and easier to nurse. The Board recommended the need for specialist psychiatric assessment before operation, careful analysis of the resulting cognitive and personality changes, and continuing follow-up. Criticisms of lack of scientific rigour in diagnosis and follow-up, though, have dogged psychosurgery ever since its inception.

These relatively positive findings encouraged further use of the operation for chronically ill hospitalised patients whose treatment options were otherwise limited. Between 1948 and 1954, around 1100 leucotomy operations were carried out each year in England and Wales. A survey of the 10,365 people who had a single leucotomy for the treatment of mental illness between 1942 and 1954 was published by Tooth and Newton in 1961. Of these, 41% recovered or were greatly improved, 28% were minimally improved, 25% unchanged, 2% worse, and 4% died. Two-thirds of those operated on had a diagnosis of schizophrenia and the rest of affective disorder; 63% of the latter were recovered or greatly improved, compared to 30% of the former. Severe frontal lobe type personality change was reported in 3.1%.

The Phineus Gage effect

The potential for long-term adverse personality changes due to frontal lobe damage caused by leucotomy was recognised from the early days of the operation. Indeed, the early reports documented many of the classic symptoms and signs of frontal lobe dysfunction, both mental and behavioural, though their clinical significance tended to be minimised or overlooked. Possibly the dramatic improvements in the mental state of previously intractibly ill patients who responded well to operation overshadowed any negative side-effects, which may have seemed a small price to pay for such a marked improvement in functioning level. In those who did not respond, the addition of an organic deficit syndrome to their psychopathology may have been regarded as of little clinical significance in people who were already severely handicapped by their chronic illness.

However, the large number of patients operated on in the late 1940s facilitated detailed psychological studies on the effect of leucotomy on frontal lobe functioning. It became apparent that although the full-blown frontal lobe syndrome was relatively rare, changes in spontaneity, drive, and level of self-restraint were common after operation, even in those with a successful outcome. One of the most systematic studies was that in 1950 by Partridge at St George's Hospital, London, who studied 300 patients over a two-year period. He found that post-operatively, almost all patients showed concreteness of thinking, a tendency to perseverate, reduced planning performance, diminished power of rapidly altering attention, and some difficulty in holding several items in the mind at the same time. He wrote:

> "It is this reduction of the psychic life to a simpler level that makes us hesitate before recommending the operation. Post-operatively, the responsiveness of the patient is reduced, and insofar as spontaneity, so-called, is a measure of responsiveness to stimuli, so is that also reduced. There is a blunting of affect, due to a reduced complexity and intensity of feeling, and therefore there is less variation and more equality of temperament. The intellectual processes are simpler, with attention to the immediate rather than to the remote, to the factual rather than deliberative, and with a restriction of the intellectual range. The total pattern of reaction is simpler, marked by an essential tendency towards avoiding discomfort and courting pleasure, with lowered standards of criticism, reduced self awareness, and diminished self control, which is considerably offset by the lessening of responsiveness in general".

Tow's monograph, published in 1955, and Crown's detailed review in the following year of cognitive and personality changes following leucotomy were also influential.

Reduced trauma, more precision?

In 1951, Fulton analysed the extent and site of the frontal lobe damage found at the postmortem examination of patients previously treated by standard leucotomy. He reported that lesions confined to the ventromedial quadrants of the frontal lobes gave the same clinical benefits, with a much reduced risk of severe personality change. These findings prompted neurosurgeons to develop modified leucotomy operations targeting the ventromedial quadrants of the frontal lobes and related areas. These operations were open in nature, rather than blind, the lesions being made in the target areas under the surgeon's direct vision with the frontal lobe exposed at operation.

The most common modified operations were the rostral leucotomy, first carried out by McKissock in 1948, orbital undercutting that was introduced by Scoville in 1949 and modified by Knight in England in 1950, and the bimedial leucotomy carried out by Schurr for over 20 years at the Maudsley Hospital, London. All targeted the ventromedial frontal areas. Ablation of the cingulate cortex (Brodmann's area 24) bilaterally was also introduced in the late 1940s and early 1950s at Oxford. The results of all the modified procedures were similar, or sometimes better, in terms of clinical improvement than the standard operation, while adverse complications were reduced both in prevalence and degree. During the mid- and late-1950s, the modified operations gradually replaced standard leucotomy. For example, in 1954, out of the total of 1094 leucotomies in Britain, 32% were modified operations, whereas by 1961, 80% of the 447 operations were modified in nature.

Decline and fall

In 1954, the introduction of chlorpromazine and subsequent antipsychotic medication provided an effective medical treatment for the positive symptoms of schizophrenia. Therefore, surgery was no longer an indication for this condition. The introduction of potent antidepressant drugs in the late 1950s also had a major impact on severe depression. In Britain, there was a consequent gradual decline in the annual number of operations throughout the late 1950s and 1960s. Similar trends occurred in other European countries. The selection criteria for surgery narrowed to focus mainly on patients with intractable depressive, anxiety, or obsessive–compulsive disorders, which in any event had always had a consistently better outcome after operation than schizophrenia. By 1961, the number of patients operated on in England and Wales had fallen by more than half, and 80% now had modified operations. The pattern throughout Britain was uneven, 45% of all operations being performed in 11 hospitals, which accounted for only 10% of mental hospital beds in the UK. In contrast, nearly half of all mental hospitals were undertaking no leucotomies at all. Of these 65 hospitals, the staff in 18 expressed their opposition in principle to the operation, while the other hospitals did not see patients that they considered suitable. The regional variations were striking: in Scotland, only a standard leucotomy, performed by a general surgeon, was available and was only carried out in two of the 13 psychiatric hospitals. Some of the local variation was due to difficulties in getting access to surgery, limited opportunity for liaison between psychiatrists and neurosurgeons, and lack of experience in the process of selecting suitable candidates for operation. Undoubtedly, the negative impact of seeing the surgical failures, who tended to become chronic hospital residents afterwards, had a significant influence on clinicians' opinions, since the destructive effects of the old standard leucotomy were not easily forgotten.

The search for greater precision

Even the modified operations, however, did not solve the adverse effects problem. For example, though rostral leucotomy produced greater clinical improvement than the standard operation, one-third of patients showed a noticeable and often persistent reduction of drive, and almost half were less restrained in speech and temper. The advent of stereotactic neurosurgery, pioneered in the USA by Spiegel *et al.* in 1947, provided neurosurgeons with the capacity to make precisely localised lesions.

In 1961, the London neurosurgeon, Geoffrey Knight, pioneered the stereotactic subcaudate tractomy (SST) operation which simulated the open, free-hand orbital undercutting procedure that had been abandoned because of a high prevalence of epilepsy. Small destructive stereotactic lesions were made in the posterior part of the substantia innominata, beneath the head of each caudate nucleus. This was done by radioactivity from arrays of implanted ceramic rods containing radio-yttrium (^{90}Y), which has a half-life of 68 hours. This proved a safe technique and well over 1000 operations were performed in London by Knight and his successors, but since radio-yttrium is no longer readily available, similar stereotactic lesions are now made by electrocoagulation.

Other stereotactic approaches have involved mainly thermal lesions; they include bilateral anterior capsulotomy, anterior cingulotomy, and limbic leucotomy. The capsulotomy operation, developed in Sweden, targets the anterior limb of each internal capsule, while the anterior cingulotomy targets the cingulate tracts on each side and is used mainly in the USA for the treatment of intractable obsessive–compulsive disorders. Finally, limbic leucotomy involves creating lesions in both basomedial frontal regions and the cingulate areas of each side; it was developed by Richardson and Kelly at St George's Hospital, London, in the early 1970s. These targeted operations have a similar, or arguably greater level of efficacy to the modified leucotomy procedure, with a low prevalence of long-term adverse effects. Though studies directly comparing the effects of the different target sites on clinical outcome have yet to be carried out, what little evidence there is suggests that the levels of efficacy are similar.

The introduction of these techniques has continued the trend for fewer, more precise operations to be carried out in specialist units on carefully selected patients — those suffering from chronic, treatment-refractory major depressive or obsessive–compulsive disorder. By 1979, the annual number of operations in the UK fell to 70, with a further gradual decline to 21 in 1985, a level that has remained roughly constant since then. Over 70% were SST procedures performed at the Brook Hospital, London. The majority of the patients operated on in the UK are suffering from chronic major depressive disorder, which contrasts with the experience in other countries such as Australia, Sweden, and the USA, where the focus is on treating obsessive–compulsive disorder patients with capsulotomy or cingulotomy.

Along with greater precision has come more regulation of the process of selection for surgery. In England and Wales, an independent second opinion is required from the Mental Health Act Commission before surgery is permitted. A similar, though less formal procedure exists in Scotland with the Scottish Mental Welfare Commission. Similar peer review processes are in place in other countries.

What of the future?

It seems likely that in several countries at least, psychosurgery will continue to have a role in the management of chronic, treatment-refractory, major depressive and obsessive–compulsive disorder. Increasingly, however, its practice will be restricted to a few specialist centres, with rigorous pre-operative assessment and follow-up. There will also be more multi-centre collaboration to facilitate comparative studies of the effects of the different stereotactic lesions. The controversy about ethics and efficacy continues; many people, both professional and lay, are still heavily influenced by memories of the 'dark ages' of standard leucotomy. Such outdated images and views need to be challenged so that the arguments can be updated to take account of modern developments. In the future, these may not even involve any damage to brain tissue. Chronic electrical stimulation through electrodes implanted in appropriate brain sites, as in Parkinson's disease, may well evolve into a viable form of treatment, and tissue transplantation may have a future in the longer term.

NEW DRUG THERAPIES

by Jean-Pierre Olié & Henri Lôo

The possibility of discovering specific drugs for treating mental illness had not been widely considered before the early 1950s. Traditional sedatives had merely symptomatic effects and 'shock' treatment, particularly ECT, was the only method that had any useful action in psychosis. Until this time, drugs such as opiates, bromides, barbiturates, and antihistamines were used in psychiatry as 'chemical straightjackets' to reduce agitation and behavioural problems, but faith in insulin coma as an effective method for the treatment of schizophrenia was beginning to erode. Between 1950 and 1952, however, a definitive turning point occurred in the use of psychopharmacological agents.

It began with the synthesis of the compound 4560 RP (chlorpromazine) by Charpentier at the Rhone-Poulenc laboratories in Paris. This substance was used in anaesthesia to induce a state of 'artificial hibernation' by the surgeon Henri Laborit, who was looking for a product with more-focused effects on the central nervous system than those of promethazine. Writing in February 1952 from an anaesthetics perspective, he envisaged its possible use "in obstetrics-related analgesia and in psychiatry", though he would probably have been aware that existing sedatives were ineffective in cases of psychosis. As a result, two French psychiatric teams achieved the following: firstly, Hamon, Paraire, and Velluz reported diminished agitation in a manic–depressive patient who was receiving a combination of ECT, pethidine, and the new 4560 RP.

Next, Delay and Deniker prescribed 4560 RP as single-drug therapy for 38 psychotic patients, and discovered that there was a general antipsychotic effect. This effect was not only on agitation, but also on hallucinations, delirium, autism, and affective symptoms (Chapter 00, p. xx). Between May and July 1952, these authors presented six papers, describing the efficacy of prolonged treatment with 4560 RP in states of agitation and acute psychosis. They wrote that this drug "was used on its own, without trying to effect a sleep cure or hibernation, and not in combination with hypnotics or analgesics". They had already noted complete resolution of excitement and confusion, as well as improvement of anxiety states and insomnia, but remained cautious as to any effect on depression. Unlike shock treatments, which they saw as acting by stimulation, psychiatry could now envisage therapeutic methods which would act "by putting the body into a state of rest... forcing the individual to suppress morbid irritating reactions".

In the following year, the first pharmacological study of chlorpromazine was published by Koetschet et al. in Paris. About the same time, clinical research began in other countries, Lehmann of McGill University, Montreal publishing the first of these studies at the beginning of 1954. In the same year, Elkes and Elkes at Birmingham University, England undertook the first controlled trial of chlorpromazine versus placebo in a mixed group of psychotic patients. The efficacy of the drug was shown conclusively.

Delay et al. had previously worked on 'shock' treatments, and experience with those certainly contributed to the interest now shown in chlorpromazine, originally presented as a drug for treating surgical shock. It therefore seemed possible that it had some effects parallel to those of shock methods, though the potentiating effect of chlorpromazine on substances affecting the central nervous system was found to be only one aspect of its activity. It neither promoted sleep nor was a form of hibernation — as was originally suggested — but demonstrated a prolonged therapeutic action in psychotic disorders.

Delay and Deniker then identified three phases of therapeutic activity: (a) initial drowsiness; (b) a psychiatric syndrome consisting of apparent indifference or delayed response to external stimulation, emotional and affective neutrality, and diminished initiative and concentration, without alteration of waking consciousness or the intellectual faculties; and (c) gradual dissipation of the pharmacological effects and attainment of a stable state during the post-therapeutic phase.

The discovery by Delay and Deniker of the value of chlorpromazine in psychosis first demonstrated the concept that a chemical agent can modify mental activity which is disturbed by a psychotic process. This was far from being generally accepted at the time, though. For example, even as late as 1965, Professor Max Hamilton in Leeds — a noted psychopharmacologist — considered that the most specific effect of phenothiazines and other neuroleptics was a reduction in the level of excitement and tension. On the other hand, he viewed these drugs as having only a modest effect on disturbed thoughts, hallucinations, and other positive psychotic features. Since he believed that they only affected behavioural problems, and to a lesser extent anxiety and emotional symptoms, the description of neuroleptics as 'antipsychotic' was held by him to be inaccurate. However, at a later stage, comparative statistical methodology confirmed that chlorpromazine and other neuroleptics did in fact have activity of a kind that was different from that of all other sedatives and tranquillisers previously used in schizophrenia. This viewpoint imposed a logical order, which is now universally recognised, on the drug treatment of psychosis. The fundamental distinguishing feature of neuroleptics is in fact their unique capacity to be able to control the symptoms and signs of psychosis, which up till then had been impervious to drug treatment. Hamilton's position was symptomatic of an active scepticism by some clinicians and researchers in the face of a revolutionary pharmacological advance. Many important medical discoveries have come up against the same inertia of thinking.

The first double-blind comparative study which was able to overcome the uncertain results of previous investigations was that of Casey *et al.* in 1960. They compared chlorpromazine, promethazine, phenobarbitone, and placebo in 692 schizophrenic in-patients over 6 months, with a crossover design. The results were clear: by the third month, chlorpromazine was superior to the other treatments. Chlorpromazine alone was found to be active against some symptoms, such as affective withdrawal, hallucinations, and cognitive disorganisation. On the other hand, its sedative effects might prevent a possibly favourable action on social withdrawal, through making the subject relatively disinterested in his surroundings.

The process of a particular compound (chlorpromazine) coming to be recognised as representing a new class of drug occurred through three significant events. The first was the isolation and clinical use of an alkaloid of rauwolfia — reserpine — which had been proposed as a hypotensive in 1953. In 1954, Nathan Kline in New York reported that rauwolfia serpentina exerted a therapeutic effect on both anxiety and obsessive–compulsive symptoms. Later that year, Delay and Deniker, as well as Noce in the USA and Steck in Switzerland, arrived at the same conclusion: that when used in the same kind of continuous administration recommended for chlorpromazine, reserpine exerted a favourable action on mania and improved its associated mental confusion. However, depressive psychoses were little affected by reserpine, which indeed was reported to have depressive side-effects of its own.

The second stage was the highlighting of neurological side-effects. At the end of 1954, Steck described the extrapyramidal symptoms observed with high doses of 500 mg or more of chlorpromazine, and with 3 to 6 mg of reserpine. The resemblance of these syndromes to the description of encephalitis lethargica and its neurological sequelae by Von Economo in the 1920s was noted. In both cases, diminished initiative, limited movement, a fixed facial expression, trembling, and abnormal movements were found, though the changes in motor behaviour, especially diminished movement, were sometimes difficult to distinguish from the catatonic features of schizophrenia.

In 1955, in a report to the French National Academy of Medicine, Delay and Deniker suggested that drugs such as chlorpromazine and reserpine should be grouped under the heading of 'neuroleptics'. This new term then came to be adopted in the European literature, replacing those used up till then such as 'neurovegetative', 'ganglion-blocker', 'ataractic', or 'neurolytic stabiliser'; American authors, however, still preferred the terms 'major tranquilliser' or 'antipsychotic drug'.

Finally, after three years of follow-up studies, it was established that neuroleptics not only acted on acute psychoses, but also had favourable long-term effects. After the initial sedative action in acute treatment, Delay and Deniker described a variable degree of improvement, sometimes resulting in resolution of the psychotic state, but more often in it becoming stable. At the same time, patients might become better adapted in behaviour towards their family or society in general. Hallucinations disappeared, either from the very start of treatment, or more often after an initial stage of sedation and loss of concern with them. The therapeutic process was thought to be a long one, though, and premature interruption of treatment likely to be followed by relapse. It was also made clear that neuroleptic treatment only controlled, rather than cured chronic psychoses.

In 1957, the psychophysiological characteristics of neuroleptics were described by Delay and Deniker, who proposed a classification of psychotropic substances which was later approved at the Third World Congress of Psychiatry in 1961, at Montreal. The three categories were: (a) psychic sedatives — hypnotics, neuroleptics, and tranquillisers; (b) psychic stimulants — drugs increasing vigilance or mood; and (c) psychic disturbants — hallucinogens. During the 1960s, European psychiatrists proposed therapeutic classifications which distinguished the following types of neuroleptic: sedative (such as levomepromazine), hallucinolytic (such as haloperidol), and disinhibiting (such as trifluoperazine). However, Anglo-American authors have criticised these distinctions, claiming that in chronic psychosis, all neuroleptics are much the same. After a period of several weeks' use, the therapeutic value of different compounds may indeed be similar.

More than half a century later, any effective drug used in schizophrenia must still conform to the criteria proposed by Delay and Deniker: (a) achieve a state of 'psychomotor indifference'; (b) be effective against states of excitement and agitation; (c) gradually reduce both acute and chronic psychotic problems; (d) produce extrapyramidal and vegetative symptoms; and (e) generate dominant subcortical effects. However, this definition of neuroleptics has subsequently been judged to be too rigid, possibly hampering research.

After the development by Janssen in 1958 of haloperidol, the first butyrophenone neuroleptic, research concentrated on the production of compounds which would have less sedative effect. In 1969, when the phenothiazines, reserpinics, and butyrophenones had been in use for a number of years, the benzamide group, of which sulpiride was the prototype, became clinically available. It was only in 1963, though, that criteria mentioning the production of extrapyramidal symptoms would be defined. Then, the antagonistic action of neuroleptics on dopaminergic transmission was clarified by Carlsson in Sweden (this chapter, p. 180). French clinicians in particular held the view that neuroleptics such as levomepromazine, which produced minimal neurological but considerable vegetative effects, are less effective in countering hallucinatory and delirium-inducing drugs than thioproperazine or haloperidol, which tend to cause marked neurological syndromes. However, the proposed link between neurological (extrapyramidal) effects and therapeutic efficacy was brought into question with the discovery of the 'atypical' neuroleptics.

From a compound to a class of drug

The definition of a separate class of neuroleptics was originally considered part of the general classification of psychotropic drugs. At about the same time, Kuhn in Switzerland was identifying the antidepressant properties of an iminodibenzyl compound — imipramine — which, due to chemical similarity, had initially been thought to have effects like those of phenothiazines. Thus, two categories of drugs became available within a very short period in the 1950s: some lowered 'psychological dynamism', according to Janet's concept (Chapter 4, p. 99), while others stimulated it and improved depressed mood. However, Delay pointed out that psychological dynamism is in fact a product of the level of vigilance and mood state. In his view, mood corresponds to the fundamental instinctual–affective feelings, which can make mental life vary between a depressive state and an expansive mood state.

Amongst psychotrophic drugs, the neuroleptics are closest to the hypnotics and tranquillisers in certain properties. While the borders between neuroleptics and hypnotics are fairly easily defined, some degree of confusion can persist when it comes to distinguishing between tranquillisers and neuroleptics — which are still called 'major tranquillisers' in the USA.

It is now accepted that neuroleptics are dopaminergic inhibitors, but progress in psychopharmacological research has also indicated that each compound has multiple effects, and may have therapeutic properties when taken as a whole. Anti-5HT$_2$, anti-sigma, anticholinergic, adrenolytic, and antihistaminic properties of neuroleptics are present in varying proportions for individual drugs.

In the early 1960s, development of the chemical series of dibenzoxazepines produced the drug clozapine. Some German authors proposed that clozapine was the first compound capable of an antipsychotic effect without extrapyramidal manifestations. Deniker's view, though, was that it was a sedative neuroleptic. For a long time, the therapeutic potency of a neuroleptic was, *a priori*, measured by the extent of the extrapyramidal effects observed. Hence, clozapine was considered to be a minor neuroleptic during the 1960s because it induced few effects of this kind. However, Kane in New York was later responsible for demonstrating the advantage of this molecule in resistant forms of schizophrenia, after it had been withdrawn from clinical use in Europe following several deaths from agranulocytosis. This provided an ultimate confirmation of the relevance of the therapeutic classification of neuroleptic and antipsychotic agents. One neuroleptic is not equivalent to another.

During the 1970s, French psychiatrists described a bipolar action of some molecules (sulpiride, pimozide, pipothiazine) according to the dosage used. This effect at low doses is mainly a disinhibiting one — counteracting psychotic autism — with a more direct effect on productive (or positive) features at high doses. Atypical neuroleptics such as clozapine, risperidone, and olanzapine do not have this bipolar action, but act in a more homogeneous manner on all psychotic symptoms — positive, negative, or of disorganisation. Whilst modern technology has advanced our understanding of the biological effects of neuroleptics, better knowledge of the clinical effects of these drugs will continue to open up new perspectives for treatment in the long run. Systematic clinical evaluation is as essential as the discovery of new compounds.

THE ORIGIN OF ANTIDEPRESSANTS

by David Healy

Imipramine

The conventional story of the antidepressants is that their discovery was second only to the discovery of chlorpromazine as a major breakthrough in the management of mental illness. The combined use of these two groups of drugs then dramatically changed the face of psychiatry. However, these impressions are misleading. Far from being interested in the possibility that imipramine might be an antidepressant, Geigy, the Swiss company which had been looking for an antipsychotic, were slow to seize the opportunity. At a time when compounds could pass from the laboratory through a clinical testing phase into clinical use within three months, imipramine took almost two years to reach the market, from the time of Kuhn's first report of antidepressant effects in February 1956. Even then, it was marketed with what retrospectively looks almost like reluctance.

Behind this reluctance lie a series of different perspectives on the antidepressant story. Imipramine was one of a series of iminodibenzyl compounds which were developed in the late 1940s as possible antihistamines. The first had been tried in a range of clinical populations, and did not appear to be of particular use. However, following the success of chlorpromazine, Geigy proceeded to try imipramine, an iminodibenzyl with the same side chain as chlorpromazine. This was done in a large group of schizophrenic patients at Munsterlingen Hospital, in the course of 1955 — with bad results. A number of patients appeared to become more disorganised, their clinical state worsened, and the company withdrew from the study. But analysing the protocols from the study, based on nursing observations, Paul Schmidlin noted that there appeared to be a mood-elevating effect in some patients. This led Geigy to re-approach Kuhn, with a view to asking him to try the drug for depressed patients. He was initially reluctant to do so, but when he did, dramatic responses in melancholic and deluded patients led to his telling Geigy enthusiastically that imipramine was indeed an antidepressant.

Against this background, it becomes difficult to sustain any absolute claim that Kuhn was the discoverer of the antidepressant effects of imipramine. Essentially, his basis for claiming priority lies in the contention that what was discovered was not the antidepressant effects of imipramine so much as the contours of a depressive syndrome that would respond to an agent like imipramine — 'vital' or endogenous depression. This distinction from reactive or neurotic depression was at the heart of the views of the Heidelberg school of psychopathology. As none of the other participants in the discovery had a knowledge of psychopathology, from Kuhn's point of view, none could have been expected to have appreciated what really was being discovered.

Geigy, however, were far from persuaded by the reports of dramatic responses within days. They had some difficulty understanding the significance of the concept of vital depression. They knew that there was already a treatment — ECT — which was available for this condition, and which was probably more effective than imipramine was likely to be. They were also faced with indicators that vital depression occurred at rates of less than one hundred cases per million. This contrasts markedly with current estimates of the frequency of depressive disorders, which is about one thousand times greater.

They were also faced with the fact that majority opinion in Europe felt that the idea of an antidepressant was almost inconceivable. Depressive disorders were considered reactive in nature or related to some form of object loss, and accordingly, a biological treatment could not be expected to remedy the problem. In addition, a range of other highly regarded clinicians across Europe, had tried imipramine in doses up to 1500 mg per day, with none reporting any comparable effects to those claimed by Kuhn.

It took an accident to further the cause of imipramine. Robert Boehringer, a shareholder in Geigy, became aware of its existence and the claims made for it. He gave it to a relative who had become severely depressed, and who responded favourably. When Boehringer advocated its further development, the company then gave it to Paul Kielholz at Basel and Roger Coirault in Paris for trial. Pierre Deniker had also been approached, but was nervous of the suicide risk associated with inadequate antidepressant treatments. Coirault and Kielholz both reported in the course of 1957 that imipramine did indeed have antidepressant effects. This, along with the emergence in 1957 of iproniazid as an 'antidepressant' finally led Geigy to market the drug in late 1957 in Switzerland. In the course of 1958, it was introduced in the rest of the world.

The imipramine story seems remarkable now, given the acknowledgement of the widespread nature of depressive disorders and the need for their treatment, along with an acceptance of the place of pharmacotherapeutic approaches in the management of these conditions. This series of events was, however, the norm for the time, rather than something surprising.

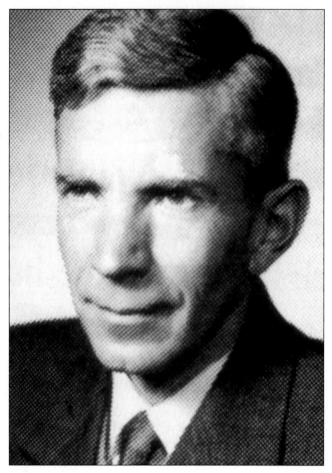

Roland Kuhn, c. 1960.

Isoniazid

In 1951, a series of hydrazide derivatives were introduced for the treatment of tuberculosis by the Roche, Squibb, and Lilly companies. The best known of these were isoniazid and iproniazid. The impact of these two drugs was remarkable. Terminally ill patients unresponsive to streptomycin were 'saved'. The most dramatic stories came from New York's Sea View Hospital. These electrifying reports captured the attention of the media, and Life Magazine ran a feature article in March 1952, showing previously moribund patients dancing in the wards. A number of psychiatrists around the United States were then tempted to try these compounds for mental health purposes, given their ability to boost appetite, cause weight gain, increase vitality, and improve sleep. It is conventionally believed that no treatment indications emerged from any of these efforts.

The first discovery in the antidepressant field was, in fact, made in 1952 by Max Lurie and Harry Salzer in Cincinnati, who began using it in out-patient and hospitalised depressive cases. They reported a first series of 41 cases in 1953 and a second series of 45 in 1955. Of these 86 cases, 42 had a previous depressive episode, 32 had had prior treatment with ECT, and 22 were bipolar depressives. Two out of three cases responded to isoniazid, and those who responded took a mean of two to three weeks to show their response.

Max Lurie was probably the person who coined the word 'antidepressant', somewhere around 1953. Kuhn did not describe imipramine as an antidepressant in the first instance. Under the influence of Jean Delay, the first tricyclic antidepressants were called thymoanaleptics or thymoleptics. Nathan Kline later discovered the monoamine-oxidase inhibitor iproniazid, but termed it a "psychic energiser", rather than an antidepressant.

Lurie and Salzer's work remained unknown for a number of reasons. First, isoniazid, while produced by Roche in 1951 from a parent hydrazide molecule, had originally been synthesised in 1912. It was therefore not patentable. Eli Lilly and Squibb also had versions of it. Second, by the time Lurie and Salzer completed their second study, chlorpromazine had been marketed. It appeared to be an antipsychotic in large doses, and an anxiolytic or antidepressant in moderate doses. Indeed, there has subsequently been a considerable body of evidence that chlorpromazine can be used in the treatment of depression, and equivalent results were found for many other antipsychotics. Against this background, the notion of a specific antidepressant did not make an impression, even though Lurie was treating outpatients — a potentially much larger market of patients than was seen by Kuhn.

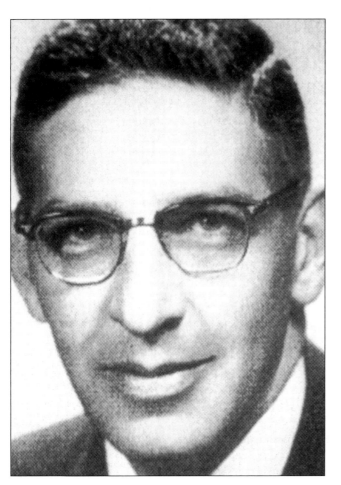

Nathan Kline, c. 1957.

A third reason for the failure of Lurie and Salzer's work to have an impact was their lack of institutional support. No university supported their work and Cincinnati in the mid-1950s was a bedrock of psychoanalytic thinking and practice. Being in private practice, they could not take the time to publicise their own work. Finally, they clearly made a mistake in publishing the second of their studies in the *Ohio State Medical Journal*. However, their work with isoniazid was replicated elsewhere, for instance by Delay and Buisson in Paris.

Reserpine

A similar fate befell reserpine. In the early 1950s, there had been reports that this drug made people feel "better than well" and that it was good psychotherapy in oral form. At the Institute of Psychiatry in London, Michael Shepherd and David Davies conducted the first prospective placebo-controlled, parallel-group, randomised controlled trial in psychiatry, using reserpine in anxious–depressive out-patients. They demonstrated clearly in 1955 that it had antidepressant efficacy. Reserpine is a neuroleptic, and most neuroleptics can be shown to be effective in depressive disorders, particularly in cases with comorbid anxiety features. Therefore, the results should not have been particularly surprising.

Yet, the evidence of reserpine's antidepressant efficacy vanished for a number of reasons. One was that there still was no such concept as an 'antidepressant' at this time. Reserpine was seen as a major tranquilliser, and its principal manufacturers were not interested in the possibility of marketing it as an antidepressant. Though the treatment of psychoses was then in the process of becoming respectable medicine, that of the less severe nervous conditions remained contentious. Secondly, by the late 1950s, there were 26 different versions of reserpine on the market, and hence no one company had much incentive to promote it for indications such as mood disorders, or to defend it when it ran into difficulties.

The third point is that reserpine did run into difficulties. It was associated with a number of suicides in patients treated for hypertension, and this was liable to occur acutely — within days of starting the drug. Doctors faced with the changes induced by reserpine reported that in some cases, it appeared to trigger a depressive or psychotic disorder. However, similar reports were being filed for chlorpromazine and other antipsychotics at the time. A review of the problem by psychiatrists such as Frank Ayd in Baltimore concluded that reserpine seemed to be doing nothing that other antipsychotics were not also doing. It was suggested that what was in fact happening was that reserpine was causing akathisia.

Iproniazid

Finally, there was the discovery of the antidepressant effects of iproniazid by Nathan Kline. This was a more successful development than those outlined above, but he also encountered the same doubts that Shepherd, Lurie, and Kuhn had met already. In late 1956, Jack Saunders, who had worked in pharmaceuticals and then joined Nathan Kline in the research department at Rockland State Hospital in New York, with Harry Loomer, a psychiatrist at the hospital, embarked on a study of the psychotropic effects of iproniazid. The subjects included 17 largely retarded and regressed schizophrenic patients, along with seven 'depressive' patients seen in Kline's private practice. By early 1957, Kline thought that the drug was promising, and approached David Barney, the Managing Director of Roche in the United States to alert him to this fact. However, Barney, it seems, was not interested, as iproniazid was a problem for Roche at the time. Its use in the treatment of tuberculosis was associated with a number of adverse mental state changes, leading the company to consider removing it from the market.

Kline, however, was in a different position from previous investigators, since iproniazid was on the market and selling well. There were no competitive companies. He also had access to the professional audiences necessary to disseminate information about the new discovery and, as the discoverer of the psychotropic effects of reserpine and a Lasker Prize winner, he had a record of achievement in this area. He was also due to chair a Research Symposium at an American Psychiatric Association Meeting in Syracuse, New York in April 1957. This gave him an opening to include the work he had done with Loomer and Saunders on the programme, and he briefed the *New York Times* about the discovery the weekend before the meeting. Within months, iproniazid was being widely used for its 'anti-nervousness' properties.

In due course, Kline was awarded a second Lasker Prize for this discovery, making him the only individual ever to receive two. As part of the award, he was invited to write an article on iproniazid and its discovery for the *Journal of the American Medical Association* in 1965. When he did so, Jack Saunders took exception to the portrayal of the discovery, and sued Kline. The issue at stake was who had made the discovery of the 'antidepressant' effects of iproniazid. Kline's case was that these effects had been discovered by him, when giving the drugs to his out-patients, whereas the rest of the patients had been schizophrenic. Saunders' claim was that he had understood that the drug was a monoamine-oxidase inhibitor and that on this basis, he expected it to have useful psychotropic effects. The case was only settled after Kline's death in 1981, with a compromise.

The tranquilliser story

In 1960, Merck, Roche, and Lundbeck all brought versions of amitriptyline to the market place, and the combined marketing powers of these three companies helped to establish the notion of an antidepressant. In the mid-1960s, amitriptyline became the best-selling antidepressant, but even so, antidepressant sales remained small compared to their current volume today. The monoamine-oxidase inhibitors ran into several crises. One was a failure to demonstrate their efficacy in a large multi-centred study run by the Medical Research Council in the United Kingdom due to inadequate doses having been selected. The second was the 'cheese effect', which compromised their safety.

There was an overarching problem, however, which was that at the time, the vast majority of nervous conditions in the community appeared to many practitioners and to the public themselves as forms of anxiety, rather than as mood disorders. Up till the 1950s, the drugs seen to be useful for these conditions were generally thought of as being sedatives. During the early years of the century, bromides had been used, but their use was eclipsed by barbiturates. In 1955, meprobamate, which had been synthesised by Frank Berger in the Carter Wallace Laboratories in New Jersey, was distributed by Carter Wallace and Wyeth. The term 'tranquilliser' was then coined as a neologism, to help distinguish meprobamate from the older sedatives. Very quickly, meprobamate and the benzodiazepines which succeeded it became known as the minor tranquillisers, in contrast to the neuroleptics, which were referred to as major tranquillisers. This usage was primarily found in the United States, but was much less common in Europe.

Berger's work with meprobamate introduced the notion that it might be possible to develop an anxiolytic. He appears to have been aiming explicitly at a drug which would produce muscle relaxation without being unduly sedative, in the hope that inhibiting the feedback from tense muscles would reduce an individual's perception of themselves as being anxious. Meprobamate, which was less sedative than the barbiturates, appeared to indicate that this was possible. This drug became a best seller, widely used in primary care and in the out-patient practice of psychiatry. Over the course of the following decade, however, it became clear that it was not much safer than the barbiturates in overdose, not much less addictive, and not dramatically less sedative. This provided an opening for the benzodiazepines, which were synthesised by Roche.

The first benzodiazepine was chlordiazepoxide, which was first synthesised in 1955. It lay unused in the laboratory for two years, until it was tested out in a routine manner and was found, surprisingly, to produce a 'taming effect'. Further research on both animals and humans indicated that it produced muscle relaxation and anxiolysis without undue sedation. This led to it being marketed in 1960. In the Roche laboratories, further work on the benzodiazepine series in 1959 led to the synthesis of diazepam. This turned out to be considerably more potent than chlordiazepoxide, in that there was a greater dissociation between its anxiolytic and sedative properties. It was marketed in the United States in 1963 and by the end of the 1960s, had become the best-selling psychotropic drug in the Western world.

BEHAVIOUR THERAPY

by Anne-Marie O'Dwyer

The decade of the 1950s was critical in the history of behaviour therapy. It was the period during which this form of treatment emerged as a formal clinical entity, moving from experimental research to the clinical application of learning theory to human behaviour. The origins of behaviour therapy significantly predate this, though, and are best understood from a historical perspective.

Early approaches

Attitudes to human behaviour have varied over the centuries. In ancient times, irrational behaviour was explained in terms of demonology, with treatment based on exorcism and seen as being in the province of priests. However, Hippocrates suggested that it had biological causes, and treatment accordingly moved into the realm of doctors, then being based on physical intervention. In the Middle Ages, demonology was again embraced as providing an understanding of behaviour, with the resultant inhumane and unpleasant treatment of those considered 'abnormal'. In the nineteenth century, as progress was made in understanding medical disorders in terms of physical pathology, abnormal behaviour was viewed as reflecting brain pathology. A key discovery was the identification in 1913 of the microorganism *Treponema pallidum* as the cause of syphilis (and thus general paresis of the insane), supporting the theory of biological causes of mental illness.

There was also a growing interest in understanding psychological factors in disordered behaviour. The work of Jean Charcot (1825–1893) and other contemporaries, demonstrating that conditions such as hysterical paralysis could be eliminated entirely through psychological means (hypnosis), intensified the interest in the role of these factors in mental illness. Influenced by the work of Charcot, Sigmund Freud incorporated hypnosis into his investigation and treatment of neurotic disorders. Ultimately, he elaborated a psychological treatment to treat neuroses, based on his own theory of personality — psychoanalysis. However, as Freud had originally trained as a physiologist, he explained psychological phenomena from a quasi-organic perspective. Freud's work was a turning point in the development of psychological therapies, since it provided a complex intellectual framework that incorporated both theories for the development of psychopathology, and strategies for treatment (Chapter 2, p. 41).

However, dissatisfaction with Freud's model gradually emerged. A scientific theory should yield readily testable hypotheses, but this was not so for psychoanalysis, which was accused of being 'immune to falsification'. In 1952, the most influential critical evaluation of psychoanalytic therapy up to that time — *The Effects of Psychotherapy* — was published by Hans J Eysenck, Professor of Psychology at London University. It examined the published data on the efficacy of psychoanalysis, and suggested that the response to treatment approximated to the spontaneous remission rate for neurotic disorders. While Eysenck's writings were subsequently the subject of much controversy and criticism, they proved central in the acceptance and development of new treatments. More importantly, he highlighted the importance of evaluation in psychotherapeutic techniques and influenced the subsequent development of psychotherapy research.

Antecedents

Though this dissatisfaction with psychoanalytic techniques provided the impetus for the clinical application of behavioural techniques, the rudiments of behavioural therapy had been established long before this.

In fact, it was the work of physiologists which produced the theoretical framework on which behavioural techniques were developed. In 1866, Sechenov, a Russian physiologist (1829–1905), published *Reflexes of the Brain* in which he emphasised the role of reflexes and learning in explaining behaviour. His work was influential on Pavlov, the outstanding Russian physiologist of the early twentieth century, as it provided a scientific explanation of the relationship between physical and psychological acts. Pavlov's work on conditioned reflexes, published in English in 1928, was the first systematic account of 'classical' (or Pavlovian) conditioning. He found that repeated pairing of an *unconditioned stimulus* (one that elicited a reflex reaction) with a neutral stimulus (one that did not elicit a reflex reaction) led to the neutral stimulus eliciting the reflex reaction, the *conditioned response*. More importantly, he established that repeated presentation of the conditioned stimulus in the absence of reinforcement, led to the conditioned stimulus losing its capacity to elicit a response (*extinction*). He also demonstrated other important principles notably '*generalisation*' (similar stimuli to the conditioned stimulus can produce the conditioned response) and *differentiation* (the conditioned response can be elicited only by a particular stimulus and not by similar stimuli).

The work of Pavlov was widely influential. He was one of the first to use objective methods of research to interpret behaviour, and also applied the scientific methods of physiology to psychology. These features of Pavlov's work — an objective, measurable approach and the application of principles of biological science to behaviour — were core issues not only in the development of behaviour therapy, but in behaviour therapy as it is practised today. One of the most direct clinical applications of Pavlovian theory was the 'pad and bell' method of treating nocturnal enuresis. In this, exposure to urine caused an electrical circuit to be completed, setting off a bell, which woke the patient (normally a child).

Pavlov's work in turn influenced John B Watson (1878–1958), an experimental psychologist in America, who introduced the concept of *behaviourism*. This emphasises the importance of the objective study of behaviour, dealing only with directly observed stimuli and responses; it rejected the concepts of conscious thoughts and imagery. Watson regarded all learning as based on reflex activity, suggesting that complex behaviour consisted of a sequence of multiple conditioned responses.

Several parallel theories of learning were now being proposed to explain the acquisition of responses. They differed in the assumptions made about the learning processes, but all focused on stimuli and responses, relied on objective evidence, and minimised the importance of consciousness.

In the 1930s, the American Thorndike, in contrast to Pavlov, concentrated on the acquisition of responses that were not initially in the repertoire of the organism under study. For example, he tested how animals learned to escape from a confined situation to procure food, and studied the effect of the consequences of this on behaviour. His work was the early beginnings of *operant conditioning*. Subsequently, another American psychologist, BF Skinner at Harvard, through the investigation of operant conditioning, studied the relationship between behaviour and reinforcement. He described such concepts as *positive reinforcement* (increase in behaviour because of reward) and *negative reinforcement* (increase in behaviour due to omission of an anticipated aversive event). He also described the reduction in behaviour consequent on *aversive conditioning* (behaviour followed by an unpleasant event) and *frustrative non-reward* (behaviour not followed by anticipated reward).

Next, OH Mowrer in America tried to integrate the concepts of both Thorndike and Pavlov. He formulated a two-factor theory of reinforcement that encompassed both these scientists' ideas. Mowrer's work was important, not only due to the integration of both these theories of learning, but also because he emphasised the importance of 'internal' events — the development of fear and anxiety. There was no conflict between learning theory and psychodynamic theory in the importance each attached to anxiety as a motivating force in neurotic behaviour, though the learning theorist might regard it primarily as a conditional fear reaction. The two schools would be equally agreed on the conception of neurotic symptoms as anxiety-reducing (or drive-reducing) mechanisms.

Emergence of behavioural techniques

Based on conditioning, Jules Masserman in Chicago and others in the 1940s began to study both the induction and treatment of 'experimental neurosis' in animals. This work was a further critical step in the development of behaviour therapy, since it applied the principles of conditioning to the induction and treatment of animal models of neurosis. He continued the tradition introduced by Pavlov of objective, measurable, scientific intervention in the manipulation and understanding of behaviour. His work not only influenced early 'behaviourists', but also constituted the foundation of contemporary behavioural techniques that were introduced many years later.

In 1920, Watson and Rayner, using the ideas of Pavlov, artificially conditioned fear of an animal in an 11-month-old child named Albert. This work suggested that learning could account for the development of abnormal fear in humans, and that conditioning provided a useful model to study it. However, they did not attempt to treat him and subsequent attempts to replicate their work failed. In 1924, Mary Cover Jones, a student of Watson, studied the effects of the therapeutic techniques suggested by this work. She found that associating a feared object with a different stimulus that was capable of arousing a positive reaction succeeded in reducing the anxiety induced by the feared object. On this basis, she hypothesised that association of a pleasant reaction with a feared object transformed the fearful response into a positive one. She also found that imitation of other people's 'normal' reactions to the fear-evoking stimulus was helpful. Subsequently, she successfully used these methods to treat a three-year-old boy with a fear of rabbits. Thus, Jones demonstrated that fear could be eliminated by behavioural methods alone, without needing to treat underlying psychodynamic conflicts, though her work was not replicated immediately; indeed, it was to be some 30 years before this model began to be widely followed.

Formal behaviour therapy

From the 1930s to the 1950s, explanations both of normal and abnormal behaviour and of psychotherapy based upon learning were gradually developed. However, contemporary behaviour therapy emerged in several continents simultaneously.

South Africa

Sometimes dubbed "the father of behaviour therapy", the work of Joseph Wolpe in Johannesburg in the 1940s and 50s was central in the formal emergence of these techniques. Influenced by Masserman, Wolpe began research on the production and elimination of experimental neuroses in cats. Initially, his work centred on the manipulation of fear in conjunction with food. He suggested that feeding might inhibit anxiety — be 'reciprocally inhibiting' — proposing that if a response antagonistic to anxiety can be made in the presence of anxiety-evoking stimuli, the bond between these stimuli and the anxiety responses will be weakened. He also developed the concept of graded presentation to the feared situation in a hierarchical fashion (graded exposure). Wolpe extended this principle of reciprocal inhibition from animals to treat neurosis in humans, but first had to develop methods to 'inhibit' anxiety. For this, he used the work of Jacobson, a physiologist, who had developed a technique of progressive muscular relaxation. Wolpe subsequently devised a system of treatment using the hierarchical presentation of fear-evoking situations in imagination, coupled with techniques of relaxation borrowed from Jacobson. He also used assertive and sexual responses to inhibit anxiety. The most frequently used reciprocal inhibition technique was muscular relaxation together with hierarchically arranged anxiety-evoking situations presented in imagination (systematic desensitisation).

Wolpe's contribution was a landmark one from several perspectives. In the tradition of Pavlov, Masserman, and other authors, it was based on scientific principles, derived from the objective observation of behavioural experiments. It combined learning concepts with the neurophysiological understanding of behaviour. The treatment was specific, relatively brief, and measurable; it proposed several hypotheses, each of which was testable, and included data on effectiveness. These features were a radical departure from the ideas and techniques of psychoanalysis, but it was primarily dissatisfaction with these more traditional methods that allowed the acceptance of such a change.

United Kingdom

In England, behaviour therapy initially emerged largely independently of Wolpe's work in South Africa. In 1945, Herzberg had published *Active Psychotherapy*, which described a graduated tasks procedure, but Eysenck questioned whether this was an effective method in its own right, as opposed to being merely an adjunct to psychotherapy. In 1952, his hugely influential paper criticising conventional psychotherapy appeared (see above). In 1959, he published the first paper introducing the term 'behaviour therapy' to England — 'Learning Theory and Behaviour Therapy' — which strongly criticised psychoanalysis. MB Shapiro, also at the Institute of Psychiatry in London, was important in introducing the concept of specific measures which were tapered to the individual's particular problem, so that any change in behaviour associated with treatment would be of clinical and research import. Behavioural techniques were applied to various clinical cases during the 1950s: one was of a female with frequent urination and anxiety in social situations, fear of going outdoors and of enclosed and crowded places, treated by a series of graduated tasks, while another was of an adult female who had multiple tics treated by negative practice. In 1960, Hugh Freeman and Don Kendrick reported the first successful case of treatment of a long-established animal phobia by desensitisation *in vivo*. These successful results led to the investigation of other techniques, including biofeedback and aversion relief, based on the works of Hull, Mowrer, and Miller. Wolpe's work was not hugely influential in Britain, however: for example, the presentation of graduated tasks was not conceptualised as reciprocal inhibition *per se*. This procedure of repeated 'scene presentations' (in which the anxiety-producing stimulus was imagined and associated with an anxiety-reducing stimulus) was labour-intensive and often tedious for the therapist. Wolpe's early claim that 90% of neurotic disorders could be successfully treated in this way did not stand the test of time.

In the 1960s, the development of behaviour therapy at the London Institute of Psychiatry gathered momentum with the appearance of Rachman, a student of Wolpe's from South Africa, who worked with Gelder, Marks, and de Silva. They were responsible for many investigations of behaviour therapy techniques, including desensitisation, flooding, modelling, and aversion therapy. These techniques were then applied to a variety of disorders including specific phobias, agoraphobia and obsessive–compulsive disorder. Success rates varied, and identification of the most effective method for particular conditions was often very slow: on the whole, exposure to the feared stimulus proved to be most important. After an apparently promising start, though, biofeedback techniques generally failed to be incorporated into successful behavioural programmes. Aversion — by an electrical stimulus or emetic drug — was extensively used in the early stages of behaviour therapy, e.g. the treatment of alcoholism by disulfiram. However, in spite of initial success in conditions such as sexual deviation and compulsive gambling, it proved difficult to obtain long-term benefit in this, while ethical objections to it became stronger.

USA

Unlike the development of behaviour therapy in England, research in the USA focused on the operant conditioning techniques of Skinner, providing opportunities for the implementation of operant methods. Since available subjects for this work were predominantly chronic hospitalised psychotic patients, such techniques were applied primarily to patients in this category, although some were also used for people with learning disabilities. For example, the *token economy system* for severely mentally ill institutionalised patients was developed by Allyon and Azrin. Token economy provides patients with reinforcers to motivate them to do specific tasks, e.g. conversing with others, taking responsibility for own medication. The reinforcers are 'tokens', e.g. plastic chips, cards, which can be exchanged for real reinforcers, such as time playing games, watching television, or other activities that the patient might want. By contrast, in London, the emphasis was on neurotic disorders, relying on classical rather than operant conditioning and concentrating on the effects of anxiety and methods to modify this.

The 1950s, then, marked a key period for the application of principles derived from scientific experimentation in animal behaviour to learning theories, and then to the treatment of neurosis in humans. The study of experimentally induced neurotic reactions suggested that conditioning was a useful perspective for understanding the development and treatment of human disorders. This research ultimately led to the discovery of such important therapeutic techniques as systematic desensitisation. As conditioning research was extended to humans, learning became increasingly important as a fundamental explanation of both normal and abnormal behaviour.

After the 1950s

Behaviour therapy grew in strength in the 1960s. The establishment of the journal *Behaviour Research and Therapy* in 1963 provided a setting for this work to be published. On the other hand, behaviour therapy was accused of borrowing terms from learning research to add 'respectability', though the actual relationship of the clinical techniques to learning theory was tenuous. Evidence of clinical efficacy was judged to be inadequate, as it was based mainly on case studies. These criticisms were strongly defended, e.g. by Rachman and Eysenck, but were useful in prompting the proliferation of research into efficacy.

The cognitive perspective

In the 1960s, another approach to learning theory was developed by Albert Badura, a psychologist at Stanford University. This included not only the principles of classical and operant conditioning, but also observational learning — the process of changing behaviour by observing the behaviour of another. Bandura's *social learning theory* emphasised the role that cognitions play in psychological functioning, including their role in the development and treatment of psychological disorders.

Cognition-based techniques — those which exploit cognitive processes to change overt behaviour — appear to be at the opposite end of the spectrum of 'rigorous' behaviour modification. This is because internal, private, implicit, or covert events, rather than the patient's environment, are manipulated to change behaviour. Most cognition-based techniques stress the individual's perception and interpretation of external events, rather than the surroundings themselves. Because behaviour therapy had its origins in dissatisfaction with psychoanalytic treatment, vigorously exhorting the objective measurement of observable behaviour, early behaviourists largely minimised the importance of 'internal' states of the individual. In fact some, such as Watson, rejected the inclusion of any covert event. Wolpe, though, had taken account of non-observable events, suggesting that anxiety (an internal variable) mediates avoidance behaviour.

The tide slowly turned again in the late 1960s and 1970s. The limitations of an approach that only considered directly observable behaviour were acknowledged, since many problems that require therapeutic intervention (e.g. obsessions, self-critical statements) are themselves based on cognition. The importance of thought processes in controlling behaviour was acknowledged. Aaron Beck in Pennsylvania developed *cognitive therapy*, while simultaneously and independently, Albert Ellis in New York developed *rational emotive behaviour therapy* (Chapter 8, p. 272). Both therapies were aimed at modifying negative and irrational thoughts, which are associated with psychological disorders. Subsequently, cognitive techniques came to be incorporated with behavioural ones, spawning cognitive–behavioural therapy. Many of the processes in treatment are in fact behavioural: the keeping of a (cognitive) diary or a diary of activity, behavioural experiments to test out the validity of the beliefs, scheduling acts of mastery and pleasure, etc. As in behaviour therapy, engagement of the patient focuses on patient-led treatment, while regular homework and structured sessions are important. Cognitive processes also gained more emphasis in behavioural techniques and so the differences between a cognitive–behavioural approach and a behavioural (cognitive) one can be minimal. The core thrust of treatment, however, generally differs — in cognitive therapy, it is on cognition, with a belief that a focus on changing cognitions will lead to an improvement in symptoms and alteration in behaviour. Behaviour therapy, by contrast, focuses on behaviour, with a belief that changing behaviour will lead to changes in cognition (the *cognitive lag)*.

Behaviour therapy in the future

Since its emergence in the 1950s, behaviour therapy has gone from strength to strength, its techniques applied successfully to a range of disorders. These include: agoraphobia, obsessive–compulsive disorder, body dysmorphic disorder, chronic pain, insomnia, social phobia, and lack of assertiveness. There are now more than 20 journals devoted exclusively to the subject, and a range of professional bodies for behavioural and cognitive therapies in both Europe and the USA. Behaviour therapy has continued its tradition of self-scrutiny with respect to the efficacy and efficiency in practice of treatment; the challenge will be to continue to scrutinise which aspects of it are essential.

A series of more recent studies have found equivalent efficacy rates for specific behavioural (exposure) and cognitive (cognitive restructuring) techniques. These findings challenge the rigorous ideology of schools of both behavioural and cognitive therapies about what is the essential focus of treatment. They provide the impetus for interesting questions about which elements of treatment in these interventions are sufficient but not necessary to mediate change — a challenge which should keep behaviour therapists occupied into the next millennium.

WILLIAM SARGANT (1907–1988)

by Ann Dally

'Will' Sargant was both one of the best loved and most hated of twentieth-century psychiatrists. He was the fifth child and second son of Norman Sargant, a rich English businessman and devout Methodist who later lost his money. Five of his uncles were Methodist preachers and his younger brother became a bishop. Sargant lost his faith early, but retained the evangelical zeal which he put into his professional work all his life. After school in Sussex and Cambridge (his chief interest then being rugby football), he read medicine at Cambridge University, where he used his sporting talents to meet influential people. He became president of the University Medical Society and won a 'football' scholarship to St Mary's Hospital, London, where he became captain of rugby and expanded his list of distinguished acquaintances.

Sargant qualified in 1929, was a house officer at St Mary's, and passed the examination for Membership of the Royal College of Physicians at his first attempt. At the age of only 25, he was appointed Medical Superintendent of St Mary's with 'complete control' over admissions, beds, junior doctors, and nurses. He then seemed very suitable to be appointed to the staff as a consultant physician, which was his ambition. For this, he needed to do some research and publish some papers, a venture which brought further success, and then disaster. He developed an idiosyncratic idea about the treatment of recalcitrant cases of pernicious anaemia and published papers recommending it in both the *Lancet* and the *British Medical Journal* (with both of whose editors he had become friendly through his Cambridge connections). In those days, clinical research was rudimentary and disorganised. Sargant's work was highly praised by uncritical seniors, but discredited by the real experts in the field. He became depressed to the point of being mentally ill and spent time as a patient in Hanwell (a mental hospital outside London). As this made him unacceptable as a future teaching hospital physician, he turned to psychiatry. All his life, he suffered from depression, for which he treated himself with a variety of drugs. It is rumoured amongst those who worked with him that he was the only person who has ever become addicted to trifluoperazine, a neuroleptic. None of this, however, prevented him from pursuing his life's interests with zeal and success.

There was a strong humanitarian side to Sargant's personality. In Hanwell Hospital, where he later worked as a doctor, he became concerned and angry about the state of patients with chronic mental illness who were housed in the back wards of the hospital, untreated, uncared for, and ignored. He was probably the only prominent psychiatrist in the twentieth century to express serious concern about the suffering of chronically mentally ill people, though

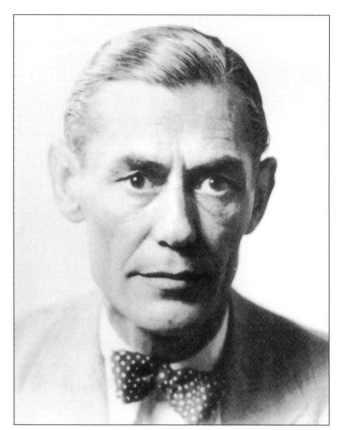

William Sargant. Reproduced with permission from Mrs Margaret Sargant. Photo courtesy of the Wellcome Institute Library, London.

he confined his interest largely to those of 'previously good personality'. His autobiography, *The Unquiet Mind*, reveals the zeal with which he set about his mission.

Sargant obtained a post at the Maudsley Hospital under Edward Mapother and devoted the rest of his life to trying to prove that psychiatry was a branch of clinical medicine, not a 'metaphysical' exercise. He was enthusiastic in using the new physical treatments in psychiatry — leucotomy, electroconvulsive therapy, and psychoactive drugs. He always disliked and despised any form of 'talking cure', though he practised a form of psychotherapy quietly and skilfully himself. His philosophy did not include self-exploration, either for himself or for his patients.

1938–1945

In 1938, Sargant was awarded a Rockefeller Travelling Fellowship to study in America. At the outbreak of the Second World War, he returned to Britain and spent the war working at Belmont Hospital, outside London, which became a centre for psychologically disturbed and injured servicemen. During these years, he worked out and refined the techniques of physical treatment in mental illness for which he became both famous and infamous. The clinical director, Eliot Slater, approved of Sargant's ideas and added many of his own (Chapter 5, p. 137). Together they wrote *An Introduction to Physical Methods of Treatment in Psychiatry*, first published in 1944, which became a standard textbook and ran into five editions.

1945–1988

After the war, he visited America and was impressed by Walter Freeman's new leucotomy technique. He also became deeply and permanently interested in the 'brainwashing' techniques he saw in some of the churches in the South, which he related to the process of religious conversion. Over many years, he made a series of films on the subject; these are now lodged in the Museum of Mankind in London. In 1948, he was appointed consultant psychiatrist to St Thomas' Hospital in London, where he remained until his retirement, apart from a period of illness from tuberculosis. He spent his convalescence in Majorca, where he became friendly with Robert Graves, who encouraged him to write his book about brainwashing, *Battle for the Mind*. Graves edited it for him and also contributed to it; it became an influential best seller.

Determined to be a 'physician' rather than a 'psychiatrist', Sargant called himself a "physician in psychological medicine", a custom followed by some others in Britain since then. He believed passionately that mental illness was a form of physical disorder, requiring physical treatments. He always extolled the virtues of dramatic and often extreme treatments, while denigrating psychoanalysis and psychotherapy. Much of his success may be attributed more to his therapeutic fervour and dominating personality than to his methods. He boasted that he could cure cases of schizophrenia, believed passionately in electroconvulsive therapy and leucotomy, did everything he could to ensure that psychiatry was part of general (internal) medicine, and predicted that by the year 1990, mental illness would have ceased to exist. He promoted the use of antidepressants, sometimes in the face of destructive scepticism, and took personal responsibility for the use of combined drugs in cases of resistant depression.

In 1956–1957, he was president of the Section of Psychiatry of the Royal Society of Medicine in London. He gave long service to the Royal Medico-Psychological Association as its Registrar, but was opposed to its proposed transformation into the Royal College of Psychiatrists, because he wanted psychiatry to remain part of medicine. However, once the new College was inevitable, he was eager to be its first President and was deeply disappointed when he was not elected. The Royal College of Physicians described him as "the most important figure in post-war psychiatry" and "huge by any standards in stature and charisma".

In 1940 Sargant married Margaret Heriot Glen (Peggy), who always supported him. They had no children. He died on 27 August, 1988.

PIERRE DENIKER (1917–1998)

by Henri Lôo

French psychiatry lost one of its foremost pioneers in clinical science and psychopharmaco-logy when Pierre Deniker died in August 1998. After receiving a medical degree at the university of Paris in 1945, he became interested in psychiatry and trained with Henri Ey (Chapter 5, p. 135). Later, he became an assistant to Professor Jean Delay at Sainte-Anne Hospital, where there was great interest in biological psychiatry. In 1961, Deniker was appointed a professor of neurology and psychiatry at the Faculty of Medicine in Paris.

After the retirement of Delay, in 1968, Deniker created a new University Department of Mental Health and Therapeutics at Sainte-Anne Hospital, where he worked until his own retirement in 1985.

He became chairman of a number of prestigious French and international scientific societies, including the Société Médico-Psychologique and the Collegium Internationale Neuro-Psychopharmacologicum (CINP). However, his name is above all associated with the discovery of the therapeutic properties of chlorpromazine. Before 1950, the lack of any effective psychotropic drug meant that disturbed patients had to be either secluded or treated with ECT or unsuitable sedatives. Chlorpromazine, synthesised by Courvoisier, was studied clinically in surgery by Laborit and later by Hamon, Paraire, and Velluz at the Val de Grâce Hospital, Paris, but in combination with other drugs. It was systematically evaluated for the first time as an original therapeutic agent in psychiatry by Delay and Deniker. Six publications of theirs between May and July 1952 explained how a psychological disturbance could be effectively treated with this chemical compound. These two clinicians realised the importance of a completely new development and provided the momentum for it to become widely used. In Pichot's view (1996), they were the "real discoverers" of the value of chlorpromazine in psychiatry. He has added, though, that to separate the respective contributions of Delay and Deniker to this discovery is almost impossible.

Pierre Deniker.

179

Having given chlorpromazine to different types of patients, Deniker's clinical expertise enabled him to delineate clearly the scope of its action. Forty-seven years later, patients around the world still benefit from this work. His discovery was rewarded with the Lasker prize in 1957.

In 1955, Delay and Deniker proposed the term 'neuroleptic' (which means taking hold of the nerves). Thereafter, a classification of psychotropic drugs was established in a collaboration which included Daniel Ginestet. This classification clearly discriminated between 'sedating anxiolytics', 'antipsychotics' (which reduce delusions and hallucinations), and 'disinhibitory compounds'. It remained the view of many French psychiatrists that some neuroleptics are more stimulating, while others are more sedative. Since then, antipsychotic drugs have improved in acceptability and in clinical specificity.

Apart from this ground-breaking advance in the psychopharmacology of schizophrenia, Deniker was active in other fields: particularly psychotropic drug abuse, which he saw as a model of experimental psychosis, and forensic psychiatry, which he taught for many years. In 1959, with Delay and Buisson, he published one of the early papers on the antidepressant actions of iproniazid and isoniazid. The psychopharmacological work of Delay and Deniker was summarised in a comprehensive book which they published in 1961. This contrasted the broadly sedative action of chlorpromazine with that of 'shock' therapies, which they regarded as stimulating the nervous system. Deniker's main interest was clinical work; he enjoyed contacts with patients, whom he described as "our best teachers in psychiatry". Whilst contributing greatly to the foundation of research in biological psychiatry, Deniker had no prejudice against psychological and psychodynamic approaches.

To his colleagues, Deniker leaves a memory of a warm, subtle, and sensitive personality, though at times masked by a facade of austerity. His judgement and remarkable intuition were always based on reality and common sense.

Generations of French psychiatrists who trained in his department or were influenced by his teaching still consider themselves as, in some sense, belonging to the same 'family'. Summarising 37 years work in psychiatry, Deniker wrote (1990) that, "the face of madness has been completely changed, not only by means of psychopharmacology but also by the development of psychotherapy, sociotherapy and the rehabilitation of patients in the community… the insane or lunatic (has changed into) an ordinary patient".

ARVID CARLSSON

by David Healy

Arvid Carlsson was born in Uppsala, Sweden in 1923. He started his scientific career in the Department of Pharmacology at the University of Lund, where his initial thesis was on the metabolism of calcium and the action of vitamin D. In 1955–56, he spent a sabbatical half-year in the laboratory of Clinical Pharmacology at the National Heart Institute in Bethesda, Maryland, headed by Dr Bernard Brodie. Carlsson took part there in the early work on the effects of reserpine on brain biochemistry, which established the field of neuropsychopharmacology.

After returning to Lund in 1956, in collaboration with Dr Nils Ake Hillarp and others, he discovered the catecholamine-depleting effect of reserpine. In 1958, he and colleagues discovered dopamine in brain tissues and identified it as a neurotransmitter, proposing a role for it in extra-pyramidal functions and in Parkinson's disease.

In 1959, he became Professor of Pharmacology at the University of Gothenberg, where with Hillarp and other colleagues he produced the first maps of monoamine neuro-

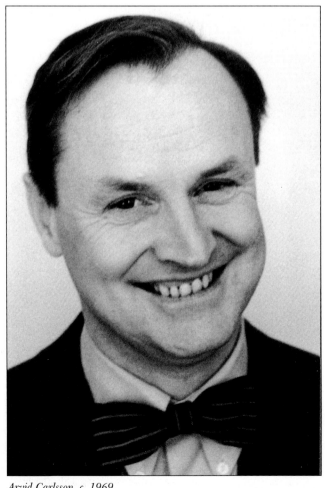

Arvid Carlsson, c. 1969.

transmitter pathways in the brain. In 1963, he published the first evidence that antipsychotic agents had effects on dopamine. This evidence later gave rise to the dopamine hypothesis of schizophrenia. In 1968–69, he proposed that, given the known effects of then available antidepressants, it would be appropriate to develop a selective serotonin reuptake inhibitor. This led Carlsson, Hans Corrodi, and colleagues to create zimelidine, the first of the selective serotonin reuptake inhibitors, in 1971. In 1975, he coined the term 'autoreceptors', inaugurating a new era in receptor pharmacology.

More recently, Arvid Carlsson has been involved in exploring the effects of glutamatergic agents in psychotic conditions. He has proposed a model of interacting neuronal subsystems which is capable of accounting for many of the beneficial effects of atypical neuroleptics. This work has opened up avenues for the development of new neuroleptic agents, as well as other new treatments in the management of both schizophrenia and Parkinson's disease. He has been honoured with a variety of awards including the Anna Monika Prize and the Japan Prize, as well as by a large number of societies worldwide, for his research relevant to both psychiatry and neurology. He is generally regarded by neuropsychopharmacologists, from both basic science and clinical science domains, as one of the key figures of the second half of the twentieth century in their subjects.

FURTHER READING

European psychiatry

Bleuler M. *Endokrinologische Psychiatrie*. Stuttgart: Thieme; 1994.

Conrad K. *Die beginnende Schizophrenie. Versuch einer Gestaltanalyse des Wahns*. Stuttgart: Thieme; 1954.

Conrad K. Die symptomatischen Psychosen. In: Gruhle HW, Jung R, Mayer-Gross W, *et al.*, eds. *Psychiatrie der Gegenwart*, Vol. II. Berlin: Springer; 1960: 369–436.

Delay J. *Les Déreglements de l'humeur*. Paris: Presses Universitaires de France; 1947.

Delay J, Pichot P, Perse J. *Méthodes Psychométriques en Clinique*. Paris: Masson; 1959.

Ey H, Bernard P, Brisset Ch. *Manuel de Psychiatrie*. Paris: Masson; 1960.

Gruhle HW, Jung R, Mayer-Gross W, *et al.*, eds. *Psychiatrie der Gegenwart*, Vol. II. Berlin-Göttingen-Heidelberg: Springer; 1960.

Hoff H. *Lehrbuch der Psychiatrie*. Basel-Stuttgart: Benno Schwabe; 1956.

Janzarik W. *Dynamische Grundkonstellationen in endogenen Psychosen*. Berlin-Göttingen-Heidelberg: Springer; 1959.

Jones M. *Social Psychiatry. Studies of Therapeutic Communities*. London: Tavistock Publications; 1952.

Koechlin P. Thérapies institutionnelles et sociothérapies. In: Koupernik C, Lôo H, Zarifian E, eds. *Précis de Psychiatrie*. Paris: Flammarion; 1982: 399–404.

Le Guillant L. Le service médico-social de secteur. *Information Psychiatrique*. 1959; **35**:9–39.

Leonhard K. *Aufteilung des endogenen Psychosen*. 1. Aufl. Berlin: Akademie Verlag; 1957.

Mayer-Gross W, Slater E, Roth M. *Clinical Psychiatry*. London: Baillière Tindal; 1954.

Pichot P. *Les Tests Mentaux*. Paris: Presses Universitaires de France; 1954.

Trillat E. Une histoire de la psychiatrie au XXe siècle. In: Postel J, Quetel C, eds. *Nouvelle Histoire de la Psychiatrie*. Paris: Dunod; 1994: 339–367.

Therapeutic communities

Barnes E, ed. *Psychosocial Nursing. Studies from the Cassel Hospital*. London: Tavistock Publications; 1968.

Clark DH. The therapeutic community. Concept, practice and future. *British Journal of Psychiatry*. 1965; **111**:947–954.

Harridan T, Clark D. The Northfield experiments. *British Journal of Psychiatry*. 1992; **160**:698–708.

Jones M. *The Therapeutic Community. A New Treatment Method in Psychiatry*. New York: Basic Books; 1952.

Jones M. *The Maturation the Therapeutic Community: An Organic Approach to Health and Mental Health*. New York: Human Sciences Press; 1976.

Manning N. *The Therapeutic Community Movement – Charisma and Routinization*. New York: Routledge; 1989.

Millard DW, Oakley H. Psychotherapeutic communities: the contemporary practice. In: Clarkson P, Porkorny M, eds. *The Handbook of Psychotherapy*. London: Routledge; 1994: Chapter 18.

Rapoport RN, Rapoport R, Rostow I. *Community as Doctor: New Perspectives on a Therapeutic Community*. London: Tavistock Publications; 1960.

Psychosurgery

Crown S. Psychological changes following prefrontal leucotomy. *Journal of Mental Science*. 1951; **97**:49–83.

Freeman W, Watts JW. *Psychosurgery: Intelligence, Emotion and Social Behaviour Following Prefrontal Lobotomy for Mental Disorders*. Springfield: Charles C Thomas; 1942.

Fulton JF. *Frontal Lobotomy and Affect: A Neurophysiological Analysis*. New York: WW Norton; 1952.

Moniz E. Prefrontal leucotomy in the treatment of mental disorder. *American Journal of Psychiatry*. 1937; **93**:1379–1385.

Partridge M. *Prefrontal Leucotomy*. Oxford: Blackwell; 1950.

Pippard J. Leucotomy in Britain today. *Journal of Mental Science*. 1962; **108**:249–255.

Pressman JD. *The Last Resort*. Cambridge: Cambridge University Press; 1998.

Shutts D. *Lobotomy. Resort to the Knife*. New York: Van Nostrand Reinhold Co.; 1982.

Swayze VW. Frontal leucotomy and related psychosurgical procedures in the era before antipsychotics (1935–1954): a historical review. *American Journal of Psychiatry*. 1995; **152**:505–515.

Tooth GC, Newton MP. *Leucotomy in England and Wales 1942–54*. London: HMSO; 1961.

New drug therapies

Casey JF, Benett IF, Lindley C, *et al*. Drug therapy in schizophrenia. *Archives of General Psychiatry*. 1960; **2**:210–220.

Delay J, Deniker P, Harl JM. Utilisation en thérapeutique psychiatrique d'une phénothiazine d'action central élective. *Ann Med Psychol*. 1952; **110**:112–117.

Delay J, Deniker P, Tardieu Y, *et al*. Premiers essais en thérapeutique psychiatrique de la réserpine, alcoloïde nouveau de la Rauwolfia Serpentina CR 52éme. *Congrès des Aliénistes et nerologues de Langue Française*. 1954: 836–841.

Elkes J, Elkes C. Effects of chlorpromazine on the behaviour of chronically overactive psychotic patients. *British Medical Journal*. 1954; *ii*:560–562.

Hamilton M. Psychological effects of antipsychotic drugs in man. *Neuropsychopharmacology*. 1965; **4**:100–102.

Kline NS. Use of Rauwolfia Serpentina Benth in neuropsychiatric conditions. *Ann NY Acad Sci*. 1954; **59**:107–132.

Laborit H, Huguenard P, Alluaume R. Un nouveau stabilisateur végétatif (le 4560 RP). *Presse Medicale*. 1952; **60**:206–208.

Olie JP, Ginestet D, Jolles G, *et al*., eds. *Histoire d'une d écouverte en psychiatrie*. Paris: Doin edit; 1992: 171.

The origin of antidepressants

Davies DL, Shepherd M. Reserpine in the treatment of anxious and depressed patients. *Lancet*. 1955: 117–120.

Healy D. *The Antidepressant Era*. Cambridge, MA: Harvard University Press; 1997.

Healy D, Savage M. Reserpine exhumed. *British Journal of Psychiatry*. 1998; **172**:376–378.

Klein DF, Fink M. Psychiatric reaction patterns to imipramine. *American Journal of Psychiatry*. 1962; **119**:449–459.

Klein DF, Fink M. Behavioral reaction patterns with phenothiazines. *Archives of General Psychiatry*. 1962; **7**:449–459.

Kline NS. The practical management of depression. *JAMA*. 1965; **190**:732–740.

Kuhn R. The treatment of depressive states with G22355 (imipramine hydrochloride). *American Journal of Psychiatry*. 1958; **115**:459–464.

Kuhn R. From imipramine to levoprotiline: the discovery of antidepressants. In: Healy D. *The Psychopharmacologists*, Vol. 2. London: Chapman & Hall; 1998: 93–118.

Loomer HP, Saunders JC, Kline NS. A clinical and pharmacodynamic evaluation of iproniazid as a psychic energiser. *Psychiatric Research Reports*. 1957; **8**:129–141.

Lurie M. The enigma of isoniazid. In: Healy D. *The Psychopharmacologists*, Vol. 2. London: Chapman & Hall; 1998: 119–134.

Salzer HM, Lurie ML. Anxiety and depressive states treated with isonicotinyl hydrazide (isoniazid). *Archives of Neurology and Psychiatry*. 1953; **70**:317–324.

Salzer HM, Lurie ML. Depressive states treated with isonicotinyl hydrazide (Isoniazid). A follow up study. *Ohio State Medical Journal*. 1955; **51**:437–441.

Smith MC. *A Social History of the Minor Tranquillizers*. Binghampton, NY: Haworth Press; 1991.

Behaviour therapy

Bandura A. A social learning interpretation of psychological dysfunctions. In: London P, Rosenhan D, eds. *Foundations of Abnormal Psychology*. New York: Holt, Reinhart and Winston; 1968.

Beck AT. Cognitive therapy: nature and relation to behaviour therapy. *Behaviour Therapy*. 1970; **1**:184–200.

Eysenck HJ. Learning theory and behaviour therapy. *Journal of Mental Science*. 1959; **105**:61–75.

Freeman HL. *Progress in Behaviour Therapy*. Bristol: John Wright; 1968.

Kazdin AE. *History of Behaviour Modification: Experimental Foundations*. Baltimore: University Park Press; 1978.

Mowrer OH. On the dual nature of learning – a reinterpretation of 'conditioning and problem solving'. *Harvard Educational Review*. 1947; **17**:102–148.

Pavlov IP. *Lectures on Conditioned Reflexes*. New York: International Publishers; 1928.

Skinner BF. *Contingencies of Reinforcement: A Theoretical Analysis*. New York: Appleton–Century-Crofts; 1969.

Thorndike EL. *The Fundamentals of Learning*. New York: Columbia University Teachers College; 1932.

Watson JB. *Behaviourism*. Chicago: The People's Institute; 1924.

Wolpe JA. *Psychotherapy by Reciprocal Inhibition*. Stanford, CA: Stanford University Press; 1958.

William Sargant

William Sargant, *Battle for the Mind and The Unquiet Mind*.

The Times, 31 August 1988.

The Independent, 5 September 1988.

The Guardian 2 September 1988.

British Medical Journal. 1988; **297**:789–790.

Lancet. 1988; **2**:695–696.

St Thomas's Hospital Gazette, Spring 1967, no.1.

World Medicine, 18 June 1975.

Desmond Kelly in Munk's Roll, *Lives of the Fellows of the Royal College of Physicians of London*, 1989, 434–436.

The late Dr John Harman, Mrs Anna Harman, Dr Peter Dally, Dr Peter Rohde, Mrs Peggy Sargant and others, personal communications.

W Sargant personal papers, now lodged in the Contemporary Medical Archive Centre at the Wellcome Institute for the History of Medicine in London.

Pierre Deniker

Delay J, Deniker P. *Méthodes Chemothérapiques en Clinique des Médicaments Psychotropes*. Paris: Masson; 1960.

Deniker P. The neuroleptics: a historical survey. *Acta Psychiatrica Scandinavica*. 1990; **82**(Suppl. 358):83–87.

Pichot P. Discovery of chlorpromazine. In: Healy D, ed. *The Psychopharmacologists*. London: Altman; 1996.

Arvid Carlsson

Carlsson A. The occurrence, distribution and physiological role of catecholamines in the nervous system. *Pharmacological Reviews*. 1959; **11**:490–493.

Carlsson A, Lindqvist M. Effect of chlorpromazine or haloperidol on the formation of 3-methoxytyroamine and normetanephrine in mouse brain. *Acta Pharmacologica (Copenhagen)*. 1963; **20**:140–144.

Carlsson A, Faxe K, Ungerstedt U. The effect of imipramine on central 5-hydroxytryptamine neurones. *Journal of Pharmacognosy & Pharmacology*. 1968; **20**:150–151.

Squire LR, ed. Arvid Carlsson. In: *The History of Neuroscience in Autobiography*, Vol. 2. San Diego, CA: Academic Press; 1998: 30–66.

1961–1970

Chapter 7
Controversy and Conflict

1961–1970 CHAPTER 7

Major world events

1961	East Germany authorities erected the Berlin Wall
1961	Soviet cosmonaut Youri Gargarine was the first man to complete the first orbit of earth
1962	Amnesty International founded by Peter Benenson and Sean MacBride
1963	Assassination of JF Kennedy in Dallas
1964	M Luther King of the USA awarded the Nobel Peace Prize
1964	Nelson Mandela sent to prison for life in South Africa
1964	Start of the Vietnam war
1965	First American bombing of North Vietnam
1966	Indira Gandhi became prime minister of India
1967	First heart transplant operation by Christiaan Barnard in South Africa
1968	Assassination of Martin Luther King (USA)
1969	Neil Armstrong of the USA was first man on the moon
1970	Allende elected President of Chile

Major events in psychiatry

1961	The London neurosurgeon, Geoffrey Knight, pioneered stereotactic subcaudate tractomy as a new form of leucotomy
1961	Founding of the World Psychiatric Association
1961	Publication of *Action for Mental Health*, the report of the US Joint Commission on Mental Health
1961	Publication of *The Myth of Mental Illness* by Thomas Szasz in the USA
1962	Michel Foucault published *Folie et déraison (Madness and Civilization)* in Paris
1962	The US Supreme Court declared addiction to be a disease and not a crime
1963	Community Mental Health Centers Act passed in the United States
1963	Arvid Carlsson showed that the neuroleptics had effects on catecholamine systems
1968	Publication of DSM–II and ICD–8
1970	Publication of *Sanity, Madness of the Family* by RD Laing and A Esterson
1970	Publication of Ellenberger's major historical work, *The Discovery of the Unconscious*
1970	Comparative study of the mental health of children in London and the Isle of Wight, under the leadership of Sir Michael Rutter
1970	Discovery of the enzyme reverse transcriptase allowing the creation of genetic probes to identify specific sequences of genomic DNA

NEW DRUG PROBLEMS AND POLICIES

by Virginia Berridge

Changes in the patterns of illicit drug use — in terms of the drugs used, the type of user, and the culture of drug use — occurred both in many western European countries and in North America in the 1960s. Britain and the United States were the two countries where such changes attracted most outside attention. They were often contrasted in published commentaries as examples of 'liberal successful' (Britain) and 'prohibitionist unsuccessful' (United States) types of policy response. Patterns of drug use in the two countries and policy responses had long been different, however. Although these patterns of use continued to be distinctively different in the two countries, the policy changes of the 1960s in fact brought increased similarities between the two treatment systems and the conceptualisation of drug use which underpinned them. Britain and the United States dominated the 'public face' of drug policy and problems during this decade, although changes were taking place in other countries.

In Britain, specific drug control legislation had been passed in the Dangerous Drugs Act of 1920, fulfilling Britain's international commitments to control under the Hague Convention of 1912. The Home Office, the justice ministry, which was the lead department in drug control policy, attempted during the 1920s to introduce a policy of prohibition whereby doctors would be precluded from prescribing to addicted patients. The Rolleston Report, of the Interdepartmental Committee on Morphine and Heroin Addiction in 1926, had overturned this emergent policy, however, finding that such prescribing did constitute legitimate medical treatment. The Report did not lead to legislation, but it was a central document in defining an essentially medical rather than criminal approach to the issue of illicit drug use in Britain. But cause and effect should not be confused. Most commentators would now agree that the Report was the *effect* rather than the *cause* of Britain's low level of drug use, both in the 1920s and over the next 40 years. The system within which medical control operated was also at one remove a legal one with criminal sanctions.

During those years, there were never more than 400–600 addicts in the whole country; there was no black market; and no drug subculture. Morphine and pethidine were the drugs most usually involved, rather than heroin. Doctors wrote prescriptions for these drugs as part of treatment, and many addicts themselves had some medical connection or had become addicted through original medical prescription. Addiction was defined as a disease — a process which had its origins in the nineteenth century, but which had been legitimised by the Rolleston Report. This informal way of responding to drug problems became characterised as the 'British system'. Foreign commentaries on this system, for example Edwin Schur's *Narcotic Addiction in Britain and America. The Impact of Public Policy* (1963) compared Britain favourably with other countries. They claimed that Britain had no major problem because of this type of policy and hence advocated a 'British system', including the prescription of opiates to addicts, as the answer to America's increased opiate problems. The correct interpretation should, in fact, have been the other way round.

Drug use did not become a major problem in Britain until the late 1950s, and then the 'British system' began to break down. The prevalence and nature of opiate problems began to change. The 1950s saw increased popularity of the recreational use of drugs: cannabis use was spreading from the black to the white population, with the first teenage cannabis smoker arrested in 1952. Use of heroin was also becoming more commonplace. In 1954, there were just 94 heroin addicts; by 1963, the number was 459. It was not until 1960 that the Home Office became aware that there were any addicts aged under 20. The new opiate users were younger, and generally male. At the same time, a wider range of drugs began to be used recreationally. There was concern about what were known as 'pep pills'. These were the amphetamines in various forms, which could be obtained without prescription up to 1956, when controls were first introduced. The best known was a combination of amphetamine and barbiturate, Drinamyl, known as 'Purple Hearts', which were popular amongst people at clubs in the West End of London. This non-medical drug use was paralleled by a 'pharmaceutical revolution' in the development of the minor tranquillisers. The benzodiazepines (Valium, Librium and other brand names) were first synthesised and marketed in these decades, Librium being the first to be synthesised, in 1955. These drugs began to be medically prescribed for a huge variety of conditions of a mental health nature.

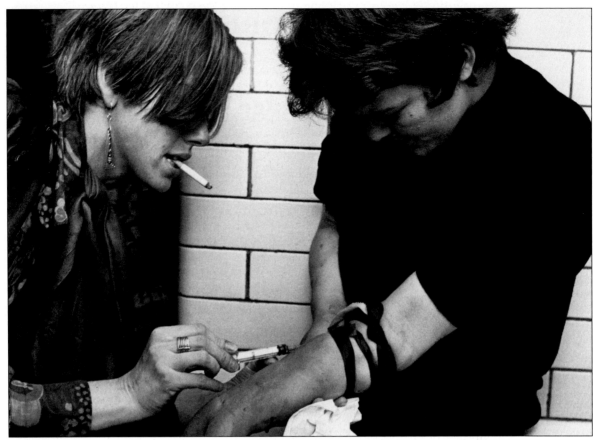

A drug addict holds the tourniquet tight as another injects him, 1969. © Corbis/Hulton-Deutsch Collection.

Clearly, this expansion of both illegal and legal drug taking had a variety of complex roots, including the establishment of the National Health Service and its relationship to the pharmaceutical industry, the post-war economic 'boom', and the emergence of a youth culture. So far as the opiates have been concerned, criticism has focused on the activities of overprescribing doctors, the development of a 'junkie' subculture, and the arrival in Britain of a number of Canadian addicts, drawn by the ready availability of medically prescribed heroin. Those involved at the time have pointed out that this was a shifting group of between six and 12 doctors between 1960 and 1969 in the inner London area, some of whom were prescribing to addicts in good faith. The activities of Lady Frankau, a central London psychiatrist who had begun prescribing in the late 1950s, caused particular concern.

New policies

The expansion of the recreational use of opiate and other drugs in Britain led to considerable activity on the policy front in the late 1950s and the 1960s. The rise in numbers of opiate users was initially considered by a new committee on drug addiction, convened in 1958. The committee, chaired by Sir Russell Brain, a neurologist and former president of the Royal College of Physicians, concluded that medical maintenance treatment should continue, and that there was no real increase in the numbers of addicts. Overprescribing by doctors was not seen as a problem. The committee's report, published in 1961, was soon seen as outdated, and a burst of legislative and committee activity followed. The first initiative concerned cannabis, when the Dangerous Drugs Act of 1964 introduced two new offences — the cultivation of cannabis, and allowing premises to be used for the purposes of smoking it. This Act also changed the legal name from Indian hemp to cannabis. In the same year, the Drugs (Prevention of Misuse) Act made it an offence to be in unauthorised possession of amphetamine drugs, or to import them without a licence. Also in 1964, the changing heroin addiction situation led to the reconvening of the Interdepartmental Committee on Drug Addiction, again with Brain as chairman.

This committee's report in 1965 recognised the changed nature of the situation; it made recommendations in three areas. The prescribing of heroin and cocaine to addicts was to be restricted to specially licensed doctors, although any doctor could continue to prescribe for medical conditions. Special clinics would be set up to treat heroin and cocaine addicts, and these would be staffed by the licensed doctors. There would be compulsory notification of heroin and cocaine addicts to a central register at the Home Office, but a fourth proposal concerning compulsory treatment never became law. The Report thus embodied significant changes in the response to addiction in Britain. It established a specialist psychiatric hospital-based system in place of the previous general practitioner-led situation. It maintained the concept of addiction as a disease requiring medical treatment, but to the individual disease model was added a population-based 'infection control' rationale. Addiction was seen in the Report as a 'socially infectious condition' which, left unchecked, could have disastrous consequences for the population as a whole. The public health model of an infectious outbreak was linked with specialist treatment under psychiatric direction.

The issue of the Report in 1965 led to a confused three-year period before the proposals were implemented. During this time, there was growing debate about the expansion of drug use of all types, and particular calls for the legalisation of cannabis. The report of a special subcommittee of the Advisory Committee on Drug Dependence, chaired by the social scientist, Barbara Wootton and published in 1968, recommended against legalisation, but suggested that penalties for small-scale possession should be reduced. However, the Report was roundly rejected by the Labour Home Secretary, James Callaghan and there was also strong opposition to the liberalisation of the law.

So far as the opiates were concerned, the late 1960s were a period of confusion and chaos as new treatment facilities failed to open and doctors who had been seeing patients withdrew from treatment. Gradually, the situation became clearer through the 1967 Dangerous Drugs Act and regulations in the following year. From April 1968, ordinary medical practitioners could no longer prescribe heroin and cocaine to addicts. The 1971 Misuse of Drugs Act consolidated the legislation of the 1960s.

Between 60 and 80% of addicts taken on at British drug clinics in 1968 were receiving heroin as part of their prescription, and the clinics initially continued this policy, which became known as 'competitive prescribing'. This was a policy of neither too little nor too much, aimed at serving the needs of individuals but also at not feeding the illicit market outside. During the 1970s, this policy changed towards one which focused more on short-term or no prescribing at all, and on increased use of oral methadone (a synthetic morphine substitute discovered by German scientists during World War II), rather than heroin maintenance. A number of reasons lay behind this change — a belief, as addict numbers initially plateaued, that the problem had been curtailed and could be dealt with; professional and staff interests who wanted more orderly clinic management; and also the impact of research comparing the two forms of treatment and their social impact. These clinic policies have been widely criticised as leading to the development of a burgeoning black market in drugs in the 1970s and 1980s. The impact of changes in the international heroin supply scene was also involved, with cheap heroin arriving from the Golden Triangle, from Iran in the wake of the fall of the Shah, and from the Indian sub-continent.

America's response to drug use

In the United States, a very different situation initially prevailed in the 1950s. American adherence to the 1912 Hague Convention had been confirmed early on in the 1914 Harrison Narcotics Act. Legal decisions under the Act criminalised doctors and pharmacists who prescribed to, or supplied addicts. Clinics supplying drugs to addicts operated for a number of years in the early 1920s, but subsequently closed. From the 1920s, America adopted a policy of prohibition of drug use; the Federal Bureau of Narcotics was established in 1930. Harry J Anslinger, head of the Bureau from its inception until 1962, was a noted anti-drug crusader against marijuana as well as opiate use. Such policies have been credited with creating a black market in drugs, driving drug use underground and down the social scale, but recent research reveals an initially more complex picture. The pattern of opiate addiction appears to have changed prior to the 1914 Act and to have assumed a new form. White middle-class female iatrogenic users were already giving place to lower-class urban males. The transformation of the addict population was accelerated, but not caused, by the new legal situation. Therefore, the policies of the inter-war period caused further acceleration of trends which were already apparent.

The 1950s marked the peak of this repressive American response to drug use. A rise in heroin use in the immediate post-war years heightened fears about its spread. The use of heroin amongst urban young people, especially blacks and Puerto Ricans, generated new fears. The new addicts were predominantly young black males and from urban ghettos, especially in the North East. They were reputed to steal to finance their habits, often lived in tough street gangs, and had no desire to be part of mainstream society. This pattern of use was distinctively different from that in the UK, and the ethnic element in patterns of use and in the formation of policy has remained an important and distinctive variable in US drug control policy. But in other respects, some trends were similar. Reports indicated that teenagers of all backgrounds were experimenting with a variety of drugs, reflecting the growing rebelliousness of youth culture. The dominant typology of the drug addict as an 'abnormal personality', in operation since the inter-war years, began to change as apparently 'normal' people came to use drugs.

On the surface, the repressive response to drug use was strong as ever. The Narcotic Control Act of 1956 provided lengthy mandatory sentences or even the death penalty for drug traffickers. But forces stressing medicalisation and liberalisation of policy were also gathering strength. The American medical profession had never been as involved with iatrogenic addicts as some of the British profession had been since the late nineteenth century. But in the 1950s and 60s, arguments for medical maintenance treatment began to be advanced, as more 'respectable' young people were found to be using drugs. The drug issue began to develop a 'multiple constituency' with the medical profession, but also psychologists, sociologists, and public health personnel who were involved. After a White House conference on Narcotics and Drug Abuse in 1962, which generally took a more medical view, the American Medical Association (AMA) seemed to soften its stand against maintenance, although its statements still held that this was acceptable only in treating withdrawal. In 1962, the Supreme Court declared addiction to be a disease and not a crime. In 1965, the sociologist Alfred Lindesmith's influential *The Addict and the Law* argued that American addicts were both more numerous and more demoralised than elsewhere in the Western World.

Treatment and rehabilitation

The 1960s saw the development of a clinic system, using methadone rather than heroin as a maintenance drug. Drs Vincent Dole and Marie Nyswander in New York pioneered methadone maintenance as a medical option, arguing that addiction created a permanent biochemical change in physiology which made such treatment necessary. Methadone also had distinct advantages in terms of the social reintegration of the drug user, though it was criticised for simply exchanging an unacceptable addiction for a form which was acceptable. President Johnson had initiated the 'war on poverty' in the mid-1960s, and methadone was seen as the 'magic bullet' to lessen the demand for costly anti-poverty programmes. Other forms of treatment and rehabilitation also gained popularity. Self-help and drug-free programmes, such as Synanon and Phoenix House built on the American ethic of work and individuality.

Such developments had their parallels in developments in the British treatment system. The general expansion of American drug use also paralleled that in Britain and other countries. The mid-1960s saw new concerns about the use of hallucinogens and the spread of drug use outside ghetto areas. Cocaine emerged as a drug of experimentation in the late 1960s and early 1970s. By the mid-1960s, amphetamines had entered the drug black market and were known as 'uppers', used by hippies in districts such as Haight-Ashbury in San Francisco. Escalating marijuana/cannabis use led the 1972 US National Commission on Marihuana and Drug Abuse to recommend the relaxation of the law — a move which led various States in the 1970s to adopt lenient laws against the possession or use of small amounts. The use of LSD by Timothy Leary and his circle of colleagues at Harvard, and the participatory 'acid tests' staged by Ken Kesey and his Merry Pranksters, attracted widespread attention.

With the advent of the Nixon government in 1969, methadone maintenance continued, but allied with a foreign policy which had a greater emphasis on law enforcement and the 'war on drugs'. The twin goals were to cut off the foreign supply of heroin and at the same time increase the availability of drug treatment programmes so that all who wanted help could find it. Nixon's 'war on drugs' has always attracted more historical attention than the expansion of treatment and research which accompanied it at home. The White House Special Action Office for Drug Abuse Prevention (SAODAP) was headed by a drug 'czar', Dr Jerome Jaffe, who was a psychiatrist and researcher familiar with methadone maintenance treatment. The early 1970s saw an unprecedented expansion of treatment facilities, new legislation in 1970 which represented a partial transition to a therapeutic approach, and the establishment both of the Drug Enforcement Administration (DEA) for law enforcement, but also the National Institute on Drug Abuse (NIDA) for drug research. Research on returning Vietnam veterans and their drug use (funded by the SAO) demonstrated the importance of culture and setting in establishing continuing drug use. Most drug-using soldiers did not continue drug use on their return to the US.

The contrasts, and increasing similarities between these two systems, dominated consideration of drug policy during the 1960s. But these patterns of policy change also affected other populations. In Europe, many countries had passed laws against drug use and/or dealing in the 1920s, in line with international requirements. A long fallow period was then followed by a spate of legislation in the 1950s; and then by the expansion of drug problems and a further spate of legislation in the 1970s. Switzerland, Germany, Spain, Belgium, and others followed this general pattern. But methods of control within European countries could vary considerably. In Norway, the 1928 Opium Act introduced a medically focused system, with illegal handling of both alcohol and drugs being treated with similar penalties. But with fears of the impact of drugs on youth culture, this system changed in the 1950s to a more penal one. In France, a dual response was maintained — both health and penal. With the exception of the United States, the Netherlands was the country whose drug control policies were most often contrasted with those of the UK. Here, a prohibitionist policy in the 1950s and 60s led to greater liberalisation in the 1970s. The Act of 1976 introduced the policy distinction between 'soft' and 'hard' drugs and instituted treatment programmes. Some commentators have located this change in a desire on the part of Dutch policy-makers to avoid the failures of both the British and the American systems. It should not be forgotten, though, that these variations in domestic systems of control operated under the overall umbrella of the international control system established in the early part of the century. The 1961 Single Convention and the 1971 Vienna Convention bringing amphetamines, barbiturates, tranquillisers, and hallucinogens under restriction, form the backdrop to national control systems in this period.

THE DIMINISHING MENTAL HOSPITALS

by Kathleen Jones

Mental hospitals were not, as some revisionist historians would have us believe, the deliberate invention of asylum doctors determined to enhance their own professional standing. The nineteenth-century literature makes it plain that they were developed to rescue mentally ill people from the workhouses and prisons where they were a nuisance to the management, and often treated little better than animals. Medical men were appointed to manage the new institutions because many of their patients came in suffering from chronic poverty and malnutrition, often dirty and infested with vermin, afflicted by a variety of physical ailments from eczema and open sores to tuberculosis. It was remarkable what could be achieved by a bath, a regular if basic diet, and a little medical attention; and if patients appeared openly demented, wept in corners, or talked to their 'voices', they were treated with a good deal more tolerance and understanding than in the outside world.

In the mid-nineteenth century, the asylum doctors had to battle with considerable public prejudice, some of it from within the medical profession; but asylum populations rose steadily for more than a century. Even as late as the 1950s, a high admission rate was regarded as an index of efficiency, not of society's failure to make alternative provision. The mental hospital had become the standard solution to the problems of mental illness. Professor Talcott Parsons, the eminent American sociologist, writing in 1957, concluded that the mental hospital was a "social organization" with four main functions: custody, protection, therapy and socialisation. It protected society against people whose behaviour might be dangerous to others, and it protected vulnerable individuals against exploitation. It provided therapy (i.e. clinical treatment) for mental illness, and socialisation to restore patients to the capacity for normal living.

But even at the time when Talcott Parsons wrote, his analysis was dated. Hospitals, which had been small and relatively humane in the days before the great population increase of the late nineteenth century, had become large and dehumanised. The aim of 'asylum' or 'sanctuary' for the vulnerable was not easily combined with that of custody for the potentially dangerous, and the clinical resources of psychiatrists were remarkably limited. Medical superintendents did their best. In Britain, Scandinavia, and parts of the United States, many were pioneers in social initiatives, blurring Parsons' distinction between treatment and socialisation. Specialist staff were recruited to provide education classes, occupational therapy, drama, music, art, physical training, and sports activities. Concerts, films, card games and outside trips were regular features of mental hospital life.

In England, some hospitals experimented with the 'open-door system', unlocking some ward doors, and allowing patients a graduated freedom: 'hospital parole', 'grounds parole' and even 'town parole'. (The use of prison terminology was perhaps unfortunate.) The experience of psychiatrists in the Second World War, particularly with patients who had spent years in prison camps or concentration camps, led to the development of therapeutic community régimes, emphasising democratic decision-making, group support, and a new respect for the individual (Chapter 6, p. 155).

In the years after the war, mental hospital populations continued to rise. The only countries which reported a reduction were those which had been under Nazi rule: in Germany, Austria, Poland, and Czechoslovakia, many thousands of patients from the back wards had been sent to the gas chambers with Jews and gypsies in what was chillingly known as 'the final solution'. It is not surprising that elsewhere, a large mental hospital population was regarded as a sign of medical and social progress.

Then, by the early 1960s, the situation changed dramatically. The reasons for the changes were complex, and can be classified under four main types of initiative: humanitarian, pharmacological, libertarian, and economic.

Humanitarian initiatives

'After-care' following hospitalisation had already begun to develop in the 1930s. Some people talked of 'pre-care', which involved providing support for the patient before admission; but the idea of 'alternative' care — avoiding hospitalisation altogether — was new. When the immediate problems of destruction and human misery caused by the war were dealt with, it was time for social reconstruction and fresh thinking. In 1953, a report from an Expert Committee of the World Health Organization outlined a blueprint for a "modern mental health service" in which the hospital would be only one 'tool in the hands of the community'. The members of the committee, included psychiatrists from the United States, Britain, Europe, South America, India, and Thailand, and their proposals were intended to be applicable to any country: a framework for a new psychiatric age. Clinics, day hospitals, social clubs, and other facilities would gradually take over much of the hospitals' work. Massive public education programmes would ensure that general practitioners, teachers, ministers of religion, employers, and other key figures played a part in creating a supportive community. Psychiatric hospitals would not cease to exist, but they would become very much smaller and more dynamic, dealing only with those patients who (for a limited period of time) required residential care.

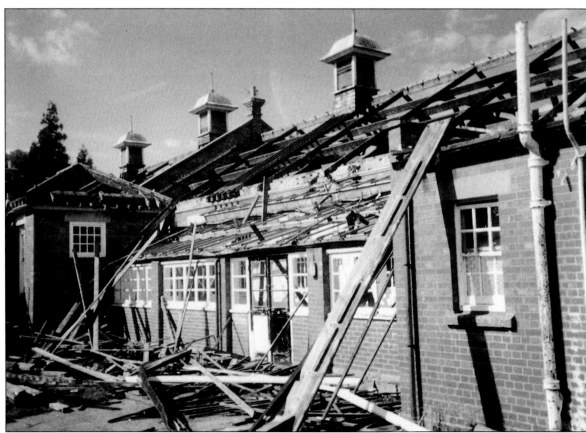

Demolition of wards at the Manor Hospital. Reproduced with permission from Bourne Hall Museum, Ewell, Surrey.

In the United States, a series of high-level consultations on the future shape of the mental health services was initiated in 1955, and culminated in the publication of a Federal Government report, *Action for Mental Health* in 1961. This initiative went further than the WHO report, which had proposed a variety of agencies, but had paid no attention to the questions of how they were to be administered or coordinated. The American proposal was a bold one: the psychiatric hospitals were to be supplemented, and in time virtually replaced for all but the most seriously and chronically ill by new agencies, comprehensive Community Mental Health Centers, supported financially by federal pump-priming. The mental health initiative became part of the wider Kennedy–Johnson human rights movement, sharing in the idealism and enthusiasm which inspired the Poverty Programs and the Campaign for Racial Equality (this chapter, p. 197).

The pharmacological initiative

The phenothiazine derivatives (Chapter 6, p. 166) were first developed by a French pharmaceutical laboratory in the winter of 1953. The WHO report was published in September of that same year. Both initiatives must have been in preparation for some years: international committees with members drawn from many countries do not report overnight, and pharmacological testing is a long and rigorous scientific process. Probably the two developments were inter-related. By 1960, it was widely recognised that the new drugs could be of benefit in suppressing florid symptoms, and rendering many patients accessible to counselling. The potential was enormous, and it became possible to think of solutions to the problems of mental illness other than that of the large and overcrowded mental hospital.

The development of the phenothiazines introduced a revolution in psychiatric practice: psychiatrists acquired a new clinical armoury, a method of treatment very similar to that of their colleagues in general medicine, by which they could prescribe medication, adjust the dosage as necessary, and look for fairly speedy results. Many found this infinitely preferable to the hit-and-miss methods of electric shock treatment and fairly superficial psychotherapy which were all that they previously had to offer to most of their patients. It was scientific; it was precise; and it relieved them of the necessity of trying to understand the morass of human emotions and human problems which faced them in their daily work. Most patients preferred a prescription to long and searching personal enquiries; and most of their relatives preferred a medical form of treatment, because it carried no stigma. Even if new patients needed hospitalisation, they could often be assured that this was only for observation purposes, and that it would amount to no more than a brief interlude in their normal lives.

The phenothiazines represented a genuine and major breakthrough in psychiatric treatment; but there were some unexpected repercussions, which were little appreciated at the time. Some governments began to think that the new 'wonder drugs' could act alone, without the need for specialist mental health services. Psychiatrists drew closer to general medicine, and some abandoned attempts to use the insights of the social sciences. Social scientists, visiting mental hospitals in which nearly all the patients appeared 'normal' — no longer openly demented, weeping or hearing voices — came to the conclusion that the hospitals were a form of social tyranny invented by psychiatrists.

The libertarian initiative

A curious assortment of writers attacked mental hospitals in the name of liberty in the 1960s. Some came from the medical profession, some were social scientists; some were hard-line conservatives, while others came from the increasingly vocal ranks of the radical Left. What they shared was a hostility to liberal humanitarianism, which they regarded as paternalistic, leading to an extension of state control over the lives of citizens. One of the medical conservatives was Dr Thomas Szasz, who voiced the alarm of American psychiatrists in private practice, insisting that fee-for-service was the only proper basis for treatment. Szasz argued, in a series of highly readable and very popular books beginning with *The Myth of Mental Illness* (1961), that mental illness was not illness at all, because there was no identifiable disease entity. If people cared to consult a psychiatrist privately for help with their 'problems in living', that was their own affair; the cash nexus preserved their human dignity, and the relationship could be terminated when they no longer wished to continue it — or when they failed to pay their bills. But State services (whether hospital or community-based) were agencies of social control, inimical to the rights of free Americans. When Szasz compared State psychiatry with mediaeval witch-hunts or the activities of the Spanish Inquisition, many of his readers seem to have failed to notice that he was himself in private practice — and a Professor of Psychiatry.

Erving Goffman, an anthropologist turned sociologist, approached the problems of psychiatric hospitals from the other end of the political spectrum in a special application of the newly developed ideas of deviance theory. It was argued that deviance was a social construct: in Kai Erickson's words, "not a property inherent in certain forms of behaviour" but "a property *conferred* upon these forms" by social control agencies and the general public. To label people as 'mentally ill', 'criminal', or 'inadequate' was to set in motion a process of 'deviancy amplification' in which they increasingly conformed to the label. In *Asylums* (1961), Goffman described the operation of what he termed "total institutions", taking mental hospitals as his main example, illustrating the ways in which the institutional process could attack and destroy personal identity, violating the individual's right to privacy. Goffman's skill in identifying and naming pathological mechanisms in psychiatric hospital life, such as 'binary management', 'the mortification of the self', and 'the betrayal funnel' earned him a massive reputation amongst radicals in the social sciences — many of whom were to staff the new community mental health services as they developed. He had less influence on psychiatrists, who were more impressed by the 'anti-psychiatry' arguments of the Scottish RD Laing and his colleagues (this chapter, p. 202) or the powerful Gallic blasts of France's Michel Foucault, self-styled 'Professor of the Archaeology of Knowledge' (Chapter 8, p. 245).

These writers laid the groundwork for a 'Literature of Protest' which was to remain active in the work of later revisionist historians. They articulated a public mood of revulsion against the old nineteenth-century asylums, which were still the most common centres for psychiatric treatment; unfortunately, they had no practical proposals to make on what might take their place.

The economic initiative

By the 1960s, it was clear that the population of psychiatric hospitals had begun slowly to decrease in the industrialised countries. Nobody knew how far this trend, which contradicted all previous trends, was due to the success of the phenothiazines, to the success of the more active hospital programmes, to the development of community alternatives such as day hospitals, clinics, and social clubs, or to adverse publicity which made patients unwilling to seek hospital treatment, and psychiatrists reluctant to commit them against their will. All four factors worked in the same direction, and they were to be reinforced by a fifth. The post-war social euphoria had worn thin, and governments were counting the cost. Health service costs were rising steeply, and public expectations of health care were rising even faster. Most psychiatric hospitals were in nineteenth-century buildings, unsuitable for modern treatment. The cost of replacing them would have been astronomical — far more than any government could contemplate. The proposition that the mental hospital system could simply be obliterated without replacement was attractive to governments anxious to cut public expenditure. It was with this in mind that the British Minister of Health, Enoch Powell, announced in 1961 that "the mental hospital is to go". He forecast that within 15 years, the number of psychiatric in-patients would have been cut by half. Powell's attack on the psychiatric hospital system did not include a social analysis of how the services were changing: it was based purely on a forecast of statistical trends. Whatever the causes of decline in resident populations, it was happening and would continue.

Other countries, particularly those in the British Commonwealth, followed the British lead. In Australia, New Zealand, and Canada, psychiatric hospital populations were steadily contracted. Experiments in new forms of community-based care in the Netherlands and in Nigeria were widely publicised, but these and other administrative models, like the later 'Italian experience' (Chapter 8, p. 257) achieved only local and usually temporary success. Attempts to provide satisfactory alternative systems of care were in general half-hearted. Governments assumed either that these were not necessary, or that the existing framework of medical and social care could take the strain. Even in the United States, the Community Mental Health Center movement began to falter once the flow of federal money stopped, and the costs fell on the individual state budgets. Health officials in countries in Asia, Africa, and South America which had never even developed a psychiatric hospital system began to congratulate themselves on the paucity of their provision, and to reduce the few beds they had to the minimum required for the custody of those patients who represented a threat to the public. They saw no reason to build up an expensive system which more highly developed societies were hastening to abandon.

By the end of the 1960s, psychiatric hospitals, faced with a chorus of disapproval from politicians, psychiatrists, social scientists, and the general public, had suffered badly in morale, and had lost much of their therapeutic impetus. The 'revolving door' of short-stay care turned faster and faster, involving fewer and fewer beds; but some two-thirds of all psychiatric beds were occupied by long-stay chronic patients, ageing and institutionalised. Many progressively minded staff left to work in community agencies.

Consequences

The contraction of mental hospital care presented no problem for patients who were not too severely ill, who had good, supportive family backgrounds and networks of friends, and whose financial resources were adequate. With the aid of medication, they were usually able to cope in the community, but it created acute social problems for many who suffered from serious mental illness. Though no government or funding agency has been willing to support major research projects on the failures in community care, small-scale projects have been eloquent about the plight of profoundly alienated patients who drift down the social scale, live alone, are unable to sustain any kind of employment, exist from one welfare payment to the next, and resist contact with the psychiatric services.

The 1960s began the landslide. Between 1960 and 1985, the resident population of mental hospitals in the United States dropped from 535,500 to 116,800 — only 21.8% of the previous total. In England and Italy, numbers dropped to 51.5% and 43.8% of the 1960 figure in the same period. The huge long-stay populations were discharged with very little more community support than the short-stay patients had received, and many hospitals were closed. The sites were often sold hastily to speculators, and the proceeds applied to meet the increasing deficits of general health-service budgets. Those mental hospitals which remained had only a very limited function — and their services were scaled down to match. As numbers began to drop, buildings ceased to be maintained, gardens and sports pitches became overgrown or were turned into car parks, and many of the activity programmes ceased to operate. The hospitals were running down like clocks that nobody wanted to wind.

The aims of protection to the vulnerable, a range of therapies, and socialisation had been abandoned, but the hospitals' custodial role had sharply increased. They had become places of last resort. Instead of being encouraged to enter hospital for treatment, patients were threatened with hospitalisation. They were no longer given an opportunity to work out their problems, or to express their turbulent emotions. A hospital stay, in the run-down psychiatric hospitals, became a penalty for non-compliance and anti-social behaviour — a new, perhaps unintentional, but very effective form of social control.

The anti-psychotic drugs made possible a considerable advance in pharmacological treatment; but improvements in medication have not been complemented by advances in social care. Policy-makers have been primarily influenced by financial considerations, and the psychiatric services have become scattered and splintered. One of the most serious effects of this diversification is that it is no longer possible to collect mental health statistics with any meaning; and as a result, there is no effective feed-back on whether services are efficient or inefficient.

Nobody wants the old-style mental hospital to become again the standard solution to the problems of mental illness. We have learned some useful lessons about the power of staff in closed institutions and the pathologies of institutional life; but no government has yet tackled the difficult issues of providing effective community services on a national basis.

AMERICAN PSYCHIATRY

by Gerald Grob

American psychiatry entered the decade of the 1960s with confidence and optimism. Indeed, contemporaries were fond of referring to a third or fourth 'Psychiatric Revolution', equal in significance to the first one when Philippe Pinel allegedly broke the chains of Parisian lunatics in 1793. Robert H Felix — the first director of the US National Institute of Mental Health (NIMH) — approvingly observed in 1957 that the pendulum had swung "from concentration on improved mental hospitals to outpatient and preventive programs". The new policy that seemed to be taking shape included a virtual end of traditional mental hospitals, the creation of community alternatives, a more active role in prevention, and the promotion of broad social changes that would optimise mental as well as physical health.

In the previous two decades, a series of fundamental changes had reshaped psychiatry. The Second World War in particular inaugurated a period of dramatic innovation. Between 1940 and 1945, the specialty doubled in size in the USA. More significantly, wartime experiences transformed both the structure and nature of psychiatry. Psychiatrists became familiar with the high rejection rate for neuropsychiatric disorders during the operations of conscription, as well as the disabling psychological effects of both training and combat situations. Slowly, they learned what their predecessors had observed between

1917 and 1919 — that environmental stress played a major role in mental maladjustment. The psychiatric 'lessons' gleaned from wartime experiences had significant policy implications. The greatest successes in treating soldiers with psychological symptoms occurred at the battalion aid station near the front line. Conversely, the therapeutic success rate declined in facilities further back. A logical conclusion followed: treatment in civilian life, as in the military, had to be provided in a family or community setting, rather than in a remote or isolated institution.

The implication of wartime experiences for psychiatry appeared clear: community and private practice would replace employment in mental hospitals. Concern with social and environmental determinants also implied a radically different role for psychiatry. Not only would the community become the focal point of psychiatric practice, but practitioners would become active in promoting appropriate social and environmental changes that presumably optimised mental health. Moreover, psychiatrists believed that it was possible to identify individuals experiencing psychological distress and to provide early treatment, thus preventing the onset of more serious mental disorders.

The new psychodynamic (or psychoanalytic) psychiatry that took shape after 1945 reflected the triumph of environmentalism in American social thought generally and the social sciences in particular. Increasingly, the attention of psychiatrists shifted away from a concern with the institutionalised severely mentally ill and towards a preoccupation with those interpersonal, social, and environmental factors that promoted mental illness and maladjustment. Mental illness, the influential psychoanalyst Karl A Menninger insisted, was "personality dysfunction and living impairment". The dominance of psychodynamic concepts was formalised and perpetuated by many medical school departments of psychiatry that were chaired by individuals within the psychodynamic tradition.

The shift in the nature of psychiatric practice was reflected in a variety of developments. One was the movement away from careers in mental hospitals, so by the 1960s, psychiatry was largely a non-institutional specialty. Another was the rise of social psychiatry, which embodied a touching, if naïve, faith that the specialty had an important role in resolving social and economic problems. Equally revealing was the emergence of a new kind of psychiatric epidemiology that was preoccupied with the role of socio-environmental variables and the relationships between social class, diagnosis, treatment, and mental disorders.

Psychodynamic psychiatry from the 1940s to the 1960s was virtually synonymous with the psychotherapies and, to a lesser extent, milieu and other psychosocial therapies. The function of practitioners was to interpret the inner meaning of symptoms, which would presumably lead to a resolution of the problem. To be sure, the introduction of the psychotropic drugs in the 1950s had added to the psychiatric armamentarium. Though most practitioners tended to be eclectic in actual practice and employ drugs, their primary concern was with the psychodynamic aspects of dysfunctional individuals. Unlike their institutional colleagues, psychodynamic psychiatrists did not for the most part deal with the severely and persistently mentally ill; their clientele had much less serious problems.

In the optimistic atmosphere of the 1960s, mental health rhetoric and ideology paralleled newly enacted federal social and economic programmes. Both grew out of the faith that the origins of most social problems could be found in a deficient environment. The term 'community psychiatry' perhaps best defines some of the distinguishing characteristics of the 1960s. Because of its all-encompassing nature, community psychiatry defied precise definition. Whatever its meaning, however, it was identified with social and political activism, 'prevention', and a clientele quite different from the severely mentally ill in mental hospitals.

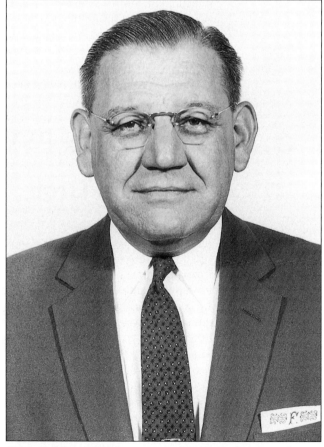

Robert H Felix, 1958. Photo courtesy of the National Institute of Mental Health.

Influence of the political environment

By 1960, advocates of fundamental changes in the delivery of mental health services were confident that they stood on the threshold of success. Their goal was to end the traditional reliance on mental hospitals, which they perceived to be the vestigial remnant of a bygone age. Public policy, they argued, had to rest on the provision of care and treatment in the community and preventive programmes; confinement in custodial institutions was counter-productive and did little to integrate severely mentally ill persons into society.

In the post-war decades, a broad coalition of psychiatric and lay activists began a campaign to transform mental health policy. The initial success came in 1946 with the enactment of the National Mental Health Act. This novel law (which also created the NIMH) made the federal government an important participant in an arena traditionally reserved for the States. In the 1950s, a number of States attempted to create community institutions to supplement rather than replace traditional mental hospitals. Their ideal, at least in theory, was an integrated system that included preventive services, treatment, and care in different kinds of settings, depending upon the severity of the illness or problem.

The Joint Commission on Mental Illness and Health

Psychiatric activists, however, found that the decentralised nature of the American political system meant that the struggle to transform public policy had to be fought in each individual State. They therefore came to the conclusion that the time was ripe for a new initiative that would shift, at least in part, authority and responsibility for mental health policy to the federal government, thus making possible a single unified national effort. The result was the creation of the Joint Commission on Mental Illness and Health in 1955.

During the six years of its existence, the commission sponsored 10 studies that would serve as the basis for the preparation of a final report. Wide-ranging in scope, the studies, conducted by individuals from a variety of disciplines, covered a broad range of topics: manpower, patterns of patient care, the role of schools in the attainment of mental health, community resources, epidemiology, research, popular attitudes, economics, and concepts of mental health. Most of the investigators shared the belief that the pervasiveness of psychological and environmental stress mandated an expansion of therapeutic services both within and without institutions; that early intervention would prevent the onset of more serious illness; that the efficacy of social and psychological therapies was a matter of fact rather than a subject to be investigated; and that a concerted attack on the problems posed by psychological disturbances and mental illness required the creation of a broad coalition of professional and lay groups. Most significant, the thrust of the reports — though little noticed at the time — further blurred the distinction between individuals experiencing problems on the one hand and the mentally ill on the other.

In 1961, the Commission issued its final report, *Action for Mental Health*, which offered a comprehensive national programme composed of four distinct but related elements. First, it called for larger investments in basic research. Second, it offered a series of recommendations relating to manpower and services. The supply of professional mental health personnel had to be increased, and other occupational groups (including doctors, teachers, clergy, social workers, and nurses) had to be trained to assume the role of mental health counsellors. Emergency services in general and hospitals for the acutely mentally ill had to be expanded. Each population of 50,000 should be served by a community mental health clinic, which was a main line of defence in reducing the need for hospitalisation. No State mental hospital with more than 1000 beds should be constructed, and existing institutions with more than 1000 beds should be converted into centres for the long-term and combined care of chronic diseases, including mental disorders. Third, there was a need to disseminate information about mental illness that would reduce stigmatisation. Finally, the Commission urged a doubling of expenditure for mental health services in five years and a tripling in 10. Its members also envisaged a leadership role for the federal government, which would provide the bulk of funds necessary to implement all of their recommendations.

Action for Mental Health was not released until John F Kennedy had entered the White House in early 1961; the assumption was that a Democratic president would be more favourably inclined to act than a Republican. Despite the publicity generated by the document, its recommendations were not unanimously endorsed. Some psychiatrists felt that the emphasis on psychotherapy and social therapy overlooked the importance of pharmacological and biological therapies. Others felt that the recommendation expanding the type and number of institutions, as well as a greater fiscal and leadership role for the federal government, was unrealistic. Nor did implied criticism of public mental hospitals go unanswered.

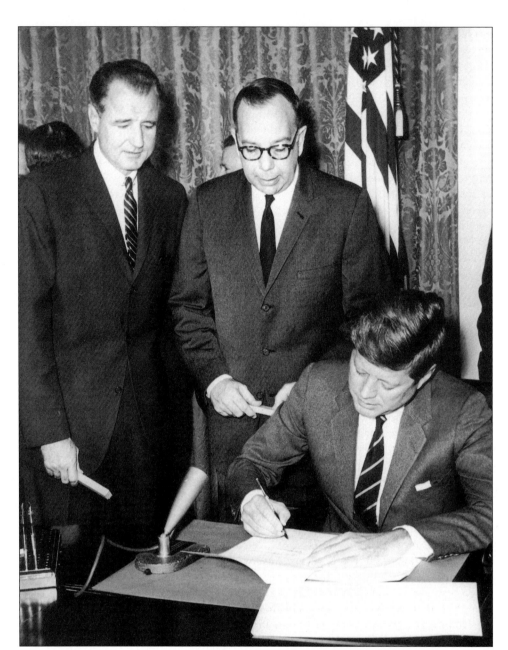

John F Kennedy signing into law the Mental Retardation Facilities and Community Mental Health Centers Construction Act, October 31, 1963. Representative Paul Rogers (centre) and Senator George Smathers (left). Photo courtesy of the John F Kennedy Library.

Nevertheless, the persistence of such disagreements did not dampen enthusiasm for some sort of positive action; the political climate was sympathetic and public sentiment appeared supportive. Concern for the mentally ill through much of American history generally had been confined to two groups: families with members whose behaviour threatened the existence of their household, and public officials responsible for providing some form of care. In the post-war era, however, psychological interventions, notably psychotherapy to deal with personal problems, had become increasingly popular. The attractiveness of a psychological model stimulated pressure for an expansion of psychiatric and psychological services for individuals experiencing personal difficulties. All of the elements for a new policy appeared favourable; what remained was to tap the massive financial resources of the federal government.

Despite the enthusiasm for action, there was no clear agreement on a clear and coherent policy that could serve as the basis for specific legislation. The recommendations of the Joint Commission were extraordinarily broad, and many remained controversial. Moreover, by 1961, advocates of mental health were in competition with the mental retardation lobby. Faced with a variety of pressures, President Kennedy created an Interagency Task Force on Mental Health. Felix played the key role; he was privately opposed to many of the recommendations of the Joint Commission, and felt that the focus of policy should be on the prevention of mental illness and the maintenance of mental health. Felix and his NIMH staff were also intensely hostile toward mental hospitals, and ultimately developed the concept of the community mental health centre. "A complete mental health center", noted an NIMH staff document, "is a multi-service community facility designed to provide early diagnosis and treatment of mental illness, both on an inpatient and outpatient basis, and serve as a locus for aftercare of discharged hospital patients". Such a centre provided a broad spectrum of services: diagnosis and evaluation; in-patient care;

day and night care programmes; 24-hour emergency services; rehabilitation; consultative services to community agencies; public information and education; and supervision of aftercare. Ultimately, all services within communities and regions would be absorbed into comprehensive centres serving a designated population within a specific geographical area.

Felix's views prevailed and in early 1963, Kennedy forwarded to Congress a message dealing with mental illness and mental retardation. Calling for a "bold new approach" based upon "new knowledge and drugs", Kennedy urged Congress to authorise grants to subsidise the construction and staffing of comprehensive community mental health centres that would provide treatment for the mentally ill in their own communities. Congress eventually acceded to this recommendation, but rejected funds for staffing. Shortly before his death, Kennedy signed the Mental Retardation and Community Mental Health Centers Construction Act, which provided a three-year authorisation for substantial grants.

Hailed by many as the harbinger of a new era in the care and treatment of the severely mentally ill, the creation of a system of novel institutions did not give rise to the anticipated consequences. Indeed, the entire context of policy-making during these years was not based on empirical data. The claim that mental hospitals were 'warehousing' patients, for example, ignored available information. Between 1914 and 1948, the rise in the number of resident aged patients with mental diseases of the senium had moved from 24 to 42%. This development, however, reflected declining mortality rates — a favourable development that simply created new problems. Mental hospitals, in other words, were serving as old-age homes for dependent aged persons, at a time when other alternatives were not available. During this same period, lengths-of-stay of schizophrenic patients had been declining sharply. In 1914, 33% were discharged within 12 months; by 1948, the figure had risen to 58%.

Other data raised even more serious problems. A community policy was based on the expectation that patients could be treated in non-institutional settings. Underlying this belief were several assumptions: that patients had a home; that each had a sympathetic family or other person to act as caretaker; that the organisation of the household would not impede rehabilitation; and that the patient's presence would not cause undue hardships for other family members. In 1960, however, 48% of the mental hospital population were unmarried, 12% were widowed, and 13% divorced or separated. A large proportion of patients, in other words, may have had no families to provide care. The assumption that most patients could reside in the community with their families while undergoing rehabilitation was hardly supported by such findings. Such data, although known by those pushing for a community policy, were barely considered during the political and legislative deliberations, even though they were crucial to the implementation of the new policy departure.

Community Mental Health Centers Act

The Act of 1963 was designed to create a novel institution — the comprehensive community mental health centre (CMHC) — that would be the foundation for a new departure in mental health policy. What is striking in retrospect, however, was the ill-defined nature and function of 'centres', as compared with existing clinics (which had more focused if limited goals). The potential clients of centres were described in global and protean terminology, which included individuals with personal problems as well as the severely and persistently mentally ill. More important, there was no provision for linking centres and traditional mental hospitals, nor was serious consideration given to the ways in which centres would or could assume the caring functions of those hospitals. Finally, there was no effort to deal with the problem of staffing the projected 2000 CMHCs. Indeed, the goal of dramatically increasing the number of psychiatrists might have the inadvertent effect of reducing dramatically the supply of general practitioners and specialists providing services to the general population, thereby exacerbating other health problems.

In the end, CMHCs neither replaced mental hospitals nor did they serve the needs of the severely and chronically mentally ill. The number that were created under the Act of 1963 fell far short of the projected goal; the fiscal pressures generated by the Vietnam War shifted resources away from the civilian into the military sector. More importantly, centres devoted much of their attention and many of their resources to individuals experiencing less serious psychological disturbances or problems in living. Unlike mental hospitals, they rarely provided an integrated system of care and treatment. Moreover, within a relatively short time, centres were staffed by clinical psychologists and social workers — groups that in general had neither the interest nor the experience to deal with the severely mentally ill.

Medicare and Medicaid

If the Community Mental Health Centers Act did little for severely mentally ill persons, the passage of amendments to the Social Security Act of 1935 was destined to have a major impact upon them. Two programmes in particular, Medicare and Medicaid, were in their origins designed to provide medical care for the aged and poor. But their impact on mental health policy was profound and paradoxical. Since the late nineteenth century, mental hospitals had served in part as geriatric institutions for aged and senile persons. In 1962, for example, 30% of the half a million patients at public mental hospitals were 65 or older; this group constituted an even larger proportion of first admissions. However, the passage of Medicaid led States to redefine senility in non-psychiatric terms. By sending such individuals to chronic-care nursing facilities, they shifted the costs of their support to the federal government. The result was a lateral transfer of patients from mental hospitals to other facilities. Inadvertently, the reduction in the admission of elderly long-term patients had the result of improving the quality of acute care and treatment in public mental hospitals. The decline in custodial functions improved the internal institutional atmosphere and fostered a more hopeful outlook. That a variety of factors played a role in institutional improvement was clear: recognition of the negative consequences of long-term hospitalisation; a greater emphasis on therapy (somatic and psychological); enhanced efforts to prevent chronicity and reduce lengths of stay; and improved staff–patient ratios. Whatever the reasons, mental hospitals were changing in significant ways by the end of the 1960s.

Challenge to psychodynamic psychiatry

Although the psychodynamic school shaped and dominated the psychiatric scene in the post-war years, a series of disquieting elements were already eroding its foundation by the 1960s. The challenges to its authority came from a variety of sources. Within the specialty, the hegemony of psychodynamic and psychoanalytic psychiatrists came under attack from more biologically orientated colleagues. To internal controversies were added sharp criticisms of both the theory and practice of psychiatry by individuals and groups from without.

Admittedly relegated to a minority position, an older biological tradition persisted in one form or another in the post-war decades. Indeed, the introduction of the psychotropic drugs during the 1950s gave a more biologically orientated psychiatry a foundation on which to build. The application of randomised clinical trials tended to strengthen the claims of biological psychiatrists and to weaken those of their psychodynamic colleagues. Two studies begun in 1961 suggested that the new drug therapies were particularly effective in dealing with severe mental disorders. Firstly, a double-blind study of the phenothiazines demonstrated the effectiveness of drug therapy with schizophrenic patients. Secondly, in a classic randomised study with appropriate control groups extending over six years, Benjamin Pasamanick and his associates found that excellent results could be achieved with drug therapy in a home-care setting. Yet, as he observed, most psychiatrists were still being trained in psychodynamic concepts that were "already obsolete, utilising knowledge and skills which daily approach obsolescence".

Another challenge to psychodynamic legitimacy came from other mental health professionals without medical degrees. Such groups were hostile toward the presumption that mental disorders were necessarily medical and biological in character. The growing significance of alternatives to mental hospital treatment — including out-patient clinics, community mental health centres, and private practice – as well as the liberalisation of third-party insurance regulations to include psychiatric coverage, gave new meaning to an older controversy about the practice of various psychotherapies and sociotherapies by non-medical practitioners.

Psychologists in particular were irritated by a medical model that in their view was deficient. During the 1950s, they came into conflict with psychiatrists on the issue of licensing and certification, and later began to challenge directly the validity of the medical model. The psychodynamic tradition was especially vulnerable to criticisms by psychologists. Having argued that environment played a crucial role in the aetiology of mental disorders, psychodynamic figures were not in a particularly good position to defend themselves from those who insisted that medical training was inadequate to deal with problems that were largely social and psychological in nature.

During the 1960s, psychiatric control over the psychotherapies became more tenuous. Several studies had made it abundantly clear that the proposed increases in the number of community mental health centres would more than drain the pool of qualified psychiatrists needed to staff them. Moreover, psychotherapies were time consuming and labour intensive, and therefore could not be used to treat the hundreds of thousands of seriously mentally ill persons. These facts alone accounted for a jurisdictional expansion of such non-medical specialties as clinical psychology, whose members offered psychotherapeutic services independently of medical supervision. As the role of mental health professionals without medical training grew, the arena of psychiatric expertise correspondingly diminished. Such developments strengthened biological psychiatry, given the fact that somatic therapies — particularly drugs — remained under medical control.

The attack on psychodynamic psychiatry was not limited to other mental health professionals, since the social activism of the specialty created a dilemma. Like virtually all professional groups during these years, psychiatrists were of two minds. On the one hand, they were aware of the effects of poverty, substandard housing, unemployment, malnutrition, prejudice, discrimination, and inadequate schooling — all harmful to emotional well-being, much as air and water pollution were to physical well-being. On the other hand, they were cognisant of the distinction between their role as professionals and that as citizens. To conflate the two could either damage professional authority or could imperil democratic and representative government. The resolution of this dilemma was by no means obvious, and disunity was common. Joseph Wortis, a prominent biological psychiatrist, was critical of many of his activist colleagues. "Jung defended the Nazis.... Freud ascribed war to aggressive instincts and took sides with the Germans in World War I; psychiatry has been invoked to support individualism and collectivism, progress and reaction, and to smear or incarcerate political opponents". Psychiatrists, he added, could direct "attention to the basic social forces that can cause or aggravate mental disorder, and by treating their patients in accordance with these insights, but it is presumptuous for psychiatrists to base their claims for leadership in the broader arena of social action on their technical credentials".

Internal disagreements, however, were overshadowed by critiques of psychiatric legitimacy and authority that were offered by a disparate group of individuals whose only common thread was their opposition to psychiatry. The best known psychiatric critics included Thomas S Szasz, RD Laing (this chapter, p. 202), Erving Goffman, Thomas J Scheff, and Michel Foucault (Chapter 8, p. 245). Politically and ideologically diverse, their writings nevertheless challenged the very foundations of the specialty. A more subtle but equally significant critique came from both the legal profession and civil rights advocates. Both raised fundamental and troublesome questions about involuntary commitment and patients' rights. If society had authority to enforce involuntary commitment, did it not have a commensurate responsibility to provide treatment, as contrasted with custodial care? What circumstances justified involuntary commitment, and who was qualified to make such decisions? Should hospitalised patients retain certain basic rights, including a right to treatment, a right to refuse (within certain limits) treatments that were controversial or had undesirable side-effects, and confidentiality of records? Although the precise impact of these critiques was not always clear, there is little doubt that they tended to weaken the legitimacy and authority of both psychiatry and mental hospitals.

Conclusion

In 1960, the influence of psychodynamic psychiatry had reached seemingly unprecedented heights. The specialty's concepts had permeated popular culture; its prestige was at an all-time high; it had close ties with the nation's political leaders; and it seemed on the verge of transforming mental health policy by shifting the focus from institutionalisation to the community. Within a few short years, by contrast, the specialty was in disarray. Psychodynamic concepts appeared increasingly irrelevant; the psychotherapies were no longer under strictly medical jurisdiction; the number of medical graduates selecting psychiatry as their career choice was falling rapidly; and the public image of psychiatry had become negative. The result was a marked transformation in the character of American psychiatry. As psychodynamic leaders who had dominated the specialty for nearly a quarter of a century retired, their places were taken by those more committed to a biological explanation of mental disorders. Less concerned with the role of broad environmental and psychological factors in the shaping of personality, these individuals stressed the importance of integrating psychiatry and medicine, as well as exploring new medical technologies that might eventually illuminate the biology of mental disorders. Psychiatric attention increasingly was riveted on problems of pathology and diagnosis; interest in psychosocial rehabilitation declined; and somatic therapies increasingly became the norm.

The growing significance of biological psychiatry, however, would give rise to new dilemmas. To be sure, the preoccupation with pathology and diagnosis shifted attention back to severe mental disorders. Nevertheless, biological psychiatrists were more likely to compartmentalise the medical and social aspects of mental illnesses; they often remained remote from psychosocial rehabilitation or community support systems, both of which were vital to a population whose illnesses created disability. The continued existence of severe and persistent mental illnesses would continue to pose a serious problem for American society as it entered the twenty-first century.

RD LAING AND ANTI-PSYCHIATRY

by Digby Tantam

RD Laing was for a brief while a celebrity — an unusual position for a psychiatrist. Like many other celebrities, he was a larger-than-life figure (though not literally; he was in fact shorter than average). He had 10 children by three wives, became notorious for being drunk at public occasions, and published books of poems, autobiography, and philosophical reflections. None of these activities are responsible for his reputation as a psychiatrist, and I shall not consider them further.

Ronald David Laing was born in October 1927 in Glasgow, Scotland. His parents had been married for nine years before his birth and never had another child. Both were musical, his father being an accomplished amateur singer. His father was an electrical engineer for the Glasgow Corporation, but his mother was the dominant influence in her son's life. He remained locked in an ambivalent relationship to her to the end of her, and nearly to the end of his own, life. She died at the age of 85, he at 61, two and a half years later; her last letter to him was to tell him not to come to her funeral. His last to her was a single piece of paper with the words "I promise", enclosed by a heart. When he heard about her death, Laing found the music of the song "A Boy's Best Friend is his Mother", and played it through with a friend.

Laing's education

Laing won a scholarship to Hutcheson's Grammar School, and stayed there until going on to a place at Glasgow University. He had asthma, but did not allow this to stop him competing successfully in school sports; physical activity remained important to him throughout his life. At school, he read widely and voraciously in the public library and learnt to play the piano, becoming an associate of the Royal College of Music. His father developed an agitated depression when Laing was 17 and this may have influenced his own decision to read medicine, even though he had had a primarily classical education up to then. At university, he founded a debating society for which Bertrand Russell agreed to act as patron, and was soon grappling with some of the paradoxes of life as a medical student, for whom the life of the soul and the demands of the body are all too often opposed. Laing became interested in existentialism, psychiatry, hypnosis, and other fields of study that concerned some of the otherwise hidden aspects of medical practice. He came across the poetry of Antonin Artaud, then an in-patient in a psychiatric hospital in Rodez in the Massif Central region of France, and was much affected by Artaud's view that "A lunatic is also a man society does not wish to listen to and whom it is determined to prevent from uttering unbearable truths".

Laing initially failed his medical finals but then passed them six months later, having spent the time working as a student locum in a city psychiatric unit that, at the time, mainly housed victims of encephalitis lethargica from the inter-war period. Laing had also performed less well in his university entrance examination than was expected of him. This pattern of not quite finishing off, of not quite achieving has been noted by those who knew him as recurring throughout his life. Various explanations have been given for it. One is that he was simply following his father, who had also quailed before the big moments. Another is that Laing struggled throughout his life with his mother's expectations of him — at one and the same time rejecting them and yet also being bound by them. She certainly reacted strongly to his examination failure, losing weight until he finally graduated, by which time she was only about five stones (just over 30 kg).

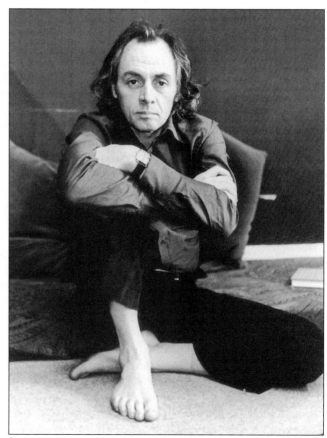

RD Laing. Reproduced with permission from Colin Davey/Camera Press, London.

Career in the army

Laing's first medical post was in a neurosurgical unit, where he met Schorstein, a literate neurosurgeon steeped in middle European culture. Laing became particularly interested in the work of Karl Jaspers, whom Schorstein had met, and planned to go to Switzerland to study with him. However, conscription was still in force, and he was called up. He then chose to pursue a career in psychiatry rather than neurology, and was posted after initial training to the army psychiatric hospital at Netley, where insulin coma was widely used. His experiences there confirmed him in his view that, like ECT and leucotomy, it was barbaric. He began to talk to patients, visiting them sometimes in their padded cells, and even took one patient to his parents' home with him when he was on leave, so that this man would not be given physical treatment in his absence. Laing became preoccupied by the possibility that psychiatry might make people worse rather than better. He also developed an interest in the problem of how to distinguish feigned from authentic illness, and wrote a paper on Ganser syndrome which was published in the *Journal of the Royal Army Medical Corps* — his first publication.

After the first year of his service, Laing was posted to the Military Hospital in Catterick, North Yorkshire. Here, he had to decide whether or not some patients were malingering, and this sharpened the interest in deception that had begun in Netley. Laing concluded that "I could not tell whether someone was lying, or telling the truth, or somewhere in between. I did not know anyone who could, or how one could". That Laing did not go on to consider what the experience of deception might be for the patient is surprising, given that self-deception is one of the central themes of the existentialist philosophy that more and more influenced his thinking. Perhaps this was because, in the final analysis, he was concerned more with the self than with others. In his autobiography, he described knocking a younger boy down with his bike. "The incident arrested my attention and has stayed vividly in my mind's eye. It showed me as clearly as possible that in an emergency, when I was simply reacting, I had no immediate concern for the boy whatever".

'Talking treatment'

Laing left the Army in 1953, and became a registrar at Gartnavel Royal Mental Hospital in Glasgow. Here, in the pre-neuroleptic era, he had to care for long-term patients for the first time. He knew that he wanted to talk to patients (although it was contrary to the policy of the hospital to do so) and that he did not value physical treatments. He got permission for 11 of the most severely disturbed women patients to spend the day with two members of the nursing staff in a newly decorated room, reserved for their use. Laing would spend time in the room, and also spoke to the two nurses once a week. He summarised the results of this experiment laconically: "Within eighteen months all original eleven patients had left. Within a further year, they were all back". By that time, he had been appointed a senior registrar at the Southern General Hospital, partly so that he could reproduce his experimental work with schizophrenia there. He had already begun to write *The Divided Self*, reading first drafts to colleagues, who met regularly to discuss intellectual issues. This was to continue to be Laing's preferred method of developing his ideas.

Out of this group also grew a paper on the theologian, Tillich which Laing sent to JD Sutherland, the then editor of the *British Journal of Medical Psychology*, who accepted it and invited him to join the training programme at the Tavistock Institute in London. This happened in 1957, and Laing simultaneously began psychoanalytic training at the Institute of Psycho-Analysis. He was analysed by Charles Rycroft and taught by some of the most celebrated British analysts including Melanie Klein, RW Winnicott, and WR Bion. His attendance at lectures and seminars was less than expected, however, and there was resistance amongst the Institute staff to his qualifying, although he was allowed to do so in 1960. This was also the year of publication of *The Divided Self*, which had previously been turned down by numerous publishers. It sold slowly at first, but received the approval of the analysts who were Laing's main teachers.

Family research project

Laing had now become more interested in the views of the American psychoanalyst Theodore Lidz, the anthropologist Gregory Bateson, and others, that families caused schizophrenia. He began a five-year study (1958–1963) of families of people with schizophrenia — a project again growing out of a study group which included new formative influences: Aaron Esterson, David Cooper, and Dennis Scott. Cooper went on to organise a therapeutic community at Shenley Hospital, 'Villa 21', and Scott to collaborate with the sociologist, Elizabeth Bott, and develop a home-based alternative to hospital treatment from Napsbury Hospital, outside London. The project studied the families of 25 women with schizophrenia who were resident in two London psychiatric hospitals, but only 11 of whom were considered in detail. The case histories appeared in the book, *Sanity, Madness & the Family* (1970), which argued that psychosis was a direct result of the way that vulnerable individuals were treated by their closest relatives.

Another strand of this work was family therapy in schizophrenia, but the absence of a control group vitiated the results of these studies — a criticism that Laing was aware of, but never managed to rebut. In fact, many years later, he admitted that data were collected on the families of controls, but that he found in them "reams and reams and reams of nothing". No further analysis of these data was ever done.

Laing's work brought together many of the current aspects of thinking in what was becoming known as 'alternative' circles. Bateson's group in California had focused on communication in families of people with schizophrenia, taking a more behavioural perspective, and had concluded that 'double bind' communication might cause the disorder. Goffman's sociological study of *Asylums* had indicated in another way that people with chronic mental illness were denied a *locus standi* in society — by confinement in a 'total' institution. Szasz had castigated the *Myth of Mental Illness* in 1960, while Harold Searles and others had proposed methods of family intervention. Several social psychologists including Timothy Leary at Harvard and Fritz Perls had been trying to develop methods of social and personal understanding that used insights from the phenomenological method. Laing's work of this period, therefore, was not particularly original and its limitations seem now to loom larger than its achievements.

The *British Medical Journal* paper of 1965 with Cooper and Esterson was Laing's last one in a medical journal; it described the results of family-orientated therapy for schizophrenic patients in Villa 21, which were claimed to be good. This year can be said to mark the end of his scientific period, but also the beginning of Laing's career as celebrity and activist, for it was in 1965 that *The Divided Self* was republished in paperback, with immediate success. Its exposition of what it is to be 'schizoid' is that, "Such a person is not able to experience himself 'together with' others or 'at home in' the world, but, on the contrary, he experiences himself in despairing loneliness and isolation". There were many people, not all of them psychotic, who experienced themselves in this way, and Laing spoke to them directly. Although he wrote as a psychiatrist, and therefore in the third person about 'them', his style was sympathetic and understanding. Laing wrote from the heart, but coupled this with an intellectual understanding that suggested that the 'schizoid' experience has a long and distinguished history and that it is by no means a nonsensical way of 'being in the world'. The tools that Laing used to find a voice for a psychotic person experiencing this alienation were mainly derived from existentialism.

The chapter of *The Divided Self* explaining how psychosis might supervene on a schizoid adjustment is the least satisfactory, relying on psychoanalytic arguments and written more obviously than the rest from a privileged position of the sane contemplating the insane.

Intellectual limitations

At the end of the twentieth century it appears that psychoses, or at least the several incapacitating disorders that Laing describes, have a biological basis. Laing's inability to account for why some people found family and other situations intolerable, while others survived — as he did himself — without becoming psychotic, is therefore understandable, since he did not accept the biological contribution. We may also say that his readiness not

---

Laing's argument

1. All of us struggle with the dilemma of both being together and being separate.
2. There are no objective truths about our relationships with each other.
3. Life is really fraught with danger.
4. The sensitive vulnerable person may be more in touch with 'reality' than someone who is more 'normal'.
5. Other people do things to one that make sensitive individuals deeply and chronically anxious, 'ontologically insecure'.
6. If the anxiety is too great, then the only way to survive is to conceal oneself — giving away, if necessary, one's body or one's personality to remain on the other side of a divide between the real and the false.
7. Other people see and interact with the false self, or the dissociated body whilst, if the divide cuts too deeply, the real self dies through inanition.

just to talk, but to exchange thoughts and feelings with people who are psychotic, was exemplary. However, it is now possible to see that Laing was caught in presumptions about the world that limited his intellectual framework. Two of these stand out particularly.

The first was the nature of reality. Laing moved from a positivist view, fully consistent with his medical background, through a brief contact with Marxism and the notion that reality was a product of the ruling class, to a mystical notion in which there were no conditions of truth for distinguishing between various interpretations of the world. The elision of the worlds of the mystic, of the psychedelic, the psychotic, and the normal was accomplished without any clear boundary markers between them. But he also knew that people who are psychotic are more at risk of homelessness, rape, and premature death; any understanding of psychosis cannot afford to lose sight of these and other contingencies.

The second presumption was that there could be an 'ontological security', which was the foil to the insecurity that he believed underlay the schizoid condition. A key point of existentialism is that all of us live under the shadow of death, of illness, of war, or of madness, and that an attitude of anxiety about the future is appropriate. Security is not the static product of early relationships, but a prize to be gained in the face of these and other insecurities. Laing often took the view that someone or something was to blame for insecurity: that its presence indicated a failing or a neglect in what a person had been given by life. Life could let a person down through giving them a bad mother, or an engulfing family, or a particularly serious birth trauma — all these were aetiological factors that concerned Laing at different times in his career. But whatever it was, he believed that a person had the right to complain — that peace of mind was a right and not an achievement.

Celebrity and activist

Towards the end of the family research project, Laing went to the USA, where he met Bateson and Goffman. On his return, he unexpectedly went into private practice as well as leaving his wife, a nurse, and his children, for a new and much younger woman, a journalist. He began to use the still-legal LSD, attracting many patients who were in the media or the arts. His writing took on a more polemical tone, much of it critical of family life, and he began to appear regularly on television and to give public lectures. When he revisited the USA in 1964, he met a more radical and more fashionable group: Leary, who had turned into a propagandist for drugs; Allen Ginsberg, the beat poet; and Ray Birdwhistell, the author of an influential book on kinesics.

Laing also met two doctors who were to become some of his first disciples: Joe Berke and Leon Redler. With Esterson and Cooper, Laing was planning to create a therapeutic milieu for people with schizophrenia. It would not be contained in a hospital, as Cooper's Villa 21 was, but in the community. It would provide the opportunity for people with schizophrenia to find their own ways back to sanity without the use of medication. In the USA, Laing had met John Rosen who was using controversial confrontational methods, which often produced regression; opportunities or even encouragement to regress were an important part of this therapeutic plan.

Kingsley Hall

Back in London, Laing had met the sister (Mary Barnes) of a young man with schizophrenia who suspected that she might also have that illness. She wanted an opportunity to find a safe haven in which she could overcome her problem. Eventually, premises were found in the East End of London, at Kingsley Hall and Barnes was one of the first to move in. The young American psychiatrists that Laing had met were then the first and the most committed of many international visitors. Laing himself moved there six months later, together with Jutta Werner, who was to become his next wife.

Mary Barnes' extreme regression has been amply documented in the book that she wrote with Berke, who had become her therapist, and in a play by David Edgar. Regression was fostered in Kingsley Hall not just as a matter of policy, but by the lack of clarity about boundaries or expectations, the reliance on individual residents to know what was best for them, and the dependence on Laing himself as a focus for the enterprise. It is not at all clear how successful it was as a therapeutic environment, though, particularly in relation to schizophrenia. Most commentators do not consider Mary Barnes herself to have suffered from the condition, but a few other residents may have done so. Kingsley Hall was only open for five years, during which time it had a total of 115 residents, but probably few of these were schizophrenic. Its most important role was as a symbol of 'liberation' from an ill-defined 'oppression' by psychiatrists. It became one of the icons of 'liberation', being visited by media stars, many young people, but rather fewer therapists (e.g. Fritz Perls) or psychiatrists (e.g. Franco Bassaglia, the founder of Psychiatria Democratica).

The Kingsley Hall experience involved long discussions late into the night with residents, visitors, associates, and Laing himself. He was then writing fluently, perhaps fuelled by these discussions. *The Politics of Experience* and *The Bird of Paradise* were published (in one volume) in 1967, setting up 'society' and not the family as its target. Laing's thesis was that society alienates individuals and seeks to destroy those who do not conform. Becoming mad is one type of destruction, but the mad are not really destroyed, for madness may be a voyage to a new conception of reality, free of alienation. If this voyage can be completed successfully (and Laing never suggested that it could always be), a person may find a new spiritual understanding. *The Politics of the Family*, written with David Cooper was published in 1969; it covered much the same ground as previous work, but was more polemicised. *Knots* appeared in 1970; this was a book of paradoxes similar to the koan of Zen, designed to sharpen the reader's awareness.

The 1970s and 1980s

The books that Laing produced during this period were short and episodic; the arguments were eclectic, but not integrated. He was being exposed to more stimulation than he could digest, and after Kingsley Hall was closed, followed the celebrity trail to Sri Lanka to find spiritual refreshment for himself. He was away a year, during which time his Philadelphia Association split, with Morton Schatzman and Joe Berke founding the Arbours. Both associations started new therapeutic communities, some of which continue today, and both have gradually moved towards a stronger psychoanalytic emphasis. No formal evaluation of their work has ever been published, nor is it clear what proportion of their clients have experienced psychoses, or even any formal mental illness. Laing was much less productive during the 1970s, and more involved in the alternative culture, speaking at conferences involving political activists, religious adherents, and those espousing the 'New Age'. *The Facts of Life* (1979) was even thinner than his previous books and even more anecdotal. Its new idea was that the birth trauma is the cause of much later unhappiness, but the real subject was that "Laing is no longer talking about the people who come to him in trouble, but about himself". He had many personal troubles then, which may have concerned him more than those of his patients.

These began to get the better of him in the 1980s. His connection with the Philadelphia Association was severed when he was accused of having sexual relations with a resident in one of its communities, though this was never proved. There was then a protracted breakdown in his second marriage. In 1983, a patient made a complaint against him that led ultimately to Laing voluntarily withdrawing from the Medical Register. In 1984, he was arrested for disorderly conduct and found to be in possession of cannabis, for which he received a non-custodial sentence. In his last two years of life, Laing seemed to find some peace, but he remained a rebel to the end. Having been advised that it would be 'mad' to play tennis on a hot day in St Tropez, he did in fact play fiercely until he collapsed and died shortly after.

The Laing of the 1970s and 1980s is often written off as a shadow of his former self. It is true that his interests were now mainly in the discontents of the sane, rather than those of the insane. Lectures by him would involve long silences, spontaneous and sometimes angry interactions with the audience, and frequent drunkenness. Yet when he was accepted and encouraged, he could nudge people into a deeper understanding of themselves, in a way that left a life-long impression. At his best, he had achieved the liberation from language that the poet Artaud, who had so influenced him many years before, had sought.

Laing himself had personal experience of psychological disorder. His mother may well have suffered from a postnatal depression. His father recovered from agitated depression, but developed dementia in his last 10 years. One of Laing's daughters was diagnosed as having schizophrenia, and one of his sons with psychological problems. Laing himself suffered life-long despondency, and once told Gregory Bateson that he had "mild anorexia nervosa". He may well have had a physical dependency on alcohol in later life. In spite of his denunciation of conventional psychiatry, he made no attempt to prevent his close relatives being treated in mental hospitals.

Despite these difficulties, Laing had an extraordinary ability to make contact with people with psychoses. Though he may have felt greater sympathy for mania than for schizophrenia, he succeeded in reaching people in states of considerable withdrawal or disturbance. This understanding was not put at the service of psychiatry, but fuelled Laing's increasing rejection of the psychiatric paradigm. He was not, therefore, a great psychiatric reformer, or even theoretician of the discipline.

Anti-psychiatry

Laing's name is inevitably linked with the 'anti-psychiatry' movement, which was strongest in the 1960s, particularly in Western Europe and the USA. This maintained that psychiatrists and psychiatric institutions, as agents of social control, were responsible for doing 'violence' to people; physical treatments such as ECT and leucotomy were particularly condemned, as well all compulsory hospitalisation. The movement contemptuously dismissed psychiatric diagnoses as mere 'labels', and may well have contributed indirectly to the international refinement of diagnosis that began in the 1970s. Anti-psychiatry claimed that conventional psychiatric practice alienated people from their humanity, and that this should be overcome by alternative therapy, self-help, abolition of the distinction between professional and patient, and the levelling of hierarchies. This critique appealed strongly to many non-medical mental health professionals who resented psychiatrists' medical monopoly over diagnosis, drug treatment, and involuntary hospitalisation. The work of Michel Foucault appeared to give historical support to the critics of psychiatry and was very influential in the intellectual discourse of this time (Chapter 8, p. 245).

Such criticisms were embedded in a highly polemical discourse, which often appealed to the mass media, for instance in the films, *Family Life* and *One Flew Over the Cuckoo's Nest*. Since any critics of this position were denounced as 'enemies', acceptance of anti-psychiatric views had to be an act of faith. Anti-psychiatric writing tended to be a promiscuous mixture of fact, imagination, and fiction, which made scientific debate with it largely impossible, although its proponents often came off best in any public contest. This was because of their use of moral arguments and appeals to a repugnance, shared by many of the public, towards some aspects of psychiatric practice. Denis Martin, a reforming British psychiatrist of the 1960s, described Laing's position in this respect as "random accusation and sloganized virulence, which destroys the possibility of discussions". In most countries, psychiatrists and their professional organisations were ill-prepared for such open confrontations and either let their case go by default or made replies which had little impact against the seductive verbal pictures painted by anti-psychiatrists.

Anti-psychiatry was eagerly taken up by sociologists and is still to be found influencing the teaching of medical sociology. It also penetrated the training of social workers in many countries; they emerged eager to confront and nullify the work of psychiatrists, rather than to cooperate in multi-professional teamwork. Political interests were also aroused; anti-psychiatrists were often committed to Marxism and saw their role primarily as taking part in the overthrow of bourgeois society. In theoretical terms, this position was quite illogical, and communist countries had no sympathy with it; their mental health services remained not just conventional, but determinedly old-fashioned. Whilst Laing himself flirted with Marxism in the 1960s, he never had any serious interest in politics. It was in Italy, however, under the influence of Franco Bassaglia, that this political involvement was most marked, underlying the Psichiatria Democratica movement and the reforms of 1978–1980 (Chapter 8, p. 257). Yet paradoxically, those Italian professionals who tried to practise along the lines approved by the reforming ideology found little support from communist regional governments.

The legacy of anti-psychiatry was a very mixed one. On the positive side, it could lead to the liberalisation of institutions, to greater sensitivity to the dignity of patients, and to a more scrupulous concern with the appropriateness of professional practice. Negatively, it devalued scientific knowledge, aroused inter-professional hostility which damaged the effectiveness of mental health services, and told relatives that severe mental illness was caused by their own actions, as if they were not already feeling enough guilt. By the 1980s, anti-psychiatry had lost most of its influence, though echoes of it continued to appear in the media and in the actions of some professionals, which might not be in the best interests of people suffering from psychiatric disorder.

What, then, is Laing's most lasting contribution? His celebrity came from the fact that, perhaps for 10 years, he was able to surf on the wave of change surrounding conceptions of madness. Previously, the mad had been isolated and the sane insulated from them, but in the early 1960s, deinstitutionalisaton was beginning to have a significant effect; the sight of someone gesticulating to the air or talking to no-one visible become almost commonplace in cities. Psychedelic drugs were becoming widely available, and their hallucinatory effects were enthusiastically described, e.g. by Aldous Huxley. For a time, the worlds of madness and of sanity seemed to converge, and then merge. Laing's work reduced the surface tension between these two worlds, but this did not last long. The '*évènements*' of Paris, the Vietnam War, and the economic downturn of the 1970s shifted cultural concerns from perception to politics. However, the 'normal' world was not unscathed by its encounter with madness. Cultural conceptions of psychosis are now very different from what they were in the pre-Laingian era. Gone is the frightening image of the madman with the strength of ten; it seems that the image of madness in the twenty-first century will rather be one of dilapidation and waste. Society has largely stopped fearing madness. One might say that with the rare exception of the psychotic murderer, people have become largely indifferent to it.

For all Laing's faults, he had the fierce determination that psychosis mattered, and for a while, persuaded many other people that it did. For that, we should honour him.

PSYCHIATRIC NURSING

by Peter Nolan

The 1930s was the decade when those in the forefront of mental health nursing began to explore what constituted its professional identity (Chapter 4, p. 93). In 1956, a WHO Expert Committee had concluded that, "Psychiatric nursing has developed in an uneven, erratic manner, leaving many gaps in the care of the mentally ill and in programmes of mental health, even in the most highly organised countries. These gaps present many of the central problems in the field today". During, the 1960s, in some countries at least, efforts were focused on clarifying the role of the psychiatric nurse. However, the rise of the anti-psychiatry movement fuelled increasing public and professional discontent with institutional psychiatry (this chapter, p. 202). This and other developments led to an acknowledgment that the community, once seen as brutalising and threatening to vulnerable people, might in fact be a better location for the treatment of many mentally ill patients. The passing of the 1959 Mental Health Act in the UK and the 1963 Community Mental Health Centers Act in the USA gave nurses confidence that they could have a significant part to play in assisting patients in community settings. However, mental health nurses still lacked a robust and well-articulated theoretical basis to which practitioners could refer, to support their claim for greater involvement in community care.

Some studies of the work of the psychiatric nurse were undertaken in the UK at this time, most significantly by Maddox and John. Both concluded that this role was difficult to define, and that only some of its aspects could be described as 'therapeutic'. However, the seminal work in formulating the theoretical basis of mental health nursing was that of Hildegard Peplau in the USA. She provided much-needed scholarly leadership for psychiatric nurses in the English-speaking world, but such was her influence that it helped to raise intellectual awareness of psychiatric nursing worldwide. *Interpersonal Relations in Nursing*, first published in 1952 and grounded in the interpersonal psychology of Harry Stack Sullivan, provided the first coherent theoretical framework for psychiatric nurses to describe their work. Peplau emphasised the interpersonal nature of nursing care and the need for nurses to understand psychodynamic concepts and to use counselling techniques in their practice. Her theme was further developed by Ida Jean Orlando's book *The Dynamic Nurse–Patient Relationship*, published in the USA in 1961, which argued for the centrality of interpersonal relationships in all fields of nursing. In a later publication, Peplau proposed that the counsellor role should be the psychiatric nurse's primary mode of engagement with patients and clients.

The increased strength of psychiatric nursing's intellectual base was seen in the publication in 1963 in the UK of the first psychiatric nursing journal, *Perspectives in Psychiatric Care*. Later the same year, the *Journal of Psychiatric Nursing and Mental Health Services*, was inaugurated to publish clinical research papers written by psychiatric nurses. By 1969, the first psychiatric nurse had moved into private practice in the USA. In the UK, nurse training in psychiatric hospitals began to embrace psychology to assist students in understanding relationships and in acquiring the skills to be able to relate to people with severe mental illness. Sociology also became part of the national training curriculum, as psychiatric nursing developed an appreciation of the importance of understanding the nature of communities and of the social context in which people live, as well as returning to society after discharge from hospital.

The wealth of new concepts, insights, treatment, and care approaches in psychiatry and in psychiatric nursing in the 1960s nurtured a climate in which change could be implemented. Nursing reflected the mood of Britain at large. This was the first post-war decade to witness an intake of student nurses with no first-hand experience of the war. Many of them identified strongly with the new libertarianism; they were keen to challenge traditional practices and sources of authority. Even where young nurses had relatives who were still working in the psychiatric institutions, since there was often a family tradition there, they often had no inclination to revere or preserve the past. They were uneasy about the lack of accountability of the psychiatric hospitals and wanted to assume the role of advocate for patients.

The medical administrative stranglehold on the British psychiatric hospitals that was exercised by the descendants of the Victorian Physician Superintendents gradually weakened at this time. This was largely as a result of psychiatrists gaining more autonomy and being appointed to work between general and psychiatric hospitals. In consequence, a new era dawned: wards were unlocked, military-style male uniforms were abandoned, and paid workers were recruited to take over the domestic work formerly done by nurses and patients. The hospital farms, pride of the nineteenth-century asylums, were run down and

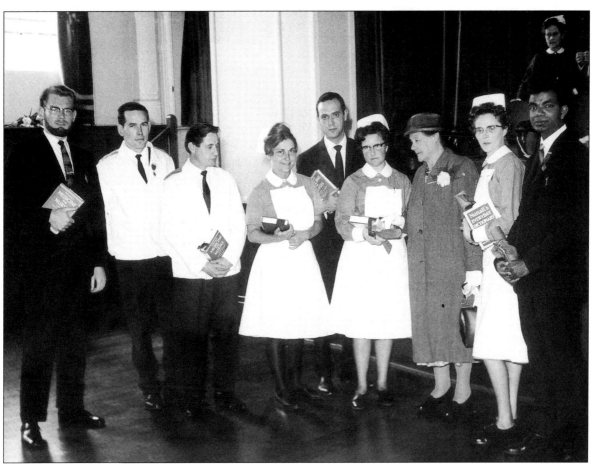

Group of psychiatric nurses (the author is the first on the left) who successfully passed their RMN (Registered Mental Nurse) examinations in 1965 at Tooting Bec Hospital, South London.

eventually sold off, while the deployment of selected patients and nursing staff in gardens and maintenance departments gradually ceased. A new emphasis on therapeutic relationships and environments became evident in many hospitals, though it has been argued by some that these changes were mainly cosmetic. On the whole, relationships between patients and staff, and between junior and senior staff, continued to be characterised by 'control' and 'authority' to varying extents. Male nurses were especially reluctant to accept new working practices and to implement innovative approaches to the care of patients. They were fearful that any threat to the traditional psychiatric hospitals would also threaten their own promotion prospects and their economic security. Similar processes occurred in the mental hospitals of most industrial countries, particularly France, Scandinavia, and Switzerland, though in Central and Eastern Europe, changes were much slower.

In several countries at this time, the policy of diversifying the locations of care for mental health clients was impeded, not only by resistance from practitioners but also by the greater expense of combining services that were provided by different authorities into a new cohesive whole. In the UK, the Government attempted to remedy this difficulty by creating new layers of health service management. Nursing officers were appointed who had the responsibility of providing 'clinical supervision' and 'management' (terms that were poorly understood at the time), as well as education, for junior staff. By doubling the number of nurses in management positions, there was an attempt to create a better career structure for nurses. In doing so, however the more experienced were thereby removed from direct contact with patients. There was no formal evaluation of what this change achieved, although it undoubtedly contributed to increased mobility amongst the nursing workforce and to psychiatric nurses being less likely to remain at the same hospital for the whole of their careers. Management positions in British psychiatric hospitals were finally opened up to outside competition, and promotion no longer depended on staying in the same place until a vacancy occurred through retirement or death.

The relocation to general hospitals of services such as radiography, pathology, and surgery, which had formerly been provided within mental hospitals, contributed further to the demise of these specialised institutions. Many treatments with which the mental hospitals had been associated were abandoned altogether; malarial treatment for patients with general paralysis of the insane (GPI) was replaced by penicillin; while leucotomy and insulin coma therapy were largely abandoned, as neuroleptics became the preferred treatment. Some somatic conditions, which had once been widespread and treated in mental hospitals became

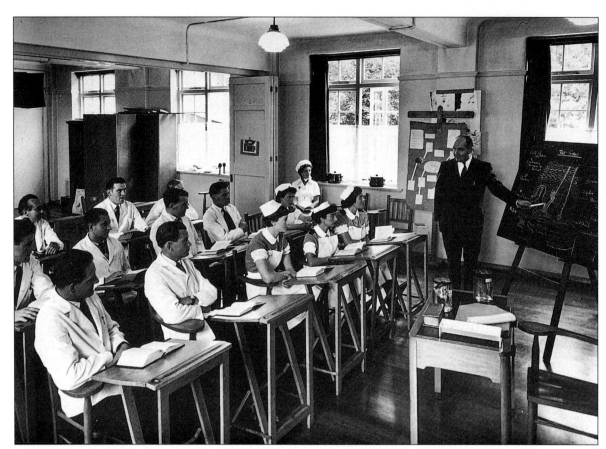

A nurses' classroom (c. 1950s). Reproduced with permission from the North East Essex Mental Health NHS Trust.

extremely rare as a result of the development of new drugs which could cure or control diseases such as tuberculosis and epilepsy. From the mid-1960s, patients with psychiatric disorders were increasingly admitted to general hospitals, many of which now provided psychiatric wards or units. Ambitious and able mental health professionals, both doctors and nurses, generally opted to work in these new settings, leaving the less able in the psychiatric hospitals to manage as best they could. Nurses working in therapeutically orientated community settings, either inside or outside the psychiatric hospitals, now put more emphasis on the individual needs of patients. Nurses working in traditional settings, on the other hand, tended to believe that the smooth running of the institution took precedence over everything else.

Inevitably, the staff left behind in the psychiatric hospitals could not provide a high quality of service for patients; standards of care fell, and critics of institutionalised psychiatry found it increasingly easy to attack them. In Britain, the stage was set for the series of hospital inquiries, which took place during the 1960s and 1970s. Individual nurses and psychiatric nursing in general were fiercely criticised during these investigations and by the time they had run their course, the morale of the profession was much weakened. It was not improved by attempts to bring psychiatric nursing closer to general nursing, such that it became almost a prerequisite for British psychiatric nurses who wished to progress in their career to train as general nurses as well. The implication was that the skills required by each group were interchangeable.

From such developments sprang a widespread view, promoted by sociologically minded critics, that mental illness was often exacerbated and even made intractable within the walls of an institution. This acceptance was given grudgingly by nurses whose lives and those of their families had for several generations been lived within the grounds of psychiatric hospitals. It was more eagerly given by those who had moved away to try their skills in the community. Nurses began to appreciate that they had to embrace change more vigorously than hitherto, but that this would require an improvement in their professional skills, if they were to be an integral part of providing care in the community.

The literature of the time periodically reports the developments taking place in mental health nursing in various countries. The role of nurses and the extent and nature of the contribution they should make to mental health care, training and education were issues very much to the fore in Australia, New Zealand, South Africa, Finland, Sweden, France, Japan, and Russia. The picture was one of increasing international recognition of the importance of mental health nursing and of widespread similarities in its practice. Cross-

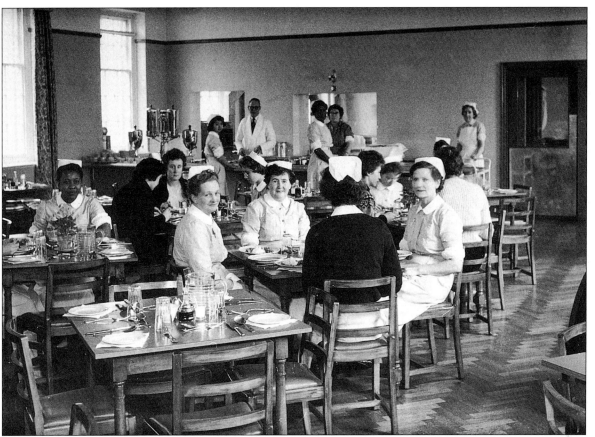

Standard dress and waitress service in the nurses' dining room (c. 1960). Reproduced with permission from the North East Essex Mental Health NHS Trust.

cultural perspectives and international collaboration continue to be pursued today, facilitated by conferencing facilities on the Internet. There is a drive in each country to improve its own practice through a better understanding of what mental health nursing means to nations across the globe.

TRADITIONAL MEDICINE AND CULTURAL FACTORS IN ASIA

by Felice Lieh Mak

The Asian continent is a land of contrast and diversity. Yet despite its diversities, Asian countries have many commonalties in regard to psychiatry and the care of the mentally ill.

By the turn of the twentieth century, Asia's population will have grown to 3.75 billion, which means that six out of every 10 people on this planet will be from Asia. But the vast majority of these people will not have access to any type of modern psychiatric service. There is a dearth of trained personnel to staff the mental health system, while in many public dispensaries there is an inadequate supply of psychotropic medication. Even when basic medication is available, there is a lack of medical personnel trained in the rational use of such treatments. Thus, the provision of psychiatric treatment as part of the primary health care system is obstructed by lack of training and an excessive workload.

The paucity of resources devoted to psychiatric care is not only due to economic constraints, but also to the lack of sustained public investment. This reflects the low priority given to mental illness by both national governments and international agencies. Notwithstanding these shortages and neglect, the prevalence of psychiatric disorders do not seem to be significantly different when Asian countries are compared to each other, or indeed when Asian are compared to Western countries. These similarities are evident both in population-based and primary health care-based surveys using standardised (ICD–9/10, DSM–III/IV) diagnostic criteria. The data seem to indicate that there are no cultural protective factors against psychiatric disorders. The myth that some Asian countries do not have certain disorders of this kind has finally been laid to rest.

Stigma of mental illness

One of the most serious obstacles to the development of modern psychiatry in Asia is the stigma attached to the mentally ill. There are a number of beliefs relating to and attitudes towards mental illness that may contribute to the propagation of this stigma:

- It is a punishment for the misdeeds of ancestors visited on the present generations of the family.
- It is associated with bizarre, violent, and deviant acts in societies that value conformity.
- It indicates hereditary defects which renders finding a spouse difficult for members of the family.
- It is incurable.
- It is due to weakness of will, lack of moral courage, or frailty in character.

Since stigmatisation also applies to those who work with the mentally ill, it not only prevents patients from being treated, but also discourages health care professionals from specialising in psychiatry.

The frequent use of somatic presentations as expression of emotional distress is an impediment to the early diagnosis and treatment of psychiatric disorders. While somatisation is found in all cultures, many aspects of Asian tradition serve to reinforce somatisation.

Traditional medicine

The three main streams of traditional medical practice in Asia are the Yunâni system, the Ayurvedic system, and Chinese Medicine. Yunâni influence is strong in Pakistan, India, Sri Lanka, Indonesia, and other southern Asian countries. Ayurveda has impact mainly in Tibet, Nepal, Burma, and Southern Asia. The practice of Chinese Medicine is pervasive in Japan, Korea, Singapore, Thailand, and also parts of Southern Asia. Yunâni is essentially Galenic medicine from Ancient Greece that was adopted by Islamic countries, and ayurveda is of Indian origin. These three systems are formulated from generic physiological and cosmological concepts; all are humoral theories and do not make a distinction between mind and body. Such cultural conceptions of health and diseases set the scene for Asians to express psychic distress through bodily organ symbols.

Asian societies value the harmony of social relationships. The individual is never conceived as a separate entity and the family is still regarded as the fundamental unit of society. Confucian ethics emphasise the collective quality in the individual's life and behaviour, while Buddhism and Hinduism preach respect for authority and self-denial. The social structure built on or inherited from an agrarian tradition and religious influences are responsible for the negative valuation of the open expression of emotions and for sanctioning the use of somatic metaphors.

While social structure and medical tradition are important, other factors also account for the tendency to somatisation. These include the stigmatisation of mental illness, scarcity of psychiatric services, the neglect of psychosocial factors in the health care delivery system, and the lack of training for doctors on how to handle psychological problems.

Traditional medicine and folk practices remain popular in Asia. Many psychiatric patients take herbs either to supplement or to counter the adverse effects of psychotropic medication. A significant proportion of psychiatric patients are found to have sought

Asian culture-bound syndromes	
Amok	Dissociative episode preceded by brooding and followed by violence
Dhat	Undue concerns about the debilitating effects of the passage of semen
Hwa-byung	Suppression of anger leading to a variety of somatic symptoms
Koro	Fear that the penis will retreat into the abdomen and cause death
qi-gong psychotic reaction	An acute, time-limited psychotic or dissociative state following qi-gong practice
Latah	Hypersensitivity to sudden fright accompanied by trance-like behaviour
Taijin kyofusho	Distinctive phobia in Japan resembling social phobia

help from shamans, traditional medical practitioners, or Buddhist/Taoist priests before being admitted to psychiatric hospitals. In many parts of Asia, local healers provide the great majority of treatments for the mentally ill.

Shoma Morita (1874–1938), a Japanese psychiatrist who had himself been troubled by panic attacks since adolescence, developed a unique form of psychotherapy around 1920. It combined periods of absolute bed rest with work therapy, in the setting of the patient's home. Morita sought to energise the 'desire for life' that lay behind the anxieties, whilst allowing them to be accepted as they are. In this way, he hoped to change the way-of-being of the former self, bound up with neurotic symptoms, into a healthier state. Morita therapy was claimed to be effective for obsessive–compulsive disorder, hypochondriasis, panic disorder, social phobia, and agoraphobia.

Though empirical data on the efficacy of folk and traditional healing are extremely sparse, there are some indications that these forms of treatment may be effective in alleviating symptoms relating to psychological and social distress. When psychiatric services are not available, local healers help in re-moralising their clients. By providing an explanatory model for their illness, they give patients and their families a sense of control.

PM Yap, a former professor of psychiatry in Hong Kong, coined the phrase "culture-bound syndrome" (see table opposite) to describe mixed disorders of behaviour, beliefs, and emotions which occur with particular frequency in certain cultures. These disorders are included in the appendices of both the ICD–10 and DSM–IV.

COMMUNITY PSYCHIATRY

by Hugh Freeman

'Community' has been one of the most frequently used words in psychiatry in the second half of this century, although without any general agreement about its meaning. Often taken to be the equivalent of 'outside mental hospitals', in practice it has covered anything from arrangements for low-cost psychotherapy to aspirations for the total transformation of human relationships. However, the many different approaches towards this uncertain goal fell into two broad categories. The first — 'community psychiatry' — was of comprehensive public services for the mentally disordered from a defined population, using hospital units as part of a network of integrated facilities. Secondly, there were consultative agencies, established on a public health model of prevention and operating through a variety of local organisations — 'community mental health'.

The fundamental difference was that the first category was concerned with individuals showing overt psychiatric illness or disability, particularly of the more severe kinds. It is an offshoot of medical science. The second, on the other hand, focused on the goals of primary prevention and 'positive mental health' and therefore dealt with many people who had no clinical abnormality. The first was particularly characteristic of the UK and the second of the USA. Towards the end of this century, though, an ideological change in many countries focused attention and resources further away from the hospital base towards smaller, more informal facilities.

Historical aspects

Historically, the only management of the mentally ill was by 'community care', and it was public outrage at their neglect or mistreatment in prisons, workhouses, and private madhouses that led to the foundation of public mental hospitals. Families, though, always carried the largest burden, with little or no outside help; in most of the world today, things remain in that original state. In the nineteenth century, European and American mental hospitals had optimistic early phases of 'moral treatment' and non-restraint, but eventually were overwhelmed by the demands of chronic mental illness. They tended to become fixed in a rigid, authoritarian pattern, with an internal culture of their own. In the post-war period, the largest mental hospitals in Europe were in France, where some had up to 4000 beds. This system resulted in the secondary handicaps of institutionalism being often added to the inherent effects of mental illness. Yet mental hospitals were highly selective in their admissions, mainly taking in those who lacked supportive relatives or caused unusual public disruption. The overwhelming bulk of psychiatric disorder was still left to be dealt with in the general community, either by primary medical care or without any care at all.

In the 1930s, the first development of general hospital psychiatry, child guidance clinics, and private psychotherapy in many countries showed that the mental hospital was not the only model of care for the mentally disordered. In Amsterdam, Querido organised a domiciliary emergency service, mainly designed to reduce the cost of mental hospital care. Though successful in the city, attempts to expand it nationally did not deal with people who were severely ill. Experience in the Second World War emphasised the importance of intervening early and not removing the patient from his normal setting. In the post-war world, there was greater concern with the needs and rights of all disadvantaged groups, as well as more confidence in society's ability to intervene on their behalf. An egalitarian philosophy of state intervention, general social changes such as smaller families and increased life expectancy, as well as new ideas and treatments within psychiatry were all influential in a reorientation of care away from mental hospitals. More awareness of the influence of social and psychological factors on both psychiatric disorder and the facilities to treat it was also important.

The move away from institutional care — often described as 'decarceration' — was not restricted to psychiatry, but affected other groups that had been subject to institutionalisation in the last century, such as children and the aged. This change was based both on humanitarianism and on a recognition that many institutions had ceased to be relevant to current conditions, though some sociological critics saw it in conspiratorial terms. It has often been said that the process was driven mainly by governments' wish to save money, but there is little evidence for this view. In the USA, David Mechanic believed that the change was a largely accidental by-product of the good sense and new techniques of clinicians, rather than a derivation from any consistent theoretical framework. Certainly, no system of care can be understood except in relation to the underlying social and political structures of the society it serves. In contrast to the classic mental hospital model, a broad medico-social approach had been commended in a report by WHO in 1953, though this was sceptical about the role of general hospitals.

The British concept

From the late 1950s, the UK provided an example of the use of comprehensive public services in community psychiatry, mainly because of the nature of the National Health Service (NHS). This gives every member of the population free access to primary medical care, which is one of the essential elements in an integrated service. At that time, profound changes began to be seen, including the open-door policy in mental hospitals, part-time hospitalisation, readily available out-patient care, industrial therapy, hostels, therapeutic social clubs, general hospital units, and home visits by mental health staff. The same period also saw the introduction of psychotropic drugs, though whether these made such changes possible by controlling the symptoms of major mental illness, or whether medication merely gave doctors more confidence to do new things remains a matter of dispute. Nevertheless, extending the effective use of medication became one of the primary activities of British community-based psychiatry, especially for the prevention of relapse in recurrent psychoses.

The first effects of policies which favoured extramural care were seen in a reduced need for patients to spend long periods in mental hospitals. From 1955, in both Britain and the USA, the previously inexorable rise in the national total of resident patients went into reverse, and it has continued to decline ever since. Most other countries, though, followed a more cautious and conservative policy, with their numbers of psychiatric beds continuing to increase during the next 15–20 years. In France, although the *politique du secteur* was first proposed in 1960, it was not generally put into effect for a number of years; change was similarly slow in Germany, Spain, and other countries. In Western Europe, an average of over 80% of national mental health budgets continued to be spent on in-patient services, at least until the mid-1980s.

In Britain, 'community care' was a phrase that became strongly associated with a Mental Health Act of 1959, although in fact the new law made no requirement for such a policy to be followed, but merely removed any legal obstacles that prevented it. This change resonated with anti-institutional feelings which were becoming widespread in Western societies then, and was probably the most successful slogan in the history of British social policy. It also corresponded with developments in general medical services, which were now focusing on the district general hospital as the centre of all secondary health care for a defined population. A national Hospital Plan of 1962 excluded any more new or enlarged mental hospitals; future developments were to occur only in district general hospitals. From then on, 'community psychiatry' was evolving into a national plan for comprehensive district-based services, but the problem arose of how to pay for setting up an alternative system. The mental hospitals were still very active and were even finding a new role

---

WHO's general principles of comprehensive community mental health care in 1980

1. Provide facilities for a defined population, small enough for most patients to be treated near their homes

2. Provide a range of facilities, meeting the needs of patients with all forms of illness and handicap, but with more specialised care on a Regional basis

3. Effective coordination of the agencies serving each defined population

4. Services of equal quality to be available to everyone, and not be of a lower standard than those for the physically ill

---

in caring for the growing numbers of psychogeriatric cases (Chapter 8, p. 260). This dilemma — of the cost of running two systems at the same time — affected every country with established mental hospitals which aimed to move towards community care. Italy made the change very quickly, though with variable results (Chapter 8, p. 257). Yet in the 1960s, when psychiatry came under much ideological attack, developments which up to then had been seen as progressive were somehow reframed as 'oppressive'. This applied particularly to any use of hospitals (this chapter, p. 202). Kathleen Jones pointed out that the 'community', which was now being seen as a healing force, was where the problems of psychiatric disorder had developed in the first place. It was also ironical that the virtues of communities were being rediscovered, just when modernisation was largely destroying many of them, in the traditional sense.

The Government statement of British mental health policy in 1975 assumed that "people with psychiatric disorders can be most effectively helped when links with family, friends, workmates, and society generally are maintained, and (when) preventive, treatment, and rehabilitative services (are provided) for a district". This was to be achieved by a partnership locally between the hospital facilities of the NHS and local social services, both collaborating with primary medical care (Chapter 8, p. 240). However, as in many countries, central government in the UK has relatively little power to influence the way in which local authorities provide such services. In some areas particularly, the numbers of hostels, day centres, or trained social workers have remained very inadequate, even after many years of a 'community care' policy.

British policy, though, has been closely in line with that fostered in Europe by WHO, which in 1980 described the general principles of comprehensive community mental health care, as outlined in the table above.

The last requirement (4) would obviously be a major problem where much care is provided by the private sector. Generally, insurance-based services have been reluctant to accept responsibility for long-term mental health care or for treatment methods outside conventional medical approaches. In Europe as a whole, WHO concluded that community mental health care was "not properly applied".

In both Britain and many other countries, much of the conventional dyadic relationship between doctor and psychiatric patient has been replaced by one with a multi-disciplinary professional team, reflecting the complex needs of many people in the general community. In these teams, psychiatry has been allied with nursing, social work, clinical psychology, and occupational therapy. Yet these members come from different levels in the hierarchies of their professions and so may have varying abilities to participate in decision-making. To what extent a team should have a leader has often been a controversial matter, and the traditional primacy of doctors has been increasingly challenged. In most countries, though, the responsibility of the psychiatrist has a legal basis which cannot be shared with other professions.

The American concept

No monolithic view of community prevailed in the USA during the period which began in the early 1960s (this chapter, p. 195). Sabshin, for instance, defined it as "the utilisation of the techniques, methods and theories of social psychiatry and other behavioral sciences to investigate and meet the mental health needs of a functionally or geographically defined population over a significant period of time, and the feeding back of information to modify the central body of... knowledge". This was a view very similar to that prevailing in the UK. Similarly, Serban described three aspects: a social movement; a service delivery strategy, emphasising accessibility and the acceptance of the mental health needs of a total population; and provision of the best possible clinical care, with emphasis on the major psychiatric disorders and on treatment outside institutions.

However, these were minority voices. During the Kennedy administration, abandoning proposals to modernise their State mental hospital system, the USA set out to create a totally new development in mental health care. This was additional to both the State hospitals and private out-patient practice (in which more than three-quarters of American psychiatrists were engaged). The entire country was to be served by a network of comprehensive community mental health centres (CCMHCs), each providing the five functions of: in-patient care, out-patient care, partial hospitalisation, consultative services, and information/education. The Federal Government would initially cover most of their cost, but it was assumed that money would gradually be transferred to the centres from State hospitals, as these were run down. Local communities were expected to accept the rest of the financial responsibility. In turn, these communities would have a strong voice in how the centres were run, and much of the time of their professional staff would be spent in working with general community organisations. It was believed at first that the activities of CCMHCs would achieve the primary prevention of mental illness, promote 'mental health' (whatever that may be), and even improve the general quality of life.

This movement was strongly influenced by the views of Gerald Caplan at Harvard, who maintained that intervening therapeutically in crises of human life, such as bereavement and divorce, would prevent much psychiatric disorder. He also stressed the value of 'community caregivers' for direct contact with the people affected by mental illness, while professional staff would be much occupied in training these caregivers. It was not surprising that expectations were aroused that were quite unreal, in view of the lack of aetiological knowledge about most psychiatric disorders. Alexander Leighton described the goal of providing services for everyone with a psychological or social need as "more and more like trying to drink the ocean". Furthermore, the idea of a community that could be given the task of caring for its mentally ill members seemed unrealistic in the case of populations containing many people with no social roots and few personal resources. In areas of social disorganisation, such as inner cities, the whole programme sometimes collapsed in total confusion. These failures seemed to be related to false perceptions about the nature of society itself.

Thus the American community mental health movement substituted vague objectives for practical action; how psychiatric expertise could ever lead to the ambitious goals that were advocated was never made clear. Resources were also diverted away from activities of proven value, such as the treatment and rehabilitation of those suffering from psychoses. Pursuing the ideology of community mental health to its ultimate goal could (and sometimes did) result in the virtual abandonment of actual clinical care. It was replaced by the attempted reform of society itself — as also occurred in some places with the Italian *psichiatria democratica* in its earlier period. This attempt ignored the fact that members of the mental health professions are employed to exercise the skills for which they have been trained. As reformers of society, they are no different from anyone else.

Worldwide considerations

Worldwide, it came to be generally agreed that any form of psychiatry that aims to serve the whole community must establish priorities for its inevitably limited resources. This has required some reversal of articulated demands, which are likely to be strongest from those with neurotic and personality disorders. Yet in terms of human needs, the groups that most require help must be those suffering from schizophrenia, dementia, and mental retardation. All three are predominantly chronic conditions which are difficult to treat by curative medicine and need prolonged care by relatives and/or public services. As a result, psychotherapeutic activities for the less severely ill must inevitably take second place. Yet in countries with insurance-based systems, treatment by private practitioners or in hospitals is paid for at higher rates than 'care' provided by services in the community. This has greatly handicapped the development of comprehensive services which have a broader view than that of the individual patient and take a longer-term responsibility. Voluntary organisations have also made big contributions, particularly to the care of patients with chronic disorders, in many countries.

Community-based psychiatry in Britain and most European countries has remained mostly within the conventional models of medicine, nursing, and social work. It did not develop on a theoretical basis, such as that of social networks, but rather through pragmatic action, using an eclectic but fundamentally biological form of psychiatry. It has not meant care by the community, which was envisaged in Caplan's model, but by professional services which are sensitive to the needs of populations as a whole.

Dealing with acute problems represents one important aspect of community psychiatry; their ill-effects are minimised and relationships of the service with the public are enhanced if there is a rapid response to them by trained staff. In Holland, since 1982, mental health centres have been established which are open 24 hours a day and seven days a week, but these do not include residential care. In other places, crisis intervention teams, usually with members of at least two professions, have been reported to be effective. Where their resources are provided permanently, and not just as part of a time-limited project, they can play a valuable part in a comprehensive community-based service. The services in Dane County, Wisconsin and in Sydney, Australia have become particularly well known. In several places including Boulder (USA), conventional hospital accommodation has been largely replaced by the use of family homes where a small number of patients are cared for by the owners, with intensive support from visiting professional staff. Not enough evaluation has been done yet to judge if this is a successful model.

However, chronic problems may be equally important. Where community-based services exist, surveys have shown that large numbers of people with psychiatric disorders are in long-term contact with them, but are not long-stay in-patients (although many would have been so in the past). In fact, the socio-demographic characteristics of these people are very similar to those of long-stay hospital in-patients. They usually have an extensive clinical history, often associated physical disability, and behavioural problems such as social withdrawal and embarrassing behaviour. Much of the burden of their care is carried by relatives in most cases. For many people like this, community care will not only be inappropriate but — if of a reasonable standard — will be no cheaper than institutional care. But comparing the effectiveness and costs of different kinds of services is a very complex process, for which reliable methods are still being devised.

Very often, as Douglas Bennett and Isobel Morris pointed out, in the dismantling of institutions, "the notion that some patients might require no less than long-life support in some sort of sheltered, protected setting was either ignored or denied". This is still the case in many countries; politicians, administrators, and financial planners remain unwilling to accept responsibility for the severe, chronic disability caused by mental illness. In Britain, smaller facilities that have been provided to replace mental hospitals have often been inadequate in both size and levels of staffing — for acute as well as for chronically ill patients.

Because of the large numbers affected by psychiatric disorder in any community, questions of coordination and administration require much greater attention than they have generally received. One example is ensuring that maintenance medication is actually continued over the long periods in which it is needed by people with chronic psychoses. This has been made more difficult by the dispersal of institutional populations into very large numbers of smaller community settings, often privately run, which presents an enormous problem for monitoring standards of care. No country has yet found a solution to this problem. In dispersed systems, it has also become much more difficult to monitor the activities of that very small minority of people with psychiatric disorders who have a tendency to violent behaviour. Such people often have unstable living arrangements and tend to be uncooperative with mental health services. It is very easy for them to become 'lost' between different facilities and personnel, each of which has a limited area of responsibility. Community-based services may not have any place in which a person with disturbed behaviour can be treated with some degree of security. This was one function of mental hospitals which has often been abandoned when new services have been established.

In Britain, one new professional group emerged in this field — community psychiatric nurses (CPNs). Many CPNs have had a special link with a primary care centre where they may administer depot neuroleptics, hold supportive groups, and assess patients referred by GPs (Chapter 8, p. 240). Psychiatrists are also becoming increasingly involved in the activities of primary care, and this devolution of specialist skills represents an important aspect of community psychiatry. Nevertheless, an unresolved problem is that of training for community work; as far as psychiatrists in most countries are concerned, this must be regarded as having scarcely begun. To achieve the necessary shift in attitudes away from traditional institutional practice, some common training of psychiatrists with GPs, public health physicians, and probably other professions seems essential.

One of the most rapid processes of deinstitutionalisation in the world occurred in Finland, where the use of psychiatric beds decreased by one-third between 1980 and the mid-1990s. Yet the development of other residential settings outside hospitals meant that the total amount of residential care did not change significantly. Re-admissions to hospitals increased, particularly for patients with a long duration of illness, but it seems that the well-developed social services have generally been able to adjust available resources to the needs of patients now living in the community. In many other countries, though, these alternative services have not been provided at an adequate level.

However defined, community psychiatry should mean much more than merely transferring activities from psychiatric hospitals. As an ideology, it has often been successful in encouraging the development of a broad spectrum of facilities — from secure hospital provision at one extreme to help within primary medical care at the other. Worldwide, there is now no serious challenge to its principles, though interpretations of the policy and attempts at its implementation vary enormously from country to country. At the end of the twentieth century, it is no exaggeration to say that, except for individuals treated in private practice, most psychiatry is 'community psychiatry' in the broadest sense. Yet it would not be in the interests of the mentally ill or their families for this to mean a rejection of residential care — whether in hospitals or other facilities — for those who need it. Too much of a dispersal of psychiatry from the mainstream of medicine into small community settings could mean that it once again becomes under-valued and neglected.

ALCOHOLISM

by Bruce Ritson

An understanding of alcoholism and alcohol-related problems during this century requires a backward glance to earlier attitudes. Societies have known about the physical and social hazards connected with alcohol since records began. But they have also been aware of its benefits, both to the individual, the producer, and — with the advent of trade and taxation — to the national economy. The tomb of an Egyptian king who lived approximately 5000 years ago carries the first known epitaph to a problem drinker: "His earthly abode was rent and shattered by wine and beer. And the spirit escaped before it was called".

Drunkenness as a disease of the mind

Whilst the medical consequences of alcohol misuse were recognised from early times, the belief that habitual drunkenness was in some way an affliction of the mind, rather than just evidence of weakness or sinfulness, arose in the eighteenth century. This was during the Enlightenment, when freethinkers were challenging the assumptions of religion. A crucial concept in what was to become a medical and psychological model of alcohol dependence was articulated by Dr Thomas Trotter in Edinburgh, who in 1804 published *An Essay Medical, Philosophical and Chemical on Drunkenness and its Effects on the Human Body*. His advice to a doctor treating a patient with a drinking problem was, "Whatever his disease may be whether stomach complaints with low spirits, premature gout, epilepsy, jaundice or any other of the catalogue, it is in vain to prescribe for it 'til the evil genius of the habit has been subdued. The habit of drunkenness is a disease of the mind". This notion that alcohol problems arise from habit has a very contemporary ring about it. Benjamin Rush was promoting similar concepts in the USA, and Magnus Huss in Sweden first introduced the term 'alcoholism', later in the nineteenth century. Many patients were admitted to psychiatric hospitals and retreats with the effects of alcohol, particularly delirium tremens and brain damage. By the start of the twentieth century, the belief that inebriety was a pathological disorder based on hereditary factors was widely held. In the UK, the Society for the Study of Inebriety was formed and promoted a scientific interest in the topic; one of its most prominent members, Dr Kerr, published a seminal work entitled *Inebriety or Narcomania — Its Aetiology, Pathology, Treatment and Jurisprudence* in 1888. The view that there was something wrong with the habitual drinker which separated him or her from other drinkers was thus well established by the end of the nineteenth century. Although alcoholism might be a disease, it was also seen even more clearly as a major social problem.

Whilst some individuals with alcohol-related problems were being treated in psychiatric hospitals and private clinics, at the start of the century there was little specialist medical interest in this area. Around this time, a number of 'homes for inebriates' were established in Britain as a result of the Inebriates' Acts which had been introduced to control compulsorily those who were recognised as habitual drunkards. These institutions emphasised rehabilitation through work and moral influence, but they were not particularly popular. One reason for this was that the cost of the facilities rested with the local authorities, who were disinclined to invest in such ventures. Echoes of this experience are evident in more recent, but largely ill-fated British attempts to set up detoxification facilities for habitual drunken offenders in the 1970s.

Temperance and prohibition

If a rudimentary scientific interest in the biological and psychological aspects of alcohol dependence was evident at the start of the twentieth century, it was of minor importance, compared with the overwhelming prominence in many countries of the Temperance Movement and the debates which it engendered. This movement had the very active support of many doctors. Particularly with the rapid growth of urbanisation, the effects of drunkenness on public order, the quality of public life, the integrity of the family, and people's capacity to work effectively became a prominent public theme. This was particularly evident at a time when alcohol was generally plentiful and cheap, and levels of consumption were prodigiously high. Because alcohol production is taxed, it has been possible, over the centuries, to record the patterns of consumption in several countries, including the UK. These records show that there is nothing fixed or unchanging about a nation's drinking habits.

The Temperance Movement, which was prominent in Northern Europe and the USA, was very aware of the social problems associated with alcohol. Their endeavours to increase the price of alcohol, reduce its availability, and improve the provision of alternative sources of entertainment where alcohol was not available, met with varying success in different parts of the world. Alongside other socio-economic changes, the Temperance Movement's activities certainly led to a marked reduction in the level of consumption in several countries, during most of the first half of this century. It was extremely effective in Scandinavia, where it continues to have a significant political influence, e.g. in maintaining state alcohol monopolies and restricting outlets for purchase. In the USA, the movement led to the introduction in 1919 of Prohibition, which was only repealed in 1933. Although Prohibition resulted in a decline in alcohol-related deaths and social problems, it ushered in a wave of gangsterism whose consequences are well known. Some individual States remained 'dry' for many more years, as did some Canadian provinces. In the 1980s, the former USSR demonstrated the benefits which could follow reducing the availability of alcohol, but more recently, releasing controls on alcohol in Russia has contributed to both a growth in alcohol-related problems and declining life expectancy. The balance between control policies in the interests of the public good and *laissez faire*, with widespread availability of alcohol, still runs through the debate on these questions throughout the world.

The work of the great neurophysiologist, Pavlov, in St Petersburg on conditioned reflexes eventually led to understanding that when alcohol is stopped, the addict may experience further withdrawal symptoms or cravings, when exposed to environmental stimuli that were previously linked with drinking. Cues that recall memories of the pleasure produced by alcohol may particularly re-awaken craving for it.

A new interest in treatment

The demise of Temperance and the repeal of Prohibition occurred at a time when the level of alcohol consumption and of scientific and medical interest in its problems were at a low ebb. Signs of a reawakening of interest, though, came in the late 1930s with the establishment of the Yale Center for Alcohol Studies in the USA; it studied the relationship between drinking and social problems, such as homelessness and crime. The self-help organisation Alcoholics Anonymous started in 1937 in the USA and gradually spread to gain world-wide significance. It is the most successful of all self-help groups, and its influence on the subsequent thinking about alcoholism has been immense. Jellinek, an educationalist working at the Yale Center, introduced its ideas into the scientific literature. In 1950, he moved to WHO in Geneva, where a series of extremely influential documents were promulgated. *The Disease Concept of Alcoholism*, his most famous book, was published in 1960. At this stage, the widely accepted view was that there were unfortunate individuals who, for biological and possibly genetic reasons, were psychologically and physically susceptible to an abnormal extent, or even allergic to alcohol and had become 'alcoholic'. In contrast, the majority of the population could drink with relative impunity. It was also stressed that these individuals suffered from a disease which merited and deserved treatment. Both WHO and a small body of experts advocated the need for properly organised specialist services for alcoholics which would help them regain abstinence and, with suitable psychological help, adopt a sober way of life.

Treatments in common use at that time included group psychotherapy; its popularity was probably influenced by the techniques of AA and also by the view that alcoholics could learn a lot from each other and, through their experience, could help sustain those who had relapsed. The therapist's task was to use the group process to aid patients gain a better understanding of the way in which their past life experiences were contributing to their reliance on alcohol, and help them to find new ways of coping and adapting to an abstinent lifestyle. Aversion treatments were also popular (e.g. the use of apomorphine to induce vomiting), as was hypnosis and a variety of psychological therapies. However, more explorative psychodynamic and psychoanalytic approaches were often thought to be poorly utilised by alcoholics, because of the destructive effect of their drinking on the ability to respond to therapy. In the 1950s, disulfiram (Antabuse) was introduced in Denmark and, with varying degrees of popularity at different times and in different countries, has remained an important part of treatment. It is a drug which has no effect provided the patient does not drink. But if alcohol is taken, it produces a toxic substance, acetaldehyde, in the body, making the patient feel thoroughly ill. It is therefore a helpful deterrent, particularly in the early months of abstinence.

Specialist units

Dr Max Glatt, a psychiatrist, inaugurated the first unit for the treatment of alcoholism at a mental hospital in Britain in 1951; between then and 1973, more than 20 such units were established by the National Health Service. They were set up in response to a series of both WHO and national government reports which recognised that alcoholism was a disease and argued that specialist in-patient facilities, staffed by multi-disciplinary teams, were required for its treatment. The underlying view was that alcoholism is a product of pre-existing psychopathology, further exacerbated by physical damage or vulnerability. The British Ministry of Health had recommended that as far as possible, treatment for alcoholism and alcoholic psychosis should be given in specialised units. It proposed that "each region of the country should establish a unit that should have between eight and 16 beds". This would be a convenient size for group therapy, which was then regarded as being the most valuable form of treatment. The Ministry also thought it necessary for the special units to run out-patient clinics and to cooperate in the aftercare of patients with Alcoholics Anonymous and other treatment agencies in the general community. However, in 1968, a further memorandum gave more prominence to the merits of out-patient treatment, which enabled the individual to retain contact with the family, work, and the community. Benzodiazepines, which came into widespread use in the 1960s, established themselves as standard medication in the detoxification process, and have largely retained that role.

It had long been recognised, both in the USA and Europe, that the process whereby habitual public drunkenness was dealt with by a 'revolving door' of arrest, court appearance, fine, failure to pay the fine, and brief periods of imprisonment, was both totally ineffective and extremely costly to the taxpayer. Throughout the century, attempts have been made in various countries, with varying degrees of success, to divert habitual drunken offenders to some other health/welfare system. In Britain, calls for the decriminalisation of drunkenness offences and the use of detoxification centres have been a recurrent theme of the last 30 years. Yet relatively few centres have been established, partly because of cost and doubts about their longer-term efficacy, although few would doubt their humanitarian and economic advantages over management by the penal system. In 1969, the US Congress recognised the need for greater attention to the problems of alcohol by establishing the National Institute on Alcohol Abuse and Alcoholism in the National Institute of Mental Health. Particularly high rates of alcohol problems were found among Native American and Inuit populations.

Evaluation

Research in the 1970s began to cast doubt on the need for prolonged specialist in-patient treatment for the majority of alcoholics. A series of carefully controlled studies had shown that many could be improved by out-patient treatment alone, and often by relatively brief interventions. A further debate, which at times was extremely acrimonious, was that concerning controlled drinking. It had always been a tenet of Alcoholics Anonymous and of most treatment agencies that for the alcoholic, abstinence was the only feasible goal for recovery. A number of studies, though, challenged this belief and showed that in some circumstances, a return to controlled drinking was possible. This view was particularly promoted by clinical psychologists, who were utilising psychological and cognitive–behavioural approaches in their treatment. Gradually, a broader view was accepted, extending treatment approaches and applying them to a much wider range of alcohol problems.

By 1978, a government advisory committee on alcoholism in Britain acknowledged that alcohol-related problems were both widespread and diverse in their manifestations. The new, broader concept of alcohol-related problems required an equally wide range of different professionals — general practitioners, social workers, and voluntary agencies — to recognise problem drinkers and respond to their needs. But to achieve this, they needed specialist support and training. The emphasis was now on the need to recognise alcohol-related problems in their early stages and to move away from an exclusive clinical focus on 'alcoholism' as a disease entity.

Thus the notion of building supportive networks which would deal with a range of alcohol-related problems was established — at least in theory. Voluntary agencies grew up which provided free counselling and advice to individuals with alcohol problems and their families. Alcoholics Anonymous and its sister organisation, Al-Anon were still the best known agencies in the field. Social service agencies developed hostels for homeless problem drinkers and habitual drunken offenders. Clinical psychologists promoted behavioural techniques to help patients relearn less maladaptive drinking patterns or find an abstinent way of life. While group treatments remained prominent, the importance of prolonged in-patient treatment began to decline. It has, however, continued to flourish in some countries, particularly in the private sector under the influence of the Minnesota model of 28-day residential treatment. This places considerable emphasis on the value of Alcoholics Anonymous and the support of its fellowship in aftercare, but has also added both family and individual counselling techniques. AA has been a much greater influence on treatment philosophy in the USA than elsewhere.

Public health perspective

In the 1970s, despite the growth in treatment services, consumption of alcohol rose in most parts of the world, and the public health approach, which had been dormant for the past 50 years, became prominent again. In 1977, WHO produced a report on *Alcohol-Related Disabilities*, which gave much more prominence to the range of problems caused by injudicious drinking in any population. A number of scientific centres began to produce information about the epidemiology of alcohol and alcohol-related problems and to look once more at the broader picture, pointing to the relationship between per capita consumption and the level of alcohol-related harm in the community. The work of epidemiologists such as Pequignot in France, who demonstrated the relationship between consumption and liver disease, and the activities of research centres such as the Addiction Research Foundation of Ontario and the Finnish School of Alcohol Studies in Helsinki began to examine the way in which socio-economic factors, particularly price and availability, influenced consumption. In 1979, Kendell in Edinburgh emphasised

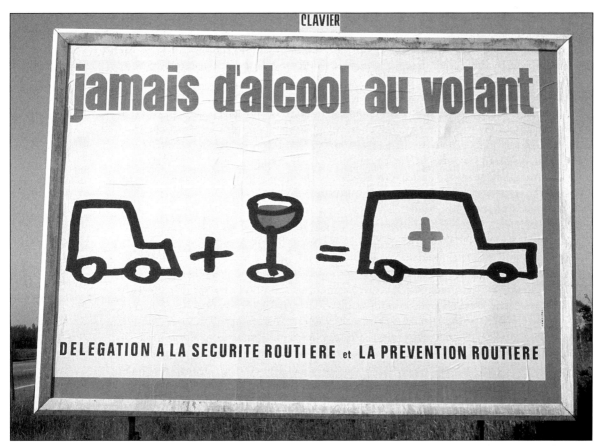

A French anti-alcoholism poster. It reads: "Don't have alcohol behind the wheel. The Delegation of Highway Security and Prevention".
© *Corbis/Paul Almasy.*

the limitations of a purely treatment response to what in fact was a socio-political issue. Yet the influence of both governments and the worldwide drinks industry in either promoting or reducing the size of the problem depended on their willingness to accept legislative controls and a public health element in alcohol taxation. Influential in this viewpoint was the Ledermann hypothesis (developed in France), which proposed that "the proportion of any population drinking in a harmful way may be calculated from the average consumption of that population". Though many have criticised the concept in detail, it remains generally true that the more a population drinks, the greater level of harm it will experience. This model provided scientific grounds for controlling the supply of alcohol, without the need for moralistic considerations.

The population approach to alcohol misuse had implications not only for national policy, but also for the organisation of treatment services. These were now required to respond to a very broad spectrum of alcohol problems, starting from health promotion activities directed first at all those who consumed alcohol, and then at those who were in the early stages of drinking in a hazardous way. This led to a search for guidelines about sensible drinking and to education directed at all health professionals, to make them fully aware of the importance of alcohol in relation to health. The fact was emphasised that alcohol is a psychoactive drug, and one which causes far greater social harm than that attributed to other more newsworthy drugs such as cannabis and heroin.

While the alcohol industry might have assumed a compassionate response to a disease concept of alcoholism, its *raison d'être* was much more threatened by the public health approach. This showed clear incompatibilities between a desire to maximise profits and increase consumption world-wide on the one hand, against the evidence that greater per capita consumption was associated with rising levels of harm. In several countries, the industry therefore formed groups who could work with governments to find areas where harm could be reduced, without seriously impeding the primary task of the industry. The responsibilities of both national and local governments for reducing the levels of alcohol-related harm was spelt out by WHO in a European Alcohol Charter and Action Plan (1995, revised 1999). This included targets for reducing alcohol consumption by adopting ten specific strategies; amongst these were public education, discouragement of drink-driving, controlling advertising, and supporting self-help movements.

Broadening the base of treatment

A small number of studies have examined the natural history of alcoholism, as well as the longer-term consequences of treatment. These have shown that a significant proportion of problem drinkers move in and out of this category over the course of years, often in response to social changes. Therefore, in evaluating treatment, the natural history of the condition needs to be taken into account. Any anxiety that this might lead to therapeutic nihilism was misplaced, though, because it was also evident that the long-term outcome was significantly improved by treatment. Both in terms of subsequent health and in costs to healthcare, treatment was significantly better than no treatment at all. This information led to a renewed optimism about the benefits of treatment, with an emphasis on simpler and earlier intervention wherever possible. Though project MATCH, a major evaluation of treatments, in the USA demonstrated both the value of treatment and the benefits of properly defining the treatment offered, it largely failed to demonstrate either the value of one method as against another or the feasibility of tailoring treatments to the characteristics of patients. Favourable outcomes were produced equally well by three different treatment approaches: 12-step facilitation (in preparation for AA), cognitive–behavioural therapy, and motivational enhancement therapy (a form of motivational interviewing in four sessions over a 12-week period). Long-term follow-up showed that even though all the therapists had been trained to a comparable standard, differences in outcome between the three treatments were minimal.

The design of services in the past has often been insufficiently attentive to the needs of certain groups such as young people, women, the elderly, and ethnic minorities. However, many treatment networks now make special provision for these groups. It has also become increasingly clear that detoxification (medically supported withdrawal from alcohol), which at one time was thought to require in-patient care, can be effectively achieved in most cases in the patient's own home or on an out-patient basis. The spread of domiciliary detoxification and community treatment has further reduced the need for specialist in-patient care, and in the UK, there has been a steep decline in the number of specialist beds for treating individuals with alcohol problems. A current concern, though, is that this trend may have 'gone too far', particularly because of the rising number of patients with dual diagnoses of alcohol problems and psychotic illnesses, who are extremely difficult to care for in a community setting. In the USA, specialist teams are being developed which work with this group, but in other countries it seems more likely that a collaborative approach between general psychiatric services and specialist services will become more common.

Conclusion

The tendency to dichotomise medical thinking about alcohol problems between a public health approach and a biological/psychological approach has now reached a more sensible accommodation. Most specialists would both see the importance of socio-political factors in the genesis and prevention of alcohol problems and acknowledge the need for policies that are conscious of the environmental impact on the use of alcohol. Treatment methods may sometimes utilise social network approaches, in addition to individual psychological intervention. There has also been a significant development in understanding the biological basis of alcohol dependence. Genetic studies have resurrected an interest in inherited factors in determining the individual's susceptibility to dependence and their vulnerability to certain forms of damage, e.g. to the liver or brain. The relationship between molecular cellular change and excessive stimulation of receptors in the brain appears to be the basis of many aspects of addictive behaviour. It has been known for some time that some Asian groups have a genetically determined variation in the activity of enzymes that metabolise alcohol — alcohol dehydrogenase and aldehyde dehydrogenase — is common in some Asian populations. This results in high levels of acetaldehyde when alcohol is ingested, causing an unpleasant flush reaction.

Current brain imaging techniques, coupled with better understanding of brain chemistry, herald a new era of biological understanding of the basis of alcohol dependence. Such better appreciation of the neurophysiological basis of dependence points the way for innovative drug treatments. These will focus first on the relief of craving, but in the future, may perhaps tackle the biological basis of excessive appetites. It is significant that genetic factors that increase the liability to misuse of alcohol may represent a more general vulnerability to drug dependence.

FURTHER READING

New drug problems and policies

Albrecht HJ, van Kalmthout A, eds. *Drug Policies in Western Europe*. Freiburg: Max Planck Institute; 1989.

Berridge V. European drug policy: the need for historical perspectives. *European Addiction Research*. 1996; **2**:219–225.

Berridge V. *Opium and the People. Opiate Use and Drug Control Policy in 19th and early 20th Century Britain* (revised edn). London: Free Association Books, 1998.

Courtwright D. *Dark Paradise. Opiate Addiction in America before 1940*. Cambridge, MA: Harvard University Press; 1982.

Musto D. *The American Disease. Origins of Narcotic Control* (expanded edn). New York: Oxford University Press; 1987.

Schur EM. *Narcotic Addiction in Britain and America. The Impact of Public Policy*. London: Tavistock; 1963.

Spear HB. The growth of heroin addiction in the United Kingdom. *British Journal of Addiction*. 1965; **64**:245–256.

Stimson G, Oppenheimer E. *Heroin Addiction. Treatment and Control in Britain*. London: Tavistock; 1982.

Wayne Morgan H. *Drugs in America. A Social History 1800–1980*. Syracuse: Syracuse University Press; 1981.

The diminishing mental hospitals

Bynum WR, Porter R, Shepherd M. *The Anatomy of Madness: Essays in the History of Psychiatry*, 3 Vols. London: Tavistock; 1985-7.

Erikson KT. Notes on the sociology of deviance. In: Becker HS. *The Other Side*. New York: Free Press/Collier Macmillan; 1964: 9–22.

Goffman E. *Asylums: Essays on the Social Situation of Mental Patients*. New York: Doubleday; 1961.

Joint Committee for Mental Health. *Action for Mental Health*, Vol. 1. Washington, DC: US Department of Health, Education and Welfare; 1961.

Jones K. *Experience in Mental Health*. London: Sage; 1988.

Jones K. *Asylums and After*. London: Athlone; 1993.

Jones K, Fowles AJ. *Ideas on Institutions*. London: Routledge and Kegan Paul; 1984.

Parsons T. The mental hospital as a form of social organisation. In: Greenblatt D, Levinson DJ, Williams R, eds. *The Patient and the Mental Hospital*. Glencoe, IL: Free Press; 1987: 108–129.

Szasz TS. *The Myth of Mental Illness: Foundations of a Theory of Personal Conduct*. New York: Dell; 1961.

World Health Organization. *Third Report of Expert Committee on Mental Health, Technical Report Series No 73*. Geneva: WHO; 1953.

American psychiatry

Foley HA. *Community Mental Health Legislation: The Formative Process.* Lexington: Lexington Books; 1975.

Grob GN. The origins of American psychiatric epidemiology. *American Journal of Public Health.* 1985; **75**:229–236.

Grob GN. *From Asylum to Community: Mental Health Policy in Modern America.* Princeton: Princeton University Press; 1991.

Joint Commission on Mental Illness and Health. *Action for Mental Health: Final Report of the Joint Commission on Mental Illness and Health 1961.* New York: Viking Press; 1961.

Kahn AJ. *Studies in Social Policy and Planning.* New York: Russell Sage Foundation; 1969.

Kramer M, Taub C, Starr S. Patterns of use of psychiatric facilities by the aged: current status, trends, and implications. *American Psychiatric Association, Psychiatric Research Reports.* 1968; **23**:89–150.

Musto D. Whatever happened to 'community mental health'? *Public Interest.* 1975; **39**:53–79.

National Institute of Mental Health Psychopharmacology Service Center Collaborative Study Group. Phenothiazine treatment in acute schizophrenia. *Archives of General Psychiatry.* 1964; **10**:246–261.

Pasamanick B, Scarpitti, FR, Dinitz S. *Schizophrenics in the Community: An Experimental Study in the Prevention of Hospitalization.* New York: Appleton-Century-Crofts; 1967.

RD Laing and anti-psychiatry

Esterson A, Cooper D, Laing RD. Results of family-orientated therapy with hospitalised schizophrenics. *British Medical Journal.* 1965; *ii*:1462–1465.

Laing RD, Esterson A. *Sanity, Madness, and the Family: Families of Schizophrenics.* Harmondsworth: Penguin; 1970.

Laing RD, Phillipson H, Lee AR. *Interpersonal Perception: A Theory and a Method of Research.* London: Tavistock; 1966.

Mullan B. *Mad to be Normal: Conversations with RD Laing.* London: Free Association Books; 1995.

Sedgwick P. *Psychopolitics.* London: Pluto; 1982.

Szasz TS. The myth of mental illness. *American Psychologist.* 1960; **15**:113–118.

Tantam D. The anti-psychiatry movement. In: Berrios GE, Freeman HL, eds. *150 Years of British Psychiatry,* Vol 1. London: Gaskell; 1991.

Psychiatric nursing

Caine TM, Smail DJ. Attitudes of psychiatric nurses to their role in treatment. *British Journal of Medical Psychology.* 1968; **14**:193–197.

Carpenter M. *Working for Health – The History of the Confederation of Health Service Employees.* London: Lawrence and Wishart; 1988.

Department of Health and Social Security. *The Salmon Report – The Report of the Committee on Senior Nurse Staffing Structure.* London: HMSO; 1966.

John A. *A Study of the Psychiatric Nurse.* Edinburgh: Livingstone; 1961.

Maddox H. The work of mental nurses. *Nursing Mirror.* 1957; **105**(12).

Martin JP. *Hospitals in Trouble.* London: Basil Blackwell; 1984.

Nolan P. *A History of Mental Health Nursing.* London: Chapman & Hall; 1993.

Orlando IJ. *The Dynamic Nurse–Patient Relationship.* New York: Putnam Press; 1961.

Peplau HE. *Interpersonal Relations in Nursing.* New York: Putnam Press; 1952.

Peplau HE. Interpersonal techniques: the crux of psychiatric nursing. *American Journal of Nursing.* 1962; **62**:50–54.

Rafferty AM. *The Politics of Nursing Knowledge.* London: Routledge; 1996.

Webster C. Nursing and the early crisis of the National Health Service. *The History of Nursing Group at the RCN, Bulletin.* 1985; **7**:12–24.

Wilson HS, Kneisl CR. *Psychiatric Nursing,* 3rd edn. California: Addison-Wesley Publishing Company; 1988.

Wing JK. The function of asylum. *British Journal of Psychiatry.* 1990; **157**:822–827.

Traditional medicine and cultural factors in Asia

Desjarlais D, Eisenberg L, Good B, Kleinman A, eds. *World Mental Health: Problems and Priorities in Low-Income Countries.* New York: Oxford University Press; 1995.

Gaw AC, ed. *Culture, Ethnicity, and Mental Illness.* Washington, DC: American Psychiatric Press, Inc; 1993.

Kleinman A. Depression, somatization and the "New cross-cultural psychiatry". *Social Science and Medicine.* 1977; **11**:3–10.

Leslie C, ed. *Asian Medical Systems: A Comparative Study.* Berkeley and Los Angeles: University of California Press; 1976.

Yap PM. Mental diseases peculiar to certain cultures: a survey of comparative psychiatry. *Journal of Mental Science.* 1951; **97**:313–327.

Yap PM. The culture-bound reactive syndromes. In: Caudil M, Lin TY, eds. *Mental Health Research in Asia and the Pacific.* Honolulu, HI: East-West Center Press; 1969.

Community psychiatry

Bennett DH, Freeman HL. *Community Psychiatry: The Principles*. London: Churchill Livingstone; 1991.

Better Services for the Mentally Ill (Cmnd 6233). London: Her Majesty's Stationery Office; 1975.

Caplan G. *Principles of Preventive Psychiatry*. London: Tavistock; 1964.

Goodwin S. *Comparative Mental Health Policy*. London: Sage; 1997.

Leighton A. *Caring for Mentally Ill People*. Cambridge: Cambridge University Press; 1982.

Mechanic D. In: Stein LI, Test MA, eds. *Alternatives to Mental Hospital Treatment*. New York: Plenum Press; 1977.

Sabshin M. In: Roberts LM, Hallack SL, Loeb MB, eds. *New Trends of Psychiatry in the Community*. Madison: University of Wisconsin Press; 1966.

Serban G. *New Trends of Psychiatry in the Community*. Cambridge, MA: Ballinger; 1977.

World Health Organization. *Third Report of the Expert Committee on Mental Health*. WHO: Geneva; 1953.

Alcoholism

Cook T. *Vagrant Alcoholics*. London: Routledge and Kegan Paul; 1995.

DHSS. *The Pattern and Range of Services for Problem Drinkers. Report by the Advisory Committee on Alcoholism*. London: HMSO; 1978.

Edwards G, Grant M, eds. *Alcoholism — Treatment in Transition*. London: Croom Helm; 1980.

Faculty of Public Health Medicine, Royal College of Physicians. *Alcohol and the Public Health*. London: Macmillan; 1991.

Glatt MM. The English drink problem: its rise and decline through the ages. *British Journal of Addiction*. 1958; **55**:51–65.

Harrison B. *Drink and the Victorians*. London: Faber and Faber; 1971.

Holder H, Edwards G, eds. *Alcohol and Public Policy*. Oxford: Oxford University Press; 1995.

Jellinek EM. *The Disease Concept and Alcoholism*. New Haven: Hillhouse Press; 1960.

Institute of Medicine. *Broadening the Base of Treatment for Alcohol Problems*. Washington, DC: National Academy Press; 1990.

Kerr N. *Inebriety, its Etiology, Treatment and Jurisprudence*. London: HK Lewis; 1889.

Royal College of Psychiatrists. *Alcohol: Our Favourite Drug*. London: Tavistock; 1986.

Vaillant GE. *The Natural History of Alcoholism Revisited*. Cambridge, MA: Harvard University Press; 1995.

World Health Organization. *European Charter on Alcohol*. Copenhagen: WHO; 1995.

1971–1980 CHAPTER 8

Major world events

1971   Hounsfield (UK) and McLeold Cormack (USA) introduced the scan into medicine
1972   Meeting between Mao Zedong and Nixon
1973   Cohen and Boyer in the USA modified bacteria by introducing foreign genes: the beginning of genetic engineering
1974   Watergate
1975   Maupay discovered vaccine against hepatitis B in France
1977   Hewlett-Packard launched a laptop computer
1978   Camp David agreement
1979   Mother Teresa won Nobel Peace Prize

Major events in psychiatry

1971   The British Misuse of Drugs Act was passed
1971   Carlsson, Corrodi, *et al.* developed zimelidine, the first of the selective serotonin reuptake inhibitors
1972   Research Diagnostic Criteria (RDC) formulated in the USA
1973   The Child Abuse Prevention Act (1983) — the Mondale Act — passed by the US Congress
1975   Arvid Carlsson coined the term 'autoreceptors', inaugurating a new era in receptor pharmacology
1975   The first Professor of Forensic Psychiatry in the UK, TCN Gibbens, appointed to the Maudsley Hospital
1976   The Netherlands introduced the policy distinction between 'soft' and 'hard' drugs
1976   Computer assisted tomography used by Dr Eve Johnstone *et al.* at Northwick Park Hospital, London
1978   Law 180 passed in Italy, introduced a new system of psychiatric care
1978   An insider's description of life in a Russian political hospital and of its mode of operation in Vladimir Bukovsky's book '...*et le vent reprend ses tours: Ma vie de dissident*'
1979   Professor Gerald Russell in London described bulimia nervosa
1980   DSM–III published by the American Psychiatric Association
1980   Death of Franco Basaglia, the charismatic leader of 'psichiatrica democratica' in Italy

CONVULSIVE THERAPY

by Max Fink

By the early 1960s, psychotropic medication had replaced ECT in most Western countries. But the drugs were limited in their efficacy, and with a greater number of applications, their risks became clear. The growing number of pharmacotherapy-resistant and pharmacotherapy-intolerant patients drove the profession to seek alternatives. Amongst the reports that ECT had merit when medication failed, a particular cogent one was the translation of an earlier Italian study. It reported that an impressive number of depressed patients who had failed to improve with adequate doses of imipramine responded well to ECT.

Many reasons, however, impeded the revival of interest. The history of the forceful use of ECT and leucotomy against the will of patients was the most infamous of these. Recollections of the difficulties in the first two decades of ECT use also discouraged some psychiatrists. But it was the overt economic and philosophical competition between the advocates of biological and psychological treatments amongst psychiatrists that was the most negative and persistent influence.

Complaints of abuse

A notorious example of abuse was depicted in Ken Kesey's book *One Flew Over the Cuckoo's Nest,* and in its highly successful 1975 film, in which the protagonist was subjected to bilateral leucotomy against his will. Thomas Szasz in the United States, RD Laing in Great Britain (Chapter 7, p. 202), Michel Foucault in France (this chapter, p. 245), and Franco Basaglia in Italy (this chapter, p. 270) contended that mental illness was a social phenomenon, secondary to economic and political problems, not to biological effects. The presentations of these men coloured the public's view about ECT's safety and efficacy, subjecting to disdain any suggestion that the treatment had changed and was not as pictured.

The movement known as the Church of Scientology was another source of anti-psychiatry sentiment. Its leaders argued that the use of psychotropic medication, ECT, and

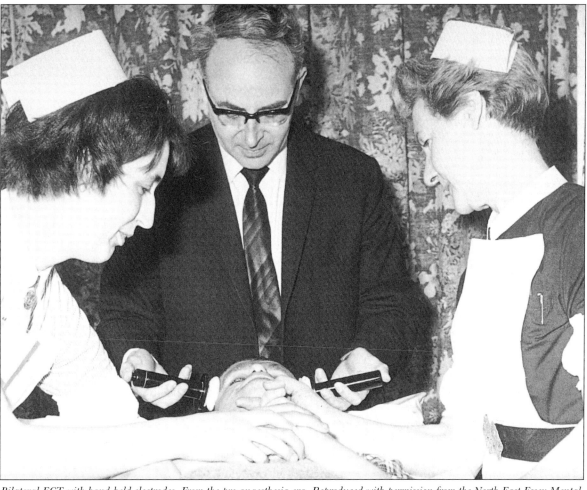

Bilateral ECT with hand-held electrodes. From the pre-anaesthesia era. Reproduced with permission from the North East Essex Mental Health NHS Trust.

leucotomy damaged the brain, and that no person should agree to a treatment that might alter the mind. The adherents of this sect have been energetic in seeking legislative prohibition of somatic treatment of the mentally ill, both in the United States and in Europe, and their lobbying has led to many legislative restrictions on the use of ECT. In Germany, Japan, and Italy, recollections of the cooperation of doctors with the experimentation and extinction of minorities stifled those few who were willing to reintroduce the treatment. Student protests intimidated academically based psychiatrists who considered the recall of ECT, and effectively inhibited its use. A similar situation occurred in Holland.

Because drugs were expensive imports to the Soviet Union and to Asian and African countries, doctors continued to use unmodified ECT as an inexpensive way to sedate and to treat psychosis and depression. It is still a feature of practice in these countries. The advances in the techniques of ECT in the 1960s and 1970s that made its application singularly effective and safe came from academic clinicians in the Scandinavian countries, where ECT continues to be used in both practice and research. In Great Britain, Ireland, Canada, Australia, and New Zealand it remains in widespread use.

In the United States, proposed restrictions on psychiatric practice by the Massachusetts legislature in 1971 led the Commonwealth's Commissioner of Mental Health to establish a psychiatric task force. It concluded that the indications for ECT were well defined for patients with affective disorders, but regarded as unproven its benefits for patients with schizophrenia and for pre-pubertal children. Regulations that defined the indications for ECT, requiring adherence to reporting and consent procedures, and limiting the numbers of treatments that could be given to an individual patient in any one year were then issued, forestalling legislative restrictions in that State. In other States, notably California, Colorado, Tennessee, and Texas, legislatures issued regulations to record all treatments with a governmental agency, and limited the age of adolescents and children who may be given ECT.

Following restrictive California legislation in 1975, the American Psychiatric Association established a Task Force on Electroconvulsive Therapy. Its report supported the use of ECT for patients with major depressive disorder and with mania, particularly for those who had not been helped by psychotropic medication. The panel recommended a formal consent procedure to ensure that ECT was administered only to consenting patients. Its report was widely adopted by American hospitals in re-establishing ECT.

A similar survey of ECT practice in Great Britain was undertaken in 1980. Its conclusions about indications, risks, and guidelines were similar to those in the American report. The British National Health Service authorised some expenditure to improve the practice of ECT, but a follow-up survey a decade later by one of the original surveyors found that practice had improved very little. An examination in Ireland found the use of ECT and the professional opinions to be similar to those in Great Britain.

The recurrent outcry against ECT led the US National Institutes of Health and of Mental Health to convene a consensus conference in 1985. Its report found ECT demonstrably effective for severe psychiatric disorders, and encouraged its continued use. Support also came from the American Medical Association and several national mental health associations.

Improvements in practice

Difficulties in its safe administration were a second impediment to the revival of ECT. When first developed, ECT had been given without anaesthesia, and each treatment elicited anxiety and dread, even panic. Reports of fractures and of death naturally made the public wary. Anaesthesia, muscle relaxation, and hyperoxygenation were answers to the problems, but they were not accepted as routine measures in developed countries until the mid-1950s, after 20 years of unmodified ECT.

Unmodified treatments temporarily affect memory, so memory loss was even seen as an inherent part of the treatment. However, this negative effect had been sharply reduced by technical changes — of continuous oxygenation, unilateral electrode placement, brief-pulse energy currents, and monitoring of the duration of seizures — that allowed minimum energy currents to be used for effective treatment. The introduction of succinylcholine as muscle relaxant did away with the risk of fractures, and the routine use of barbiturate anaesthesia diminished both the fear of treatment and the likelihood of recurrent seizures. But these improvements were not known to the public, and fears of the risks of treatment and detrimental effects on memory remained as impediments to its use.

The renewed interest in ECT in the 1980s stimulated the US government to support two programmes to evaluate the effects of the form of electrical energy and placement of electrodes on memory and efficacy. Brief-pulse currents were found to be as effective as and safer than alternating currents, leading manufacturers to develop devices that deliver only that form of current. While unilateral ECT had lesser effects on memory, it was also associated with lesser efficacy; to improve efficacy, the energy delivered in treatment had to be materially increased. Energy-dosing tactics, therefore, were needed to realise the benefits of unilateral ECT. Monitoring the duration of the seizure — first of the motor convulsion, then of the EEG, and recently the characteristics of the EEG — have been the criteria for evaluating a satisfactory treatment. These modifications of treatment, established in the United States, are being accepted in other Western countries.

Once the safe delivery of treatment was ensured, practitioners explored other applications. Though seen primarily as a treatment for resistant depression, ECT has been recognised as also effective in treating psychotic depression, mania, catatonia, schizophrenia, neuroleptic malignant syndrome, and parkinsonism. Treatment is safe even for patients with complex systemic disorders and mental retardation, and at all ages from adolescents to the elderly. Indeed, the broad application of ECT across a diverse range of diagnoses has led some authors to question the diagnostic splitting of mental disorders into ever smaller entities in classification schemes that, for the most part, have no basis in biology or therapy.

Conflicts within the profession

A third impediment to the ECT's revival was put in the way by the profession itself. The benefits of both psychological and somatic treatments were often grossly overstated, so for some psychiatric disorders, it was unclear which treatment, if any, was appropriate. Psychoanalysts, particularly in the United States, focused their attention on patients with neurotic symptoms, having a facility in expressing their thoughts, and ability to still live and work in the community. But some analysts did also seek to treat patients with schizophrenia, manic–depressive psychosis, and the more severe delusional disorders. They claimed that their methods would raise unconscious conflicts to consciousness, and that, in 'working through' these conflicts, the patient would be able to get rid of the causes of his disorder. Psychoanalysts deprecated the efforts of psychiatrists who used medication and electroshock, accusing them of burying the patient's dynamic conflicts by impairing memory and deepening repression.

This hostility between disciplines intensified after the Second World War, when American psychoanalysts established the elitist Group for the Advancement of Psychiatry (GAP), whose aim was to establish psychodynamic practice as the core discipline of psychiatry. A continuing challenge to their pre-eminent position in psychiatric practice was

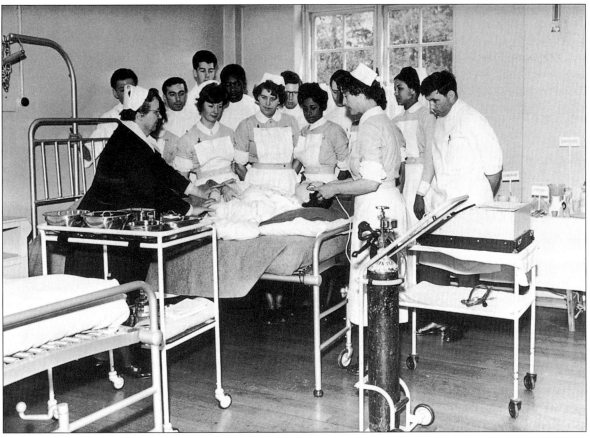

ECT treatment demonstrated in the pre-anaesthesia era. Reproduced with permission from the North East Essex Mental Health NHS Trust.

the reliance of both patients and psychiatrists on ECT. GAP considered this a direct philosophical and economic affront, stating in a 1947 broadside that, "overemphasis and unjustified use of electroshock therapy short-circuits the training and experience which is essential in modern dynamic psychiatry. Abuses in the use of electroshock therapy are sufficiently widespread and dangerous to justify consideration of a campaign of professional education in the limitations of this technique, and perhaps even to justify instituting certain measures of control". The group's antipathy, echoed by followers of psychodynamic philosophy in psychology, social work, and child and adolescent psychiatry, remains a principal obstacle in North America to the broad and useful acceptance of ECT in clinical practice.

The availability of ECT is uneven and generally sparse in most nations. While 8% to 12% of adult in-patients at academic hospitals in the USA receive ECT, fewer than 0.2% of adults admitted to non-academic centres profit from its benefits. Such a discrepancy reflects the continuing social stigma and philosophical bias against the treatment. Many hospitals licensed to admit the mentally ill are not properly equipped to deliver ECT, and relatively few psychiatrists are skilled in its use.

The techniques of ECT should be taught in postgraduate psychiatric training, along with psychotherapy and psychopharmacology, but often this is not done. Practitioners of electroshock are generally left to develop their experience while treating their first patients; no-one examines their skills in the now complex techniques. In Great Britain and Ireland, prolonged efforts by the Royal College of Psychiatrists to improve this situation have had limited success.

However, within the past decade, there has been a revival of interest in the clinical use and study of ECT; this resurgence has been most marked in the United States, but renewed interest is also manifest in the Scandinavian countries, Australia, and New Zealand. In Germany, Japan, Italy, and the Netherlands, though, use is still limited by the perceived stigma. Where ECT is paid for through insurance, e.g. in Canada, Japan and, more and more, the United States, low reimbursement rates hamper its use. Both the unavailability of modern equipment and expense of anaesthetics discourage its use in Africa, Asia, and Eastern Europe; the patients in these countries who do receive ECT are subjected to the same unmodified and risky treatments that were delivered in the 1930s and 1940s.

In spite of such financial restriction, an assessment of the outcome of treatment of patients discharged from American general hospitals with a principal diagnosis of depressive disorder has found that the initiation of ECT within five days of admission leads to shorter and less costly in-patient treatment than for those treated with medication alone or delayed ECT. Other studies showed that the antidepressant effects of ECT occur earlier and are more robust than those of antidepressant drugs.

The discovery of convulsive therapy was an important milestone in the history of modern psychiatry. Its revival, from amongst the long list of desperate experimental treatments, reflects its unique efficacy in relieving the severe mentally ill, as well as the progress that has been made in ensuring its safe administration. We know little more about the causes of mental disorders than did our forebears. Until the mechanism of ECT is further explored and understood, and its actions replaced by gentler methods, its use must continue.

PSYCHIATRIC ASPECTS OF PAIN

by Harold Merskey

By the 1970s, discussions of pain included much writing about psychological contributions to its understanding and origins. Psychoanalytic views were still respected and it was thought there were patients who were pain-prone in whom pain developed together with resentment as, in some way, a response to early feelings of guilt and humiliation and the need to suffer.

In 1973, The International Association for the Study of Pain (IASP) was founded by Dr JJ Bonica as a multi-disciplinary organisation comprising both basic scientists and clinicians, and including a wide range of disciplines. Psychology and psychiatry figured quite prominently amongst the different disciplines, along with neurology, physiology, biochemistry, pharmacology, anaesthetics, neurosurgery, and physical medicine. Bonica, who was already a distinguished anaesthetist, organised a conference attended by some 100 specialists from different fields, all of whom he believed had made a contribution to pain, along with another 150 participants. At the end of the meeting, it was agreed to form the IASP as a scientific and professional body. Most international medical organisations have arisen out of single disciplines, e.g. neurology or psychiatry, that already had their own national bodies. The IASP was unusual in its mode of founding and spread of disciplines, and probably unique in their extent and variety.

In 1979, the IASP adapted an earlier version of a definition of pain and approved the following: 'An unpleasant sensory and emotional experience associated with actual or potential tissue damage, or described in terms of such damage'.

Bonica had previously established the model of a comprehensive pain clinic with multiple professional participation. Concomitantly with the foundation and growth of the IASP, many clinical psychologists participated in the work, using behavioural techniques. However, in isolation, their methods were controversial. They were quickly modified, though, such that a cognitive behavioural approach is now standard in clinical psychology and is also often used in psychiatry, together with other techniques. Psychotropic medication proved effective, particularly amitriptyline, which was only later shown to be analgesic, even in patients who were not depressed. Most psychiatrists and psychologists came to emphasise the multi-modal approach that involves the use of all available techniques of physical, psychological, and psychiatric treatment.

The 1970s also saw increased awareness of the impact of chronic pain on the individual. It was recognised that such pain causes numerous psychological changes based upon inability to work, loss of earnings, loss of dignity, loss of the satisfaction of work, expenses for medical costs, frequent inability to manage domestic responsibilities, impairment of sexual relationships, depression, and even suicidal thoughts. There were also impairment of memory and concentration due to pain or to medication, and the debilitating effect of insomnia. These features were not always found in association with chronic pain, but tended to depend upon its severity, and some of them were affected by the ability of the individual to recover and be retrained.

In the 1970s, rheumatologists began to put together the idea that there were sometimes patients who had diffuse musculo-skeletal pain associated with a characteristic pattern of tender points. This pattern of 'fibromyalgia', as it is now called, recognised earlier as generalised fibrositis by Hugh Smythe, was found by Moldofsky and Smythe to be associated with an alteration of sleep EEG rhythms. Although their finding was later shown to be non-specific, it was the starting point of a renewed recognition that diffuse musculo-skeletal pain, whether or not it was accompanied by psychological changes, could be based upon physical dysfunction.

At the end of the 1970s most of the present-day treatments or attitudes connected with pain were well established. However, the principal controversy of the decade — namely the place of behavioural measures or their justification — is still very strong.

DSM CLASSIFICATION

by Charles H Cahn

This section deals with the Diagnostic and Statistical Manual (DSM) of the American Psychiatric Association. It is useful to take a look at how their system of classification of mental disorders has developed, and how it correlates with other systems, especially with the International Classification of Diseases (ICD) of the World Health Organization (WHO) (Chapter 9, p. 302). DSM is an important aspect of the way that American psychiatrists have succeeded in the post-Second World War years in becoming so influential in international psychiatry.

Purposes of classification

Some of the reasons why the classification of disorders is useful are that it is used:

• To promote the understanding and organisation of thought about the nature of mental disorders

• To study the morbidity and mortality caused by these disorders

• For statistical purposes, including reimbursement of professional services, particularly in the USA

• For the systematic recording of clinical and pathological observations

• For developing scientific epidemiology and other systematic research

• For the indexing of medical records, to predict outcome and for other purposes.

In summary, classification fosters unambiguous communication. However, no classification of mental disorders has so far been altogether satisfactory, in spite of great efforts by many psychiatrists to make it so.

The DSM system

DSM is a system that contains all the diagnoses used by American psychiatrists, specifies the symptoms required to make a particular diagnosis, and organises these diagnoses into a system of classification. There is a particular need for such a process in psychiatry because the aetiology of most of its disorders is unknown and there are no specific bodily tests which can contribute to making a diagnosis, except for the relatively few conditions with a known organic basis. This makes it essential that a patient's symptoms and clinical history should be fitted into some formal structure that is widely accepted. The DSM system is fundamentally atheoretical, therefore, in relation to aetiology, with a few exceptions such as post-traumatic stress disorder.

Since its first appearance in 1952, DSM has undergone three major changes, while ICD has changed four times since the first publication of its mental disorders section in 1948. All have moved in the direction of greater complexity and specificity, but not always along the same lines. Differences of opinion and at times considerable controversy have characterised their evolution.

For example, there are the 'lumpers' and 'splitters' or, put more elegantly, the 'gradualists' and 'separatists'. These expressions indicate that patients who are mentally ill cannot often be put into neat diagnostic categories — they have a range of overlapping symptoms, such as manic behaviour and delusional ideas, or anxiety states and depressive mood. The gradualists prefer to speak of spectrum disorders, where symptoms range across a broad clinical field, e.g. from schizophrenia to schizo-affective disorder, to bipolar mood disorder. On the other hand, separatists distinguish between different syndromes in trying to identify distinct disease entities, such as dysrhythmia, reactive depression, endogenous depression, and involutional melancholia. So long as we do not have more precise data concerning the aetiology and underlying pathology of psychiatric disorders, these arguments will continue.

History of the DSM

Before 1950, there was no clearly identifiable classification system used in American psychiatry. The pioneers who had been most influential over the years in developing psychiatric terminology and putting it into practice were mostly European. They included Emil Kraepelin (Chapter 2, p. 49), Eugen Bleuler (Chapter 2, p. 52), Sigmund Freud (Chapter 2, p. 47), Adolf Meyer (Chapter 4, p. 103), and Karl Menninger. They and many others tried to apply to classification the theoretical concepts they had developed in their individual ways. In most countries, mental disorders were broadly grouped together under the main headings of neuroses, psychoses, personality disorders, and mental deficiency, but there was no internationally accepted system.

After the Second World War, psychiatry was no longer largely confined to mental hospitals, but was developing extramurally in out-patient services, child guidance clinics, general hospital units and, in the USA especially, veterans' hospitals and community mental health centres. Furthermore, the private practice of psychiatry had become much more popular, particularly in North America and Western Europe. During this time, too, neurology and psychiatry became more distinct medical specialties, having previously been practised jointly in many countries.

DSM–I

Although the approaches of Sigmund Freud and Adolf Meyer to the patients they treated, lectured on, and wrote about were very different, the influence of both had become very strong in the USA in the 1930s and 1940s. They and their followers stressed both early and later events in patients' environments as the most important factors in their attempts to explain the causes of psychiatric disorder. Genetic factors, which had previously been considered of great aetiological importance, were then placed in the background. On this theoretical basis, DSM–I came into being in 1952, describing many categories of mental disorders nosologically as 'reaction types'. This also fitted well with sociological and anthropological concepts that had begun to be integrated into the field of psychiatry. At the same time, a considerable distancing — almost estrangement — developed between psychiatrists and other medical practitioners, especially in German-speaking countries. Physicians there who had been practising neurology and psychiatry together for a long time found it more and more difficult to combine both specialities. Moreover, psychiatrists were either working in psychiatric hospitals that were often situated at some distance from academic centres, or had decided to be trained in and practise psychoanalysis, whereas neurologists were more clearly integrated into faculties of medicine and general hospitals.

DSM–II

In the late 1960s, DSM–II was prepared in response to the expressed need to bring this system into line with the eighth version of ICD, for which representatives of the American Psychiatric Association had been consulted. Both DSM–II and ICD–8 were put into effect in 1968 (see table below). At this time, medical students in almost all countries learnt relatively little psychiatry, and what they were taught was generally quite inadequate, superficial, and often biased. Even postgraduate students in psychiatry were subjected to many different schools of thought on the question of diagnosis. In the USA, patients were thought to have 'schizophrenia' as soon as a thought disturbance such as tangentiality or any ideas of reference were elicited, whereas in the UK, the same patients would not have been considered schizophrenic if they also had a mood disorder or personality disorder.

This was brought out very clearly when in 1969, research workers in London and New York compared diagnostic habits in their two countries by showing videotapes of patients to audiences of American and British psychiatrists respectively. One of these cases, an emotionally unstable, loud-mouthed complainer with a history of alcohol abuse, who blamed everybody but himself, was diagnosed as having schizophrenia by more than 60% of the American, but less than 5% of the British psychiatrists. Most of the latter diagnosed a personality disorder. The same exercise was conducted at the McGill University Department of Psychiatry in Montreal, at which about 40 psychiatrists and residents in psychiatry participated (including the author of this section). There, about 30% diagnosed schizophrenia — a reflection of the fact that about half the participants had an American, the other half a European background in psychiatry.

DSM–III

A consequence of this cross-national study was that during the 1970s, a group of American psychiatrists led by Robert Spitzer decided that the time had come to overhaul DSM–II and prepare DSM–III. After intensive multi-centre testing, the final version was approved and published in 1980, revealing that the vocabulary had been considerably changed. The word 'reaction' had disappeared. The concept of 'neurosis' was to have been abolished, but after protests by psychoanalysts it was restored in parentheses, after the more generally descriptive word 'disorder'. Some of the many changes in terminology are listed in the table that follows. It was claimed that with DSM–III, the method on which a psychiatric diagnosis could be based was made relatively clear for the first time.

A new feature of DSM–III was the addition of five axes, on each of which patients were to be evaluated:

Axis 1 — reflecting clinical syndromes

Axis 2 — reflecting developmental and/or personality disorders

Axis 3 — accounting for physical disorders and/or conditions

Axis 4 — measuring severity of psycho-social stressors. This is based on an assessment of the stress that an average person, with similar socio-cultural values and circumstances, would experience from the same problems.

Axis 5 — globally assessing the highest level of adaptive functioning during the last 12 months. Functioning is seen as being composed on three major aspects — social, occupational, and psychological.

The multiaxial evaluation was an abbreviated version of the previously recommended psychodynamic diagnostic formulation, but did not truly replace it. It no longer incorporated defence mechanisms or any of the concepts of unconscious mental functioning derived from psychoanalysis. In Axis 1, the most important features of the clinical picture of psychiatric symptoms were condensed into one or more descriptive terms. In Axis 2, the underlying developmental or personality disorder (if present) was recognised. When two important syndromes (such as depression and substance abuse) coexisted, the expression 'dual diagnosis' came into use.

In line with ICD, each diagnostic item in all editions of DSM has been given a specific code, consisting of three major digits, followed by two minor digits for the subtype of the disorder. The code numbers are supposed to facilitate modern data processing and statistical compilations. Up

Time correlation between DSM and ICD		
Year	DSM	ICD
1948		6
1952	I	
1955		7
1968	II	8
1975		9
1978		9 *
1980	III	
1987	III–R **	
1992		10 ***
1994	IV	

* Clinical modification
** Revised
*** See Chapter 9

Changes in terminology	
Old term	**New term**
Melancholia	Depression
Manic–depressive disease	Bipolar mood disorder
Hysteria	Dissociative disorder
Paranoia (or paranoid state)	Delusional disorder
Organic brain syndrome	Cognitive disorder (not until DSM–IV)
Senile dementia	Alzheimer's disease
Psychosis with cerebral arteriosclerosis	Multi-infarct or vascular dementia
Psychopathy	Personality disorder
Mental deficiency	Mental retardation
– idiot } three degrees of	– profound } four degrees
– imbecile } severity	– severe } of severity
– moron }	– moderate }
	– mild }
Mongolism	Down's syndrome

to ICD–9, the codes for ICD and DSM were the same. In ICD–10, the codes have been completely changed, but in DSM–IV, the DSM–III and ICD–9 codes have so far been retained. Of course, since human beings do not function as mathematical entities, something is always lost when a patient's mental condition is reduced to a mere numerical symbol or evaluated by means of a rating scale.

DSM–III recognised the fact that American psychiatrists had begun to realise that they had been diagnosing 'schizophrenia' too readily. It was also introduced during a period when chlorpromazine was no longer the only effective antipsychotic agent. Drugs such as lithium that helped to control manic symptoms had come into greater use, making it easier to control the 'highs' and 'lows' on the emotional scale, and a number of antidepressants had become clinically available. From then on, mood disorders were diagnosed more frequently and schizophrenic disorders less frequently by those using the DSM system. It was claimed that the reliability of the system was relatively good, in that two different clinicians were likely to agree on what they found in examining a patient. However, the validity of the system was more doubtful, whether one took a psychodynamic or a biological viewpoint. To be valid, it would have to be useful in making clinical predictions, and these were not well established by research.

The specification of symptoms that had to be present before a diagnosis could be made appeared to make this process very objective. Similarly, the absence of other clinical features helped to rule out alternative conditions, thus facilitating differential diagnosis. At the same time, it has to be acknowledged that many aspects of the system are based on fairly arbitrary criteria; not enough data were available to make these wholly scientific. In the absence of better aetiological and pathophysiological knowledge, the diagnoses themselves can only be provisional. Nevertheless, they are intended to be based on a professional and scientific consensus at the time of their publication.

DSM–IV

In 1987, DSM–III–R was introduced as a revision and refinement of DSM–III; it made the diagnostic inclusion and exclusion criteria more precise, and more useful for both clinical and research purposes. However, since this enterprise still did not satisfy many psychiatrists, DSM–IV was published in 1994, listing a total of 297 mental disorders. But does bigger mean better? This latest version gives guidelines for describing the severity of a disorder as 'mild', 'moderate', or 'severe'.

Although DSM–IV separates 'mental disorders' from 'general medical conditions', this does not imply that there is any fundamental distinction between the two. Most importantly, the system is not intended to be used by individuals who have not had appropriate training and experience. From the clinician's point of view, ICD–10 is considered by many to be more user-friendly than DSM–IV, which has a stronger orientation towards research.

The question of homosexuality

During the second half of the twentieth century, Western society had gradually come to realise that homosexuality was not to be regarded as a 'disease'. Previously, it had been called 'a sexual perversion', but then became a 'sexual deviation'; it was still retained in the current classifications of mental disorders. But finally, in 1973, the American Psychiatric Association members in charge of revising DSM decided to exclude it as such altogether, retaining it only as one of the categories for people who had consulted psychiatrists because they had been unhappy with their sexual orientation.

Other classifications

The ICD had been developed primarily for statistical purposes, and had already undergone five revisions before a section was included on mental disorders, independent of other diseases and injuries, in 1948 (Chapter 9, p. 302). The next four revisions of ICD were undertaken by psychiatrists working with the World Health Organization (WHO) and so had to include mental disorders not or only rarely encountered in the USA. A worldwide epidemiological study by the WHO of schizophrenic disorders had not disclosed any great differences in prevalence, although the prognosis appeared to be better in developing than in developed countries. The next revisions of DSM (DSM–IV–R or DSM–V) and of ICD (ICD–11) will have to consider further what is and what is not schizophrenia. Another consideration is that with the great advances in psychopharmacology and other psychiatric research in the second half of the twentieth century, it becomes more important than ever for all concerned to speak the same (psychiatric) language.

The Research Diagnostic Criteria (RDC) were formulated in the USA in 1972 with the intention of standardising diagnoses and thereby improving the quality of psychiatric research. In the case of schizophrenia, RDC took a somewhat different view from DSM–III, requiring that the illness should be of at least two weeks' duration, but not limiting the diagnosis to chronic cases only. In this way, brief situational psychoses were excluded.

Nevertheless, there were still many psychiatrists in other countries and some also in the USA who were not satisfied with the by now fairly widely accepted nosology of ICD, DSM, and RDC. One very different version was that of the Wernicke-Kleist-Leonhard school in Germany, in which a much greater differentiation was made between various endogenous psychoses. In other countries, e.g. France and Russia, different classifications continued to be used throughout the 1970s and into the 1980s. With better international communication, though, and the continued support of the Mental Health Division of WHO, some of these differences have gradually diminished.

Conclusion

During the 1970s and after, American and, with it, world psychiatry became reintegrated into the mainstream of medicine, as knowledge of the biological, neuroscientific, and pharmacological aspects of central nervous system function developed greatly. Contemporaneously, the DSM system and psychiatric practice derived from it emerged from a somewhat ambiguous and simplistic way of looking at mental disorders. A much more precise and sophisticated approach became possible.

Further efforts at integrating this new knowledge have helped to promote the concept of the 'biopsychosocial model'. This is a philosophy of diagnosing and treating the mentally disturbed person not merely as a genetic, biological, psychological or social misfit, but as a whole human being in need of expert assistance.

MENTAL RETARDATION

by Mark Jackson

Introduction

The history of people now referred to as having 'learning difficulties' or 'learning disabilities' has been dominated in the twentieth century by segregation in special schools and large purpose-built mental deficiency institutions. In the decades following the passage of legislation in Britain in 1913–14 (Chapter 2, p. 55), increasing numbers of people labelled initially as 'mentally defective' (and subsequently as 'mentally subnormal', 'mentally handicapped', 'mentally retarded', and 'educationally subnormal') were admitted to institutions. These institutions were run by local mental deficiency committees until their incorporation into the British National Health Service in 1948 as part of the psychiatric services.

By the 1960s, approximately 60,000 publicly provided beds were available for adults with mental handicaps in Britain. Although a similar number of people were also being cared for under supervision in the community during the middle decades of this century, institutions remained the prime site for the diagnosis, treatment, and management of mental defectives in most countries. In addition, institutions offered opportunities for increasingly detailed scientific research into the causes and prevention of deficiency.

The 1970s, however, witnessed a transformation in the provision of psychiatric and educational services for the mentally handicapped on both sides of the Atlantic. As the result of a number of decisive critiques of institutions and of changing understandings of the causes and manifestations of deficiency, there were many calls for the replacement of institutionalisation with care in the community. As many hospitals began a prolonged period of phased closure and as children with special educational needs were increasingly taught in ordinary, rather than special, classes and schools, the institutional population in most developed countries gradually declined. From the 1970s and through the 1980s, therefore, the pessimistic policies initiated in the 1910s underwent radical revision.

Social context

During the middle decades of the twentieth century, many of the assumptions that underlay earlier legislation were challenged. Scientific support for dominant beliefs that mental defectives constituted a distinct and intrinsically pathological section of society also diminished. In addition, doctors and others, increasingly suspicious of the motives and methods of eugenics, no longer regarded the feeble-minded as a social danger to be policed. Instead, mental defectives were construed as suffering from a sickness that needed to be treated. At the same time, the financial burden of running ever larger institutions was becoming more apparent, leading politicians to search for effective alternatives to long-term segregation. Although sterilisation remained on the political agenda at least until the 1930s (and was carried out well into the post-war period in some countries), it was not adopted as a significant option in Britain. There, as elsewhere, institutionalisation continued to constitute the central policy for the mentally retarded.

Between the 1940s and the 1960s, the institutional system was put under further strain. The emergence of parent support and pressure groups raised public concern about the treatment and rights of mentally handicapped people and their families. In addition, there was increasingly strident criticism of the shortcomings of mental handicap hospitals, culminating in highly publicised official inquiries, such as those set up by the British Ministry of Health in the 1960s into conditions at several institutions. The widespread alarm caused by the inquiries' findings of malpractice, ill-treatment, and neglect at mental deficiency hospitals was raised further by Erving Goffman's seminal critique of the deleterious effects (on both patients and staff) of long-term institutional life, first published in 1961.

The effects of growing dissatisfaction with institutional policies and their legitimating ideologies became increasingly apparent. Following a Report of the Royal Commission on the Law Relating to Mental Illness and Mental Deficiency, published in 1957, the English Mental Health Act of 1959 attempted to replace the old stigmatising labels ('mental defective', 'idiot', 'imbecile', and 'feeble-minded') with the term 'mental subnormality', and initiated a shift both from compulsory to voluntary admission and from institutions to community mental health care. This process continued in the 1960s with the search for supposedly more neutral labels and clearer classifications. 'Mental retardation', 'mental handicap', and 'educational subnormality' began to replace 'mental deficiency', and doctors of all nationalities advocated using either 'Down's syndrome' or 'trisomy 21' as less racist terms for what had routinely been referred to as 'mongolism' since John Langdon-Down's first description of the syndrome in 1866. In 1968, a World Health Organization expert committee on mental health set out elaborate international guidelines for classifying mental retardation on the basis of intelligence quotient (IQ) measurements in conjunction with social factors.

In Britain, a government report entitled *Better Services for the Mentally Handicapped*, published in 1971, marked the start of a major shift away from institutions towards community care, with social services departments (and social workers) primarily responsible for the provision of services. There were associated changes in the organisation, provision, and evaluation of services, including the founding of an official National Development Group in 1975 with a remit to advise on policy and practice. Within the realm of medical practice and research, an Institute of Mental Subnormality, which later became the British Institute of Learning Disabilities, was established.

Significantly, there was a corresponding shift in educational philosophy and practice. Under the terms of the British Education Act 1970, all children were to be regarded as 'educable' and the education of all mentally handicapped children was transferred from the National Health Service to education authorities. At the same time, educationalists began to argue more forcefully for integrating children with special educational needs into mainstream schools, rather than segregating them in special schools, a process given statutory authority in 1981.

The outcome of these ideological, political, and economic trends became apparent in many Western countries in the next twenty years or so. Increasingly, monolithic mental deficiency institutions discharged their patients, often into purpose-built hostels, and closed their doors forever.

Medical understanding and aetiology

Transformation in the provision of services for the mentally handicapped in the middle decades of this century was accompanied by and sometimes closely linked to changing scientific and medical understanding of deficiency. Early twentieth-century beliefs in the inheritance of mental deficiency as a Mendelian character were undermined in the 1920s and 1930s by increasingly sophisticated studies of aetiology and transmission. Much of this research was carried out in laboratories at large institutions. The most significant study of this nature in the inter-war years was Lionel Penrose's work, carried out at the Royal Eastern Counties Institution in Colchester, England. In addition to clarifying the aetiology of 'phenylketonuria' (or PKU, a term coined by one of Penrose's collaborators) and Down's syndrome, Penrose's study, published under the title *A Clinical and Genetic Study of 1280 Cases of Mental Defect*, suggested that most cases of mental deficiency were the product of a combination of genetic, pathological, and environmental factors (Chapter 5, p. 138).

By the 1970s, the authors of medical textbooks and research papers generally classified mental handicap according to the supposed aetiology and pathogenesis, i.e. broadly on the basis of whether the condition was primarily the product of genetic or environmental factors. In the first instance, some cases of mental handicap were known to have genetic origins. Such cases included conditions thought to be caused by single gene defects (phenylketonuria, galactosaemia, Tay–Sachs disease, epiloia, von Recklinghausen's disease, Apert's syndrome, Crouzon's disease, Lesch–Nyhan syndrome, etc.), and those produced by chromosomal abnormalities (such as Down's syndrome, Patau's syndrome, and Edward's syndrome). In addition, there was a range of conditions known to be the result of various environmental insults. In general, these were further divided into pre-natal causes (such as congenital syphilis and rhesus incompatibility), natal causes (birth trauma or hypoxia), and post-natal causes (such as tuberculous meningitis, whooping cough, lead poisoning, and head injuries).

In the light of this increasingly complex array of aetiologies, clinical diagnosis and classification of handicap in the 1970s depended not only on meticulous assessment of a child's physical and mental abilities by doctors and educational psychologists, but also on a range of laboratory tests. Amongst these karyotyping to detect chromosomal abnormalities and biochemical tests to determine metabolic disturbances were notable.

Treatment

Although a growing recognition that people with mental handicaps could also exhibit various psychiatric symptoms led to the increased use of psychotropic drugs to control behavioural disturbances, there remained few pharmaceutical agents capable of alleviating or curing the mental and physical features of handicap in the 1970s. Essentially, treatment in individual cases consisted of early diagnosis, followed by the introduction of appropriate diets (as in phenylketonuria) or the use of suitable education and occupational therapy or training to encourage work and independence.

As institutionalisation diminished in appeal, these services were increasingly provided in day centres to which people travelled from hostels and houses in the community. This process of transferring people with learning difficulties from large institutions to shared houses in the community has not been unproblematic. Although they perpetuated isolation, stigmatisation, and sometimes mistreatment, institutions could offer people with learning difficulties company, facilities, and activities. Without appropriate financial support to provide suitable training and facilities and without the adequate organisation of services, care in the community has in some cases proved no more effective than institutional care in integrating people with learning difficulties.

From a medical perspective, most attention was paid to developing means of lowering the incidence of handicap within the population. Improvements in maternity and child care services were aimed at reducing the presence of pre-natal, natal, and post-natal causes. In addition, the introduction of pre-natal screening for chromosomal abnormalities in this period was coupled with the expansion of genetic counselling services and the possibility of therapeutic abortion. Although these services were sometimes criticised on moral grounds and on the grounds that they devalued the lives of people with learning difficulties, they have become a major feature of medical approaches to these difficulties in the late twentieth century.

Conclusion

In the 1970s, there was a major international policy shift in the treatment and education of people now referred to as having learning difficulties. Driven by significant and well-founded anxieties about the shortcomings of institutions, policy makers in many developed countries increasingly advocated care in the community, in line with similar (but slightly earlier) developments in the field of mental illness. The implementation of this policy incorporated both the integration of children into mainstream schools and the transfer of adults with learning difficulties from large hospitals into smaller hostels and houses. These transformations in the therapeutic and educational landscape were accompanied and in part driven by significant efforts on the part of people with learning difficulties and their families to reduce the stigma associated with their circumstances and to rehabilitate themselves politically and socially. Critically, although the closure of long-term institutions has been regarded by many as a significant advance, it is now becoming apparent that, without sufficient government funding, care in the community can also present substantial obstacles to effective integration of both children and adults with learning difficulties. For populations in many parts of the world, though, this problem is only one of many that still has to be managed within families, with little or no help from public services.

PSYCHIATRY IN PRIMARY CARE

by Greg Wilkinson

Psychiatry in primary care is predominantly a British contribution, arising from the unusual evolution of public health services and general practice in that country, from the middle of the twentieth century. Other parts of the world, though, particularly English-speaking countries, took up the theme, as national health care systems were developed over the following decades. The consequence is that the early clinical experience and research on this topic is mostly published in English, though by the mid-1980s, a substantial number of publications had accumulated by authors working outside Anglophone countries. In the 1980s, Harding *et al.* published their World Health Organization collaborative study based in Colombia, India, Senegal, Sudan, the Philippines, Egypt, and Brazil on strategies for extending mental health care. What emerged from this work is that where psychiatry is involved in primary care, the principles and practice are probably universal, with relatively minor variations within and between countries.

At a symposium on British mental health services in 1965, a well-known London general practitioner, HN Levitt, lamented the failure of communication between psychiatric hospitals and primary care. If a patient was going to be in hospital for several months — which was quite common at the time — the GP should receive a progress report. When discharge finally took place, the hospital's letter was often brief and uninformative, so the continuity of care was difficult; it might be greatly improved if the GP was informed before the discharge actually took place. Yet on their side, psychiatrists complained that letters referring patients to them were often miserably inadequate and that GPs tended to reduce the maintenance doses of medication, without any consultation. Patients who were at serious risk of relapse without their treatment might even be told that they "shouldn't get too used to taking their tablets". Failure of routine communication seemed to underlie many of these problems, though the poor level of knowledge of psychiatric disorders amongst GPs was also important.

In the 1960s, the introduction of the benzodiazepines, which were much less toxic than barbiturates, led to a steady increase in psychotropic drug prescribing within primary care. In one later British study of people taking these drugs, 45% were using hypnotics, 30%

taking minor tranquillisers (mainly benzodiazepines), and 14% taking antidepressants. Of the patients who had been given a psychiatric diagnosis, about two-thirds had had medication prescribed for them. Patients with chronic — but not acute — bodily conditions are more likely than average to be taking psychotropic drugs in addition to any specific treatment for their somatic disorder. Most psychotropic drug prescribing in general practice is relatively short-term, though in many countries, benzodiazepines continue to be prescribed at a huge rate in primary care. In the UK, this was greatly restricted in the mid-1980s.

The Classic British Study

In London, Professor Michael Shepherd and his colleagues first published their seminal work, *Psychiatric Illness in General Practice* in 1966. This established that:

- psychiatric morbidity was one of the more common reasons for consulting a general practitioner in Britain. This morbidity consisted mainly of neurotic conditions, with only 5% psychoses;
- treatment in general practice consisted largely of drugs and/or discussion, but almost one-third of patients with psychiatric disorders received no treatment. General practitioners dealt with the bulk of identified psychiatric morbidity by themselves, referring only 5% to specialist psychiatric services.

The second edition of *Psychiatric Illness in General Practice* was published in 1981, outlining more recent developments in measurement, screening, diagnosis, intervention, and classification. Overall, this work pointed to one main conclusion: "the cardinal requirement for improvement of the Mental Health Services in Britain is not a large expansion and proliferation of psychiatric agencies, but rather a strengthening of the family doctor in his therapeutic role".

Estimates from the Epidemiologic Catchment Area study in the United States indicated that at least 15% of the population is affected by psychiatric disorders in the course of one year, and work in other countries has yielded comparable findings. Both British and American research demonstrates that about half this morbidity is chronic, with a duration of over one year, but that only a small proportion of the mentally ill who consult general practitioners reach the attention of psychiatrists. However, in the community-based service in south Verona, Italy, the referral rate in the 1980s was much higher: 22% of patients who were identified with conspicuous psychiatric morbidity by general practitioners were referred to a specialist.

A survey of the European situation by a WHO group in 1973 reached this verdict: "The crucial question is not how the general practitioner can fit into the Mental Health Services, but rather how the psychiatrist can collaborate most effectively with primary medical services and reinforce the effectiveness of the primary physician as a member of the mental health team". The role played by general practitioners in mental health care was seen to be important for a number of reasons, as outlined in the table below.

In the Third World, psychiatric disorders make up a significant proportion of the morbidity seen in primary health care. In that setting, there are two main issues. Firstly, although primary health workers in developing countries see mental disorders regularly amongst their patients, they recognise only a minority of them; they need to improve their diagnostic skills so that they may recognise and provide appropriate management for such patients. Secondly, improved diagnosis is not sufficient to reach those patients with severe psychiatric disorders who do not normally present themselves at primary health facilities — educational contact with the community is also needed to change attitudes and to show that such patients can be helped by treatment.

Why is the GP so important?

- Patients with psychosocial problems are high users of medical care and tend to be well known to their GPs, who may be able to utilise this relationship for psychotherapeutic intervention

- Patients with emotional disorders experience less stigma when treated by a GP than by a psychiatrist

- Physical and psychiatric complaints tend to co-exist and are often difficult to separate in diagnosis and treatment, which makes the GP, who is well placed to treat the whole person, the first choice as doctor

- GPs are best placed to provide long-term follow-up and be available for successive episodes of illness

Primary health care

In 1976, a monumental review on *Primary Health Care* — defined as the care provided outside the precincts of any hospital — was published for the British Department of Health by Donald Hicks. His account of mental health at the level of primary care began, somewhat surprisingly, with a review of psychotherapy, referring to the earlier contribution of Michael and Enid Balint in London, which fostered dynamic understanding amongst GPs. However, that work, although the subject of much discussion and writing, affected only a small minority of British GPs directly, and the importance of its impact in the long term is uncertain. Similar developments in other countries have been very limited.

At that time, a study by Peter Brook of psychiatrists in training in three regions of England, showed that from the point of view of primary health care, the most serious shortcoming was that two-thirds of the senior trainees felt they were getting inadequate experience of psychiatry in a community setting. Contact with the community social services was also very restricted for these young psychiatrists. That situation is unlikely to have improved greatly since then, either in Britain or other countries.

Hicks pointed out that national mental health policy was mainly concerned with seriously mentally ill adults. It required hospital treatment to be as short as possible, and the majority of patients to be dealt with in the community by out-patient services, day hospitals, hostels, and rehabilitation services. Teams of psychiatrists, psychologists, social workers, nurses, and occupational therapists were each to serve a population of about 60,000 people. On average, between 20 and 30 general practitioners and their co-workers in primary health care teams would also be serving the same population. However, the problems that would have to be overcome to make collaboration effective between hospital-based units and primary health care were unsolved; for instance, how best to manage the aftercare of discharged patients, especially if they required surveillance by a community psychiatric nurse and the periodic attention of the consultant psychiatrist. The point at which responsibility for the patient would formally be handed back to the general practitioner was another critically important decision. Each year, seven million people in Britain consulted their general practitioners about psychiatric illnesses, and as attitudes to medical care changed, substantial undisclosed morbidity could well be brought to the attention of the primary care team. Yet the knowledge, practical skills, and concentrated effort needed to deal adequately with psychiatric disorders at that level did not exist — even in the country which then had probably the best developed system of primary care in the world.

A very useful classification of people with diagnosable psychiatric illness who are seen by primary medical care services was made by Tantam and Goldberg in 1991.

Group 1. Requiring specific medical treatment

Patients with major psychotic disorders are sometimes seen in primary care settings, particularly in the early stages; but they represent only a very small percentage of the people with psychiatric illness who are seen by GPs. The great majority of these either have depressive or anxiety disorders, or a mixture of the two. The discovery of antidepressant drugs in the late 1950s was a revolutionary development for people in this category, since before that, GPs could do little for them other than offer reassurance and sedation (Chapter 6, p. 169). Anxiety states rarely require specific medical treatment, but obsessive–compulsive disorder became treatable later, with the discovery of drugs such as clomipramine and the selective serotonin re-uptake inhibitors (SSRIs).

Group 2. Benefiting mainly from specific psychological treatment

These patients may be suffering many types of anxiety and phobic states, some forms of insomnia, eating disorders, and some sexual problems. Until the 1960s, management in primary care was mostly a matter of sympathy and the prescription of sedative drugs, mainly barbiturates, which were of diminishing effect as time went on. The discovery of the benzodiazepines removed some of the dangers of existing drugs, but did not greatly reduce the risk of tolerance and dependence for many sufferers. Different countries varied in their response to these benzodiazepine problems, Britain taking a particularly firm line in the early 1980s.

From the 1960s, behavioural and cognitive treatments offered a completely new approach to many of these disorders, though trained practitioners have remained relatively few in most countries (Chapter 6, p. 173 and this chapter, p. 272). Counselling by family doctors has also been shown to be effective for recent anxiety states, and has become practised by a variety of personnel, particularly in the USA and Britain. In the 1990s, psychopharmacology has made a bigger contribution to some of those conditions, with SSRIs found to have efficacy in social phobia and bulimia, for instance.

Group 3. Requiring supportive therapy and social intervention

Patients in this group may have personality disorders, chronic social stress, mild cerebral impairment, or interpersonal problems such as marital conflict. Their situation is often complicated by material social problems of physical ill-health. Chronic dysphoria was included amongst these conditions, but the identification of dysthymia, particularly by the work of Akiskal in America from the late 1970s, has shown that long-term antidepressant treatment can often be effective for patients of this kind. Sometimes, what had seemed to be an intractable personality problem can in fact be greatly improved in this way.

Otherwise, medication has little part to play. The traditional role of the sympathetic and supportive family doctor remains as important as ever, though often in collaboration with other professionals, such as social workers and nurses. Medical school training has not always equipped doctors well for this role, although it has improved in many countries since the 1960s.

Group 4. Requiring only recognition and discussion of problems

Patients of this kind may be better described as 'distressed', rather than psychiatrically ill; some may have suffered an adverse life event, but have not developed a diagnosable depressive illness. Others may have longer-term problems, but can be given encouragement to cope with these by discussion, reassurance, and perhaps the prescription of a psychotropic drug in low dose for a short time. The doctor's role with people of this kind has not significantly changed, but better medical training should have made GPs more sensitive to recognising these problems and separating them from more serious conditions.

The detection of psychiatric illness by questionnaire

One of the most significant psychiatrists in this worldwide context in the 1970s was Sir David Goldberg who, in 1972, published *The Detection of Psychiatric Illness by Questionnaire, A Technique for the Identification and Assessment of Non-Psychotic Psychiatric Illness*. Since then, the General Health Questionnaire in its various forms has stimulated a vast body of research as a screening tool. This was both for the detection of psychiatric disturbance in general practice populations, and in the assessment of the prevalence of minor psychiatric morbidity in the community. In addition, Goldberg and Huxley's (1980) influential contribution, *Mental Illness in the Community, The Pathway to Psychiatric Care*, stemmed from work with that questionnaire. It employed the concepts of levels and filters to describe both the wide range of severity of disorder and the pathways that people with psychiatric disorder take to reach specialist care.

Goldberg and Huxley's model comprised five levels and four filters; to move from one level to the next implied passage through a filter (see following tables). The characteristics of levels and filters can shed light on both patients' morbidity and decision-making about its management; both of these are influenced by different medical and cultural settings.

Pathways of referral from primary care to specialist services vary widely in different countries, and have been studied by WHO. Direct referrals from the community to psychiatric services without involving the GP are relatively common in the USA; this may be a feature of any insurance-based service in which the patients can select their own doctor at any level. A similar pattern is present, to a lesser extent, in Spain, Portugal, Mexico, Pakistan, India, and some other countries.

The interface with psychiatry

In the 1970s, the main interface between general practice and psychiatry in most countries was the out-patient clinic. In the United Kingdom, up to half of GPs used psychiatric out-patient clinics as a primary source of advice, without first treating or investigating patients; as a result, psychiatrists tended to regard themselves as largely responsible for the total care of out-patients. Yet a study of the specialist care provided in British out-patient clinics suggested that fewer than half the patients attending really needed to remain under the direct supervision of consultants. Even fewer required special facilities or treatments which were available only at a hospital. This situation is likely to have resulted mainly from inadequate psychiatric education of GPs, lack of interest by many of them in psychiatric illness, and overall pressure of work in their practice.

At the out-patient clinic, there was a high degree of uniformity in the diagnostic categories recorded, the treatments prescribed, and the further arrangements made for patients. At initial specialist consultation in Britain, three-quarters of the patients were prescribed continued out-patient treatment. Yet in fact, some two-thirds of these were seen

---

Goldberg and Huxley's model

Level 1 Refers to psychiatric and emotional disorder in the community, as measured by community surveys. A proportion of people with psychiatric disorder in the community consult a GP. To do so, they pass through filter 1, which is the decision made by the person to seek help and the act of consulting

Level 2 Comprises the total of all psychiatric morbidity in general practice. However, a proportion of level-2 morbidity remains unrecognised by a GP, and this is referred to as 'hidden psychiatric morbidity'. These people do not pass through filter 2 and fail to reach level 3

Level 3 The morbidity identified and recognised by the GP

Level 4 Consists of all people with psychiatric disorder referred to psychiatric services

Level 5 Refers to those who are admitted to hospital

---

on fewer than four occasions; this rapid decline in attendance appeared to be due equally to high rates of discharge and of lapse from care. After three months, less than half of patients referred were still attending the clinic, one-quarter were receiving psychiatric treatment from their GP, and the rest were not receiving any treatment. Those who decided to stop treatment themselves tended to make relatively poor progress. It was in the 1980s, however, that different forms of consultation–liaison between general practitioners and psychiatrists developed more widely.

Whether an educational programme on depression could influence the attitudes towards and ability to treat depressive disorders was investigated by Rutz *et al.* on the Baltic island of Gotland, which contained 56,000 people and 18 GPs. A course of lectures on suicide and related topics was given three times to the doctors. There were useful results in the short term, with a significant fall in the number of suicides in the first year, but this was not maintained. The conclusion was that educational activities of this kind would have to be repeated every two to three years, if the management of depression in primary care was to be significantly improved.

Further developments

In 1979, the US National Institute of Mental Health produced an annotated review of the literature on mental disorder and primary medical care which comprised more than 350 publications, bearing witness to the widespread and growing international interest in the subject.

Shepherd, in his preface to the second edition of *Psychiatric Illness in General Practice*, had commented that "What was originally expected to be a small island of psychiatric morbidity has turned out to be a large unchartered continent... the notion that all you would find in general practice was what was left over from the designated mental health services in hospital was clearly absurd. Nonetheless... the publication of our monograph... in 1966 attracted little serious attention". When I asked Shepherd if primary care psychiatry could become as successful internationally as in Britain, he responded: "The subject is now recognised as a top priority by WHO. It appeals to many individual workers, in many other countries but they are often handicapped by the fact that their system of medical care does not lend itself to this type of investigation. In this country, it has been creeping into the system... and it has had to overcome opposition from both hospital psychiatrists and general practitioners for quite different reasons".

In Britain, the GP remains the first point of contact for most people who receive mental health care, but in some other countries, a greater proportion of primary care is provided by specialist professionals — psychiatrists, psychologists, or social workers. Probably the greatest variety of such types of service delivery is to be found in the USA, where ministers of religion also play a significant role. In the USA, Australia, and some other affluent countries there are more psychiatrists, relative to the size of population, than in the UK or most places outside Western Europe. However, even in the USA, data from the Epidemiologic Catchment Area Study in 1978 showed that less than half the people in a study population with an identified psychiatric disorder were referred to a mental health

Goldberg & Huxley's Levels and Filters				
	Community		**General practice**	**Specialist services**	

Levels	1	2	3	4	5
	Morbidity in random samples	Total morbidity	Conspicuous morbidity	Psychiatric patients	Psychiatric in-patients
Filters		first	second	third	fourth
Manchester*	250–315	230	101.5	20.8	3.4
Groningen*	250–303	224	94	34	10
Verona*	227	34	23	4	0.7

* Period prevalence rates for total population mortality at all 5 levels in three European cities (Manchester/ Groningen — annual rates; Verona — weekly rates).
Adapted from Goldberg D, Huxley P. *Common Mental Disorders. A Biosocial Model*. London: Routledge; 1992.

specialist. The same study found that 15% of patients seen by non-psychiatric medical specialists had a psychiatric disorder, and so most people with a psychiatric problem who seek medical advice will initially see a doctor whose main work is with bodily illness. In the USA, the comprehensive community mental health centres set up under the Kennedy legislation of the mid-1960s were originally thought of as places where primary psychiatric care would be obtained. The extent to which this was achieved in practice, though, is uncertain.

A WHO working group on psychiatry and primary medical care stated in 1973 that the primary medical care team is the keystone of community psychiatry. Its non-controversial recommendations were: (a) more evaluative studies; (b) more training of GPs in psychiatry; (c) more research into diagnosis and classification; (d) extension of primary health care teams; and (e) closer communication and cooperation between specialist and primary health care services. The last of these recommendations was thought to be particularly important, but there has been no agreement since as to how it can best be achieved. The WHO group thought that the responsibility lay more with the psychiatrist to collaborate effectively with primary medical care, rather than with the GP to fit his contribution into the mental health service. In Britain particularly, a large proportion of psychiatrists have arranged to devote some of their time to working in primary care settings, and this integration has taken several different forms. It is still not known, however, whether this kind of arrangement is cost-effective, compared with other ways in which the psychiatrist might spend his professional time.

It has often been said that GPs do not primarily concern themselves with diagnosis, but follow a pragmatic, problem-solving approach, which is more likely to involve symptomatic treatment. Diagnosis may then come afterwards, to justify the clinical management decisions which have already been made.

Acknowledgements

Parts of this contribution have been modified from Tantam D, Goldberg DP. Primary medical care. In: Bennett, DH, Freeman H, eds. Community Psychiatry. *Edinburgh: Churchill Livingstone; 1991.*

MICHEL FOUCAULT (1926–1984)

by Chandak Sengoopta

Michel Foucault (1926–1984), author of a series of historical analyses of subjects ranging from madness to sexuality, was a philosopher who found his greatest fame outside the discipline of academic philosophy. Foucault's influence has been seminal in many areas of historical, social, and humanistic studies, especially the history of medicine and psychiatry. This does not necessarily mean that psychiatrists, doctors, and historians agree with whatever he had to say on their subjects — far from it. But whether one agrees with Foucault's contentions or not, their force, sweep, and philosophical depth compel one to approach them with respect.

When he died suddenly in 1984, Foucault held a chair in the 'History of Systems of Thought' at the Collège de France. By then, he had become a familiar and controversial figure in international academia; his books *Histoire de la folie à l'âge classique* (translated in abridged form as *Madness and Civilization*, 1965), *Les mots et les choses* (translated as *The Order of Things*, 1970), *Naissance de la clinique* (translated as *Birth of the Clinic*, 1973), *Surveiller et punir* (translated as *Discipline and Punish*, 1977), and *Histoire de la sexualité, I: la volonté de savoir* (translated as *The History of Sexuality*, Vol. 1: *An Introduction*, 1978) were read, interpreted, and vigorously debated by scholars from a broad range of disciplines. Foucault did not single-handedly create the current vogue for scholarly studies of behaviour and attitudes that were traditionally dismissed as deviant. But the trend could not have survived, let alone flourished as luxuriantly as it has, without stimulation from his works. Foucault made deviance a respectable and challenging subject for academic research — a royal road to understanding the true character of modern Western civilisation. Even sympathetic biographers, however, have suggested that his own lifestyle — he was homosexual with apparently a strong preference for sadomasochistic relationships — played a significant role in shaping his scholarly interests.

Whatever be the relation between Foucault's personal life and his scholarly work, his lifelong quest was to understand the evolution of the twin concepts of 'Normal' and 'Deviant' across history. Consequently, the history of concepts of reason and madness was prominent in his project. Foucault's first, rather slight book, *Maladie mentale et personnalité* (1954; translated as *Mental Illness and Psychology*, 1987) was not of much importance to his general endeavour. However, his doctoral thesis — published as *Folie et déraison* in 1961, subsequently abridged by the author himself as *Histoire de la folie à l'âge classique* in 1964, and translated in this form into English as *Madness and Civilization* in 1965 — was a major text generating seemingly endless streams of new research, responses, and critiques. When the English translation was first published, RD Laing observed that it was a work of such "sustained intensity and verbal momentum" that it took a while to "come to terms with the measure of its truth". Thirty or more years on, scholars are still grappling with it. How can one book on the *history* of ideas of madness have had such an effect?

The answer lies in the sheer innovativeness (not necessarily the accuracy) of Foucault's interpretation of how certain people came to be seen as mentally ill, and therefore in need of supervision and treatment from a special kind of doctor who came to be known as the psychiatrist. The heroic story of the laudable if slow progress from condemning madness as diabolical possession to recognising it as mental illness, told in so many histories of psychiatry by clinicians, was turned completely on its head by Foucault. Whatever else *Histoire de la folie* presented to its reader, it was not a triumphant tale of the rise of compassionate, scientific psychiatry.

The narrative of the book commenced in the Middle Ages and ended in the early nineteenth century. Virtually every 'advance' of psychiatry that had occurred in between came in for a thoroughly revisionist analysis. Foucault was more interested in establishing how 'madness' was first divided from 'reason' than in the science that developed on the basis of this fundamental distinction. It was his conviction that the birth of psychiatric medicine, instead of bringing succour to the insane, had actually resulted in the exclusion of the insane from society. The Middle Ages, he argued, had treated madness as a vice, whereas in the Renaissance, madness and the mad 'invaded' everyday life as an ever-present threat, as well as a reminder of the fragility of reason. (It is characteristic of Foucault's arguments that he posits sharp breaks in ideas and practices without ever pausing to analyse why such breaks might have occurred.) From the seventeenth century, however, this omnipresence of madness was on the wane. The mad were now being enclosed within institutions of incarceration, in a process which

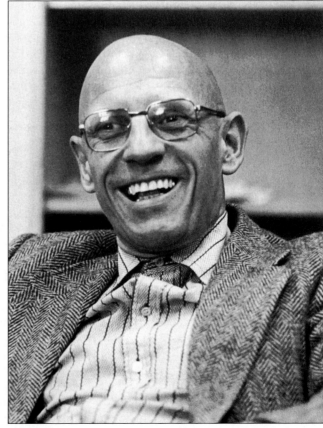

Michel Foucault, 1979. © Corbis/Bettmann.

Foucault called the 'Great Confinement'. This process initially had nothing to do with medicine and lumped the indigent mad with the bad, the idle, and the redundant in one great mass — a group replacing the older excluded category of 'leper'. Once confined, they were put to work, since all unreason was deemed to be inseparable from sloth, and work was the panacea for all social ills. Madness, then, was no longer irrational or purely vicious: it was undesirable because the madman had transgressed the bourgeois imperative of industriousness. 'Madness', declared Foucault, "was thus torn from that imaginary freedom which still allowed it to flourish on the Renaissance horizon. Not so long ago, it had floundered about in broad daylight: in *King Lear*, in *Don Quixote*. But in less than a half-century, it had been sequestered and, in the fortress of confinement, bound to Reason, to the rules of morality and to their monotonous nights". The Age of Reason, he claimed, ended the dialogue of sane and insane, replacing it with "the language of psychiatry, which is a monologue of reason *about* madness".

Foucault argued that before the seventeenth century, no matter how violent or despicable it might be, evil was dealt with and punished in the open, thus authenticating the power of the ruler — usually an absolute monarch. But after the seventeenth century social conscience changed. The most shameful forms of evil were now feared as sources of moral contagion, and therefore shut away. Madness was not necessarily evil, but nor was it a form of Unreason with which society felt at all comfortable. Hence, said Foucault, it continued to be exhibited in controlled settings (in the notorious trips to Bedlam, for instance), but never again was it to be a part of everyday life, as it had been during the Renaissance. During the eighteenth century, the undifferentiated confinement of all varieties of Unreason gave way to a more specific confinement of the insane alone. In this way, madness became "the very symbol of the confining power and its absurd and obsessive representative within the world of confinement".

The mad were now synonymous with the asylum, but the asylum itself was to undergo reforms soon. All psychiatrists and historians of psychiatry have grown up with what Foucault called the 'myths' of Pinel and Tuke and their 'moral treatment', which emphasised that the behaviour of the insane must be controlled, not by chains but by reawakening their reason and sense of responsibility. In what was perhaps the most controversial section of an already provocative thesis, Foucault argued that moral treatment was anything but a liberation. The Tukes' famous Retreat and its well-ordered, compassionate life did not simply protect the inmates from cruelty and exploitation. Rather, in the new setting, the mad were turned into their own guards and tormentors: the old routines of observation, restraint, and punishment were now placed within the minds of each insane individual, whose good behaviour was no longer a voluntary choice but one issuing from the threat of guilt. The old systems of restraint, in short, had been substituted by a no less coercive self-restraint. Foucault also maintained that the Tukes established medical authority over the asylum, a claim made apparently in ignorance of the fact that the founding father of the Retreat was a tea merchant, not a doctor of any kind. Since observation, or rather surveillance, was fundamental to the new-style asylum, it was only natural that asylum psychiatry was based exclusively on observation and classification, unlike psychoanalysis, which much later would at least try to establish a dialogue with Unreason. The asylum doctor did not have a scientific role, but one of paternal and juridical authority, such that asylum psychiatry was "no more than a complement to the old rites of Order, Authority, and Punishment".

Few could fail to be fascinated by certain aspects of this complex and challenging analysis of the rise of psychiatry. One would, however, have to be a member of the Foucauldian Cult (an ever-expanding group in today's academia) not to find quite a few of his arguments perverse, poorly researched, sophistical, or downright meaningless. His almost romantic idealisation of Renaissance ideas of madness, for example, has been questioned seriously by historians, who dismiss Foucault's assertion that this condition was a part of everyday life during that period. Foucault's postulation of an undifferentiated Great Confinement of the mad and the bad all over Europe during the seventeenth century has also come in for severe criticism.

In one of the most persuasive critiques, Roy Porter has shown how inapplicable the notion of a Great Confinement is to Britain, where during the seventeenth and eighteenth centuries, there were few large institutions for incarceration. Even the few institutions that did exist did not follow Foucault's pattern. For instance, Bethlem, perhaps the best-known repository of the mad, and Bridewell, the London institution for the 'bad', shared the same governors for a time. Those governors, however, did not believe in the undifferentiated confinement of the mad and the bad, postulated by Foucault, and were careful about consigning the former to Bethlem and the latter to Bridewell. It is hard to dispute Porter's conclusion that while Foucault's model might conceivably have some relevance in the context of French history, his claims for its pan-European applicability simply cannot be sustained.

Foucault's defenders have countered all empirical critiques with assertions that such deficiencies characterise only the abridged version of *Histoire de la folie* and the English translation that was made from it — a contention that some historians have challenged. His study, in any case, was not really a work of history, but rather a philosopher's abstract analysis of how psychiatry *might* have evolved. Moreover, it was written during the 1960s, when psychiatry was demonised as an oppressive force in modern society (Chapter 7, p. 202). For the intellectual radicals of that era, mental illness was a category invented to imprison the human spirit; Foucault's work resonated well with such sentiments. Laing and the British anti-psychiatry movement, expectedly enough, held *Madness and Civilization* in high esteem — it carried a foreword by the renegade psychiatrist David Cooper — and ever more marginal countercultural voices tried to speak in Foucault's voice. Madness, it seemed, could be written out of existence by a radical Parisian philosopher. Whether the anti-psychiatry movement and its countercultural associates understood Foucault correctly or not, critics of anti-psychiatry ever since have considered him, perhaps unfairly, to be one of its spiritual mentors. Somewhat similarly, Foucault, without being a committed Marxist, was involved on several occasions with projects and protests inspired by Marxist groups and as a result, Marxist scholars have not treated him with quite the disdain they reserve for mere liberals. Anti-Marxists, on the other hand, regard his work as yet another example of the Red menace in modern scholarship.

There are other reasons why Foucault's approach to madness has faced criticism. Clinical psychiatrists in particular find his condemnation of moral treatment highly frustrating. If compassion is as oppressive as chains, then what indeed could the psychiatrist do to improve his work? It is not the job of a historian or philosopher to offer clear-cut alternatives to systems he criticises, and Foucault himself denied the negativity imputed to him. "My point", he asserted, "is not that everything is bad, but that everything is dangerous, which is not exactly the same as bad. If everything is dangerous, then we always have something to do. So my position leads not to apathy but to a hyper- and pessimistic activism".

Though Foucault's flaws were legion, his achievements must not be overlooked or underestimated. There are many reasons why, over the last three decades, the history of psychiatry has been transformed from the somewhat antiquarian hobby of practising clinicians into a field at the leading edge of historical research. One of those reasons (and not the least important one) was the stimulus of Foucault's work. Even though his analyses and factual research left much to be desired, his fundamental questions have been unrivalled in stimulating a whole generation of scholars. Some of the work he has inspired has undoubtedly been opaque, tedious, or amateurish, but more than a few of his successors have produced excellent scholarship on the history of different forms of deviance in Western history. Much high-quality research in this area, moreover, has resulted from successful attempts to refute Foucault's assertions. In overall terms, Foucault incontestably extended and remapped the boundaries of historical research. He raised questions few historians or clinicians ever thought of raising before him, and his works helped transform apparently narrow medical issues into matters of broader scholarly concern.

POST-TRAUMATIC STRESS DISORDER

by L Stephen O'Brien

Post-traumatic stress disorder (PTSD), as a defined condition, was born with the publication in 1980 of the *Diagnostic and Statistical Manual of Mental Disorders,* Third Edition. It appeared with a definition which was very different from previous official American Psychiatric Association (APA) attitudes to post-traumatic mental health problems. They had then assumed that reactions to extreme trauma were necessarily transient in persons of normal personality, chronic disability being the representation of character defects and/or the colouring of constitutional disorders.

However, the condition had a rather longer gestation. For hundreds of years, there had been recognition that some of those people exposed to the severe trauma of either man-made or natural violence suffered psychiatric or psychological reactions. What appear to be traumatic reactions can be seen both in ancient myths and legends, and in more recent historical records. From his diary, it seems that Samuel Pepys may have suffered PTSD after the Great Fire of London, and reports of cases have been identified following an avalanche in Italy during the eighteenth century.

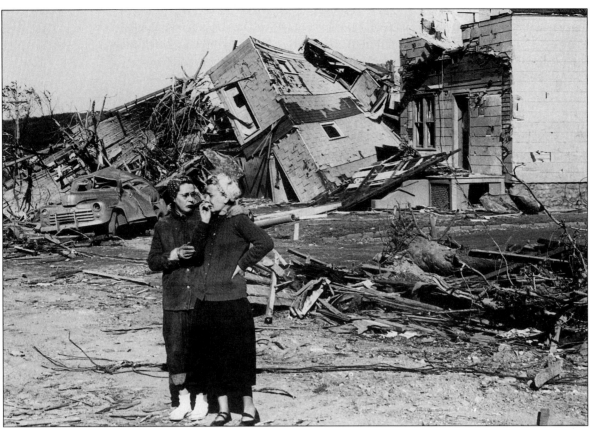

With the wreckage of her home in background, Mrs Alice O'Donnell weeps over her loss while her neighbour, Mrs Florence Long tries to comfort her as officials and residents of Worcester, Massachusetts today began to assess the damage done by a tornado, 1953. © Corbis/Bettmann.

However, the development of PTSD undoubtedly owes much to the history of warfare. In this volume, Shephard considers shell-shock and the legacy of the First World War (Chapter 2, p. 33). Interest diminished, though, when peace broke out, and a major study of traumatic stress, discussed at the Fifth Psychoanalytic Congress of 1918, was abandoned after the war ended. Those lessons were largely forgotten and then relearned in the Second World War. Despite the fact that there were real attempts not to forget this knowledge again in Vietnam, it is clear that the critical stage of development in the gestation of PTSD occurred towards the end of and following that War. This involved predominantly American investigators, vigorously assisted by the press and public. Though it has been widely recognised that war is not the only stressor causing psychological trauma, a succession of wars have been associated with increased interest in, and advances in knowledge about, the subject.

An acknowledged condition

But what were the influences which led to the development of PTSD as an acknowledged condition? How did the war with the lowest known rate of psychiatric casualties lead to the growth industry which is now PTSD — said to have a lifetime prevalence of up to 8%?

Some of the other sources of stress considered in the pre-PTSD era included rape and industrial accidents. Burgess and Holstrom published an important paper on 'Rape Trauma Syndrome' in 1974, based on a study of 92 adults and 37 children attending hospital after rape or sexual assault. The features they described included nightmares and 'traumatophobia', the latter being essentially a description of both distress at reminders of the incident and avoidance of these. A number of authors continued to study the psychological effects of trauma at work, while Fellner's 1968 publication, *Post Traumatic Neurosis — Theme and Variations*, suggested that psychedelic drugs such as psilocybin might be used in the treatment of chronic post-traumatic patients, although this method was not generally accepted. There had already been publications on psychiatric injury following road traffic accidents. In 1938, Farber had used the panic of an estimated one million people when Orson Welles' version of the *War of the Worlds* was broadcast on radio in New York to consider the psychological effects of mass disasters. A number of publications concerning medico-legal aspects of what was described as 'traumatic neurosis' had already appeared.

Since the end of the Second World War, interest had continued in Holocaust survivors and their psychological problems. Krystal, after 30 years treating survivors, wrote a series of papers examining psychoanalytic theories of trauma, and reviewing work from Freud and Breuer onwards. His conclusion was that the "final common path" of various sorts of traumatisation was "the development of overwhelming affects", as Freud had originally indicated. While Rappaport, himself a concentration camp survivor, called upon the much older work of Rado to support the differentiation of the psychological sequelae of concentration camp experience from war neurosis, others used the work of Chodoff and Strom to support the similarity of the response. This difference of opinion was not resolved.

Contribution of the Vietnam War

But what of Vietnam? What was it about this foreign war, involving more than three million Americans in the 1960s and early 1970s, which led to the definition of a new disorder? It also led to a turning away from the existing view that traumatic responses were either short-lived or else represented the establishment of other recognisable disorders.

Studies of the mental health of American soldiers in Vietnam consistently showed markedly lower rates of psychiatric breakdown than in other wars. Tiffany contrasted a 5% rate with 23% in the Second World War, while others described how effective the preventive strategies of forward psychiatry were in dealing with combat stress reactions. In spite of, or perhaps because of the contrasts between Vietnam and other wars, this difference in rates of breakdown appears to be a genuine one. In the years after that war, however, it was gradually acknowledged that survival without breakdown during conflict did not mean the absence of psychiatric problems in the long term. A study by Haley of soldiers who had participated in atrocities emphasised that while the rate of breakdown in Vietnam was lower than in previous wars, this did not mean that they would not become psychiatric casualties later.

This was a change to the current received wisdom at that time. While it had been accepted since the First World War that some of those who suffered shell shock would have problems for many years, there had been a tacit assumption that those who came through the conflict apparently unscathed would remain well. Towards the end of the Vietnam era, though, people began to realise that many of the veterans who had apparently not had psychiatric breakdown during their service nevertheless had significant 'readjustment' difficulties on their return to the USA.

The Vietnam veterans began to be seen as a people apart — as 'psychological time bombs'. Braatz et al. were amongst those who regarded Vietnam veterans as different from the survivors of other foreign wars. Horowitz, the creator of the Impact of Events Scale, who had previously developed the concept of a stress response syndrome, predicted that there would be large numbers of veterans who would present with delayed symptoms and would not be dealt with effectively by mental health services. Borus, however, was one of a minority who tried to demonstrate that Vietnam veterans had no greater incidence of maladjustment than other soldiers, claiming that "Because of substantive public and political interest in this area, the professional literature has chronologically lagged behind often sensationalised media accounts that have emphasised detrimental psychological and behavioral effects of the war experience of the returning veteran".

Vietnam was considered to be different from other conflicts — an unpopular, prolonged, relatively low intensity, distant, guerrilla conflict which did not involve the majority of the people and, unprecedentedly, was lost by the Americans. Returning Vietnam veterans were not welcomed as heroes. At best, they were ignored and at worst were vilified for the part that they had played in an unpopular war. Fleming, though, a Vietnam veteran and Associate Professor of Psychology, was unusual in questioning the uniqueness of that conflict. He compared it with the Indian Wars and the Philippine Insurrection, saying that each of these was equally brutal. These too were guerrilla wars, there were demonstrations against the Philippine intervention, and the average age of combatants in the American Civil War was only 18, compared with 19 in Vietnam.

Both public and political interest led to a Veterans Administration Study into the particular problems of the young veteran. Van Putten and Emory published the emotively entitled 'Traumatic neurosis in Vietnam returnees — A forgotten diagnosis?', in which they accepted that veterans "reject authority and mistrust institutions". This described five case histories of patients who had been diagnosed as suffering from definite or probable schizophrenia, all of whom had either had clear 'breakdowns' in Vietnam or had sustained physical wounds there. It was concluded that much that had been learned in previous wars had been forgotten, with the result that cases of traumatic neurosis were not recognised. Finding a predominance of diagnoses of schizophrenia in 50 'random psychiatric admissions', Zarcone et al. commented on the "unusually impulsive, disruptive, distrustful, and violence-prone" nature of their patients, and differentiated them from other veterans. Their cases were said to have a characteristic symptomatology, presentation, and response, and it was suggested that a significant proportion of Vietnam veterans were disabled but untreated.

An oft-quoted study is that of Figley, who studied veterans at university, comparing those returned from Vietnam with other G.I. students. Of approximately 1200 subjects circulated, only 120 responded and 101 of those responses were usable. Although the title of the paper refers to "symptoms of delayed combat stress", the conclusions refer to "interpersonal adjustment", and the low response rate raises questions about the findings that non-combatants had better subsequent interpersonal adjustment than combat veterans. These early studies were generally on a small scale and had significant methodological problems. However, they were followed by two very large ones, the Vietnam Experience Study and the National Vietnam Veterans Readjustment Study, which involved the face-to-face assessment of thousands of randomly selected veterans across America. These confirmed that PTSD was a real problem in many thousands of veterans who had not shown evidence of psychiatric disturbance while they had been in Vietnam.

One of the principles of combat psychiatry, as developed in Vietnam, was that of 'proximity' — that sufferers should be treated as near the site of the trauma as possible. In military terms, since the individual does not leave the area of potential further danger, the symptoms are not reinforced or perpetuated by the reduction of anxiety associated with escape from the feared situation. This principle does not normally apply to civilian trauma, but accident victims often experience significant delay in obtaining symptomatic relief from pain, shock, and distress. It is possible that this delay contributes to the development of persistent PTSD symptoms.

It was not just Vietnam, though, that was being studied during the 1970s. 'Combat neurosis' was described in teachers at American inner-city schools, and there was a report on the survivors of the IRA bombs in Birmingham, as well as studies of the floods at Buffalo Creek, West Virginia, and elsewhere. As well as developing the Impact of Events Scale, Horowitz described a brief psychodynamic therapy for the stress response syndrome. Interest in post-traumatic illness continued to grow: the US Congress agreed to the funding of 'shop-front' services for Vietnam veterans with 'readjustment problems' in 1979, although it did not formally accept that their problems were different from those of previous wars. This allowed immediate walk-in access to services in some areas for veterans with emotional problems.

By this time, through the APA Task Force set up to consider a possible post-Vietnam syndrome, PTSD emerged in DSM–III. It was not defined as specific to Vietnam, but as a response to a "recognisable stressor that would evoke significant symptoms of distress in almost anyone", and examples such as concentration camp experience, violent crime, and natural disasters were given. This was significant, because it was accepted that the pathological response to all major stressors was essentially common, rather than event-specific. PTSD was included amongst the anxiety disorders; the symptom criteria were basically those still in use today — intrusive, avoidant, and arousal symptoms.

Stressors

Since then, the concept of PTSD has continued to develop. The nature and significance of the stressors preceding PTSD have been the subject of constant discussion, and its definition has changed over time. While clinicians began to attribute PTSD to a wider and wider range of 'stressful' events, DSM–III–R in 1987 actually tightened the stressor criterion significantly to events "outside the range of usual human experience". Yet before DSM–IV, there was serious discussion about doing away with that criterion altogether. It had been recognised that a similar syndromal pattern was seen without catastrophic events and that relatively little of the variance of symptomatology could be explained by the severity of the stressor. Though the stressor criterion was not in fact removed, the importance of the individual response to the event was now emphasised.

PTSD was also included in the *International Classification of Diseases, Tenth Edition* (ICD–10) but there are some differences (Chapter 9, p. 302). While DSM–IV emphasised the individual experience or meaning of the stressor, ICD–10 retained a view of PTSD being the consequence of 'catastrophic' events. In addition, it described the intrusive symptoms as being central and essential, with avoidant and arousal symptoms as additional, but not necessary features. ICD–10 also introduced the concept of a permanent change in personality as a consequence of extreme and inescapable stressors, though this view was not founded on empirical data and it could well be modified in the future.

The creators of PTSD initially opposed the earlier view of stress reactions as greatly influenced by constitutional factors or inherent weakness, but there has been a resurgence of interest in other factors, including personality, previous history, and social support. In 1972, for instance, Bloch and Bloch had claimed that, "A traumatic neurosis is a process neurosis. Past, present and future take part in its course".

On the other hand, adverse psychiatric consequences of an accident which do not fulfil the complete criteria for PTSD are not uncommon. They can usefully be described as 'post-traumatic illness'.

Pathology, aetiology, and treatment

Other major developments since the 1970s have been in the pathology of PTSD, with neuroendocrine, physiological, and neuro-imaging studies extending the initial view of a psychological response to overwhelming stress. Abnormalities in the hypothalamic-pituitary-adrenal axis have been convincingly demonstrated, while physiological responses, such as change in heart rate following exposure to reminders of the stressor have been used as diagnostic tests. There is a preliminary suggestion of positron emission tomography changes in PTSD patients, with a change in the ratio of cortical to sub-cortical blood flow ratio, and peak activity in the thalamus.

The recognition of objective changes in PTSD has fuelled the debate about aetiology. Most people no longer see it as a purely psychological or psychodynamic response to traumatic events. There is increasing support for the hypothesis of it representing a neuroendocrine abnormality, with detectable evidence of pathology and of physiological change. However, the aetiology of the disorder is thought to consist of a complex interaction of: the type and severity of trauma, prior personal and family history, personality, pre-existing illness, and subsequent experience. The view that PTSD is entirely a consequence of trauma, and that individual differences are essentially irrelevant is no longer tenable.

There have been many attempts to find objective measures of PTSD, but these have generally been developed for specific groups of subjects, and not validated more widely. Physiological measures, particularly changes in heart rate on exposure to stimuli recalling the stressor, appear promising but are difficult and expensive to apply. Psychometric measures may give an impression of objectivity, but it has not been demonstrated that their scores necessarily measure clinical sensitivity, or that small changes in these scores represent significant clinical change. Severity needs to be assessed in clinical terms and with reference to both observed and reported disability. So far, there is no evidence that the findings of a conscientious clinical interview can be made more accurate by available tests.

Children, even at very young ages, have been shown to develop PTSD, though the reported rates have varied widely. Witnessing a violent assault — particularly to a parent — seems to be particularly likely to cause disorder, and those involved in war have shown intermediate levels of disturbance. Whilst child sexual abuse causes much emotional disturbance, the evidence for it as a cause of PTSD is very variable.

Much work has centred on treatment of this increasingly diagnosed condition. There is some evidence for the efficacy of psychodynamic therapy, but better support exists for a range of behavioural treatments based upon exposure. These include eye movement desensitisation and taped imaginal exposure to memories, as well as cognitive–behavioural treatment. A growing body of evidence exists for the value of drug treatment, including antidepressants, which seem to have an effect on PTSD symptoms as well as strictly depressive features. Many specialist centres use a combined approach, adopting all modalities of treatment together with a problem-centred approach to specific individual difficulties such as anger control and interpersonal relationships.

It is perhaps surprising that after the lessons of the First World War, the lessons of Vietnam, and thousands of subsequent studies, we still need to know what exactly causes PTSD, to develop a simple diagnostic test for it, and to have a clear view of the natural history and prognosis.

Symptomatic presentations which are apparently indistinguishable from PTSD have been reported after a bewilderingly wide range of events, including childbirth, the onset of mental illness, general medical conditions, and chronic situations such as being bullied at work or at school. Mayou *et al.* at Oxford showed that five years after being involved in road traffic accidents, 10% of the victims (who had not suffered head injuries) were still suffering from PTSD, though the course of the disorder was very varied. Post-traumatic symptoms were associated with a very considerably impaired quality of life. Since road traffic accidents and accidents in the workplace are common precipitants of PTSD, it is inevitable that questions should be asked about the role of litigation and compensation in the development or perpetuation of symptoms. However, the available evidence indicates that PTSD does not usually clear up when the litigation is over. Prolonged disability may occur in a minority of people who experience an accident, whether or not they receive any compensation for it. It seems that we still have much to learn about this condition, and particularly about the role and significance in it of the stressor.

REHABILITATION

by Jim Birley

During the 1970s, the numbers of patients in psychiatric hospitals fell in most Western countries. In the USA, from a peak of 559,000 in 1955, it had fallen to 340,000 in 1970 and to 132,000 in 1980. This was the era of 'deinstitutionalisation' to a more complex and stimulating, but confusing and risky environment: first for the patients and for those looking after them; second, for those researching the development of new forms of care; and third, for those trying to coordinate the different agencies involved in providing a wide spectrum of services. Would this spectrum produce a guiding beam of light or merely a fitful sparkle?

1970 was the year in which Brown and Wing's classic *Institutionalism and Schizophrenia* was published in Britain. They had compared three mental hospitals of differing standards, and found that the social environments — for instance the attitude of staff, the amount of privacy, space for personal possessions, and opportunities for meaningful activity — had a considerable effect on the mental states of patients suffering from schizophrenia. The more deprived the environment, the worse the psychiatric outcome. Thus, the 'natural history' of schizophrenia had acquired an ecological dimension. The 'better environment', while requiring the vision, energy, and power of psychiatrists to bring it about, was actually provided by non-medical staff: nurses, occupational therapists, and supervisors with domestic or industrial skills.

However, schizophrenic patients do badly in response to both extremes in levels of stimulation — very high or very low — and both positive and negative symptoms can be increased then. In rehabilitation, the appropriate level of stimulation needs to be found for each patient. If the expectations of staff and relatives are too optimistic, this may result in too much pressure for change, causing a relapse of acute symptoms. A well structured environment can help patients to re-learn any normal habits of life that may have atrophied — getting up, washing and dressing, preparing food, and going out to some regular activity.

By 1970, many 'acute' psychiatric units had become sited in general hospitals, where psychiatrists were happy to work in a more attractive environment than that of traditional mental hospitals. There were complaints of 'revolving doors' — but this was not a new phenomenon; for years, some 70% of all 'acute' admissions had in fact been readmissions. While patients suffering from chronic mental illness required special attention to help them to benefit, rather than suffer from deinstitutionalisation, most psychiatrists were too busy and neither inclined nor trained to take a leading role in the community. But there were notable exceptions, and sometimes other professionals such as psychologists, nurses, or social workers filled the gap.

This was the arena in which rehabilitation was performed from 1970 to 1980, the year of publication of another classic — Stein and Test's evaluation of their 'Daily Living Program' in Madison, Wisconsin.

Nature of rehabilitation

From the early post-war period, a central focus of rehabilitation had been the resettlement of patients from long-term care in psychiatric hospitals to alternative homes outside. In practice, though, deinstitutionalisation was largely a process of relocation, often a 'transinstitutionalisation' to other deprived environments such as boarding houses or nursing homes. Many people ended up spending most of their time — sometimes all of it — on the street or in ramshackle shelters. This process was not rehabilitation, although some 'street people' preferred this existence to their previous hospitals. But for most, it was a degrading experience and as obvious a social exclusion as the mediaeval pillories.

From the late 1950s, rehabilitation of patients in psychiatric hospitals had been seen as a process of gaining increasing competence and independence in a step-by-step process. Eventually, it was hoped, the patient would emerge as an independent person, able to cope with the essential activities of daily living. To help in this process, transitional hostels or half-way houses were developed in several countries, with the purpose of providing a supportive environment for a limited period. Optimistic ideas that residents would move on fairly soon to independent accommodation were not fulfilled in practice, though, and the permitted lengths of stay often had to be extended. Similarly, the hope that residents would become self-supporting by getting paid jobs increasingly failed to be ful-

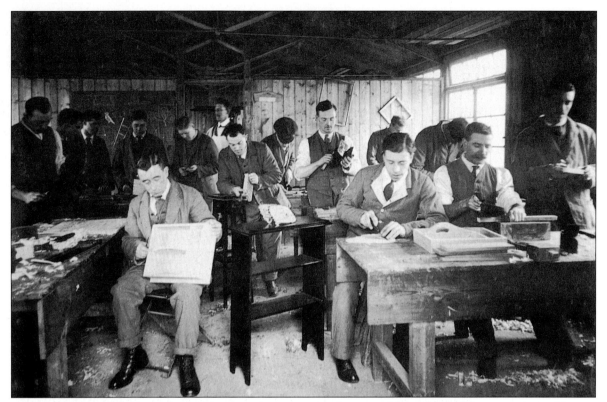

Patients in the Carpenter's Shop at the Maudsley Hospital, 1918. During the First World War the Maudsley was requisitioned for use as a military hospital treating 'shell-shock' cases. Reproduced with permission from the Bethlem Royal Hospital Archives and Museum.

filled, as economic problems increased. Those who could respond to more active rehabilitation and gain autonomy proved to be relatively few. On the other hand, a range of supportive residential settings were needed for people who had difficulty in functioning but were very varied in their handicaps. In most countries, such facilities were not provided on any large scale in the community.

Rehabilitation is a complex process. Douglas Bennett at the Maudsley Hospital, the doyen of rehabilitation in the UK and beyond, called it "a process concerned with the individual person in the context of the environment". This aims to bring about "improvements in adaptation which enable the disabled person to make the best use of residual capacities in as normal a social context as possible". Relocation might be included in this process, but it was not essential — "Although not every handicapped person can be relocated, few cannot be rehabilitated". Because schizophrenic patients are often unable to generalise from learning situations, that learning needs to be in situations which are as similar as possible to the circumstances of real life in which the skills will be needed, e.g. shopping near the person's home. It is also necessary to provide continuous reinforcement of the newly re-learned behaviour by praise, encouragement, or practical rewards. Otherwise, this behaviour will be likely to atrophy again.

Rehabilitation diagnosis involves making careful assessment of an individual's capacities — skills, interests, and strengths — and of his disabilities. These handicaps could be classified according to whether they were: (a) present before the person's illness; (b) acquired as a direct effect of the illness; or (c) an indirect effect — from treatment, reactions to illness, or being a patient. Equally important were the attitudes of significant others — family, friends, employers, and the professionals involved in treatment. Such a classification is helpful in deciding on the most appropriate approaches to rehabilitation.

It became increasingly clear that the individual had to be both assessed and treated in their own environment, but that there was not just one environment to be assessed. Rehabilitation diagnosis divided the patient's 'environment' into different settings, each of which required different roles and different performances. These settings, and the person's responses to them, had to be assessed and treated first-hand. Community psychiatry might be practised from a psychiatric unit, but for rehabilitation in the community, psychiatry had to leave its base. The methods of rehabilitation include training for specific tasks, enhancement of skills, monitoring of goals, and making use of feedback from others.

Unlike schizophrenia, the rehabilitation of people with chronic depression had received relatively little attention, and not much has been written about it. Paykel and Marshall pointed out that in depressed patients, some lasting handicaps may result from the process of having been ill, rather than from the consequences of persistent symptoms. These handicaps include, "the effects of institutionalisation, loss of employment, and the damage done to social and personal relationships during the period of impaired health". In affective disorder, severe handicap develops much less often than in schizophrenia, but amongst the long-stay population of mental hospitals, there were nearly always some patients with severe depression or recurrent mania. Such patients needed the facilities which had been developed for the rehabilitation of people with chronic functional psychosis. For those living in the community, a range of services was also needed — day hospitals or centres, sheltered workshops, drop-in facilities, and self-help organisations. Scientifically, though, this area continued to be neglected, so the changes achieved by rehabilitation programmes for depression remain unevaluated.

Psychiatrists and sticklebacks

Were psychiatrists fitted for this task? In many countries, there was resistance amongst them to taking on the burden of treating those suffering from chronic mental illness. Psychiatrists, like most doctors, prefer to look after patients who get better, and especially those who appear to improve as a result of the treatment they receive. Psychiatric departments of medical schools, where most psychiatrists were trained, felt that they required a regular supply of acute and preferably 'new' cases for teaching. Chronic patients provided only old information; they were seen, when in crisis, in casualty departments, but sent elsewhere for treatment. Thus, many psychiatrists and their trainers had not been educated in the treatment and management of the chronic mentally ill, who were often seen as unattractive in their appearance, hygiene, and behaviour. They might have a depressing effect both on other less ill patients at the clinic and on the psychiatrist's income from private practice, in countries where that exists.

Psychiatrists lay great weight on 'diagnosis'. This indicated the illness or disorder which they should treat, and was a judgement which only they could make, or change; it was one which increased in value during the 1970s, with the rise of biological psychiatry. But diagnosis was much less significant in the assessment of patients for rehabilitation. Like Manfred Bleuler, many psychiatrists recognised the importance of "being in touch with the person behind the psychosis", but rehabilitation assessment put the person in front and the psychosis behind. In his pioneering work in Gorizia during the early 1970s, Franco Basaglia (this chapter, p. 270) argued that it was necessary "to place in brackets the patient's diagnosis, since the diagnostic label hung fixedly on the patient like a preformed value judgement" — creating potentially disabling attitudes in the minds of both the patient and of those concerned with the case. Research studies had indicated that in terms of the outcome of rehabilitation, diagnosis was not an important predictor. A study by Presley *et al.* in 1982 had found that only 'domestic skills' predicted outcome for survival outside hospital. This was not surprising, but domestic skills were not a matter about which psychiatrists inquire with the same interest as they do about the first-rank symptoms of schizophrenia.

In addition, like other hospital staff, psychiatrists were used to working on their own territory — in hospitals and clinics, with their own personal space. To be out and about, assessing patients and relatives in an environment which was not their own, and depending on an array of staff with different outlooks but requiring extra training — was quite a challenge. Paul Polack, who pioneered a very innovative community-based programme at Denver, Colorado, was moved to comment that "like the male stickleback, the courage of the mental health professional decreases in direct proportion to the distance from the nest". But their lack of courage was the same as that of a non-swimmer on being told to jump into the deep end of the pool; they lacked the appropriate skills and attitudes for the task in hand.

The basic sciences that were most relevant and useful to rehabilitation were largely social and behavioural— fields more familiar to psychologists than to doctors. Their kind of thinking was more in terms of altering behaviour and assessment of disability, rather than making a diagnosis and treating an illness. In many rehabilitation schemes, as well as in the development of the theory and practice of rehabilitation, clinical psychologists took a leading role.

Experimental schemes developed in a number of countries, differing in their leadership, staffing, and style. Yet their aims varied less — to help patients to develop the skills and attitudes which would allow them to have a more independent life, and either to produce new environments or else adjust current ones to be suitable to patients' levels of disability. Some of these schemes were based on established after-care facilities such as club-houses, but others, e.g. at Denver, Madison, and Trieste, were quite new. Some made use of either experientially skilled volunteers or paid 'enablers' to assist patients with their problems of daily living and teach them appropriate skills. Autonomy was encouraged, but it was recognised that continued medication was also essential for many people.

Alternatives to hospitals

At Denver, much use was made of community-based intensive care, using six carefully select-ed families who could accept up to two clients at one time, with 24-hour nursing available and psychiatric assistance on call. In Italy, in a more radical development (this chapter, p. 257), the law of 1978 abolished further use of the mental hospitals – generally agreed to be in a very degraded state there. Instead, intensive community treatment was to be provided, aiming to liberate patients from their victimised roles and help them assume their rightful place as citizens in their communities. This approach, based on British and Dutch models but pushed to extremes, had mixed success, according to the leadership and facilities pro-vided locally. In Trieste, which was the model service, the staffing ratio was twice as high as in the rest of northern and central Italy and 11 times higher than in the south.

By the end of the 1970s, a number of alternatives to the mental hospital were becom-ing available. In many countries, the use of in-patient beds was considerably reduced, while patients were learning skills and attitudes that helped them to live a more satisfy-ing life. Most relatives were also pleased, provided that they had ready access to appro-priate emergency care when a relapse occurred.

But several problems remained. In most countries, the hospital wards were still by no means empty. Some of the remaining patients were old and frail, but others were mainly disabled by continuing severe psychiatric illness. These were now being joined by 'new chronic patients' with an age-range of 20 to 50 years, some of whom seemed to need 24-hour residential supervision, but not necessarily in a hospital. They were certainly not well cared for in acute admission wards, where they were regarded as 'blocking' beds. They were also expensive to treat, but when psychiatric beds were reduced, the money that was 'saved' tended not to go into community services, but into improving hospital facili-ties. In some cases, it was being diverted to other branches of health care altogether, includ-ing the hard-pressed and increasingly expensive medical and surgical wards.

Changes in society

There were changes, too, in society as a whole. The post-War economic recovery with its high levels of employment was beginning to wane. This affected both employment prospects for the mentally ill and the commercial viability of the workshops that provid-ed sheltered work. In the 1960s, individual rehabilitation had encouraging results, but as the better functioning patients were discharged and economic conditions worsened in the 1970s, this approach became less effective.

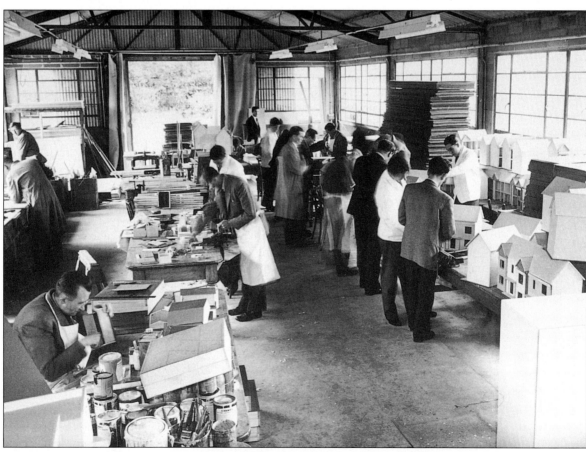

Male industrial unit making dolls houses, c. 1960s. Reproduced with permission from the North East Essex Mental Health NHS Trust.

Psychiatry itself had come under fierce attack for its alleged abuse of human rights, its failure to be 'scientific' and to provide effective treatments, and its alleged 'invention' of mental illness. In particular, there were loud voices from both patients and their relatives demanding representation and change. Their views often disagreed profoundly, but they were united in their criticism of psychiatry, which they saw as failing to meet their needs and sometimes blaming parents for causing their children's illnesses.

Psychiatrists responded to these criticisms — much enjoyed by the media — in various ways. A positive approach was to view critics as potential allies and to engage or negotiate with them, both politically and clinically. Another reaction was to strive to make psychiatry more scientific — an admirable aim, but turning to medical sciences was likely to omit the social and behavioural disciplines. The siren voices of medical respectability tended to lure psychiatrists away from the deep waters of rehabilitation, to the shallows and rocks of DSM diagnosis. But the 'call for science' did provide a challenge to assess the processes and outcomes of rehabilitation in ways which were more rigorous, in terms of validity and reliability, yet remaining meaningful for those working in the field. Stein and Test's 1980 papers, in assessing their Madison scheme and its costs, provided an important example, pointing the way to evidence-based rehabilitation. Supervised work experience came to be seen as an important strategy for social and vocational rehabilitation, but was never evaluated in a reliable way.

The 1970s had produced enough leaders and sufficient theory and methodology to provide an agenda for the next 10 years. But in any country, the number of comprehensive schemes was quite inadequate for the total population of chronic mentally ill. Taken together, they did not provide a network, but rather a few outstanding services, surrounded by poor provision. As in the past, the sheer numbers of the chronic mentally ill and their need for intermittent or permanent help had been seriously underestimated. Or rather, this underestimate was a symptom of not facing up to the costs involved in providing the required help — a symptom of the continued stigmatisation of the mentally ill. The problems for succeeding years mainly concerned the needs for both quality and quantity of services. Yet planning by governments was limited by insufficient knowledge of the extent to which rehabilitation programmes actually improved social adjustment and economic self-sufficiency — a deficit which still largely remains.

THE ITALIAN PSYCHIATRIC REFORM

by Michele Tansella & Lorenzo Burti

In most Western countries, mental health services are undergoing substantial changes. A common element of these changes is the transition from a system of care which is largely hospital-based to one which is predominantly community-based.

In 1978, Italy introduced one of the most innovative and radical changes in mental health legislation, based on a model of community psychiatry that was designed to be alternative to, rather than to complement the old hospital-centred services. The new system was intended to provide care and support to all types of patients, without back-up from the public mental hospital, where only old long-stay in-patients could continue to be accommodated.

Shortly after the approval of this psychiatric reform, the Italian parliament also passed legislation that established the Italian National Health Service (NHS). This was to provide health care to all citizens through local administrations — '*Unità Sanitarie Locali*' (USL), or local health units, each responsible for a catchment area of 50,000 to 200,000 inhabitants. USLs administer all health services in the area, excluding large hospitals in big cities, which have had an independent administration since 1995.

The main characteristics of the 1978 Italian psychiatric reform are summarised in the following table. These sudden and radical changes in the law must be considered in context. In particular, three main issues need to be examined:

- Before the reform, the quality of care provided was very poor, being delivered almost exclusively in large, old-fashioned, and custodial mental hospitals. For a long time, they had been subject to stringent criticism by psychiatric professionals, as well as by lay people and the media;
- Substantial social changes, with the related cultural aspects of the 'anti-institutional movement', had occurred in Italy in the 1960s and 1970s, prior to the reform. Therefore, it became urgent to fill the gap between these rapid political, social, and cultural upheavals and the conventional practice of psychiatry;

- The principles and practice of the reform had been tried out, in the 10 preceding years, achieving apparently good results in selected areas of the country (e.g. Arezzo, Perugia, Trieste). This had been under the leadership of Franco Basaglia, a charismatic and influential psychiatrist (this chapter, p. 270).

Slow transition

Evaluation of the reform has been difficult because of the lack of regular nation-wide collection of data. At the same time, only few regions (e.g. Lombardia, Emilia-Romagna, and Lazio), have so far set up mental health information systems to monitor the input and process of care. However, in 1984, the Ministry of Health appointed the Centro Studi Investimenti Sociali (CENSIS) to carry out a nation-wide survey on the implementation of the new psychiatric services. This was done by interviewing key persons, usually the administrators and directors of various kinds of facilities.

A more recent inquiry was then completed by the Istituto Italiano di Medicina Sociale (IIMS). It found that a slow but consistent reduction of the in-patient population had been achieved mainly by closing the front door of the old mental hospital, without abrupt discharge of old long-stay residents. This policy — a slow transition — had the advantage of avoiding any large-scale transfer of patients to the community. This helped to achieve a gradual shift of the focus of care from the traditional hospital to the new community-based services. On the other hand, the main disadvantage was that, for a long time, elderly long-stay patients gained little or no advantage from the reform. Both systems — the elderly and the new — had to be maintained at the same time.

The impact of the reform on the Italian psychiatric system can be considered in a number of ways. First, the number of mental hospital in-patients (both public and private) in the whole country has decreased by about two-thirds, from about 60,000 (105 per 100,000 inhabitants) before the reform to 17,068 (30 per 100,000) at 11 November 1996. There were then 11,882 in-patients in public mental hospitals and 5186 in privately owned institutions.

Since this decrease was gradual, the dramatic adverse effects of mass deinstitutionalisation, seen in some other countries, did not occur in Italy. However, the process and outcome of discharge from mental hospitals have not been systematically studied. Except for crude figures published by the National Institute of Statistics, no reliable data on patients discharged following the psychiatric reform are available nationwide. A political commitment to the final dismantling of the public mental hospitals was planned to take place during 1998.

Characteristics of Italian psychiatric reform

(i) Gradual closure of public mental hospitals by blocking all new admissions, with immediate effect, as well as readmissions, two years later (i.e. from 31 December 1980). The aim was to have, in due course, a psychiatric system that would be able to function without the mental hospital. It was to be not just the addition of new services, which usually risk recruiting only new, more 'attractive' patients instead of serving the severely mentally ill and removing the need for their admission to the mental hospital. Since no abrupt discharge of current in-patients was prescribed by the reform, it implied their progressive rehabilitation, rather than a sudden deinstitutionalisation, with the well-known adverse effects of such a process.

(ii) New community-based services (community mental health centres, day hospitals, and residential facilities) were to be established to provide all types of psychiatric care to the population of a given area. Initially, such services had to be staffed mainly through the relocation of mental hospital personnel.

(iii) Hospitalisation, when necessary, had to take place in general hospital psychiatric wards (GHPW). These wards were not to exceed 15 beds, in order to avoid an excessive concentration of psychiatric patients — a characteristic of the mental hospital that was considered detrimental to its patients' well-being.

(iv) Compulsory evaluation and treatment had to take place in GHPW. The criteria for involuntary admission were: (a) an emergency intervention was needed; (b) the patient refused treatment; and (c) alternative community treatment was impossible. Dangerousness was not considered a criterion, because the Italian psychiatric reform was intended to be a public health law, and thus dealing only with treatment, not custody.

Some of the premises formerly used as mental hospitals wards have been used as general medical wards, medical out-patient departments, health centres, or rehabilitation facilities. Some have been converted into hostels or nursing homes to offer a better quality of care than before to former mental patients, who have been given a new status. The personnel now looking after these residents belong to the social services, rather than the health sector, but psychiatrists and nurses provide a consultation–liaison service to these former patients. The extent of these changes is not uniform throughout the country; in general, it is more satisfactory in the north. In areas where the mental hospitals were mainly private (even if supported by public funds), these hospitals show a strong resistance to the changes.

Second, the block on admissions to State mental hospitals has prevented the long-term institutionalisation and reinstitutionalisation of patients. This has been associated with a related increase of short-term admissions to general hospital wards, but without any significant shift of such cases to private hospitals.

Third, a comprehensive network of both in-patient and out-patient community services has been implemented all over the country, now serving more that 80% of the Italian population in their own USLs. However, 64% of acute psychiatric beds are presently provided by private institutions, *'convenzionate'*. These have a contract with the NHS and are therefore funded with public money, rather than by public services developed according to the reform. Moreover, the quality of care provided in some GHPW and community-based services is relatively poor, as was shown by a study on the use of psychotropic drugs that was carried out in all mental health services of Piedmont, in north-west Italy.

Fourth, remaining problems are essentially due to delayed or incomplete implementation of the law. This has resulted from the limited resources made available for the process of change or their inadequate reallocation from the mental hospitals to the new services. Also, the development of new services has become more difficult in recent years because of the overall reduction of financial resources available for mental health. Many community-based mental health services remain severely understaffed. Mediocre integration of services and insufficient training of the personnel are also relatively common problems. The current political climate, though, seems more sympathetic to increasing these resources.

Moreover, the reform law was essentially a guideline: it provided recommendations for the development of new services, but without either assigning an *ad hoc* budget or prescribing sanctions for non-compliance. A National Mental Health Plan was only approved in 1994, and has been revised in 1998; the revisions essentially confirm the community-based system of care. Where services have been appropriately developed, the reform has proved to be successful, but poorly served areas still do exist, especially in the south.

As mentioned above, the reform did not include special provision for dangerousness. After 1978 forensic psychiatric hospitals, which are administered by the Ministry of Justice and which are separate from the NHS, continued to admit those patients who had committed a crime. In-patients in these hospitals, who numbered 1256 in 1975, increased slightly in numbers in the first few years after the reform to 1424 in 1980, and then consistently decreased in the following years to 1109 in 1998.

Children and adolescents are normally treated in out-patient and community services that are separate from those for adults. Also, elderly patients with dementia are admitted to geriatric institutions and hostels which are not part of the mental health system of care; psychogeriatric wards are few.

No data on the homeless mentally ill are available, but it is generally believed that their number did not increase after the reform and that they represent a less severe and less visible problem than in some other countries, particularly the USA.

Data at the local level

The implementation of the reform has been monitored with greater accuracy in some areas, such as South Verona, where a psychiatric case register has operated since 1978. South Verona is a mainly urban, relatively affluent, predominantly middle-class area, with a low migration rate. The total population is about 75,000. It should be emphasised that the South Verona community-based mental health service is not just an experimental programme. It was implemented 20 years ago, shortly after the legislative approval of the psychiatric reform, and has been in operation ever since. It provides all kinds of psychiatric intervention and care to all South Verona residents who require them, including the most severely ill. Therefore, it avoids restrictive selection procedures for patients and includes a comprehensive and well-integrated series of programmes. It provides in-patient care, day care, rehabilitation, out-patient care, and home visits, as well as a 24-hour emergency service and residential facilities (three apartments and one hostel) for long-term patients.

Case register data show that in 1998, the total number of beds occupied in both public and private hospitals in South Verona was 41 per 100,000 adult inhabitants. If those patients who are in hostels or sheltered apartments are excluded, the rate of occupied hospital beds is 25 per 100,000, a figure that has been constant for some years. The point-prevalence rate of long-term patients (those who were not long-stay patients but continuously in contact, for one year or more, with some psychiatric service, with no period between two contacts exceeding 90 days), is consistently increasing. In 1998, this rate was 309 per 100,000 adult residents. The implication of this increase is that more resources have to be dedicated in future to long-term patients. Since they already absorb 60–70% of the resources available to the mental health service, it will be necessary to increase the total budget for mental health if any further shift of resources from less severe cases is to be avoided.

The South Verona Outcome Study is a project designed to assess the effects of the new system of care on psychopathology, social performance, satisfaction with services, and other measures including costs. It has found that this service essentially meets the needs of patients, including those with the most-severe psychotic disorders. However, this experience can be generalised only to other areas in Italy where the reform has been fully implemented.

Conclusions

Four lessons can be learned from the Italian psychiatric reform, when considering both the sudden and radical changes introduced in the legislation and the slow implementation of those changes in the following two decades:

1. The transition from a hospital-based to a community-based service cannot be accomplished simply by closing the mental hospitals. Appropriate alternative facilities must be provided, and this requires adequate time for planning and implementation. The time needed is often longer than expected.
2. Political and administrative commitment is necessary, since effective community care is not, and never will be a cheap solution. Indeed, if it is to be effective, appropriate investment has to be made in buildings, staff, and supportive facilities.
3. Monitoring and evaluation are important aspects of change.
4. A reform law should not only be a guideline (as the Italian law was), but should be prescriptive and include both minimal standards for care and mandatory timetables for implementing the new services.

It would be simplistic to think that the Italian model of community-based mental health care can be exported elsewhere, or simply copied. In implementing community care, general principles and guidelines are useful, but the practice needs to be adapted to the particular context in which it is to be applied. In some areas of Italy, the psychiatric reform was not adequately implemented and therefore has not been successful. The number of these areas is not yet accurately known. However, it is necessary to distinguish clearly between the failure of community care as a principle and the failure to implement and properly implement it: this distinction represents an essential key to full understanding of the 'Italian psychiatric reform'.

Acknowledgements

The preparation of this contribution was supported by a Fondazione Cassa di Risparmio di Verona Vicenza Belluno e Ancona, Progetto Sanità 1996–1997 Grant to Professor M Tansella. Dr Giovanni de Girolamo (Istituto Superiore di Sanità, Roma), read an early version of this chapter and made helpful comments.

PSYCHOGERIATRICS

by Tom Arie & David Jolley

Psychogeriatrics, or the psychiatry of old age, is a new speciality which arose over the last decades of this century. Its origins were in demographic change, in concern for welfare and in growth in public expectations. It was inspired and informed by the 'social psychiatry' movement, by the medical speciality of geriatrics, and by the post-war growth of effective treatments in psychiatry. Through its National Health Service, Britain played a leading part in shaping this activity (and was first to designate the new branch as an official speciality within psychiatry). Inevitably, much of this account is concerned with the British experience, but the psychogeriatric movement is worldwide — and is not confined merely to industrialised countries.

Origins

Until the 1960s, activity in the mental disorders of old age had been clinical, and in nosology, pathology, and (more recently) epidemiology. Names such as Felix Post (clinical and prognostic studies), Martin Roth and David Kay (clinical and nosological studies and epidemiology), and Nicholas Corsellis (pathology) stand out in the literature of the 1960s, as do the studies of burden on carers of Grad and Sainsbury, also in England. Post had established a clinical teaching unit in London at the Bethlem and Maudsley Hospitals, in which several of the later workers were trained, but there were few local services directed to the needs of old people. RA Robinson of the Crichton Royal Hospital in Scotland was one of few forerunners of those who developed such services.

In 1965, a London conference of the World Psychiatric Association was devoted to 'Mental disorders in the Aged' — a novel topic for the WPA. Contributors included all the above names, as well as VA Kral from Canada, and Alvin Goldfarb from the USA. That meeting, and the book which derived from it, had a catalytic effect. Six years later a volume from the predecessor of the Royal College of Psychiatrists on *Recent Developments in Psychogeriatrics* showed both the growth of activity and the new familiarity of the term 'psychogeriatrics'.

Alongside professional developments came a series of 'scandals'. The book *Sans Everything* by Barbara Robb and others appeared in 1967, documenting abuses in public institutions for the aged. In 1969 came the Report on Ely Hospital, an institution for the mentally handicapped, chaired by a lawyer who later, as Sir Geoffrey Howe, became Foreign Secretary. A previous Minister of Health had hesitated to publish the Ely report, fearing that the abuses revealed would be too damaging to health service morale. His successor, Richard Crossman, decided to publish the report and at the same time established the Hospital (later Health) Advisory Service. The purpose of this organisation was particularly to inspect long-stay institutions and to spread knowledge of good practice.

Publications of further reports of enquiries into similar scandals, many in units for old people, contributed to public awareness that things were not well in their care. The mental health service was feeling the pressure of receiving many more referrals of very aged patients. Few psychiatrists were confident that they knew how best to cope with a state of affairs foreseen, as a consequence of demographic change, by the leader of British psychiatry, Sir Aubrey Lewis, as far back as 1946.

Towards a national pattern of services

In the late 1960s, a group of some eight younger psychiatrists began to organise a part of their local psychiatric services to meet the special needs of old people. Psychiatry was then operating mostly in large mental hospitals, and its status was low even without the addition of 'geriatrics', which was also of low status in medicine. The new 'psychogeriatricians' began to meet regularly as a 'coffee house group', for exchange of experiences and for mutual support. They were conscious that their work was often seen as unattractive, reflecting the stigma of what Robert Butler in America called 'ageism', while Alex Comfort, a British gerontologist, poet, novelist, and later, sexologist wrote of 'gerontophobia'. Yet they felt that despite the negative resonances of ageing, much of the lack of appeal to brighter members of the health professions reflected apathy and the shabby settings in which much of the work had to be undertaken, rather than of lack of inherent interest. It became an intriguing challenge to test whether this work, if done well, in good accommodation and with reasonably adequate resources, would give intellectual and professional satisfaction to some of the best people in the health professions.

The small group became a focus for contacts with the Ministry of Health (or Department of Health and Social Security, as it had become), which was itself trying to confront the problems of meeting the needs of the growing numbers of aged users of health and social services. Publications had been appearing which drew attention to the mixed physical–mental nature of many disorders of old age, and to the unfavourable consequences of admitting such patients to inappropriate units. In 1970, the government urged that 'Psycho-geriatric Assessment Units' should be established in general hospitals, run jointly by psychiatrists and geriatricians, and designed to assess, classify, and treat the mixed disorders which are typical of old age. This official pronouncement reinforced the importance of these matters in the public and professional agendas.

In the course of their dialogue with the new psychogeriatricians and other professions, the government issued guidance on other aspects of the psychiatric care of old people. It moved gradually towards public recognition of the new, but still informal specialism. The psychogeriatricians' numbers began to grow, as did the published reports of their services and of the principles of practice which were evolving.

Following the publication of pieces in *The Lancet*, the *British Medical Journal* and elsewhere in the early 1970s, professional visitors came to the new units, meetings were held, and younger colleagues began to seek opportunities for training. Though unfashionable, mental hospitals which housed these units became international foci for training and for visitors, many of whom became professional leaders in their own countries. The hope that the work would appeal widely was soon borne out.

The principles evolved in these early days of psychogeriatrics have proved remarkably enduring. The first was non-selective responsibility for the whole range of mental disorders in old people within defined populations. These populations were initially huge: one psychiatrist and multidisciplinary team might initially serve up to 50,000 elderly (over 65 years) people; the present UK target is 10,000. The policy was, and generally remains, to make the first assessment at home, and whenever possible to bring the service to people's own homes, or into other 'community' facilities (such as day hospitals and health centres). Rapid response, with deployment in people's own homes of all staff, particularly community psychiatric nurses, is paramount, as is teamwork, and close working with primary care staff. In more recent times, cooperation with voluntary and private agencies has been important. The base is now most often in a general hospital, close to the geriatric service, with a network of outreach facilities.

Initially, the service was also responsible for long-stay care, mostly in large mental hospitals, but this has now almost disappeared from hospital settings in Britain. Much smaller units, often more pleasant and more appropriately designed, mostly in private hands, have taken over, but they present greater problems of surveillance and of the regulation of standards.

Meanwhile, psychogeriatrics, which became an official speciality in the British National Health Service in 1989, has hugely expanded, and is now one of the largest branches of psychiatry. Nearly every district now has a service, and some 450 consultant psychiatrists, with their trainees and teams are involved. The table below gives a picture of that growth, whilst the range of functions and facilities is summarised in the table opposite.

In Nottingham University, where the first UK professor was appointed in 1977 (there was at least one earlier established professorship, in Berlin), a joint department of Health Care of the Elderly was developed. This included both geriatrics and psychogeriatrics, reflecting the interdependence of the two.

Education and the international dimension

Professional activity abounds, especially, but not exclusively in the 'Western' world. The European Association of Geriatric Psychiatry, originally formed as a group from German-speaking countries, now embraces the whole of Europe, including Scandinavia, the UK and the Mediterranean countries, and increasingly, the countries of Eastern Europe. In the Czech Republic there is a higher qualification in old age psychiatry, though Vojtechovsky reports that in 1995, this was held by only 15 out of the 50 active members of the Czech Psychogeriatric Association (the latter dating as far back as 1968 — the year of the Soviet invasion).

Academic posts are widely established in the USA and in Canada; in Ontario Kenneth Shulman, after training in England, was particularly influential in encouraging development of local services. The American Board of Psychiatry and Neurology offers a qualification in geriatric psychiatry, and Canada has an advanced programme of training in the speciality. Academic posts are increasingly being established in Europe. In the UK nearly every medical school has academic posts, and there are full professors in some 10 schools.

In Australia and New Zealand early pioneers were Kingsley Mortimer of Auckland and Herbert Bower of Melbourne; both were influenced by developments in the UK. Mortimer came to this work in his sixties after a career as a medical missionary, and he was honoured in the late 1970s with a decoration for 'services to psychogeriatrics' — an early official recognition. A Section in Psychiatry of Old Age in the Royal Australian and New Zealand College of Psychiatrists was established in 1988; in 1999 this became a full Faculty of the College, with a formal programme of advanced training.

UK consultants in psychogeriatrics	
1969	8
early 1970s	30–40
1980	120
1984	180
1989 (specialty status granted)	circa 280
1991	362
1993	405
1999	450+
Source: surveys and estimates.	

In the UK, old age mental disorders feature now in the curricula of relevant health professions — and in the interests of many other groups, e.g. architects, designers, lawyers, clergy, police. An international course, run through the 1980s and early 1990s in Nottingham for the British Council, brought together workers from over 30 countries. It contributed both to starting developments throughout the world and to making continuing links between them. Later, versions of that course was 'exported' to Poland, Israel, and Australia, and more recently, by Edmond Chiu of Melbourne, to Hong Kong, Singapore, and Beijing. The International Psychogeriatric Association was started by members of the Nottingham course, but grew as a hugely successful independent organisation, now spanning both Western and developing countries, and numbering attenders at its congresses in thousands.

The World Health Organization has long been active in this field. Latterly, it has collaborated with the Geriatric Psychiatry Section of the World Psychiatric Association in drawing up three consensus documents (on Content, Services, and Education). The meetings in Lausanne (the base of a university-related service) from which these documents derive brought together a range of organisations which included the University of the Third Age. National professional bodies exist in many countries, most of them with a multi-disciplinary membership; the most recent was founded in 1998 in Hong Kong.

In some respects, the most influential organisations have been those based on users of services. Prominent amongst these are the national Alzheimer Disease Societies, and their international federation (ADI), which have not only been very effective in supporting their members, but have been a force for education and understanding, and some even sponsor research. They have gained the ear of governments, who recognise that dementia touches almost every family and thus the bulk of voters. No doubt it is also hoped that support of voluntary effort will reduce the cost of public services, but in fact, better public services are a prime purpose of these organisations.

Clinical developments

The elderly have benefited from virtually all the advances in psychiatry and medicine, including pharmacotherapy and social and psychological treatments. Non-invasive brain imaging is a particularly welcome and powerful new tool. But in general, few new thera-

---

What does a psychogeriatric service do?

- Home assessment; community outreach and liaison with primary care
- Hospital out-patient, day patient, and in-patient assessment, diagnosis, investigation and treatment
- Collaboration with the geriatric service, and 'liaison psychiatry' with other specialties
- Day care, respite care, 'rehabilitation', long-stay care (including care of people dying with dementia)
- Special services: e.g. 'Memory Clinic'

- Support for carers

- Service planning and development

- Advocacy / liaison / fund raising / in relation to
— other statutory services
— voluntary, charitable and commercial bodies / individuals
— other professions (e.g. architects, designers, educators, lawyers, clergy, police)
— local and national Government and members of parliament; 'the public' (including public speaking)
— the media

- Advice:
— financial (e.g. State benefits, enduring power of attorney)
— legal (e.g. assessment of mental capacity, or of fitness to drive, or of allegations of abuse)
— ethical (e.g. difficult treatment decisions, advance directives, research on patients who lack capacity)

- Education – of others, of trainees and own continuing education; attendance at conferences

- Research and audit

pies have been specific to older people. The wish to reduce as far as possible unwanted effects of drugs, which are generally most troublesome with increasing age, has been a source of motivation in the development of new generations of medication for all ages. Recently, specific anti-Alzheimer drugs have been licensed in many countries, but which patients are most likely to benefit and for how long is still unclear.

The main progress has been in development of services. Here, in its emphasis on bringing services to patients' homes, psychogeriatrics has sometimes led the rest of psychiatry. Also, in its necessarily close links with medicine, it has contributed to the growing reintegration of psychiatry with the mainstream of medicine. Many trainees, rotating through a placement in psychogeriatrics, have commented with satisfaction on finding that psychiatric work with old people calls greatly on the skills of the general internal medicine in which they were trained.

The personal pressures on psychogeriatricians have grown, as demand rises and resources fail to keep pace in most places. The closer association of this work with academic centres has meant that research activities are increasingly expected of many psychogeriatricians — both because of the 'research ethos' of modern times and because funding of universities increasingly depends on it. Making priorities between research and the expanding demands of clinical practice and teaching is a dilemma with which psychogeriatricians are not alone in wrestling.

Changing emphases

Early developments were shaped by the self-evidently unmet need of gross morbidity in older people. In most of the world, this is still the case, but particularly in countries where services have already developed, new issues have become prominent. Important amongst these are consumerism, the retraction of the welfare state, ethico-legal debates, and the growth of biological research, especially in molecular biology. These are less disparate than may appear at first sight.

In developed countries at least, expectations have grown, and users of services expect to be heard, rather than rely just on paternalism of the professions. Yet political ideologies at the end of the century have everywhere veered towards the retraction of public provision, even though most older people are poor, and so depend on public services. In Britain, great aspects of care which formerly were provided by the State have been made over to the commercial sector; amongst these, long-stay care in old age is especially important. The maintenance of standards in long-stay care is a big issue, though this need does not apply only to long-stay care.

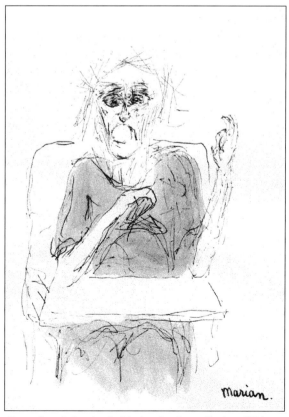

Pen and wash drawing by Marian Carolus, collection of T.A.

INSTITUTIONAL CARE OF A PATIENT WITH ADVANCED DEMENTIA — AS IT OFTEN WAS AND SHOULD NOW NEVER BE

She is locked in a so-called 'geriatric chair', a substitute for human care, intended to prevent her from falling or wandering away, for which staff might incur criticism. Trapped, she is terrified and repeatedly calls out, and therefore is considered 'disturbed'; she will be further sedated. She cannot see clearly, for she does not have her spectacles, nor are her dentures in place. Her hair is unkempt. She wears a drab, institutionally-issued garment. The combination of dementia and lack of toileting, together with sedation, ensure that she will be incontinent.

The 'rationing' of public provision is now pervasive around the world, and most rationing affects the old most sharply, especially when, as often, it is age-based. Examples are access to 'high-tech' procedures, despite the fact that the relative benefits are often greatest for the old, and the need for expensive anti-dementia drugs or drugs to enhance sexual potency. Questions of ethics and equity in these matters have to be dealt with by psychogeriatricians every day.

'Ethics' is now high on the agenda of debate in regard to old age. These questions include 'euthanasia', advance directives made before serious or terminal illness, and questions of research on subjects who are incapable of giving valid consent. A recent ('Bournewood') judgement of the House of Lords in Britain has made it clear that while we have a well-developed law of mental illness, the law of incapacity is primitive. And the questions which arise, and will arise from the explosive growth of molecular biology and genetics are quite new, and some no doubt still scarcely to be imagined. Already, psychogeriatricians are pressed to advise younger healthy people on the difficult questions surrounding genetic tests for the risk of Alzheimer dementia. One thing is sure, though: the public will be much more insistent than ever on being informed, and on having a say on all these fast-changing matters.

FORENSIC PSYCHIATRY

by Peter Snowden & Hugh Freeman

Fear of the mentally ill or personality-disordered offender is not a recent phenomenon; neither is the reaction of politicians and the judiciary in most countries. The principle that a madman lacks reason and does not know what he is doing emerged in the law of many countries and has continued down to the present day, though more strongly in Europe than in the Anglo-American courts. The history of forensic psychiatry can be best understood by following the responses of both medicine and the law to human catastrophes perpetrated by mentally disordered offenders, as well as by the impact of a number of important pioneers.

France

In France, some kind of role for the doctor as the ancillary of justice had arisen at a very early period, through witchcraft cases. During the later eighteenth century, the Age of Enlightenment, interest developed in the psychology of deviant individuals, including criminals. According to Michel Foucault (this chapter, p. 245), it came to be assumed that a calculating rationality was at the origin of all criminal acts. Therefore, unless the act was rational, there could be no offence. This was recognised by Article 64 of the Napoleonic Penal Code of 1810.

Etienne Esquirol, disciple of the great reformer Philippe Pinel, introduced the concept of 'homicidal monomania', based on Pinel's *manie sans delire*. In England, James Prichard described a similar condition as 'moral insanity'. For French early nineteenth-century cases, disposal to asylum or prison depended mainly on whether or not monomania was thought to be present. Supplemented by the Law of 1838 on insanity, Article 64 regulated for well over a century the way in which criminal responsibility was removed from those who were insane. It required the accused to be either in a state of 'dementia' when the criminal act was committed or else to be constrained by a force they could not resist. 'Dementia' covered all serious mental disorders which adversely affected intellectual and moral judgement, but the need to categorise accused individuals as 'demented' or normal was described by Ey *et al.* as an 'all or nothing' principle. Belgium also adopted the French view that no matter what the extent was of any illness involved, the mentally ill person should not be punishable.

In 1905, the possibility of diminished responsibility was introduced into the French legal system, though many psychiatrists there believed it was impossible to judge the extent to which an individual's responsibility had been reduced by mental disorder. A new *Code de Procédure Pénale* in 1958 removed this question from forensic assessments, but added others, such as 'can the accused be cured or rehabilitated?'.

It was not in fact until 1994 that a new Penal Code finally removed Article 64 of 1810. Severe mental disorder now continued to exclude penal responsibility, but where judgement and control over one's actions are impaired, these factors are to be considered when the length of a sentence and choice of institution are being decided. Decisions on discharge are to be made jointly by administrative, medical, and legal representatives. Proposals for the compulsory treatment of sex offenders, either in addition to or as an alternative to prison, were approved in 1997.

Britain

In England, Daniel M'Naghton, tried in 1843 for killing the Prime Minister's private secretary, was found 'not guilty by reason of insanity'. The defence had relied on the American Isaac Ray's *Treatise on the Medical Jurisprudence of Insanity*, though its arguments were not accepted by the judges. This judgment led to the 'M'Naughton Rules', which are still the basis for the British insanity verdict today. In Scotland in 1851, Alexander Dingwall, who had a long-standing alcohol problem, killed his wife. Reviewing the case, the Judge considered that although the defendant was sane, the crime was the result of 'extenuating circumstances'. Over time, this became known as the defence of 'diminished responsibility', and was later adopted in England, but only in 1957. Other cases during this same period highlighted the lack of suitable hospital provision for what were then known as 'criminal lunatics'.

Bethlem Hospital in London had developed a purpose-built wing for offenders as early as 1816; by 1844, it housed 85 criminal patients, and there was a total of 224 such cases in various asylums in England. However, Broadmoor Hospital, in Berkshire had to be opened in 1863 because of overcrowding, caused by the growing population of criminally insane in-patients. Two others were added — in 1914 and 1933 — an additional one in 1974, and also one in Scotland. These Special Hospitals have not only been 'special' because of the security provided and the nature of the high-risk patient group they contain, but were managed and funded directly by the central government, instead of through the normal structure of the National Health Service. Even the nurses have been unusual, in that many still belong to the prison officers' trade union, as they do in similar institutions in some other countries. Together, these factors have allowed the Special Hospitals to function separately from mainstream service developments, but there has been severe criticism of them by a number of inquiries because of poor patient care and security lapses. The next decade should see them increasingly integrated with local forensic psychiatry services, and general mental health services, if the necessary resources are provided.

However, the conventional mental hospitals in Britain and many other countries, which were largely locked until the 1960s, always contained some patients who had been convicted of criminal offences. It was only the more difficult and dangerous offenders who would be sent to the Special Hospitals for mentally ill criminals.

Professor Paul Bowden in London has identified two broad developmental themes within criminological psychiatry (now generally known as forensic psychiatry), which arose out of British prison medicine. One group of doctors in that system proposed the doctrine of free will, whereas another were determinists, sympathetic to psychoanalysis. In the 1930s, Hamblin Smith, influenced by psychoanalytical thinking, argued that the punishment of crime was not an adequate response on behalf of society, whereas psychoanalysis could provide both understanding and treatment. A contemporary psychiatrist at St Thomas's Hospital, London — WH de Bargue Hubert — argued from his experience of using psychotherapy in a prison that special units should be developed, to carry forward this treatment approach for selected prisoners. He was supported by another medical pioneer, Norwood East, and they jointly wrote a *Report of the Psychological Treatment of Crime* (1939). It was not until 1962, though, that Grendon Underwood Prison opened in England, to provide treatment for some prisoners along psychotherapeutic lines. Yet in the British prison service, as in most other countries, the treatment ethos has never achieved primacy; punishment and control have always been of greater importance. No other service of this kind has since been developed in England, though in Scotland, a special unit in Barlinnie Prison, Glasgow pursued a therapeutic approach for some time.

Following the 1959 Mental Health Act in England, the substantial reduction in the number of locked wards in psychiatric hospitals made worse the problems for the offender with mental health problems, since there was then little secure provision outside the special hospitals. It then took another catastrophe, to prioritise the needs of this group of individuals. Graham Young was admitted to Broadmoor Hospital at the age of 14 with a diagnosis of psychopathic disorder. He had administered poison to his father, sister, and a fellow schoolboy. Following his discharge, eight years later, he obtained a job as a 'tea boy' in a photographic warehouse, where he poisoned work colleagues, with fatal effects. On his conviction for murder in 1972, the British government set up two special committees to review the arrangements for the discharge and supervision of high-risk patients who were subject to special restrictions under mental health legislation. One of these has become a permanent body to advise Home Office Ministers on proposals for the discharge or transfer of these offenders. The second (Butler) Committee made a fundamental review of the legal provisions and facilities for the treatment of mentally abnormal offenders. It expressed concern at the 'yawning gap' in secure care provision, and recommended the development of medium-secure units that would be the focus for the development of forensic psychiatry.

At this time, there were only eight forensic psychiatrists in England, each jointly appointed between a prison and a local mental health service, but these doctors had no hospital base to treat offenders and no multi-disciplinary staff. The 1975 Butler Report, though, triggered the modern development of British forensic psychiatry, and it now includes over 150 consultants. This development was not without its critics. Dr Peter Scott, one of the founding fathers, believed that it would have been better to focus on developing specialised units in prisons. In predicting that medium-secure units would not relieve the overcrowding in the Special Hospitals, he proved to be correct. Medium-secure units soon became blocked themselves with patients who were difficult to move on to hospitals with a lesser degree of security or to the community, because of a lack of suitable facilities there. This situation is still largely unchanged.

The development and reputation of British forensic psychiatry were harmed by the response of the public, politicians, and the courts to the case in 1976 of Peter Sutcliffe, the 'Yorkshire Ripper', who had attacked and killed a number of women. All the doctors who saw him found him to be psychotic, with clear delusional beliefs, but the general view at the time was that he could not be both mad and bad. The psychiatrists giving evidence in the case were made to look foolish, and Sutcliffe was sent to prison. In time, though, after further psychiatric assessments, he was correctly transferred to a Special Hospital, with a diagnosis of schizophrenia. Though such notorious cases are rare, they do tend to shape public opinion and clinical practice. In the 1980s, following the killing of a social worker by a mentally ill individual, it became mandatory to set up a homicide inquiry whenever a killing occurred by any such person who was in contact with mental health services. As a result, all psychiatrists, and in particular forensic psychiatrists, now practice within a 'blame culture' setting, which is not likely to lead to the most positive development of these services.

In 1990, the inadequacies of British services (in both the prison and health systems) led to the setting up of a joint committee of the Home Office and the Department of Health, under Dr John Reed. Its reports, particularly on the management of psychopaths, represent one of the important landmarks in the development of British forensic psychiatry, even though many of the recommendations have not yet been implemented (see table below).

The development in London of the Institute for the Study and Treatment of Delinquency (ISTD) in the 1930s owed much to the psychoanalyst, Edward Glover. Its aim was to promote the view, already backed by scientific research, that there was a practical alternative to prison. The ISTD was the forerunner of the Portman Clinic, which trains doctors and other professionals in forensic psychotherapy, but that kind of treatment hardly exists in Britain outside London, and to a very small extent in most other countries. In fact, the 'determinists' have not had a central role in the development of British forensic psychiatry over the last 25 years. The speciality has primarily been developed by a number of charismatic clinicians based in medium-secure units, who have been more interested in practical solutions to clinical problems.

Reed Report — guiding principles

Mentally disordered offenders should be cared for:

- with regard to the quality of care and proper attention to the needs of the individual;

- as far as possible, in the community, rather than institutional settings;

- under conditions of no greater security than is justified by the degree of risk they present to others;

- in such a way as to maximise rehabilitation and their chances of sustaining an independent life;

- as near as possible to their own homes or families if they have them.

So far, academic forensic psychiatry in Britain has followed, rather than led clinical developments. The first Professor of Forensic Psychiatry was TCN Gibbens, appointed to the Maudsley Hospital in 1975. He advocated the provision of court medical services in 1951, but it was not until the 1990s that these were started, to encourage the diversion of mentally disordered offenders from the criminal justice system to the health service. Over the last few years, a number of new academic departments have been centred both in medium-secure units and in the high-security hospitals.

The British concept of psychopathy was influenced in the first half of this century by Sir David Henderson in Edinburgh. He emphasised the role of the individual constitution, shaped by heredity and environment, rather than the earlier notion of 'degeneration'. However, the concept of psychopathic disorder has had a troubled history in Britain, with at least three meanings — legal classification in terms of the 1983 Mental Health Act, a clinical diagnosis, and as a pejorative label. No consensus has been reached on the best assessment process, the role of psychiatry in management, or whether the service for this group should be a health or a prison responsibility. Whilst some of these individuals are at present managed in the high-security hospitals, many are in prison, where few therapeutic opportunities are available. However, it will not be possible to develop services in a more rational manner until there is research evidence that treatment of psychopaths is effective, in terms of both individual mental health and public safety. Political pressures have followed some high-profile crimes by psychopathic individuals, and controversial proposals for detaining them are still under discussion.

The United States

American forensic science began in the early nineteenth century with the work of Benjamin Rush, who distinguished between 'general' and 'partial' insanity. The latter was equivalent to the European 'monomania'. In 1838, Isaac Ray published *A Treatise on the Medical Jurisprudence of Insanity*, which remained the seminal work for almost a century. England's M'Naughton Rules became the criteria for acquittal on the basis of insanity in almost all American States, but this has led to much conflict between psychiatry and the law, for instance on whether knowing right from wrong might be regarded as a moral, rather than a scientific question. The influential Durham decision in the District of Colombia ruled in 1954 that if an act is a result or the product of a mental disease, then criminal responsibility does not exist. As early as 1921, the Briggs Law in Massachusetts provided for an individual who had been indicted for a capital offence or who had a previous conviction for a felony to be examined by an independent psychiatrist. William Alanson White's *Insanity and the Criminal Law* appeared in 1923, by which time the views of both Freud and Adolf Meyer had become influential in the USA. White maintained that 'insanity' was a legal term without medical meaning, and the general view had taken hold by then in the country that insanity and criminality were different facets of the same phenomenon.

A national discipline of forensic psychiatry did develop in the USA, mainly from the sociologically orientated work of Sheldon and Eleanor Glueck at Boston in the 1920s. They found statistical confirmation for the clinical view that both severe neglect and punishment favour the development of delinquent tendencies, while weakening the restrictive influence of conscience. It also emerged that delinquent boys tended to come from families with poorer than average mental health, and that they were more likely to solve their emotional conflicts by external action than by socially harmless symptoms, as neurotic boys did. However, the emergence of American forensic psychiatry was slow and formal qualifications in the subject were not awarded until the late 1970s. In New York, Melitta Schmideberg, the daughter of Melanie Klein, founded the Association for the Psychiatric Treatment of Offenders, which emphasised the need for close liaison between psychotherapists and the probation service. At the same time, it saw effective control of antisocial behaviour as essential to the rehabilitation of offenders.

In the 1930s, many American States had passed special commitment laws for mentally ill sex offenders, to provide treatment as an alternative to prison, but during the 1970s, it was increasingly felt that these arrangements had failed. Almost all of these laws were repealed or had become inoperative by the mid-1980s. At this time, following the growth of political and cultural conservatism, sentences of fixed length were becoming more common, instead of the possibility of early release on parole. More recently, new laws have been widely enacted for the special further psychiatric commitment of sex offenders who have completed a criminal sentence. These have aroused much concern as likely to create a 'psychiatric gulag' in the long run.

Holland and Italy

Holland passed a law on psychopathy in 1929 which acknowledged 'defective develop-ment or pathological disturbance' as accounting for some criminal actions. This took account of social factors, in addition to pre-existing 'defective intellectual capacities'. It introduced the concept of diminished responsibility into Dutch Law and later, a sliding scale of responsibility was gradually accepted. Dutch courts appoint a single, impartial expert on psychiatric questions, unlike the British and American practice of hearing from experts on each side. This psychiatrist has to try and quantify the degree of involuntari-ness that was present at the time of the offence. As in some other countries, Holland has experienced political pressure during the 1990s to increase the length of prison sentences — a development viewed with concern by forensic psychiatrists there.

In nineteenth-century Italy, Morel's theory of degeneracy, focusing attention on the links between crime and insanity, was further developed by Cesare Lombroso, whose work extend-ed beyond 1900. He defined a category of 'born criminals', characterised by specific forms of bodily morphology and of psychiatric and behavioural disorders. The predisposing fac-tors to this state were said to include epilepsy, syphilis, and trauma. The incarceration of such individuals was described as more a means of protecting society than a punishment, since they were not 'responsible' for their criminal behaviour. The first Italian institution for the criminal insane was opened in 1869, but advances in both neurological and psychiatric knowl-edge in the early part of this century discredited the principle of neuro-psychiatric degen-eracy. Yet later concepts of causality in forensic psychiatry owe much to Lombroso's work, with its attempts to understand criminality and its use of 'social' concepts. Increasingly, the assessment of mentally ill criminals centred on the issue of dangerousness, nothwithstand-ing the difficulties of predicting this trait. In France, the concept of *defense sociale* (social defence) evolved as a legislative response to the issue of dangerousness.

The Italian psychiatric reform of 1978 has been criticised for failing to provide, within the general mental health care system, for patients with recurrent psychotic episodes who may break the law, often in non-serious ways. This left the special (or judicial) hospitals as the only option for residential care, though they offer no real therapeutic possibili-ties, are staffed mainly by prison officers, and are unsuitably located geographically. Although two experimental centres for forensic psychiatry were opened, neither remained in operation for long. Law 180, which established the general reform, was greatly con-cerned with the civil rights of the mentally ill, but those who break the law can be con-fined on indeterminate sentences in institutions which do not offer them any appropriate help. This contrast is of concern to many mental health professionals in Italy.

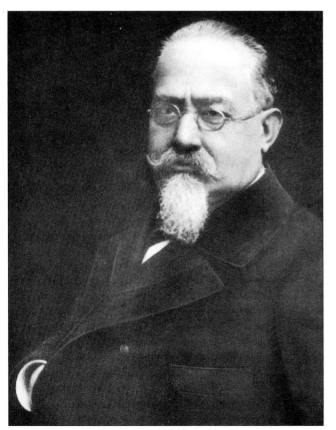

Cesare Lombroso. Photogravure. Reproduced with permission from the Wellcome Institute Library, London.

Germany

Karl Wilmanns, Professor of Psychiatry at Heidelberg from 1918 to 1933, has been regarded as one of the founders of forensic psy-chiatry in Europe because of his book, *Zur Psychopathologie des Landstreichers* (On the Psychopathology of the Vagrant), published in Leipzig in 1906. From 1910, he contributed to the proposed revision of the German criminal code, published studies of 'prison psychosis', and wrote many descriptions of criminal types and personalities. Though seen as a major figure in German psychiatry of the early twen-tieth century, his name did not become widely known outside central Europe.

Alexander and Staub published a psychoan-alytically influenced view of criminality in 1929 in Germany. The human being was said to be born asocial, but acquires social attitudes during the process of emotional maturation. As parental views are accepted and internalised, some asocial wishes — particularly aggressive and hostile impulses — are renounced. The equilibrium that is then achieved between grat-ification and renunciation is perceived as a 'sense of justice', which will be disturbed if other individuals are seen to be unpunished for anti-social behaviour. This was said to be a cause of the revenge motive, which may influence judges, juries, and the general public. Alexander and Staub proposed that all offenders who were capable of rehabilitation should receive psychotherapeutic treatment, but that those who were 'incurable' should be incarcerated, to protect society. Such a distinction between 'the sheep and the goats', though, raised issues about prediction which are still unresolved.

Conclusion

An influential force in the forensic psychiatry of the twentieth century has been that of psychoanalysis. In a paper of 1925 – 'Criminality from a sense of Guilt' – Freud proposed that guilt feelings originate from repressed antisocial cravings — primarily Oedipal tendencies — and that these cravings and feelings are often the chief determinants of criminal acts. Freud claimed that the neurotic individual is at the same time anti-social and overly social — symptoms satisfy anti-social tendencies in fantasy, but the individual atones for these in self-inflicted suffering caused by neurosis. After the punishment, though, which relieves guilt feelings, the individual with a neurotic character may feel free to offend the social order once again.

In 1967, it was the view of Alexander and Selesnick that no suitable definition of mental illness had so far been incorporated into any system of law, in spite of the dramatic evolution of psychiatry up to then. This situation had not significantly changed at the end of the century.

FRANCO BASAGLIA (1924–1980)

by Michael Donnelly

Franco Basaglia, who died in 1980, was the charismatic leader of a radical movement promoting 'alternative psychiatry' in the Italy of the 1960s and 1970s. Although sometimes linked with contemporary proponents of 'anti-psychiatry', Basaglia held rather different views; the Democratic Psychiatry movement he led, moreover, had a wider social base and wider influence than the 'anti-psychiatry' currents elsewhere.

Basaglia's early career was conventional; he trained in neuropsychiatry and gained a prestigious position in the university psychiatric clinic at Padua. In 1961, however, after 14 years there, he suddenly abandoned his academic career to become head of a provincial public mental hospital at Gorizia, a town in the extreme north-east of Italy near the Yugoslav border. Along with a hand-picked group of collaborators, Basaglia hoped to make the Gorizia hospital into a pilot experiment — a 'laboratory', as he often called it, for innovation in public (asylum-based) psychiatry.

The first steps that Basaglia and his team took were simple practical measures, designed to humanise the custodial environment and to introduce the look and feel of an 'open' hospital. In many respects Basaglia was introducing into Italy the British and American experiences with the therapeutic community. But from the outset, the team also had distinctively different and more radical goals. Drawing on phenomenology and existential psychiatry (interests which form a thread running throughout Basaglia's career), they sought to 'make contact' with the patients as subjects, criticising traditional 'positivist' psychiatry for objectifying patients in diagnostic categories. To approach a patient without prejudice or presuppositions Basaglia argued, it was necessary to "place in brackets" the patient's diagnosis, "since that diagnostic label hung fixedly on the patient like a pre-formed value judgment" (Basaglia, 1968). Such 'bracketing' was not, as later critics were to charge, a denial of mental illness; but Basaglia did claim that much of what appeared to be mental illness was more the result of institutionalism or institutional neurosis than the outcome of a disease process. The deteriorated state of the inmate in the asylum was in effect the social product or artifact of institutional conditions themselves. The therapeutic community interested Basaglia in large part as a means to destabilise the institutional regime. He saw the daily assemblies of patients and staff, for instance, as an effort both to encourage patient self-government and also to draw out individual patients, putting them "back in touch with their own biographies". The focus in the assemblies was not merely on the here and now, but also on understanding the transformations which people had suffered over time in the institution. Retracing a life history was thus (amongst other things) a way of drawing attention to the malign effects of the institution, identifying it as the problem, and thus bringing to light the patients' collective predicament as inmates.

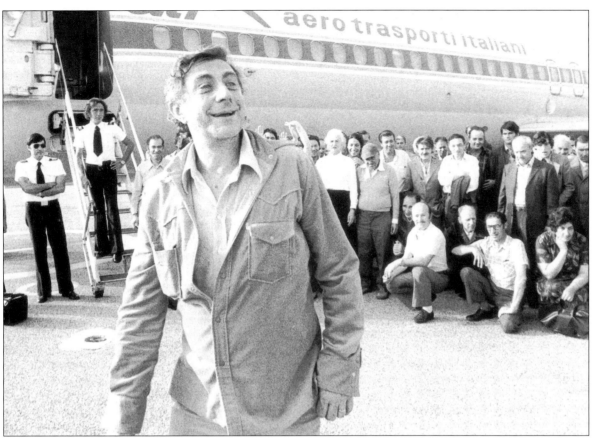

Franco Basaglia. 'Il volo', photograph by Claudio Ernè, Trieste Airport, 1974. This photo captures the first outing of patients from the San Giovanni Mental Hospital.

As the experiment at Gorizia evolved, Basaglia came to speak of the therapeutic community as only a way-station, an advance over the custodial hospital, but still an institution whose 'contradictions' would have to be confronted if the patients were ever to recover their 'subjecthood' and capacity to act as agents. To make this step, Basaglia spoke of trying to mobilise amongst the patients an 'institutional rage', which would, focus their aggressivity against the institution as both the symbol of and the practical means for their exclusion from the broader society. The real struggle, in other words, had to move beyond the asylum, beyond attempts at making the asylum therapeutic, to questioning why it need ever exist. Henceforth, at least part of the alternative psychiatrist's task would lie not in working with patients, but in a broader political and cultural campaign to change society's relation to the mentally disordered. Basaglia recounted the course of the Gorizia experiment in *L'istituzione negata* (*The Institution Negated*, 1968), which came to serve as a manifesto for the growing political ambitions of alternative psychiatrists. It also struck a wide resonance in Italian society at large, quickly becoming a key text in the radical students' and workers' mobilisations that swept Italy during 1968–69.

Basaglia began a second pilot experiment in 1971, when he was invited by the provincial administration of Trieste to reorganise the local mental health services, then centralised in a 1200-bed hospital. Basaglia's aim was to take up from where the experiment at Gorizia had ended, emphasising community-based care — not to improve the hospital, but to move outside and beyond it entirely. The number of hospital beds was fairly quickly run down, accompanied by elaborate efforts to ease and support patients' re-entry into the community. Basaglia's work in Trieste was notable also for a variety of imaginative cultural initiatives designed to mix ex-patients with community residents and both practically and symbolically break down barriers between the institution and its environing society. As a largely favourable World Health Organization (1980) assessment later summed up the Trieste experience: "The provision of mental health centres, group apartments and other parts of a supportive community system was synchronous with the reduction in hospital beds. Staff and patients moved to the community, pari passu with the closure of the hospital wards. There was no interruption of responsibility, and staff and patients were 'deinstitutionalized' together". Basaglia left Trieste in 1979 to take over psychiatric services in Rome and the surrounding Lazio region. He died suddenly the next year.

Basaglia's legacy for Italian psychiatry has been somewhat ambiguous. Although he has been widely credited as the architect and inspiration for the sweeping mental health reform enacted in 1978 (this chapter, p. 257), the so-called Basaglia Law has been only patchily implemented. The pilot experiments in alternative psychiatry may well have been remarkable achievements, but they did not provide easily repeatable or sustainable models that could be implemented through broad-gauged policies. Indeed, it is clear in retrospect that part of the success of the pilot experiments depended upon the support and cooperation (or at least non-interference) of local political authorities, and on the extraordinary energies mobilised through the course of a radical social movement. Neither of those factors could long be taken for granted, particularly as the fervour of political mobilisation in Italy began to wane. Moreover, the law mandating psychiatric reform was more a statement of principle than a blueprint for new policies. Many key details, including the financing of the reform and its implementation and monitoring, were left to be worked out. In some areas of the country they were; in others, the law has yet to be appropriately implemented. Perhaps most tellingly of all, Basaglia's legacy was in many respects a negative one: his practical accomplishment was removing obstacles to reform, clearing away the antiquated laws, institutions, and practices which marginalised the mentally disordered. The positive goals of the new alternative psychiatry, beyond its salutary concern with restoring the dignity and the agency or selfhood of mental patients, were always less clear. At the least it has proven difficult to articulate such goals programmatically into Italy's new mental health policies.

COGNITIVE THERAPY

by Jan Scott

Cognitive therapy (CT) is the most widely researched and practised short-term psychotherapy in both the USA and Europe. Prior to its introduction, the two dominant models of psychotherapy were psychoanalysis and behaviour therapy (BT). Although several individuals (e.g. Aaron T Beck, Albert Ellis, and Donald Meichenbaum) can be regarded as the 'founding fathers' of CT, the key figure within psychiatry from this point of view is Beck. The development of his model of CT is therefore discussed here primarily, with limited reference to other models.

Origins

The profession of psychotherapy is about 100 years old. Despite the vast expansion that has occurred in the number of different psychotherapies now practised, most approaches may be categorised as either 'insight-orientated' or 'action-orientated'. In the early years, insight-orientated approaches such as Freudian psychoanalysis, which emphasised the development of greater self-awareness or self-understanding, were predominant. In the last 30–40 years, action-orientated models, often referred to as brief therapies (characterised as short-term, problem-orientated, and concentrated on change in the here and now), have become the most frequently practised intervention. The paradigm shift that began in the 1950s arose because of the move within psychology towards behavioural and later cognitive models of psychological disorders, together with the failure of psychoanalysts to demonstrate a scientific basis for their approach.

The development of learning theory, which proposed that psychiatric disorders were the product of faulty learning, by behaviourists such as Skinner, Eysenck, and Wolpe, led naturally to the introduction of BT as the first brief model (Chapter 6, p. 173). Followers of Skinner used reinforcement contingencies (reward systems) to try to overcome previous inappropriate conditioning in people with severe mental disorders, whilst Wolpe focused on systematic desensitisation (imaginal graded exposure to a stimulus after the induction of a relaxed state) as a fear-reducing technique in people suffering from 'neuroses'. However, the early success of BT in treating disorders such as anxiety and agorophobia was not matched by equivalent results in the treatment of depression — a disorder with an obvious and large cognitive element. Therefore, psychologists began to explore other models of therapy that appeared to have an empirical basis. A further important prompt in the move away from pure learning theory towards cognitive science was the discontent in some quarters at working exclusively with models developed through animal experiments, when the ultimate goal was to explain human behaviour and experience.

In contrast to the 'environmental determinism' or 'conditioning' model suggested by behaviourists, psychoanalysts continued to support the 'motivational model' which proposed that behaviour was driven by unconscious beliefs. Ironically, it was Beck's attempt to convince other researchers, particularly those working in experimental psychology, of the scientific basis of this theory of psychoanalysis that led to the development of the cognitive theory of depression. At Philadelphia, Beck had originally trained as a psychoanalyst, because he believed it offered a way of viewing the whole range of human experiences and problems. Like Freud, he began by exploring the links between the environment, the individual, and their emotions and motivations, as well as how disturbances in the balance between and within these factors resulted in emotional problems and disorders. However, Beck's research experiments with depressed patients undermined rather than supported the motivational theory. The results did not suggest that internal determinism was based on unconscious motivations or biological drives, but on how the individual constructed his or her experience. He realised that a cognitive or information-processing model offered a far more powerful explanation of both the experimental data and the phenomena he observed in his own clinical practice.

A similar hypothesis had been reported independently by Albert Ellis in New York. He had identified a further implication of cognitive theory that an individual's belief system, which is important in determining the meaning given to events or experiences, could be assumed to be accessible to both the patient and the therapist. This meant that such beliefs could be approached by direct questioning, rather than indirectly through interpretations. Ellis contacted Beck to share his ideas, and so began over 30 years of correspondence. At about the same time, Beck also noted the parallels between his own ideas and the work of Kelly on 'personal construct theory', which led to the rapidly developing field of cognitive psychology.

Between 1960 and 1965, Beck wrote his seminal papers on depression and on the cognitive theory of emotional disorders; these still contain the core of his theories on psychological problems. Beck's model offers a 'continuity hypothesis', since it suggests that psychiatric syndromes are exaggerated forms of normal emotional responses. It also sees emotional and behavioural responses to events or experiences as being largely determined by the cognitive appraisal that is made of them by the individual.

The information-processing paradigm has two key elements: cognitive structures and cognitive mechanisms. The underlying structures, termed 'schemata', are defined as containing a network of core beliefs, but there is also a more accessible, but involuntary level of cognition, which Beck termed 'automatic thoughts'. These occur at the same time as or immediately prior to an emotional response to an event or experience. Such thoughts are particularly important in therapy, as they encapsulate the individual's response to a specific situation in an 'event-thought-feeling-behaviour' link. The analysis of automatic thoughts across different situations allows underlying themes to be identified, so giving clues to the content of the underlying schemata. 'Cognitive mechanisms' refer to the faulty information processing that may occur when individuals selectively screen in or screen out information from their environment that either supports or refutes their view of themselves and their world.

This model has been applied to a number of emotional disorders, but was first elaborated for depression. The cognitive theory of depression represents a stress-diathesis model which postulates that some individuals may be vulnerable to depression because, as a result of early learning experiences, they develop dysfunctional beliefs. For example, if an individual experienced physical or emotional abuse or neglect as a child, they may develop a negative belief that they are unlovable. Such beliefs may be latent for long periods, but become reactivated by events that carry a specific meaning for that person, e.g. the experience of personal rejection for an individual who already believes they are unlovable. Negative cognitions about the self, world, and future are seen as manifestations of these maladaptive beliefs. These negative automatic thoughts dominate the thinking of many depressed patients and are sustained through faulty information processing, thus contributing to further depression of affect. Beck states that whilst the vicious cycle of low mood enhancing negative thinking, which then leads to further lowering in mood, may represent a causal theory in some cases, it acts as a maintenance model for other forms of depression. Nevertheless, he also points out that intervention in the cycle can be effective in alleviating acute depressive symptoms in either group.

Outline of the therapy

Most models of CT share a common core — that since psychological distress is a function of disturbed cognitive processes, the focus of therapy is on changing cognitions. Beck's model is the most widely practised; it differs from Meichenbaum's and Ellis' approaches in important ways. Meichenbaum developed a cognitive modification model called 'self-instructional therapy'. This places importance on the modification of what people say to themselves (self-talk), but puts little emphasis on underlying cognitive structures. It therefore contrasts significantly with that of Beck, who maintains that modification of the deeper-level schemata is a necessary component of the therapy. Whilst Ellis proposes that individuals have a common set of assumptions, Beck maintains that an individual's underlying beliefs are idiosyncratic. The practice of Beckian CT also differs from Ellis' 'rational emotive therapy' in several important aspects, notably that Beck employs a 'guided discovery' approach to help the individual explore their ideas and cognitions, whilst Ellis uses rational disputation to openly challenge an individual's assumptions. For instance, Ellis may say to a patient who is affected by an adverse event — "Why should you assume that everything which happens in the world is designed to increase your happiness?".

Beck's model of CT is a collaborative 'hypothesis-testing' approach; it uses a questioning style, termed 'guided discovery', to help the individual identify and challenge their distorted cognitions and dysfunctional beliefs for themselves. At the time of the introduction of CT, there were only a few brief therapy models, and Beck largely had to forge his own therapeutic tools. As well as devising techniques to educate the individual about their problems and to explore their automatic thoughts, CT integrates interventions which are targeted at definable modes of behaviour that can be readily monitored and addressed. Although Beck acknowledges the use and importance of behavioural techniques in CT, he emphasises that they are only one of several mechanisms for producing change. Furthermore, the therapy is not simply technique-driven; the therapeutic relationship is a crucial aspect of the approach, as described below. This makes CT one of the most human and compelling versions of an action therapy.

In the course of therapy, the interventions that are proposed to help a particular individual are selected on the basis of a cognitive conceptualisation; this draws together key information about the individual which uniquely explains the onset and maintenance of their distress. If the individual shows a low level of functioning, behavioural techniques may be used to improve their activity levels and enhance their problem-solving and coping skills. However, a further goal of behavioural intervention is to identify negative cognitions and underlying beliefs. Verbal interventions are initially employed to teach the individual to recognise and challenge negative cognitions. This usually leads to improved mood, positive changes in behaviour, and a reduction in acute symptoms. The therapist never tries to persuade individuals to change their views, but rather helps them to explore their perceptions of events and experiences, and to discover for themselves the evidence to support or refute their hypotheses. This collaborative–empirical approach is crucial to the success of the therapy. Later, as the individual's acute distress attenuates, cognitive and behavioural interventions are used to try to identify and modify underlying dysfunctional beliefs. Events that hold specific meaning for the individual and that may make them vulnerable to distress in the future are also identified and discussed. The aim of this part of the therapy is to identify high-risk situations for the future and to reduce the individual's underlying vulnerability to relapse.

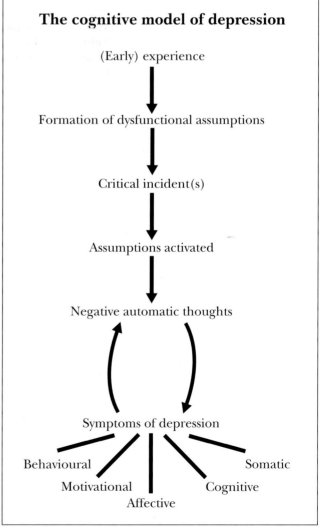

The cognitive model of depression.

Reactions to cognitive therapy

Initially, negative views of CT were expressed by radical behaviourists, who supported the environmental determinism theory. Wolpe was particularly critical of the Beckian hypothesis that the patient could consciously make a choice to change. However, the failure to develop a more sophisticated BT model based on learning theory and the rise of cognitive science increasingly led clinicians to explore Beck's writings. The process of acceptance was helped by the fact that CT also incorporated BT techniques and acknowledged the behaviourist's emphasis on empiricism. The move towards cognitive interventions in psychotherapy in the 1970s and 1980s was driven by clinical need and by the inadequacy of existing models to deal with the patient's internal dialogue. Many biological psychiatrists have been sympathetic to the use of CT, mainly because it is based on an accessible and understandable theory that is open to empirical testing. Yet the acceptability of CT is not only related to its scientific foundations, but also to the basic humanity that underpins both the theory and the practice.

Initially, clinicians in Europe seemed to embrace CT more readily than professionals in the USA, but in the last decade, Beck's considerable contribution to the development of cognitive psychology and psychotherapy has also been acknowledged in America. In analysing Beck's contribution to the evolution of psychotherapy, Sir David Goldberg suggests that Beck bears the same relationship to psychoanalysis as Gorbachev did to communism. Whilst Gorbachev vowed that all he was trying to do was reform communism, he is now seen by historians as the person who actually began the process of dismantling it. Likewise, Beck began by trying to demonstrate the scientific basis of psychoanalysis, but ended by providing an alternative, more empirical, briefer model of therapy that has demonstrated efficacy in randomised controlled treatment trials.

Recent developments

Meta-analyses of randomised controlled trials of the treatment of depression confirm that CT is an effective alternative to medication for people with mild or moderately severe disorders. Cognitive therapy is not usually recommended as the first-line treatment in more severe forms of depression, as the response to CT is slower than that achieved with antidepressants or ECT. However, CT can have significant long-term benefits, with reductions in relapse rates of depression that are equal to those achieved with prophylactic medication. Research also demonstrates the importance of referring patients with depression to trained and skilful therapists. Data suggest that the expertise of the therapist, particularly in severe or complex cases, may account for 30% or more of the variance in patients' response.

Following the successful application of CT to depression, cognitive models have been developed for most of the anxiety disorders (including panic disorder, obsessive–compulsive disorder, excessive health anxiety, and social phobia). Cognitive therapy manuals have also been developed for people with personality disorders and those with drug- or alcohol-related problems. There is a continued expansion of empirical data that support these cognitive theories, further cementing the relationship between cognitive science and CT. Research findings which demonstrate the effectiveness of CT for these disorders are also accumulating at a rapid rate.

The most recent developments in CT focus on its use in severe mental disorders, including psychosis. Although CT is used mainly in combination with medication, rather than alone, the results of early studies in schizophrenia suggest that individuals who receive the combined treatment have a better short-term outcome and are less likely to relapse than those receiving medication alone. These approaches have now been extended to individuals with bipolar disorder. Such research is in its infancy, but it is hoped that these studies will not only establish that CT can be effective, but also determine how it works.

The development of CT over the last 30 years has surprised many mental health professionals. It seems unlikely that another novel model of therapy will have such an impact on clinical or research practice in the foreseeable future. Effective new therapies will now probably arise as hybrids of established approaches, rather than de novo. Opinions vary as to whether the relationship between CT and BT represents evolution or revolution, but there is continued cross-fertilisation between these approaches, and models of cognitive–behavioural therapy have been developed. These are proving to be particularly useful in liaison psychiatry and have been successfully applied to syndromes such as chronic fatigue. As the dialogue between CT and BT seems likely to continue, the interaction between these schools of therapy should act as a model to other groups. This may lead to greater dialogue and a shared understanding of the core characteristics of effective forms of brief therapy.

POLITICAL ABUSE OF PSYCHIATRY IN THE FORMER SOVIET UNION

by Toma Tomov

At the funeral of a senior person with whom one has been closely involved, before gaining independence due to increasing seniority, there are similar feelings to those of reconsidering a controversial subject. It is a moment when one hopes that the passage of time has already made a real difference, though the feelings experienced are of both shame and sadness. By the grave, there are flash-backs of moments when revelations about one's own attitude were about to be made, but one then lacked the courage to face reality. Now the person who then needed help is dead, so it is too late to set the record right. I got to know many psychiatrists from the former Soviet Union through the Geneva Initiative of Psychiatry and the network of reformers that it developed. From this, I recognised the difficulty of deciding whether to regard oneself as somebody who avoided being bothered by the issue of abuse, or who simply managed to remain personally uninvolved.

The background

Though cases began soon after the Bolshevik revolution, presenting political dissent as a form of mental aberration in the Soviet Union dates substantially from Stalin's era; he declared that a Leninist scientific worker must strive "to be an active participant in the political guidance of the country". It was a strategy that was employed both by villains and heroes — to their very different ends — and it could be seen as either criminal, immoral, or just shrewd, depending on the individual case and one's own perspective. Some individuals manipulated their way into psychiatric institutions as a better alternative to the Gulag. During the Second World War, a psychiatric hospital was established in Kazan under the direct control of the NKVD (later KGB). However, the systematic use of psychiatry as an instrument of evil for defeating political opposition evolved further under both Stalin and Khruschev, though it was the latter's regime which provided the ideological justification for it. Students of dictatorship have documented the fact that ideology had a much greater influence than scientific or ethical arguments in regulating the practice of many professional fields in the Soviet Union.

From the late 1930s until the late 1940s , the classical frontal leucotomy of Moniz and Lima was used for the treatment of schizophrenia and severe pain. But on December 9, 1950, a special order of the Ministry of Health of the USSR prohibited the use of prefrontal leucotomy for the treatment of neuropsychiatric disorders as "contradicting the basic principles of Pavlov's physiological theory". Many psychiatrists (mostly of Jewish origin) who advocated psychosurgery were then dismissed from their jobs, and psychosurgical interventions were not performed for several decades afterwards.

For political reasons of the later 1950s, the 1960s, and 1970s, accusations of disloyalty to the Soviet system could no longer be upheld in court, because at that time, the regime had committed itself in the international arena, under the Helsinki accords, to observe individual rights and freedom. A new approach to suppressing dissent was badly needed therefore. Under these circumstances, framing the champions of democracy and human rights as mentally sick offered the advantage of allowing their elimination through a court case for statutory placement. Even the mildest divergence of behaviour or opinion could then be used as evidence of mental disturbance.

Serbsky Institute

The Serbsky Central Research Institute of Forensic Medicine, named after the Russian psychiatrist VP Serbsky (1855–1917), was established in Moscow in 1921. Although ostensibly under the Ministry of Health, it was effectively controlled by the Ministry of Internal Affairs. It was drawn into the process of political abuse through its Fourth Section, which specialised in handling cases deemed to have political significance, i.e. which appeared to dissent from the Soviet ideology and political order. Dr DR Lunts, who chaired the Fourth Section between 1948 and his death in 1977, is regarded as having masterminded the logistics of putting psychiatric technologies in the service of oppressive handling of individuals. Like some of the other leading figures in the abuse, Lunts was actually an officer at the Ministry of Internal Affairs. Professor GV Morozov was chairman of both the Serbsky Institute and the All-Union Psychiatric Society throughout the years of international protest. As a result, he stayed in the international limelight for some considerable time, coming to personify the apparatchik–psychiatrist. This was a man of great power, but all of it illegitimate, if judged by the criteria of the international psychiatric community, since it was conferred on him only for political reasons. Information about the activities of the Serbsky Institute was revealed in General Grigorenko's prison diary, but as a response to increasing international criticism, the Institute was awarded the order of the Red Banner of Labour by the Soviet government in late 1971.

Sluggish schizophrenia

'Sluggish schizophrenia' is a category in a classification of schizophrenia developed by Professor A Snezhnevsky, director of the Institute of Psychiatry of the Soviet Academy of Medical Sciences for many years. It is revealing of the kind of construct used by Soviet psychiatry, since it was developed as the result of the politically motivated thinking of a powerful doyen in the field, rather than by providing evidence of known validity. Using an extensive but entirely speculative account of causative influences, which were named 'nosos' and 'pathos', several clinical forms of schizophrenia were defined by Snezhnevsky. Having been used in an attempt to legitimise scientifically a situation in Soviet psychiatry in which political abuse was established, these categories became dominant from the 1950s. Sluggish schizophrenia then turned out to be a particularly convenient category, since it enabled schizophrenia to be diagnosed in the absence of psychotic symptoms. The behavioural changes which could be interpreted as evidence of a severe psychiatric condition could sometimes be so subtle that they were described as "seeming normality". Some of the phrases commonly used in reports on dissenters which established such a diagnosis were: "reformist delusional ideas", "over-estimation of his own personality", and "poor adaptation to the social environment".

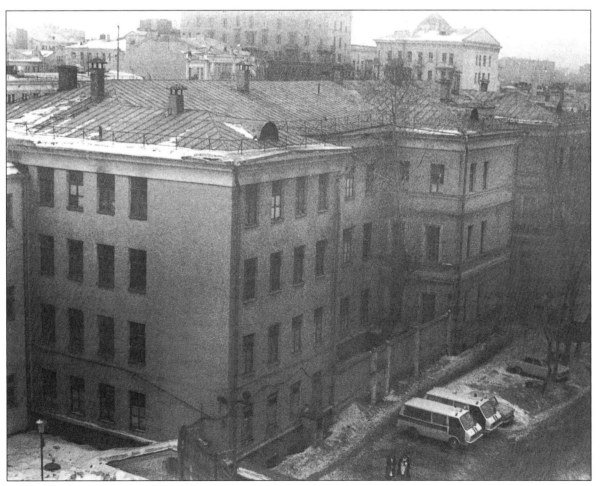

The Serbsky Institute of General and Forensic Psychiatry, 23 Kropotkin Lane, Moscow: view of the main building, which contains Section 4 for political cases (second storey from top, far right). Two nurses and two ambulances can be seen in the yard. Most of the building is occupied by Section 1 (ground floor), Section 2 (first floor), Female Section (second floor), and Section 3 (third floor). Reproduced with permission from Aid to Russia and the Republics.

Political hospitals

Political hospitals had the design of maximum security forensic wards, were under the Soviet Ministry of the Interior, and bore the official designation 'Special Psychiatric Hospitals' until 1988, when they came under the jurisdiction of the Ministry of Health. These hospitals were established to keep patients with severe mental illnesses, many of whom had committed violent crimes; most of the staff were criminals, serving their sentences in that environment, while nurses and doctors had a relatively insignificant role. Brutality was common and drugs with severely toxic effects, particularly sulphazin, were used for punitive rather than therapeutic purposes. Detention might be for several years, sometimes for more than a decade, and the detainee knew nothing about his chances of release. There were eight such hospitals, seven on the territory of present-day Russia and one in the Ukraine. An insider's description of life in such a hospital and of its mode of operation can be found in Vladimir Bukovsky's 1978 book *'To Build a Castle'*. Bloch and Reddaway classified the confined dissenters as: (a) advocates of human rights or democratisation; (b) nationalists; (c) would-be emigrants; (d) religious believers; and (e) people inconvenient to the authorities.

Unsurprisingly, there are no statistics about the total size of this operation. Political dissidence providing psychiatric grounds for disqualifying persons from normal life was, of course, never officially recognised as an identifiable category requiring treatment. However, to try and estimate how widespread was the psychiatric abuse of dissidents, some evidence could be found in the 1960 Criminal Code of the Russian Soviet Federated Republic. Soviet public prosecutors had used as grounds for detainment in special psychiatric hospitals articles 70 ('especially dangerous crimes', e.g. anti-Soviet agitation and propaganda) and 190–1 ('other crimes', e.g. slander of the Soviet State) of this code. The examination of such data has not yet been done, though. A further complication in estimating the magnitude of this activity arises from the fact that many people were detained without being officially charged with any crime. This kind of activity went hand-in-hand with an institutional culture marked by arrogance and contempt for the sick. Whenever that issue was raised, though, the cliché used in reply was that in their hearts, the common people had trust in their health service because of the self-sacrificial nature of doctors' contribution to it. To cast doubt on the devotion of such professionals to helping people might have proved very risky for that society. The estimate given by Peter Reddaway is that 300 people were affected; Andre Koppers lists over 340 names, while Robert van Voren from the Geneva Initiative of Psychiatry gives a number of 60 on the grounds of the above articles for the Ukraine only.

Emblematic of the Soviet political abuse of psychiatry were two cases in particular. Firstly, Petro Grigorenko, an army general who supported the Crimean Tatars in condemning their forceful deportation and who was eventually expelled to the United States. Secondly, Vladimir Bukovsky, a student and essayist, who was particularly active in disseminating information by way of *samizdat* — the illegal publishing used by dissident intelligentsia — and who took written medical reports out of the Soviet Union. The underground *Chronicle of Current Events* recorded various forms of violation of human rights, including the enforced hospitalisation of psychiatrically normal people, until it was eventually closed down by the KGB. Other familiar names of individuals rescued to the West are Leonid Plyushch, Alexander Esenin-Volpin, and Natalya Gorbanevskaya.

Those psychiatrists actively involved in the abuse probably did not number more than 40, but they generally had senior administrative positions in medical schools or hospitals, through which they had considerable power and influence. For whatever reason, all had an unquestioning loyalty to the Communist Party and its ideology, and were correspondingly rewarded with material benefits which were confined to the elite in the Soviet Union. On the other hand, two psychiatrists who protested against the misuse — Semyon Gluzman and Andrei Koryagin — both received long prison sentences. The average Soviet psychiatrist had very little direct knowledge of the political use of the discipline, though rebuttals in the media of Western criticism would have drawn some attention to the issue. Any failure to comply with the demands of the State amounted to professional suicide.

The international response

Information about the political abuse of psychiatry in the Soviet Union started reaching the West in the early 1970s, through channels operated by human rights activists. In 1971, Vladimir Bukovsky sent the official psychiatric reports on 10 dissenters to Western doctors, and this provoked enough momentum to enable political abuse to be put on the agenda of the international psychiatric community. The way events evolved since then has been relatively well documented, particularly by Bloch, Reddaway, and Gluzman, though the question what made Soviet psychiatry liable to abuse on such a large scale still deserves further examination.

As information about psychiatric abuse of Soviet dissidents continued to leak to the West, human rights activists, professionals concerned with ethical issues, and Western intellectuals rallied for joint political action over it. The International Association on the Political Use of Psychiatry, a group of liberal thinkers, spearheaded efforts to bring this practice to the attention of the international psychiatric community. Particularly important contributions were the two books of Sidney Bloch and Peter Reddaway: *Russia's Political Hospitals* and *Soviet Psychiatric Abuse*.

In the summer of 1973, the Royal College of Psychiatrists adopted a motion deploring "the current use of psychiatry in the Soviet Union for the purpose of political repression". Following this, a long letter was published from the Presidium of the All-Union Society of Neurologists and Psychiatrists in *The Guardian* (London) of 29 September. This referred to "malicious concoctions" that had appeared in the media of Western countries, "alleging that in the Soviet Union mentally healthy people are being placed in mental hospitals for their 'dissenting' political views". Also, it was being "falsely charged that these persons are given medicines that are damaging to their health". The signatories expressed their "indignation and emphatic protest against the slandering of Soviet psychiatry and thereby of medicine in general", while acknowledging that the urgent hospitalisation of "insane persons" was permitted under Article 36 of the Fundamentals of Legislation on Public Health of the USSR. The Serbsky Institute was described as one of the "leading clinical psychiatric institutions of the country". In a small number of cases, it was agreed, mental derangement might lead to anti-social actions "such as disturbance of public order, dissemination of slander, manifestation of aggressive intentions, etc… they can do this… with a 'cunningly calculated plan of action'". At the "open trial of the criminal case of Yakir and Krasin, who were condemned for subversive propaganda and the dissemination of malicious concoctions", Yakir had admitted that the claim that healthy people were placed in mental hospitals "was fabricated by him and accorded with the desires of some correspondents of the bourgeois press". As was usual with such Soviet activities, the letter had no less than 21 signatories. The well-known names amongst them included Georgy Morozov, Andrei Snezhnevsky, and Eduard Babayan.

The congresses of the World Psychiatric Association were then targeted as settings for the dissemination of revelations about this malpractice. At the meetings in Mexico City (1971), Hawaii (1977), Vienna (1983), and Athens (1989), the issue repeatedly emerged. Eventually, there was strong support for the proposals of some member-organisations to

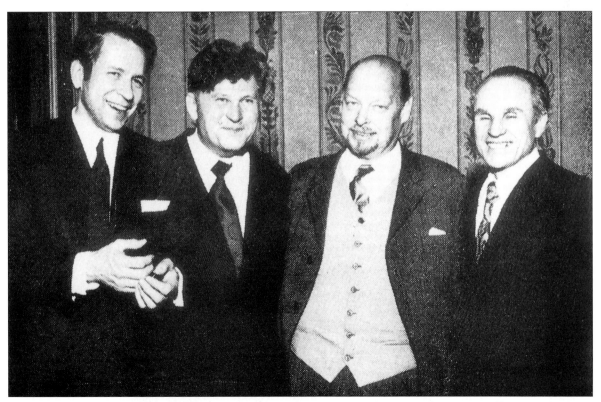

Professor Georgy Morozov (2nd from left), the top administrator of Soviet psychiatry, with his Serbsky Institute colleague N Zharikov (right) and two Finnish psychiatrists. Reproduced with permission from Aid to Russia and the Republics.

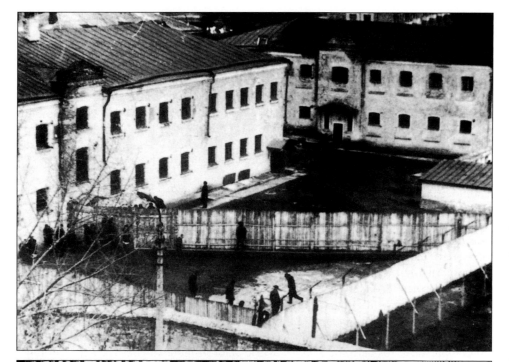

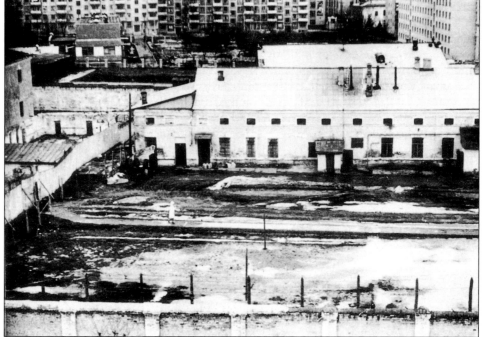

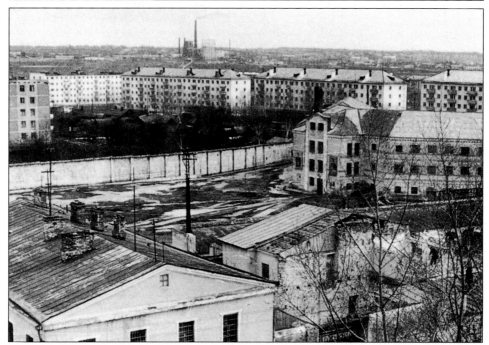

The MVD Investigations Prison and MVD Special Psychiatric Hospital (SPH) in Orel. The prison and the SPH occupy the buildings of an eighteenth-century hard-labour prison. Prior to 1970 each block housed prisoners in different categories (including one for tubercular prisoners) and had its own exercise yard. The outer wall is about six metres high, with a barbed wire fence inside. One wall has an electrified wire on top of it. The SPH is the block on the extreme left of the top photograph. Reproduced with permission from Aid to Russia and the Republics.

suspend the membership of the Soviet All-Union Society until it corrected its human rights record. In response, that Society decided to withdraw from WPA in 1983, on the pretence of 'slander'; several others, including the Czecho-Slovak and Bulgarian, followed suit. As political change began to alter the situation, however, two official visits to the Soviet Union took place. One was in 1989 by a delegation of the US Department of State's Bureau of Human Rights, led by Professor Roth, and the other in 1991 by a team from the World Psychiatric Association, led by Dr James Birley of Britain. The findings of these visits enabled the return of the All-Union Society back into the World Psychiatric Association to be re-negotiated.

The aftermath

Disqualifying opponents, rather than engaging in open contests of ideas with them, is practised to some extent in all societies. Totalitarian systems, however, apply the approach widely and indiscriminately, submitting both friends and enemies to it and managing to induce developmental arrest in individuals, groups, and organisations. The analogy with a young child who is the victim of parental abuse has repeatedly been drawn. The primitive psychological coping employed by such a child so as to come to terms with the abuse, and yet at the same time to follow the parental injunction to conceal it, leads to a bad concept of the self. If the actions of Soviet psychiatrists are considered within this frame of mind, such an interpretation seems to be a valid one. Historical evidence confirms that totalitarian regimes, by taking political control over professional bodies, render institutions like psychiatry as helpless to confront the regime as the young child is to confront the abusive parent. Complementarity of the victim–perpetrator relationship can also account for the persistent and refractory nature of the abusive pattern.

Such an approach to making sense of Soviet political abuse might suggest that with the downfall of that political system, things would tend to correct themselves. This would be convenient, since it implies that the individuals who have lived through all this need to do nothing specific about it. But the question remains — What in fact can doctors and mental health professionals of the former Soviet Union do now about this legacy? Some of the strategies offered for that purpose, in particular in the Network of Reformers, have been shown to be effective. They involve confronting the domain of authority and, more specifically, exposing those affected to a more relaxed attitude to authority than groups originating in the former Soviet Union had previously experienced.

The Network of Reformers is a major five-year international project in the ethics of psychiatric practice in Eastern and Central Europe, run by the Geneva Initiative on Psychiatry. Many international sponsors, e.g. The Soros Open Society Foundation, the Democracy Programme of the European Union, and the MATRA Programme of the Dutch Government, have contributed. The project was conceived primarily by Jim Birley and Robert van Voren, to support the efforts being made to restore and develop principles of psychiatric good practice in the region. The lack of established networks with lateral rather than hierarchical relationships was identified early on as a major deficit on the mental health scene there. The Network attempts to raise awareness amongst Eastern and Central European professionals about their communication style and the impact that this has on teamwork, therapeutic relationships, leadership, research, etc. Opportunities are generated for psychiatrists, nurses, relatives, and consumers from countries in the region to come together with Western counterparts to engage in discourse, training, and planning. These are concerned with psychiatric 'reform', in the sense of a transition to community psychiatry and the enhancement of patients' participation in society. Experience gained through the Network facilitates the establishment of independent professional and non-governmental organisations in the field of mental health. This helps to build a new professional identity, making it possible for the past practice of psychiatry in the region to be critically examined.

In the former Soviet Union, there was a 'reification' of diagnosis by psychiatrists, in the sense that this label was seen as the creation of an outside authority, rather than of a member of the professional community. Therefore, once acquired, it became very resistant to change. To contribute to a discussion group, a former Soviet Union person has somehow to internalise 'Authority' — only then is it possible to act. Such an uneasiness in dealings with authority probably results from the fact that former Soviet Union persons had little first-hand experience of that situation. This background allows one to understand the professional arrangements which still operate in former Soviet Union hospitals and mental health services. Ways of working together for clinical tasks tend to operate not through the richness of experience within the group, but through accepting the existing hierarchical order and obsequiousness of behaviour as the norm.

In the training of psychiatrists, clinical supervision is transmitted only down the power lines of administrative hierarchy. A training programme for psychiatric nurses in the

Ukraine by Z Mihova and A Fercheva hoped to enable nurses to make diagnoses and practise professional decision-making, in parallel to doctors. However, the beliefs of those nurses who received the training conflicted in a fundamental way with the philosophical underpinnings of present-day psychiatry with its move to community care, needs assessment, and case management. Delegating authority cannot happen if those who are supposed to do this have never actually had any authority.

Visualised in this way, the psychiatric scene in Eastern Europe offers endless opportunities for improvement. On the other hand, the power hierarchies, doctrinal clichés, or tokens of academic significance which are so often mistaken there for authority may well prove resistant to it. Yet as they do change, imperceptibly at first, new forms of human communication and new professional procedures will surely contribute to preventing any reoccurrence of the political abuse of psychiatry.

FURTHER READING

Convulsive therapy

Fink M. Impact of the anti-psychiatry movement on the revival of ECT in the US. *Psychiatric Clinics N.A.* 1991; **14**:793–801.

Fink M. Prejudice against ECT: Competition with psychological philosophies as a contribution to its stigma. *Convulsive Therapy.* 1997; **13**:253–265.

Fink M. *Electroshock: Restoring the Mind.* New York: Oxford University Press; 1999.

Group for the Advancement of Psychiatry (GAP). *Shock Therapy.* Report No. 1. Topeka, KS. (Quoted in full in Fink, 1979, p. 14.)

Shorter E. *A History of Psychiatry.* New York: John Wiley & Sons; 1997.

Psychiatric aspects of pain

Melzack R, Wall PD. *The Challenge of Pain.* London: Penguin Books; 1996.

DSM classification

A more detailed history of DSM between 1952 and 1994, with the prominent American psychiatrists shaping it, is found in: Shorter E. *A History of Psychiatry.* New York: John Wiley & Sons; 1997: 298–305.

Another very comprehensive account of the DSM system is found in the introduction to: American Psychiatric Association. *The Diagnostic and Statistical Manual of Mental Disorders*, 3rd edn, revised. Washington, DC: American Psychiatric Association; 1987: xvii–xxvii.

A third article by Mitchell Wilson, (DSM–III and the transformation of American psychiatry. *American Journal of Psychiatry.* 1993; **150**:399–410), vividly describes the events and prime actors in the 1970s that led to such a great change in the way American psychiatrists thought and felt about their profession.

Mental retardation

Alaszewski A. The development of policy for the mentally handicapped since the Second World War: an introduction. *Oxford Review of Education.* 1983; **9**:227–231.

Atkinson D, Jackson M, Walmsley J, eds. *Forgotten Lives: Exploring the History of Learning Disability.* Kidderminster: BILD Publications; 1997.

Busfield J. *Managing Madness: Changing Ideas and Practice.* London: Hutchinson; 1986.

Clarke AM, Clarke ADB. *Readings from Mental Deficiency: the Changing Outlook.* London: Methuen; 1978.

Gabbay J, Webster C. General introduction: changing educational provision for the mentally handicapped: from the 1890s to the 1980s. *Oxford Review of Education.* 1983; **9**:169–175.

Goffman E. *Asylums: Essays on the Social Situation of Mental Patients and Other Inmates.* New York: Anchor Books; 1961.

Jones K. *A History of the Mental Health Services.* London: Routledge and Kegan Paul; 1972.

Jones K. *Experience in Mental Health: Community Care and Social Policy.* London; 1988.

Kanner L. *A History of the Care and Study of the Mentally Retarded.* Illinois: Charles Thomas; 1964.

Kevles DJ. *In the Name of Eugenics: Genetics and the Uses of Human Heredity.* London: Penguin Books; 1986.

Morris P. *Put Away: A Sociological Study of Institutions for the Mentally Retarded.* London: Routledge and Kegan Paul; 1969.

Ryan J, Thomas F. *The Politics of Mental Handicap.* Free Association Books; 1987.

Thomson M. *The Problem of Mental Deficiency: Eugenics, Democracy, and Social Policy in Britain, c.1870–1959.* Oxford: Clarendon Press; 1998.

Trent JW. *Inventing the Feeble Mind: A History of Mental Retardation in the United States.* Berkeley: University of California Press; 1994.

Wright D, Digby A, eds. *From Idiocy to Mental Deficiency: Historical Perspectives on People with Learning Disabilities.* London: Routledge; 1996.

Psychiatry in primary care

Cawley R, McLachlan G, eds. *Policy for Action: A Symposium on the Planning of a Comprehensive District Psychiatric Service*. London: Oxford University Press (for Nuffield Provincial Hospitals Trust: 117); 1973.

Goldberg D, Huxley P. *Mental Illness in the Community. The Pathway to Psychiatric Care*. London and New York: Tavistock Publications; 1980.

Hankin J, Oktay JS. Mental disorder and primary medical care: an analytical review of the literature. *National Institute of Mental Health Series D*. No. 5; 1979.

Hicks D. *Primary Health Care*. London: Department of Health and Social Security; 1976.

Kaeser A, Cooper B. The psychiatric patient, the general practitioner, and the outpatient clinic: An operational study and a review. *Psychological Medicine*. 1971; **1**:312–325.

Levitt HN. Communication, cooperation, and education. In: Freeman HL, ed. *Psychiatric Hospital Care*. London: Bailliere; 1965.

Rutz W, Walinder J, Eberhard G, Holmberg G, Von Knorring A-L, Von Knorring L, *et al*. An educational programme on depressive disorders for general practitioners. *Acta Psychiatrica Scandinavica*. 1989; **79**:19–26.

Shepherd M, Cooper B, Brown AC, Kalton, G. *Psychiatric Illness in General Practice*, 2nd edn. (with new material for this edition by M Shepherd and A Clare). Oxford: Oxford University Press; 1981.

Tantam D, Goldberg D. Primary medical care. In: Bennett DH, Freeman HL, eds. *Community Psychiatry*. London: Churchill Livingstone; 1991.

Wilkinson G, ed. *Talking about Psychiatry*. London: Gaskell; 1993.

Wilkinson G. Psychiatry in general practice. In: Stein G, Wilkinson G. *Seminars in General Adult Psychiatry*. London: Gaskell; 1998.

Williams P, Clare A, eds. *Psychosocial Disorders in General Practice*. London: Academic Press; 1979.

Michel Foucault

Digby A. *Madness, Morality and Medicine: A Study of the York Retreat 1796–1914*. Cambridge: Cambridge University Press; 1985.

Foucault M. *Folie et Déraison: Histoire de la Folie à l'Age Classique*. Paris: Librairie Plon; 1961.

Foucault M. *Madness and Civilization: A History of Insanity in the Age of Reason*. London: Routledge; 1965.

Midelfort HE. Madness and civilization in early modern Europe. In: Malament B, ed. *After the Reformation: Essays in Honor of J. H. Hexter*. Philadelphia: University of Pennsylvania Press; 1980: 247–265.

Porter R. Was there a moral therapy in the eighteenth century? *Lychnos*. 1981–82:12–26.

Porter R. Foucault's great confinement. *History of the Human Sciences*. 1990; **3**:47–54.

Porter R. *Mind-Forg'd Manacles: A History of Madness in England from the Restoration to the Regency*. London: Penguin; 1990.

Scull A. *The Most Solitary of Afflictions: Madness and Society in Britain, 1700–1900*. New Haven: Yale University Press; 1993.

Still A, Velody I, eds. *Rewriting the History of Madness*. London: Routledge; 1992.

Post-traumatic stress disorder

Davidson JR, Foa EB, eds. *Post Traumatic Stress Disorder: DSMIV and Beyond*. Washington, DC: American Psychiatric Association; 1993.

Figley CR. Symptoms of delayed combat stress among a college sample of Vietnam veterans. *Military Medicine*. 1978; **143**:107–110.

Figley CR, ed. *Stress Disorders among Vietnam Veterans: Theory, Research and Treatment*. New York: Brunner/Mazel (Brunner/Mazel Psychosocial Stress Series, 1); 1978.

Fleming RH. Post Vietnam syndrome: Neurosis or sociosis? *Psychiatry*. 1985; **48**:122–123.

Friedman MJ, Charney DS, Deutch AY, eds. *Neurobiological and Clinical Consequences of Stress*. Philadelphia: Lippincott-Raven; 1995.

Haley SA. When the patient reports atrocities. Specific treatment considerations of the Vietnam veteran. *Archives of General Psychiatry*. 1974; **30**:191–196.

Mayou R, Tyndell S, Bryant B. Long-term outcome of motor vehicle accident injury. *Psychometric Medicine*. 1997; **59**:578–584.

O'Brien LS. *Traumatic Events and Mental Health*. Cambridge: Cambridge University Press; 1998.

Van Putten T, Emory WH. Traumatic neuroses in Vietnam returnees. A forgotten diagnosis? *Archives of General Psychiatry*. 1973; **29**:695–698.

Zarcone V, Zarcone VP Jr, Scott NR. Psychiatric problems of Vietnam veterans. *Comprehensive Psychiatry*. 1977; **18**:1–53.

Rehabilitation

Donnelly M. The implementation of the law. In: *The Politics of Mental Health in Italy*. London: Routledge; 1992: 81–94.

Minkoff K. Resistance of mental health professionals to working with the chronic mentally ill. In: Myerson AT, ed. *Barriers to Treating the Chronic Mentally Ill*. San Francisco: Jossey Bass; 1987: 3–20.

Paykel ES, Marshall DL. Depression: social approaches to treatment. In: Bennett DH, Freeman, HL, eds. *Community Psychiatry: The Principles*. London: Churchill Livingstone; 1991.

Polak P. A comprehensive system of alternatives to psychiatric hospitalization. In: Stein LI, Test MA, eds. *Alternatives to Mental Hospital Treatment*. New York: Plenum Press; 1978: 115–137.

Presly AS, Grubb AB, Semple D. Predictors of successful rehabilitation in long-stay patients. *Acta Psychiatrica Scandinavica*. 1982; **66**:838.

Stein LI, Test MA. Alternative to mental hospital treatment I. Conceptual model, treatment program and clinical evaluation. *Archives of General Psychiatry*. 1980; **37**:392–397.

Watts FN, Bennett DH. The concepts of rehabilitation. In: Watts FN, Bennett DH. *Theory and Practice of Psychiatric Rehabilitation*. Chichester: John Wiley; 1983: 3–14.

Wing JK, Brown GW. *Institutionalism and Schizophrenia*. Cambridge: Cambridge University Press; 1970.

The Italian psychiatric reform

Amaddeo F, Beecham J, Bonizzato P, Fenyo A, Tansella M, Knapp M. The costs of community-based psychiatric care for first-ever patients. A case register study. *Psychological Medicine*. 1998; **28**:173–183.

Centro Studi Investimenti Sociali (CENSIS). *Le Politiche Psichiatriche Regionali nel Doporiforma e lo Stato Attuale dei Servizi, Mimeo*. Roma: CENSIS; 1984.

Istituto Italiano di Medicina Sociale (IIMS). *L'Assistenza Psichiatrica in Italia: La Normativa e la Diffusione dei Servizi sul Territorio*, Secondo Rapporto (a cura di M. Cozza & G. M. Napolitano), Tab. 37. Roma: Istituto Italiano di Medicina Sociale; 1996.

Ministero della Sanità. *Nucleo S.A.R., Progetto 'Tutela della Salute Mentale' Istituti Psichiatrici Residuali Pubblici* (Tab. 4) e Privati (Tab. 5). Roma: Ministero della Sanità; 1997.

Mosher L, Burti L. *Community Mental Health. Principles and Practice*. New York: Norton; 1989.

Ruggeri M, Biggeri A, Rucci P, Tansella M. Multivariate analysis of outcome of mental health care using graphical chain models. *Psychological Medicine*. 1998; **28**:1421–1431.

Tansella M, ed. *Community-Based Psychiatry. Long-Term Patterns of Care in South-Verona*, Psychological Medicine Monograph Supplement 19. Cambridge: Cambridge University Press; 1991.

Tansella M, Ruggeri M. Monitoring and evaluating a community-based mental health service: the epidemiological approach. In: Smith R, Peckham M, eds. *The Scientific Basis of Health Services*. London: British Medical Journal Publishing Group; 1996: 160–169.

Tansella M, Amaddeo F, Burti L, Garzotto N, Ruggeri M. Community-based mental health care in Verona, Italy. In: Goldberg D, Thornicroft G, eds. *Mental Health in Our Future Cities*. London: Kings's Fund; 1998: 237–260.

Thornicroft G, Tansella M. *The Mental Health Matrix. A Manual to Improve Services*. Cambridge: Cambridge University Press; in press.

Tibaldi G, Munizza C, Bollini P, Pirfo E, Punzo F, Gramaglia F. Utilization of neuroleptic drugs in Italian Mental Health Services. A survey in Piedmont. *Psychiatric Services*. 1997; **48**:213–217.

Psychogeriatrics

A recent international review of psychogeriatricians and services:

Reifler BV, Cohen W. Practice of geriatric psychiatry and mental health services for the elderly: results of an international survey. *International Psychogeriatrics*. 1998; **10**:351–357.

An account of the earliest days:

Arie T. The first year of the Goodmayes Psychiatric Service for Old People. *Lancet*. 1970; **2**:1179–1182. (A commentary and retrospective on this paper is in the *International Journal of Geriatric Psychiatry*. 1995; **10**:927–932.)

A recent comprehensive review:

Royal College of Physicians of London, Royal College of Psychiatrists. *The Care of Older People with Mental Illness: Specialist Services and Medical Training*. London: Royal College of Physicians of London and Royal College of Psychiatrists; 1999.

Good major textbooks include:

Busse EW, Blazer DG. *Textbook of Geriatric Psychiatry*, 2nd edn. Washington, DC: American Psychiatric Press; 1995.

Copeland JRM, Abou-Saleh MT, Blazer DG. *Principles and Practice of Geriatric Psychiatry*. Chichester: J. Wiley; 1994.

Jacoby R, Oppenheimer C. *Psychiatry in the Elderly*, 2nd edn. Oxford: Oxford University Press; 1997.

The back-numbers of the *International Journal of Geriatric Psychiatry* and of *International Psychogeriatrics* provide a good picture of activity and developments.

Forensic psychiatry

Alexander FG, Selesnick ST. *The History of Psychiatry*. London: Allen Unwin; 1967.

Alexander FG, Staub H. *The Criminal, the Judge and the Public*. New York: The Free Press of Glencoe; 1956.

Bowden P. Pioneers in forensic psychiatry. William Norwood East: the acceptable face of psychiatry. *Journal of Forensic Psychiatry*. 1991; **2**:59–78.

Department of Health and Home Office. *Review of Health and Social Services for Mentally Disordered Offenders and Others Requiring Similar Services (the Reed Report)*, Cm2088. London: HSMO; 1992.

Ey H, Bernard P, Brisset C. *Manual de Psychiatric*. Paris: Masson; 1976.

Fitch WL. Sex offender commitment in the United States. *Journal of Forensic Psychiatry*. 1998; **9**:237–240.

Fornari U, Ferracuti S. Special judicial psychiatric hospitals in Italy and the shortcomings of the mental health law. *Journal of Forensic Psychiatry*. 1995; **6**:381–392.

Forshaw D, Rollin H. The history of forensic psychiatry. In: Bluglass R, Bowden P, eds. *Principles and Practice of Forensic Psychiatry*. London: Churchill Livingstone; 1990: 61–101.

Freud S. *Criminality from a Sense of Guilt*. Collected Papers, Vol. IV. London: The Hogarth Press; 1925.

Jones B. *Voices from an Evil God*. London: Blake; 1992. (This book is a biography of Peter Sutcliffe, the Yorkshire Ripper.)

Quen JM. The history of law and psychiatry in America. In: Bluglass R, Bowden P, eds. *Principles and Practice of Forensic Psychiatry*. London: Churchill Livingstone; 1990: 111–116.

Franco Basaglia

Basaglia's principal writings are contained in several edited volumes:

L'istituzione negata. Torino: Einaudi; 1968.

Che cos'e la psichiatria? Torino: Einaudi; 1973.

Basaglia, Ongaro Basaglia F, eds. *Crimini di pace*. Torino: Einaudi; 1975.

Morire di classe: la condizione manicomiale. Torino: Einaudi; 1976.

A selection of Basaglia's writings is available in English in: Scheper-Hughes N, Lovell A, eds. *Psychiatry Inside Out*. New York: Columbia University Press; 1987.

For a general discussion of psychiatric reforms in Italy, see Donnelly M. *The Politics of Mental Health in Italy*. London: Routledge; 1992.

Patterns in Mental Health Care. Copenhagen: Regional Office for Europe, World Health Organization; 1980 contains an assessment of the Trieste model.

Cognitive therapy

Alford B, Beck AT. *The Integrative Power of Cognitive Therapy*. New York: The Guilford Press; 1997.

Beck AT. Thinking and depression. 1: Idiosyncratic content and cognitive distortions. *Archives of General Psychiatry*. 1963; **9**:324–333.

Beck AT. *Cognitive Therapy and the Emotional Disorders*. New York: International Universities Press, Inc; 1976.

Beck AT, Rush AJ, Shaw BF, Emery G. *Cognitive Therapy of Depression*. New York: The Guilford Press; 1979.

Ellis A, Dryden W. *The Essential Albert Ellis: Seminal Writings on Psychotherapy*. New York: Springer Press; 1990.

Rachman S. Trends in cognitive and behavioural therapies. In: Salkovskis P, ed. *Trends in Cognitive and Behavioural Therapies*. London: John Wiley & Sons Ltd; 1996: 1–24.

Rachman S. The evolution of cognitive behaviour therapy. In: Clark D, Fairburn C, eds. *Science and Practice of Cognitive Behaviour Therapy*. Oxford: Oxford Medical Publications; 1997: 1–26.

Salkovskis P. Cognitive therapy and Aaron T Beck. In: Salkovskis P, ed. *Frontiers of Cognitive Therapy*. New York: The Guilford Press; 1996: 531–540.

Scott J. Psychological treatments for depression. *British Journal of Psychiatry*. 1995; **167**:289–292.

Weishaar M. *Aaron T Beck*. London: Sage Publications; 1993:16–85.

Political abuse of psychiatry in the former Soviet Union

Bloch S, Reddaway P. *Russia's Political Hospitals*. London: Victor Gollancz; 1977.

Bloch S, Reddaway P. *Soviet Psychiatric Abuse*. London: Victor Gollancz; 1984.

Bukovsky V. '...*et le vent reprend ses tours: My vie de dissident*'. Paris: Editions Robert Laffont; 1978.

Gluzman S. *On Soviet Totalitarian Psychiatry*. Amsterdam: International Association on the Political Use of Psychiatry; 1989.

Koppers AA. *Biographical Dictionary on the Political Abuse of Psychiatry in the USSR*. Amsterdam: International Association on the Political Use of Psychiatry; 1990.

Mihova Z, Fercheva A. Training in therapeutic nursing. Amsterdam: *Mental Health Reforms*. 1999; **1**:8–10.

Roth LH, Rechetov Y, Regier DA, Keith SJ, eds. The report of the US delegation and the Soviet response. *Schizophrenia Bulletin*. 1989; **15**(4)(Suppl.).

van Voren R, ed. *Soviet Psychiatric Abuse in the Gorbachev Era*. Amsterdam: International Association on the Political Use of Psychiatry; 1989.

1981–1990

1981–1990 CHAPTER 9

Major world events

1982	First miniature magnetophone (the Walkman)
1983	Identification of HIV virus by Luc Montagnier (France) and Gallo (USA)
1984	Edwards and Steptoe achieved the birth of the first test-tube baby from a frozen embryo in Britain
1986	Chernobyl disaster in the Ukraine
1987	Michael Gorbachev issued *Perestroika* in Moscow
1989	Berlin wall fell
1990	Nelson Mandela freed (South Africa)

Major events in psychiatry

1983	The Soviet All-Union Society decided to withdraw from the World Psychiatric Association, on the pretence of 'slander'
1983	New Mental Health Act in Britain
1984	The British Advisory Council on the Misuse of Drugs published a report on 'Prevention'
1988	The transfer of the 'harm minimisation policy line' to Britain was achieved in the report *AIDS and Drug Misuse*
1988	Fluoxetine (Prozac) introduced into clinical use
1988	Kane *et al.* demonstrated efficacy of clozapine in treatment-resistant schizophrenia
1988	A Section in Psychiatry of Old Age in the Royal Australian and New Zealand College of Psychiatrists was established
1989	Psychogeriatrics became an official speciality in the British National Health Service
1990	Maxwell Jones died
1990	The Reed Committee proposed new forms of management for mentally ill and psychiatric offenders in Britain

PSYCHIATRIC EPIDEMIOLOGY

by William W Eaton

The field of psychiatric epidemiology was not well developed prior to about 1975. There were relatively few epidemiological studies of specific mental disorders, and those that existed focused on measuring the extent of these conditions in the population — descriptive epidemiology. Research directed toward understanding the aetiology of disorders — analytical epidemiology — used measures of psychological distress or global impairment, which precluded integration with laboratory and clinical research. The notion of prevention of mental disorders — experimental epidemiology — was the subject of considerable controversy, but there was little empirical research in this area. In the last quarter of a century, however, psychiatric epidemiology has consolidated efforts at measuring the extent of disorders, made considerable progress in suggesting aetiological clues, and is on the brink of a revolution in prevention of disorders. What accounts for such developments?

The most important advance has been in the empirical basis for psychiatric diagnosis. In the latter half of the 1960s, several studies showed that the reliability of psychiatric diagnosis was so weak as to allow the charge, by social scientists like Scheff or psychiatrists like Szasz, that diagnoses were 'myths' or 'ideology'. Empirical work on the methods of making diagnoses, such as carefully structured examinations with rigorous training of diagnosticians, was led by epidemiologically orientated clinicians. It was driven by the need for epidemiological comparisons, as in the US/UK comparative diagnostic study in 1969. Though this study initially implied huge differences in rates of schizophrenia between London and New York, they were virtually eliminated when standard methods of diagnosis were used in both settings. These advances stimulated development of operational criteria for the whole range of psychiatric disorders, which in turn generated assessment instruments directed at a variety of specific diagnostic targets, as well as a nearly fanatical concern for the reliability of diagnosis.

The validity of psychiatric diagnosis was enhanced during this same period by developments in genetic research and in psychotropic medication. Although there had been family and twin studies of psychiatric disorders since the early part of this century, the findings had always been subject to the interpretation that the transmission within the family was cultural, not genetic. Even twin studies are open to this interpretation, since the argument could be made that monozygotic twins are treated in a more similar fashion than dizygotic twins. In the late 1960s and 1970s, however, adoption studies, including one based on a strong epidemiological design in Denmark by Kety *et al.*, presented data which were nearly immune to this interpretation. The effect was to provide credibility for the entire corpus of genetic research, as well as evidence for the validity of the diagnostic process. Likewise, during these decades, there was increasing recognition of the specificity of the targets of new psychotropic medication, again supporting the validity of the diagnostic process.

The utility of specific diagnoses was further enhanced by reviews of research around the world, such as by Dohrenwend and Dohrenwend, which suggested that each disorder had its own specific pattern of association with epidemiological risk factors, and that many disorders found in modern Western settings could also be found throughout the world. There remained many culture-bound syndromes, but even these are sometimes understood as reflecting basic physiological and cultural processes existing in humans generally. The prototypical study is the WHO International Pilot Study of Schizophrenia (IPSS), and its descendants. The IPSS applied the new standardised diagnostic procedures in a variety of settings around the world. In each of these, there was a syndrome that could be reliably diagnosed as schizophrenia. In later studies led by WHO, the incidence rate of schizophrenia was credibly established at about 0.20 per 1000 per year, and the variation in rates of incidence was well within one order of magnitude, suggesting that methodological factors which had threatened previous cross-national comparisons could be overcome successfully.

From descriptive to analytical epidemiology

During the current generation of research, new field surveys took advantage of developments in diagnosis to develop survey instruments in a format which could be administered by interviewers without medical or clinical training. These instruments relied solely on the responses of the subject, and used computer algorithms to construct diagnoses from the answers, taking advantage of the new, explicit operational criteria for diagnoses. Such verbatim instruments had the potential to link field survey diagnoses, made in house-

1981–1990

hold surveys, with diagnoses made in clinics and laboratories by psychiatrists. The Epidemiologic Catchment Area (ECA) study in the United States was followed by the National Comorbidity Survey there. Other research used verbatim instruments from these studies, in translation, in cultures around the world. These instruments were less successful where insight is a principal feature of the disorder. As a result, they did not add greatly to the understanding of schizophrenia or bipolar disorder, even in estimating their respective prevalences credibly. The diagnostic field surveys remained in the descriptive tradition, for the most part, not adding greatly to the understanding of aetiology. But by presenting basic socio-demographic information for a range of specific disorders, the ECA and related surveys provided benchmark data for a wide variety of comparisons. The figure opposite shows prevalence rates for 13 disorders. The high prevalence of phobia (more than one-tenth of the population) was surprising and has stimulated research on this condition. A striking result shown in this figure is the degree to which psychiatric disorders are not treated — less than half receiving treatment, even for disorders as serious as depression, panic, and schizophrenia. This finding led to efforts to increase recognition and treatment of disorders such as depression by primary care practitioners, in whose practices they are most likely to be found (see Chapter 8, p. 240). The ECA study stimulated the field of psychiatric epidemiology generally, providing a paradigmatic or conceptual benchmark as well as a quantitative one.

The enhanced credibility of specific diagnoses, as well as of the tools of diagnostic assessment which had been developed, facilitated the transition from descriptive to analytical epidemiology, which is the hallmark of current research. The focus now is usually explicitly aetiological, directed at the search for clues to causes of disorders. In this context, the most basic tool of analytical epidemiology — the case-control design — is far better understood and utilised than earlier. An example in this generation of research is the large body of work on the effect of disruption in the immediate social environment of the individual — 'life events' — on their risk for onset of depressive disorder. These epidemiological findings were to be integrated into models of depression that included biochemical, ethological, social, and clinical research. Another example is the series of case-control studies showing that obstetric complications heightened the risk for the later development of schizophrenia. These results were to be integrated into neurodevelopmental models of schizophrenia that include studies of brain structure.

Genetic epidemiology

Genetic epidemiology is another area of advance consistent with the newer analytical orientation. At least three specific disorders — autism, schizophrenia, and bipolar disorder— have very strong genetic components, in that monozygotic twins of diagnosed individuals have over 50 times the risk of developing the disorder as the general population. These three have the strongest potential for a simple Mendelian (single gene) model, but several major genes may explain the transmission. Genetic studies have progressed from family, twin, and adoption designs to linkage studies, with the entire genome as the object of search. Many candidate genes or markers have been identified in one or another study, but the results have not been replicated in later work. In the last decade, methods have been developed which permit immortalisation of DNA from a subject, using non-invasive techniques such as a prick of the finger, a sample of hair, or a buccal swab. Statistical methods are quickly evolving to account for the additional chance variation that opportunistic search of huge numbers of genes brings with it.

Risk factors for specific disorders

Efforts in analytical epidemiology have progressed to the point where major risk factors for important specific disorders can be enumerated, including the relative risk as compared to the general population. For example, risk factors for schizophrenia, and their respective relative risks include: (a) genetic inheritance, with a relative risk of 50 or more for monozygotic twins of schizophrenics; (b) obstetric complications, with a relative risk of 2 or more; (c) urban birth, with a relative risk of 2 or more; (d) winter birth, with a relative risk of about 1.1. What remains is the large challenge of understanding how the risk factors interact with each other. For example, is the effect of obstetric complications a common consequence of genetic background for the disorder, or does it represent an independent causal chain? The interaction of risk factors is important in elucidating aetiological pathways and in developing preventative intervention. Further progress will require understanding the entire framework of possibilities for environmental causes, as well as the effects of the genome. Gene–environment interactions will be the area of most interest.

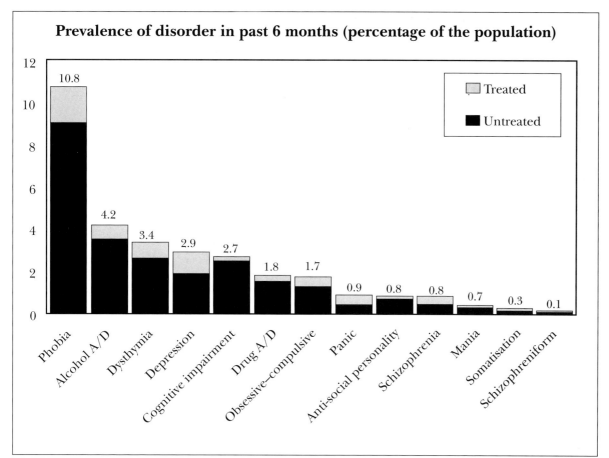

Prevalence of disorder in past 6 months (percentage of the population)

Prevalence of disorder in past 6 months (percentage of the population). Reproduced with permission from Eaton WW. The NIMH epidemiologic catchment area program: implementation and major findings. International Journal of Methods in Psychiatric Research. *1994; 4:103–112. Copyright John Wiley & Sons Limited.*

Conclusion

Progress in analytical epidemiology has set the stage for trials of forms of intervention that will prevent the onset of disorder in individuals who have no signs of it, or only prodromal signs. So far, there has been only limited success at the primary prevention of specific disorders. But enhanced understanding of aetiological possibilities has narrowed the range of potential causes for some disorders. Many such conditions develop over a long period of time, during which presumed genetic vulnerabilities interact with environmental contexts in very precise ways. Informative future epidemiological studies are likely to focus on cohorts of individuals identified at birth, whose DNA has been obtained, and whose growth and development is assessed periodically throughout their lives. However, lack of progress in the identification of important risk factors outside genetics has lowered the yield of information from existing long-term cohort studies. Current information on parameters of risk will suggest how subsamples of the larger cohorts can be identified progressively over time, for more intensive assessment. Many crucial aetiological variables may be impossible to comprehend, however, without systematic intervention trials. Such trials, in combination with genetic information on each respondent, in the context of cohort studies, may offer important advances during the next generation of psychiatric epidemiological research.

LEROS

by John Henderson

The Greek island of Leros, one of the cluster of Dodecanese islands in the Aegean Sea, lies to the south of Patmos. Originally in the possession of ancient Greece, the island was part of the Ottoman Empire from the fifteenth century until 1912, when it was ceded to Italy. After the Second World War, in 1947 it became again part of the Greek State. The island has a total area of 55 square kilometres and a resident population of about 8000.

After the Second World War, psychiatric care in Greece was based on five public mental hospitals, but by the early 1950s, the severity of overcrowding had led to an increase of beds in the existing hospitals and the opening of four additional public mental hospitals, as well as one large psychiatric institution for children and adolescents. The island of Leros was chosen as a location for one of the additional mental hospitals, partly because it offered an apparently cost-effective solution, since it had a large military and naval base, built by the Italians between the World Wars. It was chosen partly also because political leaders wished to create jobs there and foster the economic growth of the island.

The 'Psychopathic Colony of Leros'

In 1958, the 'Psychopathic Colony of Leros' was duly established to provide medical and nursing care to mental patients from the Dodecanese islands and long-stay patients from the mainland. The early residents of the new hospital came first from the large public mental hospital in Athens (Dafni Hospital), while mass transfers from most other of the public mental hospitals on the mainland of Greece took place during the 1960s and 1970s.

In 1965 alone, some 900 transfers took place and by 1971, the resident population numbered 2600 patients, though the original bed establishment had been set in 1958 at 650 places. In 1965, the 'Colony' changed its name to the Mental Hospital of Leros. Eleven years later, following an administrative merger with the 30-bed general hospital, the name changed again to the State Mental Hospital of Leros. As a consequence of these developments, some 60% of the working population of the island were engaged in supporting this hospital — 35% in direct employment and 25% in indirect support as suppliers of goods and services.

The process of selection for the transfer of patients from the mainland to Leros changed little over the years. It was based largely on a designation as 'socially unclaimed', representing those patients who, in their existing hospital, had received no visitors or whose families had shown no concern for them in the course of the past year or two. Inevitably then, the majority who were selected were those with severe disabilities, multiple pathologies, and with long-standing and enduring mental symptoms.

Significantly also, the patient population was an admixture of those with a psychiatric diagnosis and also those with a diagnosis of mental retardation. The necessary separation of these two groups and appropriately planned interventions for them became an important feature of subsequent developments. Thus on this island hospital, some 14 hours travelling time by boat from Piraeus, a mass of patients was accumulated who would normally require trained specialised medical and nursing staff, as well as experienced and competent therapists. They were exposed instead to social isolation in poorly adapted large-scale institutions, in a location unattractive for specialised professionals. Here, they were severely neglected, abandoned, and interned in an island already infamous by its history, past and present, as a place for German prisoners of war in the 1940s and as an internment camp during the Greek civil war.

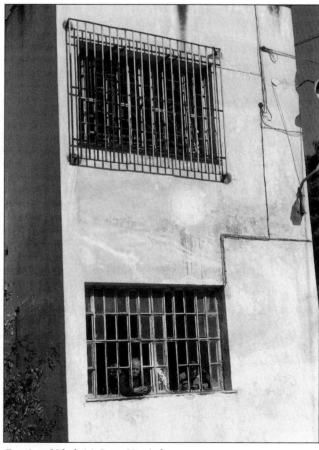

Exterior of Block 16, Leros Hospital.

Recognition of poor conditions

By the end of the 1970s, the first public expressions of concern and misgivings about the patients in this State Mental Hospital began to appear in both the local and national Greek media. In December 1981, at a Greek–French symposium on social psychiatry, a small group of doctors with experience of the conditions on Leros openly denounced the situation there and called for the hospital's early closure.

In 1982, a clandestine documentary film that was shown in Greece and also in France contributed substantially to informing the public of the internment, isolation, and therapeutic abandonment of some 2000 patients, detained in overcrowded and degrading living conditions. The film portrayed vividly the primitive and oppressive conditions of daily existence in vast impersonal dormitories, with dozens of beds crowded one adjacent to the other, living quarters without any semblance of privacy, no day halls or dining rooms, and with only rudimentary toilets and bathing conditions. Clothing was communal and rarely of a kind to give an individual any sense of personal identity.

The staff of the hospital, always lacking in quantity, was even more lacking in quality. For many years, there were but one or two doctors employed, few if any qualified nurses, and very rarely any specialised therapists. Guards or wardens formed the greatest numbers of staff, and were recruited mainly from the resident islanders. They had little education, no knowledge of professional caring or psycho-social rehabilitation, and were expected only to perform the guarding, surveillance, and enforcing duties of the archetypal 'total institution'.

In the early 1980s, Greece embraced the 'Health for All Policy' of the World Health Organization and in 1983, its parliament introduced a national health service. One important component of this policy was the integration of psychiatric care within the general health care system, for which a National Mental Health Policy was promulgated. This was based on the provision of comprehensive community-based psychiatric services, which were intended to replace the nine overcrowded State mental hospitals, unevenly distributed throughout the country.

Membership of the European Economic Community

In 1981, after Greece became a Member State of the European Economic Community, a memorandum was submitted to it by the Greek Government, which sought support for the reform of the psychiatric care system for the whole country. Based on the National Mental Health Policy, the EEC Council provided exceptional financial support to deal with the serious deficiencies of the Greek psychiatric care system. The special programme envisaged developments across the whole country, with new structures and services aimed at the social integration, vocational rehabilitation, and treatment of the mentally ill, as well as improvement of conditions for patients in the State mental hospitals. The Regulation ensured community aid, covering 55% of public expenditure on construction, equipment, and training schemes and 100% expenditure on technical assistance.

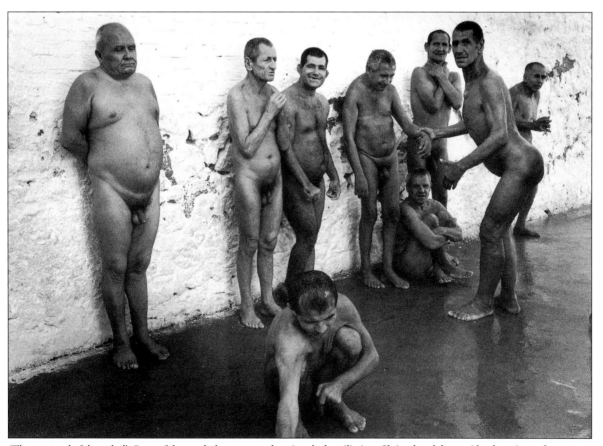

'The courtyard of the naked'. Some of these naked men are undergoing the humiliation of being hosed down with a hosepipe and sponge. This happens up to three times a day, because the patients vomit, urinate and defecate wherever they happen to be. © John Wildgoose.

The adverse national and international publicity surrounding the conditions at Leros State Mental Hospital had played an important part in the realisation of the EEC action. Although central planning for the implementation of the reform programme became heavily bureaucratised, local planning for action on Leros began on the basis of a proposal to achieve the early closure of the hospital and its replacement by the relocation of patients to their home areas, on both the mainland and the Dodecanese islands. It was assumed that 30 hostels, each with 30 places, would suffice for patients to be transferred out of Leros. The remaining patients, composed in the main of the elderly whose numbers were gradually diminishing by natural decease, would be provided for on the island in much improved villa-type and hostel accommodation. However, in the ensuing years, it proved impossible to follow the national plan of psychiatric reform, not only because of the enormous number of projects proposed, but also through their size and complexity and the limited time-frame available.

In Leros, the hospital, now with a reduced population of around 1600 patients, made valiant attempts to accomplish a few of the planned reforms. A residential villa was converted to provide a centre for rehabilitation acitivities, while a guest house project for self-care, a scheme for recruiting foster families, social rehabilitation excursions, and inter-ward social events were tried. Occupational therapy facilities were opened in the township of Lakki, and therapeutic initiatives introduced in the hospital.

Ministry reform programme

In 1987, the Ministry of Health and Welfare, in an attempt to foster wider local knowledge and understanding of the reform programme, convened a European Conference on the theme of 'Deinstitutionalisation and Professional Rehabilitation' on the island, in association with the hospital. However, this meeting actually gave further opportunity for adverse publicity about the disturbing physical and professional conditions of the hospital, which were widely publicised and commented upon in a number of European countries in the following months. The 'shame' and 'scandal' of the Leros State Mental Hospital hit the headlines in Belgium, Denmark, France, Germany, Holland, Italy, and the United Kingdom.

The practical outcome, though, was not significant locally, except in two respects. First of all, the complete cessation of all admissions to the hospital, which had first been mooted as a course of action in 1981, was finally implemented. Secondly, there was the decision to invoke financial incentives for medical staff salaries, to attract a cadre of specialist psychiatrists and ensure effective leadership for the reform plans.

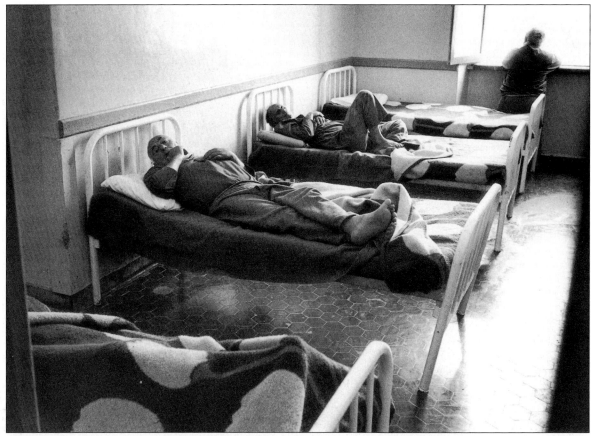

Patients in their usual state. They spend most of their time lying in bed. Some of the patients from Section 2 were tied to their beds.
© *John Wildgoose.*

In 1988, it became obvious to the hospital authorities that the island's population, including the staff itself, did not accept the reform programme, based as it was on a general assumption that the hospital would close completely. Central and local government appeared to be forever debating a regional economic development plan for the South Aegean region, including this island. A study spoke of airports, roads, water and sewage networks, and tourism infrastructure, but achieved little and certainly nothing which took account of any links with hospital reform.

By the end of 1988, the EEC Commission ascertained that within this, the final year of their support, only 20% of the overall approved budget had been absorbed. Although the EEC Council did extend the budget appropriations to 1991, the Commission suspended all action, subject to a total revision of the programme. Renewed planning by the Ministry was required so that the revised programme should include concrete, realisable, and measurable action. This was to ensure the reduction of admissions to the State mental hospitals, as well as intervention to prevent chronicity and promote the return to the community of all categories of patients. In addition, the Commission insisted on the establishment of a system for monitoring and evaluation of the programme, as well as a demonstrable effort to improve radically the conditions of Leros State Mental Hospital. In 1989, the Commission engaged an international group of experts to assist the Greek authorities in reviewing and revising their national plan. A special two-year programme for Leros hospital was approved in 1990, followed by a national programme of reform action.

During the summer of 1990, an intervention team of volunteers from Thessalonika, where the mental hospital had become a leader and exemplar of the Greek reform programme, began practical work in Leros Hospital. The aim was to humanise and de-institutionalise groups of severely institutionalised patients in the vast barrack blocks. This activity of external volunteers from Greece itself was expanded quickly to include similar teams from Italy and the Netherlands, which together made an important contribution to the reorientation and restructuring of the function and practice of the hospital.

The revised programme included plans for the deployment to the hospital of staff from the hostels which were to be established on the mainland. A selection process also began of patients from their 'place of origin', together with a preparation programme for their transfer to the mainland. In all, some 110 patients were transferred to 13 hostels, which were under the management of not-for-profit organisations in each locality.

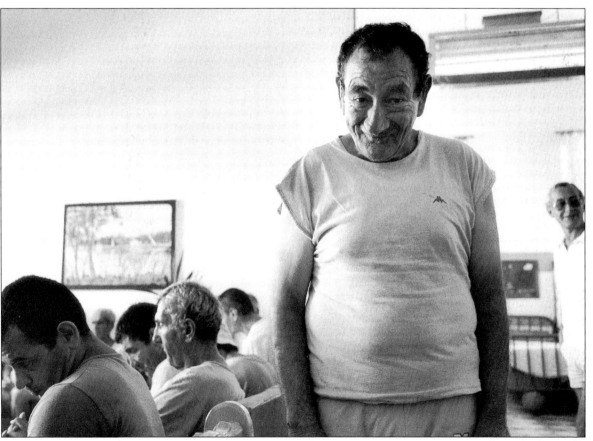

Patients often wander around in a state of deep desperation. They moan, shout and laugh in a hysterical fashion. There is no conversation, no exchange of words, no communication. Most of their movements are repetitive, which is usual for people deprived of affection. © *John Wildgoose.*

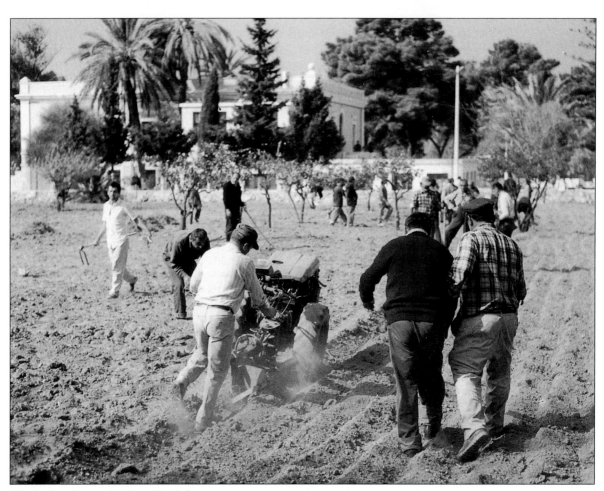

The Gardens Cooperative, Leros Hospital.

In 1991, within the hospital, an agricultural cooperative was finally established as an important outcome of an earlier horticultural activity for patients. This initiative, based on the principles established by the patient cooperatives in Trieste, promoted the principle of paid employment, together with creative activity to build self-respect, autonomy, and the means for patients to earn income to support their living in the community.

By the end of 1991, with due ceremony, a large pavilion for female patients was closed, facilitated by the renovation of residential villas in the hospital grounds. New ideas for apartments and hostels in the island itself took shape and the local council, representing a distinct change of public perception of the reform programme, gave permission for building these. By the next summer, nearly 50 patients were resident in independent family-scale apartments and guest houses, in different locations throughout the island. By now, the local planning authorities, the Ministry of Health and Welfare, and the island council had all perceived the impossibility of achieving a total closure of the hospital. It was finally appreciated that very few patients — less than 3% — had any real chance to return to their families or indeed to their 'place of origin', and that the ambition to achieve their social integration elsewhere in Greece was indeed a false hope.

Therefore, the special programme led to developing and extending rehabilitation activities throughout the entire hospital population. A strict timetable to extend the development of apartments and guest houses in the island was adopted, the community having openly accepted the prospect of many patients regaining their full rights, including pensions, as citizens and residents of Leros. In addition, the action plan programmed the final evacuation of patients from the vast and unacceptable barrack blocks and pavilions, to a series of renovated small wards, villas, and prefabricated hostels, each with a maximum of 10–15 patients.

Although the special programme for Leros was suspended, left in political limbo by reason of national elections and a change of government for some months between 1991 and 1992, extensions of the original expenditure was allowed by the Commission to the end of 1994. After the resumption of active measures to implement the reform, the refurbishment of small wards and villas then proceeded. More professional staff were hired, and the transfer of patients to apartments and guest houses continued. One other large and isolated pavilion, which originally had over 400 patients, was closed finally in May 1994. Throughout this and the following year, rapid and radical changes took place,

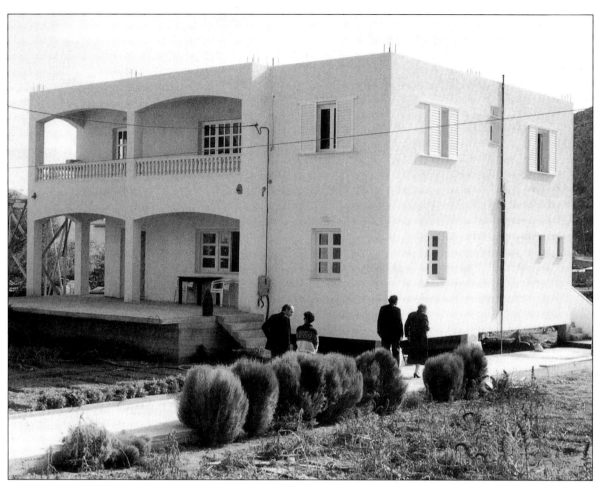

Patients' residential apartments on the island, after rennovation.

creating the conditions for a more therapeutic, rehabilitative, and caring regime throughout the service. These did not have to do with new structures and better living conditions alone, but also meant changing the culture of the institution, and above all recognising and asserting the civil, legal, and social rights of patients, both in and outside the hospital.

Success of the programmes

By the end of 1995, less than 600 patients remained, and the last of the vast barrack blocks finally closed the following year. Some 20 apartments in the island now provided residence for over 100 patients, external guest houses supported over 40, while villas, hostels, and small units in the campus of the hospital provided appropriate accommodation for the remainder.

The EEC financial support was completed by the end of 1995. The State Mental Hospital still dominates the island's economic life, but to a lesser extent than before. The institution has literally opened its doors and significant numbers of patients have found a new life in the community, albeit remaining in a hospital. There is now a regional development plan for Leros, which is part of the EEC structural funding for the region of the Dodecanese in support of further expansion of new social and economic infrastructure. The future will demand such alternative economic development of the island, in view of the hospital's ultimate and inevitable closure in the long term.

The years of experience of the reform programme for the mental hospital on the island of Leros have been instructive in a number of key areas on the process of deinstitutionalisation. The changes required in both public and professional attitudes to the process of transition from institutional to community care demand a lengthy process of public and professional information and education. The reform process itself must be given a realistic time frame, and be provided with a guarantee of the necessary human and material resources. It is also essential that both the manifest and latent functions of care and treatment of the previously closed institution are ensured. This requires a certainty and continuity of commitment to the simultaneous development of comprehensive community-based services. However, the total deinstitutionalisation of a chronic, long-term mental hospital population has not proved to be an achievable objective.

DRUGS AND AIDS

by Virginia Berridge

In the 1980s, the emergence of the human immunodeficiency virus (HIV) brought changes within drug policy in many European and North American countries. The advent of the new syndrome was initially seen as specific to homosexual men, hence the initial acronym GRID or Gay Related Immune Deficiency. In the United States, however, the initial explosive spread of infection amongst gay men, especially in West Coast cities, had given way by the end of the 1980s to a pattern of spread which affected young, poor, and black/Hispanic communities, where drug use and heterosexual transmission were more common. In 1990, the male/female ratio of AIDS cases was still high at 8.5:1, but an increasing proportion of cases was occurring amongst the female sex partners of intravenous (IV) drug users and amongst their children: 1.25% of new-born babies in New York were positive for HIV in 1988. Similar patterns of sharp rises of HIV amongst drug users, with low but accelerating prevalence amongst women and children, were recorded in other countries where the initial spread had been amongst homosexual men. In Europe as a whole, the proportion of AIDS cases attributed to drug use was only 2% in 1983, by 1985 had risen to 15%, by 1988 had reached 34%, and by 1991 almost 50%. Much of this was due to drug-associated epidemics in some southern European countries, but even in northern Europe, where the pattern of spread remained primarily homosexual, the proportion of AIDS cases amongst drug users was increasing. In the then West Germany, for example, the proportion of drug-related AIDS cases rose from 5% in 1983 to 13.2% in 1990.

In a belt of southern Europe covering Spain, southern France, and Italy, and in some countries of Eastern Europe, the key issue was the spread of HIV amongst drug users. This was also true of individual cities in other countries, such as Edinburgh and New York. The virus could spread rapidly because of the needle-sharing practices of drug users. For example, studies of drug users in Bari, Italy in 1982 revealed a 5% prevalence of HIV, rising by 1985 to 76%. HIV was first detected in drug users in Edinburgh in 1983 and by 1985, a prevalence of 51% was recorded. In New York, cases of AIDS amongst IV drug users and their partners began to outnumber those amongst homosexual men for the first time in 1988. Positivity amongst drug users was thought to be as high as 50% at the end of the 1980s, and this in turn created a problem for punitive drug control policies. If drug users were imprisoned, prisons in turn became a major location for both drug use and the spread of HIV. In New York, 20–25% of all new prison inmates in the late 1980s were found to be infected.

In some southern European countries, IV drug use was the predominant means of transmission in the 1980s. In Spain in 1989, 66% of all AIDS cases were amongst drug users, as were three-quarters of the female cases. In Italy, the appearance of HIV coincided with a rise in drug use which some argued had been facilitated by the passing of a law in 1975 legalising possession of drugs for personal use, as well as by limited treatment facilities. In 1989, 80% of cumulative cases were attributed to drug use, if heterosexual contact with users and the children of drug users were included. As in New York, prison rates of HIV were high in Italy and in Spain. In Catalonia (Spain), amongst prison inmates, HIV prevalence was 63.2% amongst drug users and 5.9% amongst non-drug users. Such an association with drug use appeared to lead quite quickly to second-generation heterosexual transmission, and also to increasing prevalence amongst disadvantaged groups and areas.

In Eastern Europe, it appeared that the epidemic started four or five years later than in the West. In some countries — Hungary for example — the initial spread was amongst homosexual men. In others, the majority known to be HIV-positive were drug users — 70% of cumulative cases reported in 1989 in Poland. By the end of the decade, other areas such as south east Asia, Thailand in particular, were seen as potential further 'flash points': numbers of AIDS cases were still low, but the potential for spread was considerable. In Thailand for example, at the end of 1990, there were only 80 reported cases of AIDS, but surveillance testing of different 'risk groups' had revealed more than 235,000 HIV-positive individuals. Two-thirds of these were IV drug users.

Harm minimisation policies

The rapid advent and spread of HIV amongst drug users presented a challenge to existing policies and practices. These varied considerably in severity between countries and were dependent on historical factors. In some countries, AIDS led to the acceleration or introduction of what became known as 'harm reduction' or 'harm minimisation' policies. The UK was a case in point. The moves towards abstention in drug treatment policy in the 1970s had been followed by the 'war on drugs' stance of the Thatcher Conservative government in the early 1980s. But other tendencies in drug policy were also apparent. The 1970s and 1980s had seen the emergence of a new drug 'policy community', which included medical and especially psychiatric personnel, but also encompassed social workers, psychologists, probation officers, social scientists, and members of the drug voluntary sector. One of its objectives was harm reduction, enunciated in the British 1984 Advisory Council on the Misuse of Drugs (ACMD) report on *Prevention*. However, this objective, while widely held in the health policy community, had little acceptability for politicians.

The advent of AIDS and the crisis brought in its train, which began with the discovery of the virus amongst drug users in Edinburgh in 1985, changed this situation. The 1986 McClelland Report on the Scottish situation, for the first time placed the threat of HIV as greater than that posed by drug use. It stated,

"There is...a serious risk that infected drug misusers will spread HIV beyond the presently recognised high-risk group and into the sexually active general population. Very extensive spread by heterosexual contacts has already occurred in a number of African countries.... There is... an urgent need to contain the spread of HIV infection amongst drug misusers not only to limit the harm caused to drug misusers themselves but also to protect the health of the general public. The gravity of the problem is such that on balance the containment of the spread of the virus is a higher priority in management than the prevention of drug misuse".

The situation in Scotland was distinct from that in the rest of the UK, in that Scotland had almost no specialist psychiatric treatment system for drug users on the English model, established in the 1960s. Most drug users were seen in general practice and the role of one such GP, Dr Roy Robertson, working on the Easterhouse estate in Edinburgh, was significant in uncovering the extent of the spread of HIV. There was also a strong tradition of injecting drugs and of repressive police action; police had been confiscating syringes dispensed to Dr Robertson's patients. These factors, it was argued, had facilitated the spread of HIV; prevalence was established by testing blood samples taken during an earlier outbreak of hepatitis B amongst drug users in the city.

The transfer of the harm minimisation policy line to England was achieved in the ACMD's *AIDS and Drug Misuse. Part 1* report published in 1988, which argued along similar lines. The acceptability to politicians and to other doubters of the harm minimisation approach was secured through the medium of research. An evaluation of a number of pilot syringe exchange projects appeared to demonstrate that they did indeed 'work'. The close relationships in the drug 'policy community' between researchers, doctors and medical civil servants meant that the matter was essentially dealt with as a technical scientific one, rather than the highly political issue which it could have become. Harm minimisation became

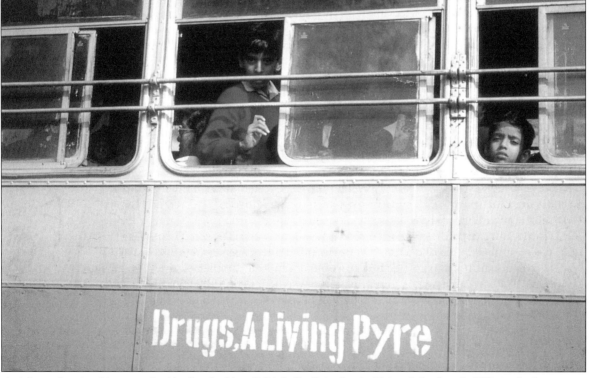

Anti-drugs educational poster on the side of a school bus, Delhi, India. Reproduced with permission from the Wellcome Institute Library, London.

the new policy orthodoxy. In practice, this meant support for syringe exchange, but also a focus on attracting drug users into treatment, rather than leaving them 'out in the cold'. It was seen as important to make contact with the population of potentially HIV-infected drug users. Prescribing methadone, which had tended to fall out of favour because of the increased stress on abstinence-orientated treatment in the 1970s and early 1980s, was back once more on the agenda. The rationale was rather similar to that of the 'competitive prescribing' bait of the 1970s. Methadone this time was the bait to bring drug users into services and away from unsafe injecting and HIV infection. It potentially undercut HIV, rather than the black market, as before. These approaches were characterised as a new 'public health' response to drug use. However, quite what public health meant in practice was unclear. Commentators pointed to a new emphasis on a medical problem of drug use and a new focus on treatment. Such developments had a dual focus — at one and the same time both curative and preventative. As in the 1960s, public health rationales for policy making were grafted onto a specialist psychiatric-led treatment system.

Harm minimisation in Europe

The harm reduction approach became an important policy stance within Europe in the 1980s. The Netherlands pointed out that it had had harm reduction policies even before the advent of HIV. One of the earliest needle exchanges had been set up in Amsterdam, by the Junkies' Union in 1984, in response to an outbreak of hepatitis B. Methadone had become freely available in the late 1970s because of Surinamese addicts in Amsterdam and the city's 'methadone buses' became famous through numerous media presentations. Other Western countries also adopted such measures. In Denmark, public needle dispensers were provided, and in Austria, needles and syringes could be purchased without restriction. In France, there were pilot exchange schemes and unrestricted access to equipment in pharmacies. Poland began a needle exchange scheme in 1989. The use of methadone in treatment programmes also became the new orthodoxy across Europe, even ultimately in countries such as France which had used only very different models of psychoanalytically based treatment before AIDS.

But there were also doubts about the apparently automatic correlation between 'liberal' policies on needle exchange and methadone on the one hand, and the success of limiting the spread of HIV amongst drug users on the other. It was pointed out that syringes had been freely available in Italy since the mid-1970s as a preventative strategy, during a previous epidemic of heroin use and of hepatitis B — yet Italy had one of the highest rates in Europe of HIV prevalence amongst drug users. The difference between the neighbouring Scottish cities of Edinburgh (with high prevalence amongst drug users) and Glasgow (with low prevalence) also led to doubts about the specific impact of particular policies. And other commentators cast doubt on the success of methadone and needle exchange in the Dutch context. It was pointed out that methadone was perhaps less important in limiting the spread of addiction in the Netherlands in the 1970s than were the cultural patterns of use amongst Surinamese in Amsterdam. Yet subsequently, methadone as a policy option to prevent drugs and HIV was widely advocated for other countries; it provided a type of 'magic bullet' solution. The paradox was also that both France, with restrictive policies, and Italy, with liberal policies, had high rates of prevalence. There were also striking similarities in prevalence between Sweden, the leading restrictive country, and the Netherlands, the 'home country' of harm reduction. It seemed that cultural and historico-social factors were more important than the impact of policies in isolation.

Harm minimisation in the United States

Harm minimisation was not the automatic policy option in all countries however. In the USA, for example, there was strong opposition to it. Needle exchange was proposed in New York as early as 1985, and its effectiveness was to be tested through the medium of a randomised controlled trial. In the British situation, the impact of research had taken the issue out of politics; and the authority of science had made it appear simply a technical matter. But the policy situation in the United States was different. The proposed trial was condemned by moral interests, by the law enforcement agencies, but also by black leaders, who saw the provision of needles as potential 'genocide' for their people. Similar arguments had been used against the provision of methadone in the 1960s and harm minimisation remained controversial. Some pilot needle exchange schemes were set up and outreach work also focused on providing bleach for disinfecting 'works', together with advice on risk reduction. US drug policy in general, however, did not move towards harm reduction as a result of AIDS.

AIDS amongst drug users promoted change in a number of different organisational locations. The self-help therapeutic communities were forced to accommodate drug users who became ill and had to deal with harm reduction policies, where previously their focus had been unequivocally on abstinence. Prison, too, was a major location of the response to HIV and drug use. More resources, both in Europe and the USA, were deployed in sending drug users through the criminal justice system and in housing them in prisons than on any other form of management. A World Health Organization (WHO) consultation on the control of AIDS in prisons in 1987 recommended the principle that health care there should be equivalent to such care outside. But in many countries, segregation of HIV-infected prisoners was common in the 1980s. In the UK, the use of Viral Infectivity Regulations (VIR) to segregate HIV-infected or drug-using prisoners was common, although there was considerable variation in practice in the locally run British prison system. Some countries introduced harm reduction measures in prisons, such as making condoms available, as in the Netherlands and Switzerland. In Spain, condoms were distributed and drug users encouraged to stop injecting or at least to clean equipment with the bleach that was provided. The provision of needles, however, was hugely controversial and was not practised anywhere. AIDS was one issue which forced change within the Prison Medical Service in the UK; this became part of the National Health Service in the 1990s rather than, as before, a section of the prison service. Methadone prescribing, rather than 'cold turkey' became available to some prisoners, although there were distinct differences between the English and Scottish prison situations. Scotland recorded a greater number of HIV-infected drug using prisoners, and so a later policy document in 1994 contained a stronger emphasis on harm minimisation in prison than did its English counterpart.

In general, AIDS served to bring about a re-negotiation of the boundaries between medical and penal approaches in policy, and apparently to introduce a policy of greater liberalisation in treatment. A larger number of players were now part of the drug policy arena. But looked at from another perspective, continuity rather than change was the dominant tendency. The new public health approach of the 1980s had strong similarities with the rationales which had animated the changes in drug policy in the 1960s. In some respects, too, AIDS did not demedicalise drug use, but rather re-medicalise it. From yet another perspective, the relationships between penal and medical approaches remained as closely entwined as they had been historically. In the 1990s, drug testing was introduced in many prisons, while pre-trial diversion into treatment, as well as treatment and testing orders, also became options in order to contain the spread of drug use and HIV in the prison system. These moves recalled the long history of attempts at medical compulsion in the drugs area and underlined the complexity of the relationships between medical and penal approaches. As in the 1960s, the 'new public health' stance for drugs in the 1980s and 1990s at one level had, in practice, amplified this compulsionist strand.

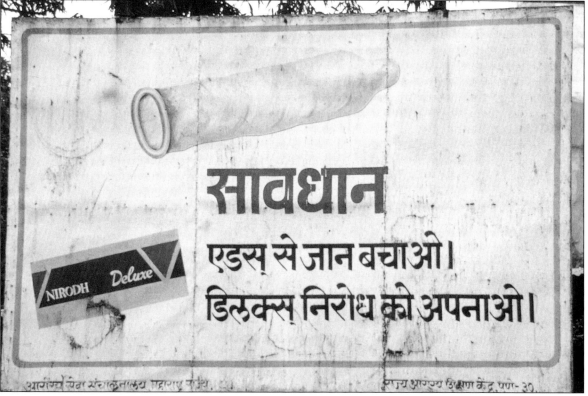

"*Prevent AIDS — Use a condom*", *educational poster, India. Reproduced with permission from the Wellcome Institute Library, London.*

ICD–10: MENTAL DISORDERS CHAPTER OF THE INTERNATIONAL CLASSIFICATION OF DISEASES, TENTH REVISION

by John Cooper

Chapter V of ICD–10 was not published for international use until 1992, but it was during the 1980s that the essential and worldwide processes of consultation and field-testing were carried out. An important prelude to the development of Chapter V itself was an international conference held in Copenhagen in 1982, jointly organised by the Division of Mental Health of the World Health Organization (WHO) and the Alcohol, Drug Abuse, and Mental Health Administration of the USA. This conference reviewed the conclusions of nine scientific working groups that had examined the latest research and developments in classification in their respective areas of interest. The future ICD–10 was kept very much in mind, together with an acceptance of the general policy that differences between it and future versions of the DSM of the American Psychiatric Association, although inevitable, should be kept to a minimum.

This initiative became known as the Joint Project, and it coordinated a variety of studies on standardised methods of interviewing and rating, in addition to other aspects of the classification and diagnosis of psychiatric disorders. In other words, ICD–10 does not stand alone; it is the central member of a family of closely related documents, produced with the aim of facilitating international communication and research (listed in the table on p. 305).

ICD–10 has a different status from that of its predecessors because of the unique efforts put into its development. It will also have a very different fate, because WHO has already stated that it will no longer follow its previous policy of ten-yearly reviews of all the chapters of the ICD. Instead, as new findings emerge that have obvious implications for the classification, it should be possible to introduce changes to limited sections without disturbing the whole.

Necessary properties

The new classification needed to be both acceptable and versatile, since it would have many different types of users, but it also had to follow the basic rules and structure of the ICD as a statistical classification. These required a finite size, and the presence of categories such as 'other' and 'not otherwise specified' alongside the groups of categories with specified meanings. Publications produced during the development process dealt with topics such as theoretical issues in classification, the requirements for an international rather than a national classification, the relationships between Chapter V and the other chapters, options for its general structure, the design of field trials, and prospects for multi-axial versions.

An extensive process of consultation was the first prerequisite, so as to achieve wide acceptability of the final document. One of the main tasks was to ensure that it reflected recent advances in knowledge, without being unduly influenced by current fashions in psychiatric practice or by potentially controversial viewpoints. These may be put forward enthusiastically by experts of the day from wealthy and influential countries, but caution must prevail in the preparation of a classification that has to achieve worldwide acceptability.

A strategy of different versions for different purposes was adopted from the start, accompanied by an equally important principle of making sure that the different versions were kept compatible with each other as they were developed. The longest version, designed for use by clinical psychiatrists and named *Clinical Descriptions and Diagnostic Guidelines*, was the first to be developed in 1992.

The table opposite outlines the consultation process, which started in 1982 and continued until 1986. A first wave of more than 50 experts in many countries were asked to provide first drafts and suggestions about the main sections of the classification, and a second wave of more than 200 experts were involved during 1983 and 1984. Through the World Psychiatric Association, the resulting document was then circulated for further comments to all its constituent associations and societies during 1985 and 1986.

Consultation and development process for ICD–10, Chapter V

1981–2 First drafts — 50 experts

1982–3 First document — 200 experts

1985–6 Circulation by World Psychiatric Association

1987–8 Field trials — 100+ centres six languages

1989 Final version

1990 Adoption by WHO

1992 Publication

Division of Mental Health, WHO Geneva

Dr N Sartorius, Dr A Jablensky

Assisted by consultants, Directors of FTCC, and collaborators in FTCs

---

Need for different versions

The consultation process just described resulted in a draft of the full version of Chapter V, aimed at psychiatrists and other mental health professionals engaged directly in clinical work. Other shorter documents required were:

1. A brief glossary, similar in length to that of ICD–8 and ICD–9, for the main ICD volume that contains all the other chapters.

2. A set of Diagnostic Criteria for Research (DCR–10). These are derived directly from the Clinical Guidelines, but contain more detailed specifications of the numbers and duration of symptoms, in addition to other points that help in the selection of comparatively homogeneous groups of patients for research.

3. A shorter and simplified version for use by health professionals in primary care.

In an international setting, it is particularly important to emphasise the differences between the needs of a clinician and those of a researcher. Lists of detailed but limiting criteria are essential for many types of research, but over-enthusiastic or inexperienced clinicians may be tempted to apply them too rigorously, if the only version of the classification is presented in this form. On some occasions, clinicians need more information than is contained in criteria for research (for instance, when trying to understand a diagnostic concept or an individual patient to whom it might apply). On other occasions, they may have to manage with less (for instance, when faced with urgent decisions about admission or the need for treatment). The policy of different versions for different purposes adopted by WHO keeps to a minimum the misuse of criteria. Clinicians are best served by a narrative account of the clinical concepts on which diagnoses are based, followed by suggestions or 'guidelines' about how to apply the concepts as required. Researchers usually need to select a group of subjects that are as similar to each other as possible, and like all other sets of criteria for research, the DCR–10 are designed to be restrictive in this way. Their use maximises the homogeneity of the group of subjects chosen, but necessarily limits the generalisations that can be made from the results.

The DCR–10 (or the 'green book') is published separately from the *Clinical Descriptions and Diagnostic Guidelines* (or the 'blue book') in a smaller document that contains only the criteria. The descriptions of the diagnostic concepts contained in the blue book are not repeated, since it is assumed that researchers will have it available.

The field trials

First, the Clinical Descriptions and Diagnostic Guidelines, and then the Diagnostic Criteria for Research were put through extensive field trials. This was done with the help of several hundred collaborators in 39 countries. They were coordinated by 12 regional Field Trial Coordinating Centres (FTCC), organised according to the main language of each group. A necessary and arduous preliminary task was the translation of the draft classification into six languages (French, German, Spanish, Arabic, Chinese, and Japanese). This was done by the Directors and Staff of the FTCCs.

More than 700 clinicians conducted more than 15,000 independent clinical assessments of patients using the draft classification, following a simple protocol provided by WHO Geneva. The results were examined for inter-rater agreement and disagreement, but much attention was given to the opinions of the clinicians about whether the categories of the classification were reasonably easy to use and understand, and whether they actually fitted the patients seen. The final draft of the new classification was produced in 1989. A further period of passage through the official processes, committees, and assembly of the World Health Organization was then required before publication in 1992.

Contents

All the categories of ICD–9, or very close equivalents, can be found in ICD–10, but the overall concepts of neurosis and psychosis were not used as basic classifying principles. This is because it has always been very difficult to obtain agreement between psychiatrists about the precise meanings of 'psychosis' and 'neurosis' as concepts, even though the words are commonly used by clinicians more loosely as adjectives in many countries, without causing problems. This last point led to the decision to retain a limited use of the adjectives (psychotic and neurotic) so that those psychiatrists who wish to continue to use these concepts can easily identify those disorders traditionally called neuroses or psychoses. (For instance, in the heading of F40 — 'Neurotic, stress-related and somatoform disorders', and F23 — Acute and transient psychotic disorders'.) The term 'disorder' is used widely, though not exclusively.

Grouping by common descriptive themes or because of evidence of relationships between disorders was used as the main organising principle. However, the broad aetiological groupings of disorders due to physical conditions, drugs, and alcohol were also retained in view of their popularity with clinicians and their importance for public health. Examples of new arrangements resulting from the use of common descriptive themes and relationships are that cyclothymia (F34.0) is placed in affective (mood) disorders (F3) (rather than in the personality disorders), and schizotypal disorder (F21) is placed together with schizophrenia and other related disorders in F2 (again, rather than in the personality disorders).

Clinicians can be reassured that there is nothing strange or controversial in ICD–10. In general, its content will be found to be familiar, since it reflects what was regarded as already established and useful to the many clinicians that advised on its preparation.

The new category of acute and transient psychotic disorders (F23) represents an attempt to recognise clinical concepts that have traditionally been recognised in several countries. There is now sufficient evidence to justify their inclusion, since this is a classification of descriptive disorders, and not necessarily one of diagnoses (using this term to imply that some abnormal processes are known that underlie the presenting symptoms).

The concept of somatoform disorders (F45) has been in the international literature for long enough to now be included in ICD–10, in spite of continuing lack of knowledge about incidence and prevalence of the disorders in this group. Reactions to severe stress and adjustment disorders (F43) have similarly become sufficiently well recognised to justify a much fuller treatment in ICD–10 than in ICD–9.

The two major categories of F8 and F9 are now devoted to disorders of psychological development, together with behavioural and emotional disorders with an onset usually occurring in childhood and adolescence respectively.

The compilers of ICD–10 made it clear from the start that justice cannot be done to the subject of F7 — mental retardation (or 'learning difficulties') — by a comparatively simple single statement about intellectual abilities. This is all that can be included in F7, but as noted later, an additional and specially designed multi-axial system has been provided for clinicians working in this discipline.

Use in primary care

In all countries, a large proportion of persons with mental health problems are dealt with by medical professionals in the primary care services, and in many developing countries, this applies even to those with severe psychiatric disorders. A shortened and simplified version of ICD–10 was therefore prepared and field-tested with the requirements of primary care workers in mind. It has only 24 categories, and is presented in a way that combines a brief description of the main clinical features that allow disorders to be identified, with a set of reminders and guiding comments on the management and treatment of both the patient and family.

Multi-axial versions

The success of the ICD–9 multi-axial schema for child psychiatry has led to the production of an equivalent version for ICD–10. A multi-axial schema for use in general adult psychiatry has recently finished its field trials, and a similar instrument for use in mental retardation (or learning difficulties) is nearing completion. It will be interesting to see whether these comprehensive instruments will achieve the popularity that they might be thought to deserve from a purely rational point of view. A number of multi-axial systems have been available in the literature for many years now, but they are largely ignored by general psychiatrists in most countries. DSM–IV follows DSM–III in having a multi-axial format, but even in the USA, the consistent use of all the axes available is by no means universal.

The rest of the family

An important part of the strategy of WHO has been to encourage the widest possible use of ICD–10 as a means of communication between health professionals. With this aim, a number of aids to the easier use and better understanding of ICD–10 are now available (see figure opposite). These include Lexicons of Cross-Cultural Terms in Mental Health and of Alcohol and Drug Terms, a Symptom Glossary for Mental Disorders, and the ICD–10 Symptom Check-List.

Another new feature is the production of 'Fascicles' that bring together those parts of Chapter V and other chapters of ICD–10 most relevant for those with a special interest in psychogeriatrics, headache, and cerebro-vascular disorders. An ICD–10 casebook has also been prepared, demonstrating the use of the Chapter V categories with a variety of patients from different cultures. Two additional explanatory documents that are not members of the official family are 'Understanding the ICD' and a pocket guide to ICD–10 Chapter V.

ICD–10 and DSM–IV

It is a mistake to regard ICD–10 and DSM–IV as competitors, since ICD–10 has to try to meet the needs of the international community of mental health workers, whereas DSM–IV is primarily directed towards the requirements of the members of the American Psychiatric Association. It is inevitable and appropriate that there will be some differences, but since both classifications are widely used, it is to the advantage of everyone if unnecessary incompatibility is avoided. With this aim, as both ICD–10 and DSM–IV approached the final stages of preparation, the collaboration of the Joint Project was continued in the form of a number of meetings between 1988 and 1992. At these, the chair-persons and other members of the task forces preparing the various sections of DSM–IV met a selection of WHO advisers for ICD–10. As far as possible, differences between the developing drafts were minimised, for both concepts and text.

Because of the remarkable increase in recent years in the international nature of all aspects of science in general, and medicine and psychiatry in particular, both the classifications had broadly similar contents from the earliest drafts onwards. The collaborative meetings increased this concordance further, and the remaining differences are almost all quite small. In fact, apart from obvious differences in the order of the main sections (which are of no consequence for the way that the categories are used), anyone outside the mental health field will probably have difficulty in detecting any differences between the two. Those variations that persist should be of interest to clinicians, but largely as interesting differences of opinion, rather than differences due to knowledge. This is because both the classifications are based upon the same internationally available literature, and they shared a number of internationally respected experts as advisers.

One such difference of opinion that could not be resolved by discussion is how best to define schizophrenia. There was no disagreement about what are the most typical symptoms by which this syndrome should be recognised, but in ICD–10 these symptoms need to be present most of the time for one month for the diagnosis to be made; in the minimal instance, no other symptoms are required. In contrast, DSM–IV requires the additional presence of either: (1) a prodrome of minor behavioural changes and complaints or (2) a set of residual symptoms, and thus the total duration of symptoms of some sort is at least six months. In other words, the DSM–IV concept of schizophrenia is that of a necessarily long-standing illness. In the absence of any objective methods for measuring the abnormal processes (whatever they may be) that underlie the presenting symptoms of schizophrenia, it remains purely a matter of opinion whether a long or a comparatively short duration is the most useful criterion to use. There are interesting but non-conclusive reasons for both viewpoints.

A second example is the absence of Neurasthenia from DSM–IV — the word is not even in the index. In ICD–10 it must have a place alongside other related conditions (F48.0) because it is a frequently used diagnosis in many countries, particularly China.

None of the other differences that remain are of great importance in clinical practice. This is because the compilers of both the classifications took care to instruct users that when making diagnoses, clinical experience and common sense should always prevail over the rigid application of the criteria and guidelines provided.

Prospects for ICD–11

At the time of writing, the World Health Organization is undergoing a major reorganisation, and until the future policy about the whole of the ICD becomes clear, it is impossible to say what might happen with respect to Chapter V. For the moment, there is a positive need for a further period of years in which the existing classification can be tested and tidied up, preferably by many workers in many different ways. ICD–10 represents a demonstration that a large measure of agreement has been reached between psychiatrists and other mental health professionals world-wide about which disorders they should be concerned with, both in their daily work and in their research.

This is a considerable achievement, but further work is needed to clarify the very different natures of the conditions that have been included under the broad concept of 'disorder'. This was chosen purposefully by the compilers of both ICD–10 and DSM–IV, and defined so as to include virtually anything psychiatrists find of interest. One consequence of this is that some of the disorders now included can be regarded as personal illnesses, whereas others are disturbances that necessarily involve more than one person. Others, such as some of the dissociative disorders and somatisation disorder, are probably better regarded as disturbances of illness behaviour and the sick role. These are only a few examples of the heterogeneity of the contents of ICD–10. A differentiation into sub-groups of various types would be one way of starting the process of trying to improve our understanding of what has been agreed to be important.

NEURO-IMAGING

by David Cunningham Owens

The need to 'see' is a well-trodden path from belief to knowledge. For much of medical history, the 'belief' amongst professionals was that major psychiatric disorders emanated from abnormalities of the brain — or what the early British psychiatrists Bucknill and Tuke described in 1858 as disturbance to its "due nutrition and repose". Swings in medical fashion shifted much opinion away from this view during the first half of this century, though for some psychiatrists, the principle remained non-negotiable. At mid-century, Kurt Schneider wrote that "our concept of psychiatric illness is based entirely on morbid bodily change".

It is only during the last quarter of the twentieth century, however, that the idea of morbid brain change as a substrate for psychiatric disorder has gained sound acceptance, though it would be premature to conclude that this as yet amounts to anything in the realms of 'knowledge'. This shift in both professional and lay opinion has been made possible by the development of new ways of 'seeing' the brain in both its structural 'repose' and its functional 'nutrition'.

The subject will be discussed here from the perspective of schizophrenia, because it was from this field that the early development of imaging research in psychiatry came. It could be argued that it is still within this field that neuro-imaging retains its vitality. However, over the last 20 years, the applications of imaging technology have spread widely, to encompass areas that even those who pioneered the methodology might have had difficulty in anticipating. These conditions include non-psychotic disorders such as anxiety states and obsessive–compulsive disorder. But in terms of using modern imaging methods to unravel the mysteries of how the brain works and to challenge old 'functional'/'organic' dichotomies, schizophrenia remains the exemplar.

Pneumoencephalography

The first attempt to visualise brain structure in life was by the technique of pneumoen-cephalography (PEG), introduced by the American, Dandy, in 1918. Though modified over the years, the method essentially involved the removal of a variable amount of cere-brospinal fluid (or in one or two 'pioneering' instances, all the cerebrospinal fluid), usu-ally via a lumbar puncture. The fluid was replaced with an equivalent amount of gas, most often air. Ascent and distribution of the gas was 'encouraged' by vigorous movement and on a standard X-ray film, this permitted visualisation of the ventricular system and of sur-face characteristics of the brain (figure p. 309, top left). PEG was first applied to the study of schizophrenia by the German psychiatrists Jacobi and Winkler, who in 1927 published an initial report on 19 patients, with a follow-up of a larger sample the following year. Using the suboccipital approach, they reported that the brains of 18 of their original sample were abnormal.

Over the next half-century, approximately 50 major studies applied the technique of PEG to psychiatric samples. Almost half of these studies focused on schizophrenia, and although not unanimous, the findings in this condition demonstrated a remark-able degree of consistency. Overall, around 60% of more than 1800 schizophrenic patients were reported as showing structural brain changes, though the figure was sub-stantially higher in studies which used the lumbar (67.3%), as opposed to the suboc-cipital (48.5%) method.

For reasons which have never been clear, this work failed to inspire other writers. One set of problems were methodological. The technique was impossible to standardise and prone to variations in the way it was undertaken. Of greater importance, though, was the lack of adequate control data. Because of the significant morbidity and a small but definite mortality associated with this method, the American Roentgen Ray Association decreed in 1929 that it was unethical to use normal subjects as controls in studies utilis-ing PEG. This ruling, while undoubtedly justified, had a catastrophic effect on its use in English-language psychiatry. But perhaps most important of all was the fact that psychi-atry's preoccupations at the time were more psychodynamic, taking the search for 'cause' of disorders to the opposite end of the theoretical spectrum. Whatever the explanation, this potentially important body of work, no matter how flawed, was ignored to a degree that was entirely unjustified.

Computer assisted tomography

The method necessary to take imaging in psychiatric disorders forward was provided in 1973 when Godfrey Hounsfield, working for Electrical and Musical Industries (EMI), at Hayes in London, demonstrated for the first time his technique of computerised axial tomography (CAT). This was the first technique that could safely and non-invasively visu-alise internal body structures, including soft tissues, without the need for injecting con-trast media. Because it was sensitive and had minimal requirements for cooperation by the patient, it was ideal for intracranial imaging, particularly in psychiatric patients.

CAT soon came to mean 'computer assisted tomography', a less restrictive term, though it was in fact widely referred to as 'EMI scanning' in the early days. The initial psychiatric applications were understandably in organic conditions, but the technique was first applied to investigate a traditionally 'non-organic' question by Dr Eve Johnstone and colleagues at Northwick Park Hospital, London in 1976. One issue to interest this group was encapsulated in the title of the full report of this work, published in 1978 — the 'dementia' of dementia praecox. Dr Tim Crow, director of the unit, had become interested in 'age disorientation' — the phenomenon whereby chronic schizophrenic patients tended to give their ages within plus or minus five years of their age at first admission, and hence presumably of their age of illness onset. This might theoretical-ly have been linked to central noradrenergic dysfunction as a 'specific' marker of the disorder, but equally might have been a 'non-specific' feature of evolving dementia in older patients. However, the new imaging technique offered the ideal means of relat-ing the *in vivo* structure of such severely ill, chronic patients to both the results of clin-ical — and specifically cognitive — test data, as well as routine laboratory investigations for dementia. The original sample comprised 17 patients from the long-stay wards of a local psychiatric institution.

The first generation of CT scanners were, in retrospect, crude contraptions, with only a 64 x 64 pixel matrix, which produced a grainy, poorly defined 'impressionist' type of image (figure p. 309, top right). Furthermore, slices were relatively thick, at an average of 13 mm. As the image produced represented an average of the absorption coefficients for all struc-tures within each unit of volume (or voxel), this resulted in imprecise delineation of the boundaries between brain substance and the naturally irregular ventricles. Although such 'partial volume effects' were a major problem, the early pictures did allow the identification of the ventricular system, and hence the possibility of measurement, though even this initially had to be improvised. In the original study, the area of the ventricles at their maximum was measured by counting millimetre squares traced onto paper. None the less, the result was clear. The ventricles of the schizophrenics were significantly larger than those of controls — a finding which was not associated with abnormalities in other investigative markers of dementia, such as routine blood parameters, B12/folate, thyroid function, specific serology, etc. In addition, lateral ventricular size in the patients correlated with general cognitive performance, which in its turn was related to 'negative' features of schizophrenia.

This relatively small investigation was to prove seminal. Although it was three years before the original finding was replicated (by Weinberger *et al.* at the National Institute of Mental Health in Washington), several hundred studies of CT findings in schizophrenia have now been published, over 50 of which represent good quality, controlled investigations. Lateral ventricular enlargement as a correlate of schizophrenia is now one of the most robust findings in biological psychiatry. It is not, however, a unanimous finding. Some of this variation can be explained by the clinical heterogeneity of patient samples, but it also undoubtedly reflects an unexpected consequence of the technique — its sensitivity. Rather than freeing us from the need to pay attention to the characteristics of control subjects, CT soon threw up the crucial impact of this aspect of design on detailed measurement studies of this type.

It was clear from the start that such a finding has two possible — and opposite — explanations. The first is that ventricular enlargement results from the loss or atrophy of originally sound cerebral substrate; the second is that some part of the cerebral substrate has failed to develop properly. In other words, either the illness promotes the changes or the changes promote the illness. This apparently simple choice was in fact a difficult one, largely because of the relative rarity of first-episode cases of schizophrenia and the very long time-scales necessary for subjects to enter the period of maximal risk. Population-based studies were clearly impractical. Furthermore, CT was not the ideal method to unravel the question. Despite its sensitivity and the great improvement in resolution that was produced within a few years of its introduction (figure opposite, bottom left), its non-invasive application did not allow for a detailed distinction between grey and white matter, such that the localisation of underlying pathology was impossible. Since the procedure also involved exposure to ionising radiation, there were continuing doubts about its safety, especially with repeat examinations.

A further difficulty was that the technology only permitted an *inference* about abnormalities of volume obtained from changes in *area* measures of the lateral ventricular system at its largest (the ventricular-brain ratio, or VBR). For the first decade of *in vivo* brain imaging research, the technology did not exist for simultaneous imaging of contiguous 'slices' that were thin enough (i.e. 1–2 mm) to allow construction of 'near-life' volumetric models. A small number of studies on first-episode schizophrenic patients did tend to support the view that structural changes were present at the onset of illness. However, the standardisation problems, especially for repeat scans, were such that the issue could never be adequately decided.

Magnetic resonance imaging

By the early 1980s, CT was rapidly being supplanted as the method of choice for *in vivo* structural brain imaging by new and powerful developments. The first was the new technique of magnetic resonance imaging (MRI). This was initially known as 'nuclear magnetic resonance' (or NMR) imaging, though this term was modified to avoid confusion with other, controversial applications of the word 'nuclear'. The physical phenomenon of magnetic resonance was first demonstrated by Purcell as far back as 1946 — a finding for which he and Bloch shared the Nobel Prize in 1952. However, it did not have a practical medical application until the engineering of the 1970s allowed the manufacture of stable magnets that were sufficiently large for the study of humans. The clinical development of the technique was spearheaded in Nottingham, where the echo planar method of rapid imaging was devised by Mansfield *et al.*, and in Aberdeen, Scotland, where Mallard's group devised the 'spin'-warp method. The first investigation of cerebral structure in schizophrenia, published in 1984, was however conducted in the United States by Smith *et al.*, with the Northwick Park group following this in 1986.

The other field of innovation was in the development of a new generation of computer hardware and software. This provided sufficient power and sophistication to make possible simultaneous imaging of contiguous slices, along with complex analysis of volumes that approximated closely to real-life anatomy (figure opposite, bottom right).

MRI has now replaced CT as the research tool of choice in studying the human brain *in vivo*. This is mainly because it does not involve ionising radiation, and hence its use

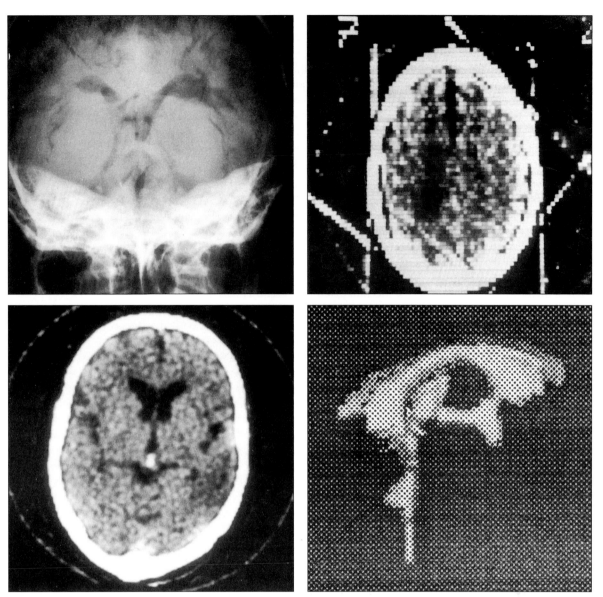

In vivo *morphometric evaluation of the ventricular system: a quarter of a century of progress. (Top, left) Pre-1973: Pneumoencephalography (coronal image) showing lateral ventricles; (Top, right) 1973: Original 64 x 64 matrix water bag CT image of lateral ventricles (axial slice); (Bottom, left) 1977: Improved resolution (160 x 160 matrix) lateral ventricles; (Bottom, right) 1998: Computer generated volumetric reconstruction of total ventricular system (MRI). PEG and CT images courtesy of Dr Evelyn Teasdale, Institute of Neurological Sciences, Glasgow.*

(and repeated use) is not associated with possible adverse health consequences. In addition, it is capable of providing flexible sequences and clear grey–white contrasts, which for the first time permit the evaluation of individual components of cerebral substance as primary sources of the pathology. Ventricular enlargement is only a secondary manifestation of this pathology.

One consequence of this pioneering period of *in vivo* research, in the early 1980s, was a resurgence of interest in post-mortem studies, particularly in schizophrenia. This field had previously been abandoned, in the words of the eminent American neuropathologist Plum, as "the graveyard of neuropathology" because of a lack of results. In suggesting that the brains of schizophrenic patients showed an absence of gliosis, and hence no evidence of a previous inflammatory response, this work supported the idea of changes that were developmental rather than acquired and that pre-dated the onset of illness. Detailed morphometric evaluations of post-mortem material from schizophrenic patients further suggested that the weight of the brain was reduced in this condition; any abnormalities were most likely localised to temporal lobe structures, especially in the region of the parahippocampus.

Recent meta-analysis of some 40 controlled volumetric MRI studies in schizophrenia has confirmed that on average, the condition is associated with volume reductions in whole brain (3%), temporal lobe (L = 6% : R = 9.5%), and amygdala-hippocampal complex (L = 6.5% : R = 5.5%), as well as increases in lateral ventricles (L = 44% : R = 36%).

While it can therefore be concluded that schizophrenia is, in general, a condition associated with structural brain changes, up to now it has not been possible to correlate such abnormalities consistently with clinical phenomena. A further pressing task for the future is clarifying the relationships between such structural changes and gender.

Clear evidence is also now emerging that structural changes (especially in the mesial temporal lobe) can be present *prior* to the onset of illness in those who, because of their family histories, are at high risk of developing schizophrenia. Such changes may not be identical to those in patients without a family history, and are unlikely in themselves to be sufficient to permit the development of psychosis. The detailed nature of their consequences on mental state function is far from being elucidated. None the less, after more than a century, the ability to 'see' the brain in new ways is starting to guide this most enigmatic and controversial of conditions — schizophrenia — slowly along the path from dogma and 'belief' to that knowledge which is the prerequisite of true understanding.

While an understanding of the brain's 'repose' is a crucial piece in the jigsaw of schizophrenia (and other morbid states), what has attracted researchers for decades has been the prospect of observing the 'nutrition'. Mental state phenomena, both normal and abnormal, could then be related to their underlying functional pathways.

Functional imaging

In vivo investigation of brain function was pioneered half a century ago in the USA by Kety and Schmidt, who measured total cerebral blood flow, using inhalation of nitrous oxide. This technique was subsequently supplanted by a 'cleaner' method, based on calculating clearance of the 133 isotope of the inert gas, xenon. This allowed assessment of regional cerebral blood flow (rCBF) in brain areas which corresponded roughly to anatomical lobes. Using this somewhat invasive methodology the Swedes, Ingvar and Franzen, in 1974 described a pattern of diminished functional activity in anterior brain areas in older chronic schizophrenic patients, which they referred to as 'hypofrontality'. However, in view of the methodological limitations of the technology and the highly selected nature of the patients (predominantly older, long-stay, medicated patients with 'negative' symptom profiles) who formed the bulk of the study samples, this remained a controversial concept. The work none the less stands as the first finding of the era of functional imaging in psychiatry.

It was not until the 1980s that the sophisticated technology necessary to study cerebral function *in vivo* became available. Two methods have been utilised.

Positron emission tomography

Positron emission tomography (or PET) requires access to a cyclotron for production of short-acting positron-emitting isotopes. It is therefore expensive and has been restricted to a small number of centres internationally. The application of complex mathematical models has, to a large extent, overcome the early problems of quantitative data analysis. This method has now produced some of the most exciting information available on: (a) aspects of normal brain activity; (b) receptor (particularly dopaminergic) profiles, both in illness and in response to drug treatments; and (c) certain phenomenological characteristics of schizophrenia in particular. It is suggested, for example, that a predisposition to auditory hallucinations may be associated with a failure to activate brain areas in the left middle temporal lobe which are concerned with the monitoring of inner speech.

Single photon emission tomography

Single photon emission tomography (or SPET) utilises radioisotopes of longer half-life and gamma capture technology. Although cheaper and more widely available, it has a less refined methodology than PET, and has been most widely applied in receptor binding studies.

Functional magnetic resonance imaging

The ultimate limitation to both these methods, however, is again the issue of exposure to ionising radiation — something that effectively limits them to single, cross-sectional application. Once again, the emphasis is shifting to magnetic resonance technology. Functional magnetic resonance imaging (fMRI) is based on mapping signal shifts which are associated with conversion of oxy- to de-oxyhaemoglobin. Because it looks at the *effects* of metabolic brain change, rather than the metabolism itself, it was the source of some early controversies. While fMRI seemed able to produce valid images with motor paradigms (e.g. a cortical response to finger movement), it was less clear that this was possible when psychological paradigms (e.g. a word generation task) were the focus of investigation. Now, however, there is an emerging consensus that the method is able to generate images that are both valid and reliable, utilising psychological paradigms that are of value in psychiatric research. The next generation of investigations will focus increasingly on this technology, which is not subject to the limitations of repeated use that have hampered PET in particular.

Magnetic resonance spectroscopy

One further application of MRI is promising, though it has not as yet realised its potential. Magnetic resonance spectroscopy (MRS) is capable of providing an evaluation of the chemical architecture of a defined brain area. It is of particular interest as a method of studying phosphorylated structures such as cell membranes, though other possible uses include *in vivo* pharmacokinetic investigations. The limiting factor to its use in psychiatric research has been the poor spatial resolution that has been possible to date. Other modifications of magnetic resonance technology, such as diffusion tensor imaging, may allow examination of the integrity of specific nerve tracts — and hence of connectivity between anatomical areas. Thereby, they may take us closer to the essential elements of brain activity.

Conclusion

Clinical applications of the principle of nuclear magnetic resonance are transforming our understanding of the human brain, shedding light in dark corners that previous generations of psychiatrists hardly knew existed. However, existing methods need to be refined towards improved spatial resolution. Also, the issue of temporal resolution — the essential next step in exploring the sequences of regional brain activation – has yet to be tackled. For this, other technologies, such as the exploitation of electromagnetic principles, may remain to be fully realised.

For most of the twentieth century, psychiatry has founded its reputation on its specialist knowledge of the nature and management of mental disorders. However, this claim has not been translated into a unified and authoritative position on such fundamentals as classification, aetiology, pathology, risk, course, and prognosis or many aspects of treatment. This has been particularly the case in relation to schizophrenia.

As the second millennium draws to its close, technology is at last offering us the tools to provide, by the application of *scientific* method, those observable facts on which genuine specialist knowledge rests. The tools still remain relatively crude and the hard data are few, but it will not be long before they allow us to settle some long-standing controversies. Was Kraepelin right when he proposed the concept of "natural disease entities" in relation to dementia praecox? Was Bleuler correct in postulating a "group of schizophrenias"? Within the working lives of many present-day psychiatrists, these imaging techniques or their successors are likely to assume routine roles in clinical assessment and the management of patients. The introduction of computerised tomographic analysis will undoubtedly be seen in retrospect as a landmark in medical science that was as profound as the invention of the microscope. The brain is no longer the 'silent organ' of classical medicine, but can now be 'seen' in both its 'repose' and its 'nutrition'. Within the mysteries of this system's incredible organisational complexity will be found the origins of much human suffering.

THE COMING OF AGE OF EXPRESSED EMOTION

by Christine Vaughn

The 'expressed emotion (EE) story' might have appeared in any of the chapters in the second half of this book, since it spans more than 40 years and mirrors in its own development the shifts in thinking and practice which occurred in psychiatry over the same period. The research began in the late 1950s with highly tentative explorations of possible environmental influences on the course of schizophrenia in discharged long-stay male patients. It eventually produced clear statements concerning the role of the family in relapse of schizophrenia, which inspired numerous replications in many different cultures. Encouraged by the consistent results and evidence of mediating mechanisms which offered some protection against relapse, researcher/clinicians initiated controlled family intervention trials with patients and their relatives. These did in fact significantly improve rates of relapse and other measures of outcome. Their success led to training programmes for community nurses, nursing staff, and others working with the seriously mentally ill. Meanwhile, the focus of EE research has shifted from schizophrenia to other psychiatric conditions, and in recent years to a variety of physical illnesses including diabetes, asthma, and heart disease.

The MRC Social Psychiatry Unit

The first of several distinct phases in the history of EE began at the Medical Research Council (MRC) Social Psychiatry Unit in London. There, a multidisciplinary team of researchers led by the sociologist George Brown was asked to consider what happened to discharged long-stay schizophrenic patients. At that time, large numbers of them were being discharged into the community after many years in hospital, and the early relapse and readmission of many raised questions about their little-known home environments. In a refreshingly honest account of his inductive approach and the almost serendipitous 'discovery' of EE, Brown has pointed out that "in 1956 there was little hint in the literature of British psychiatry that the core symptoms of a schizophrenic illness might be importantly influenced by social experience". Nevertheless, early results hinted at influences stemming from relationships within the home, rather than merely some working through of an inevitable disease process. There were links between relapse and the type of living group to which a patient returned, as well as with patterns of contact in the home, which suggested that returning to the close ties of parent or partner might not be beneficial.

The above study was the first of three major projects carried out over 12 years by Brown and his colleagues in an effort to identify more precisely elements in the 'family atmosphere' which might influence outcome in schizophrenia. The landmark second study by Brown, Monck, Carstairs, and Wing, published in 1962, stated for the first time the themes which were to be important in all subsequent research: the association between relatives' emotional attitudes and worsening of the patients' schizophrenic illness; its apparent independence of the severity of the patients' disturbance; and the apparently protective effect of social distance from the involved relative. A distinction was made between 'high-involvement' and 'low-involvement' homes, based on key relatives' verbal and non-verbal responses at interview. The term 'expressed emotion' did not emerge until the next study, which featured new measures of family life developed by Brown and Sir Michael Rutter. This third study included women as well as men, and male as well as female relatives. Its results were striking. The best single predictor of symptomatic relapse of schizophrenia over a nine-month follow-up period was the relative's EE towards the patient and the illness. This was assessed during a confidential tape-recorded interview (the patient not being present) and later scored on scales of criticism, hostility, and emotional over-involvement. Patients returning to 'high-EE' relatives who scored above threshold on any of these scales were three to four times more likely to relapse than patients returning to 'low-EE' homes. The relationship between relatives' EE and relapse was independent of all clinical variables studied, including the duration of illness, the severity of the patient's psychopathology, and any behavioural disturbance. However, regular prophylactic medication and reduced face-to-face contact with high-EE relatives afforded some protection to patients who were considered to be 'at risk' because of their home environments. Patients from low-risk, 'low-EE' homes tended to remain well, whether or not these protective mechanisms were operating.

Schizophrenia and neurotic depression

There was surprisingly little interest in the 1972 report of the third MRC study. It took yet another report — essentially a replication of a replication, by myself and Julian Leff — to generate a wave of enthusiasm amongst other research centres, who then wished to develop and extend the work. The clinical implications of the 1972 paper by George Brown, James Birley, and John Wing were enormously exciting, scientifically. This was especially true of the idea that the relationship between a highly critical, emotional family atmosphere and relapse might be moderated not only by phenothiazine medication, but also by reduced contact between patient and relative. I therefore proposed to extend the EE work by comparing schizophrenic patients with patients suffering from neurotic depression. This would test the original researchers' hypothesis that the emotional responses and reported behaviour recorded by the EE scales were not specific to schizophrenia. Indeed, they might be found in ordinary families. For this, Julian Leff and I streamlined the very long Camberwell Family Interview (CFI) developed by Brown and Rutter for rating relatives' EE. It was possible to demonstrate that the production of criticism about the patient (the main EE component) was independent of the length of interview, thereby justifying the use of an abbreviated version of the original instrument. With the exception of the abbreviated CFI, the techniques of behavioural, family, and psychiatric assessment were identical to those used in the 1972 study.

We obtained nearly identical results to those of Brown *et al.* in replicating the association between relatives' EE and schizophrenic relapse. We also were able to clarify the effects of regular prophylactic medication and low face-to-fact contact, which were identified as important in the earlier studies. Our findings suggested that either of these factors gives a measure of protection against the risks of living in a high-EE home. When they occur together, there is an additive effect, and virtually complete protection against the difficulties of a high-EE environment is achieved. As in the 1972 study, patients from low-EE homes were likely to be well at nine-months follow-up, whatever the patterns of contact with relatives and whether or not they took medication. However, regular medication did appear to confer benefit on this group over a longer follow-up period.

EE research since 1976

This 1976 EE study gave rise to a virtual 'industry' of international replications, concurrent validity studies, and clinical intervention programmes. Undoubtedly, there was great benefit from the progressive refinement of research methods over the years, and the verification of results by the repetition of studies over long periods. Also, the schizophrenia results may well have made clinical sense and offered new hope in an area of psychiatry where hope is often in short supply. We identified the patients likely to be at greatest risk and suggested guidelines for working with them and their families. The controversial nature of some of these conclusions probably also contributed to the paper's impact. In particular, there were provocative statements about the role of medication in the prevention of relapse in schizophrenia, indicating that social rather than clinical factors might account for failures of medication. The implications for the management and rehabilitation of patients were that pharmacological and social treatments must be prescribed together. Clinical support for this view came from later successful attempts in the 1980s to reduce the relapse rates of high-risk schizophrenic patients through a combination of medication, mental health education, and specific family intervention. Spearheading these efforts on both sides of the Atlantic were a number of key figures: Robert Liberman, Ian Falloon, and Michael Goldstein in Los Angeles; Gerard Hogarty in Pittsburgh; Lyman Wynne in Rochester; and Julian Leff, Elizabeth Kuipers, Nicholas Tarrier, and Christine Barrowclough in the UK.

The body of evidence from EE research since the 1976 study has gone some way toward vindicating the much maligned family of the schizophrenic patient, although this aspect of the literature regrettably tends to be overlooked. Psychophysiological experiments by Tarrier, David Sturgeon, and others have confirmed the impression that many relatives of schizophrenic patients exert a *positive* influence, aiding in the patient's recovery and making future relapses less likely. Furthermore, the depression data, interesting in their own right, demonstrated that the attitudes associated with relapse in schizophrenia were not specific to that disorder. Subsequent studies have confirmed that the constellation of responses characterised as 'high-EE' occur in many different cultures and across a variety of diagnostic groups.

In the 1980s, in addition to the schizophrenia family intervention trials carried out in the USA and UK, there were many attempts worldwide to replicate the London EE findings. These were both for schizophrenia and for other conditions, including depressive disorder, bipolar illness, learning difficulties, agoraphobia, obesity in women, eating disorders, conduct and emotional disorders, post-traumatic stress disorder, and alcoholism. Most of these studies obtained positive results. A recent meta-analysis involving an extensive literature search confirmed the importance of EE in the understanding and prevention of relapse in a broad range of psychopathological conditions. Indeed, the mean effect sizes associated with EE for mood and eating disorders were significantly higher than that for schizophrenia.

EE in physical disease

While EE is a major predictor of outcome across a range of psychiatric conditions, its role in physical disease remains to be established. Positive links between relatives' criticism and clinical outcome have been demonstrated for bronchial asthma in children and for Alzheimer's disease. In the latter study, though, EE predicted only an increase in negative behaviour and not a deterioration in other measures of functioning. High levels of relatives' emotional over-involvement have been associated with an increased frequency of seizures in epileptic patients at follow-up; with higher scores of anxiety and depression in women with breast cancer; and with a worse illness course in patients with acute myocardial infarction. However, two major studies of diabetes produced contradictory results. In America, Koenigsberg *et al.* found that relatives' criticism significantly predicted glucose control in patients. No such association was found in a comparable British study, although the authors noted the potential of a reliable standardised interview like the CFI to explore the relationships between cognitive and emotional variables in families. In the 1990s, the relevance of EE for different outcomes is being tested in a diverse range of investigations, both within and without the field of psychiatry.

A predictor of outcome

The EE concept itself and its constituent scales have received increasing attention in recent years. Forty years' research has demonstrated an association with relapse in a wide range of conditions, but why? What exactly are we measuring, and how does it operate? Initially, EE researchers were simply concerned with measuring the *intensity* of the negative emotional response of a relative or key other person to the psychiatric patient's behaviour, when ill. There was no attempt to understand or to *explain* that relative's behaviour. Explanations would involve very different questions. Current studies are examining: the relative's personality and own mental health; the presence and severity of other life stresses; cognitive attributions about the illness; and the existence of different norms across cultures for what is appropriate or inappropriate parenting behaviour. The significance of positive affect, particularly warmth, also warrants further investigation. Warmth is the least reliable of the EE scales and the most culture-bound, but it may have an important mediating role to play in the relationship between criticism and relapse.

The support and care of patients and their families remains a continuing concern. Despite hundreds of English-language papers in the past 15 years, the EE literature has generated little apparent clinical interest at the 'grassroots' level. This is rather puzzling, since there are clear guidelines for how and when to intervene, and the EE-based family intervention courses which are on offer are oversubscribed. In the UK, more than 300 nurses and other professionals have been trained to work with patients and their families. Nevertheless, many say that once trained, they have little opportunity to practise what they have learnt. Their managers expect them to do this 'special' and emotionally demanding work in their own time. The approach differs from that of traditional family therapy in certain important respects: in the aim of therapy, the roles of the family and of the therapist, the function of insight, and the concept of the illness. Yet the principal findings offer a real possibility of lessening the impact of severe illness. This will require more than summary 'high-EE' versus 'low-EE' indices, serving as risk markers for particular outcomes; the mere fact that a relative is high- or low-EE tells you very little. The planning of individualised treatment programmes calls for an understanding of the fuller response profiles and a recognition of family members' strengths as well as deficits. This is the *real* challenge to psychiatrists and other health professionals as the new millennium dawns.

CHILD PSYCHIATRY SINCE THE 1980s

by Rachel Klein

As is true of all fields, child psychiatry has proceeded in incremental steps. The era since the 1980s flourished, in large part, because of contributions made in the 1970s, a decade during which child psychiatry witnessed a major evolution as a result of the scientific work done under the leadership of Sir Michael Rutter. The first comprehensive population survey of 9- to 11-year-olds, carried out in London and the Isle of Wight, which appeared in 1970, addressed major questions that have continued to be of key importance; for example, rates of psychiatric disorders, the role of intellectual development and physical impairment, and specific concern for potential social influences on children's adjustment. This work was tremendously influential, especially since the investigators demonstrated specific continuities of psychopathology over time in their subsequent re-evaluation of the original cohort of children. It was paralleled by similarly important work on the epidemiology of autism (Chapter 5, p. 139). Although serious attention had been given in the 1960s and 1970s to the classification of childhood psychiatric disorders, and some key issues had then been well delineated, such as the distinction between neurotic and conduct disorders, the nomenclature did not parallel the growing clinical knowledge. This situation was altered in the late 1970s with the development of the DSM–III.

Diagnosis

It is not possible to envisage the evolution of child psychiatry in the decade of the 1980s without considering the impact that DSM–III has had on all aspects of child psychiatry.

Up to its publication in 1980, the childhood psychiatric nomenclature consisted of only six disorders, all defined as 'reactions', such as hyperkinetic reaction. This convention was not one of mere accidental or arbitrary semantic usage, but reflected the ethos of the times. The whole scope of childhood behaviour, normal as well as pathological, was conceptualised as the end-product of familial, and in some instances social influences. Major innovations in the DSM diagnostic system, however, irretrievably altered child psychiatry by excluding inferences about antecedents or causal mechanisms, and by providing relatively elaborate definitional standards for these disorders. This approach did not preclude the possibility of pathogenic familial or social experiences, but while keeping such possibilities open, it allowed consideration of other influential factors, without violating diagnostic conventions.

Important as this new nomenclature was, it clearly did not allow discovery of childhood psychiatric disorders. Most of the conditions included in the new manual had been described and even studied systematically before; cases in point are hyperkinesis [renamed attention deficit disorder with hyperactivity (ADHD)], conduct disorder, and infantile autism. Curiously, this work had had little impact on clinical child psychiatry, especially in North America, which in general retained divided loyalties between traditional psychodynamic or broader family models, and devalued the descriptive diagnostic process. At the same time, DSM–III introduced criteria for many new disorders of childhood, causing some consternation about the multitude of options now available to diagnose children with behaviour or anxiety disorders. Fortunately, the advent of the new system coincided with progress in research technology that allowed advances in epidemiology, statistics, and electronic data processing which could facilitate the relatively rapid validation or refutation of the newly defined disorders. Because of its purely descriptive approach to child psychiatry, a unique contribution of the DSM system rests in the ease with which, based on rigorous, empirical findings, diagnoses can be altered to reflect new knowledge without incurring the opprobrium of established dogma.

Epidemiology

The 1980s, therefore, heralded the era when child psychiatrists throughout the world could use a common language — something that had been lacking previously. This development was strengthened by the virtual overlap between the DSM–IV and ICD–10, allowing national diagnostic conventions to give way to an international system. This major event in child psychiatry has led to an explosion of epidemiological studies in diverse countries, and because of common diagnostic standards, the findings can now be compared across countries. Ultimately, this diversity may lead to a better understanding of differential cultural influences in child psychopathology, which may encompass social, familial, and biological differences.

Epidemiological studies since the 1980s have altered the clinical landscape of child psychiatry. Amongst many findings, some key ones are: (a) that major depression, as found in adults, can be identified in adolescents and incurs significant impairment; (b) that anxiety and depressive disorders are not synonymous emotional disturbances with only minor differences in clinical features, since they have different patterns of age of onset and comorbidity; and (c) that comorbidity is not an artifact of clinical status, but is also a feature of psychiatric disorders that can be identified in non-clinical groups of children. In addition, population studies have also indicated that both major depressive disorder and anxiety have considerable diagnostic specificity, as demonstrated by a differential clinical course. Thus, major depression in adolescence is a significant predictor of later depression, but importantly, is not a harbinger of other psychopathology, while on the whole, anxiety disorders predict later anxiety. These epidemiological reports confirmed the general validity of findings obtained from studies of clinical cases of depressed adolescents. The latter findings have put to rest the popular notion of 'masked' depression in children, which was based on undocumented views regarding the development of the expression of mood through childhood. Amongst the anxiety disorders, separation anxiety and social phobia appear to have different natural histories while in contrast, the DSM–III diagnosis of 'overanxious disorder' does not appear to have a specific course. Research findings have not clearly supported the validity of this diagnosis, which has not been retained as a specific childhood disorder in DSM–IV. In other clinical domains, epidemiological studies have noted that ADHD is a risk factor for conduct disorder, and may in fact be a necessary feature for the development of conduct disorder in early childhood. A key contribution of epidemiology is the identification of associated risk factors, and this is emerging as a particularly promising area in child psychiatry.

Treatment

Although prior to the 1980s, parental behaviour was generally held to be the key to child psychopathology, child psychiatric treatment in many industralised countries consisted to a large extent of individual psychotherapy of the child, with little parental involvement. An exception was family therapy, in which the family is considered to be the patient. Most practice was based entirely on articles of faith, and this situation has not changed completely, much of what is professed in child psychiatry still resting on theoretical predilections. However, more rigorous diagnosis, coupled with systematic treatment evaluation, has been a major factor in the slow process of eroding this unsatisfactory state of affairs.

The 'gold standard' of randomised, controlled clinical trials had its beginnings in the late 1950s in child psychiatry, but such investigations remained exceedingly rare. However, the frequency of rigorously designed treatment studies surged in the 1980s, and has continued to this day. A vast literature has appeared, confirming earlier reports of the marked efficacy of stimulant treatment for children with ADHD. Multiple behavioural treatments were developed for this disorder, and were tested systematically. Yet disappointment in this approach has come from findings that such improvement does not generalise to non-targeted problematic behaviour, or to situations in which the treatment is not directly implemented. Moreover, gains do not persist when treatment ceases. Another disappointment has come from much evidence that combining stimulants with behavioural treatment, even if this is intensive and broad, does not offer meaningful advantage over treatment with stimulants alone.

For the first time, the study of treatment of children and adolescents with conduct disorder met with some success, with evidence of some efficacy for social interaction skills training of the child, parent management training, and intensive family treatment that encompasses function in the community, as well as for pharmacotherapy (stimulants and lithium in selected cases). The treatment of major depression, however, provided some surprises. In spite of similarities in clinical presentation across the age-range, trials have failed to document efficacy for tricyclic antidepressants in children or adolescents. In contrast, the SSRI antidepressants appear to provide significant benefit to adolescents with major depression. Encouraging results have also been obtained for cognitive–behavioural therapy and interpersonal therapy in adolescents with depressive disorders. Though controlled treatment studies of children with anxiety disorders were initiated in the 1970s, they were not followed by a consistent research effort, and the therapeutic literature on these disorders remains sparse. Behavioural treatments appear to have efficacy for anxiety, relative to withholding any treatment, but it is not clear that the same is true in comparison with interventions that provide professional attention and care, but which lack the specific approach of the particular treatment under study.

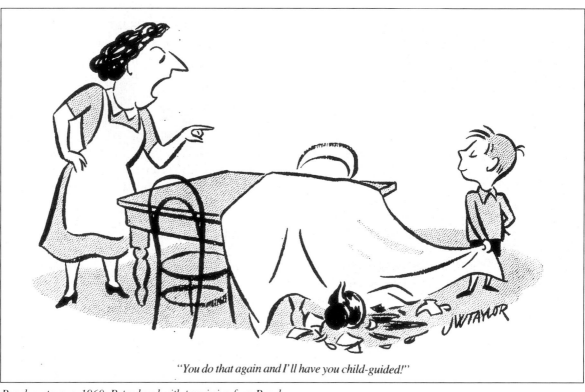

"You do that again and I'll have you child-guided!"

Punch cartoon, c. 1960. Reproduced with permission from Punch.

The unexpected finding of the inefficacy of tricyclic antidepressants in child and adolescent major depression has led to the conclusion that in keeping with the view that children are not miniature adults, treatment outcomes obtained in adult patients cannot be assumed to apply to children with similar disorders. So far, however, this phenomenon appears to pertain to depression exclusively: treatment outcomes do not differ as a function of age in schizophrenia, attention-deficit disorder, obsessive–compulsive disorder, or bipolar disorder.

Environmental factors

Since the 1980s, child psychiatry has also examined factors that may incur dysfunction, but not necessarily a psychiatric diagnosis, such as the impact on children's development of physical and sexual abuse, divorce, chronic medical illness, low birth weight, school environments, maternal psychiatric disorder, etc. There is evidence from work done in Great Britain that urban living is associated with increased rates of disorders of conduct, and that schools with multiple signs of disadvantage may contribute to this pattern. Furthermore, family adversity has also been found to be a contributor to the development and maintenance of conduct problems.

Familial concordance of childhood psychiatric disorders

Prior to the 1980s, virtually no research examined the possible familial transmission of various childhood psychiatric disorders, but there is now a considerable accumulation of data. All those conditions studied (autism, attention-deficit disorder, major depression, anxiety disorders) have yielded evidence of concordance amongst related family members, although the findings are not universally consistent. Yet the interpretation of positive findings is controversial, due to the lack of independence between environmental and genetic characteristics, as well as difficulties in disentangling the influence of parental behaviour and heredity respectively. These ambiguities notwithstanding, it is now generally held that genetic factors play a significant role in the development of diverse childhood psychiatric disorders, though ADHD is the only one for which specific genes have been implicated. Inconsistent initial findings have linked a dopamine transporter gene and a dopamine receptor gene to the disorder, but this subject remains under investigation. More recent studies of behavioural genetics are examining populations identified through twin registers — a strategy that can better disentangle the respective contribu-

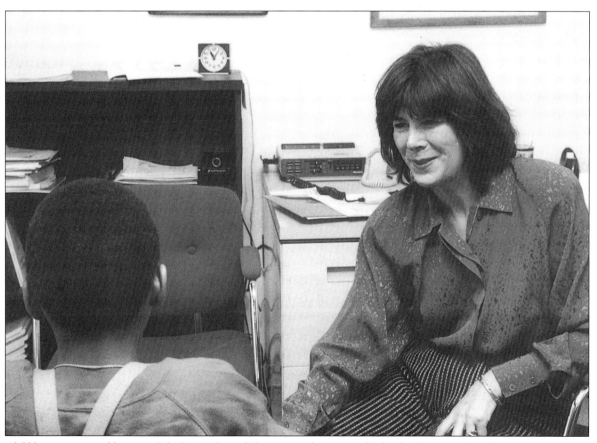

Child being interviewed by Dr Rachel Klein, College of Physicians and Surgeons of Columbia University, New York.

tions of genetic and environmental contributions to phenotypic expressions of childhood psychiatric disorders. This approach, combined with molecular genetics, is a powerful means of informing on the relationships between phenotype and genotype of child psychiatric disorders. This field very likely represents a model for the future of child psychiatric research.

Neurobiological correlates

As with family studies, investigations of the biological features of childhood psychiatric disorders were practically non-existent before the 1980s. This investigative field has closely followed approaches established in adult psychiatry, and procedures that yielded significant results there have been transferred to the study of childhood psychopathology. The most studied disorder has been major depression, where research has been aimed at serotonergic function, sleep architecture, HPA axis function, and growth hormone secretion. Findings for blunted growth hormone response and response to serotonergic challenges in depressed children are fairly reliable, but other biological findings have been inconsistent in drawing parallels between child and adult depression. This may be due, in part, to the fact that age could influence the functions studied, independent of the presence of depression; increasing age may well enhance the ability to detect abnormality in respective functional systems.

Childhood anxiety disorders also have been examined in the context of the biological study of adult anxiety disorders. For instance, respiratory abnormalities in response to laboratory exposure to CO_2 have been linked to adult panic disorder; initial studies report that CO_2 sensitivity also occurs in childhood anxiety disorders, especially in separation anxiety disorder.

Infant temperament, which is generally viewed as being a function of biological regulation, was first examined in the 1950s as an independent contributor to children's development. Yet although the study of temperament has been actively pursued in research on child development, it has received relatively little attention in clinical studies, in spite of its potential relevance to psychopathology.

Brain imaging techniques are being applied to a number of conditions, such as autism, attention deficit disorder, obsessive–compulsive disorder, and childhood schizophrenia. In children, these procedures are often precluded because they incur exposure to radiation, except for MRI whose application has been very limited. Attention deficit disorder/hyperactivity is the best researched of these conditions. Recent anatomical MRI studies report abnormalities in basal ganglia, globus pallidus, caudate, and the posterior portion of the cerebellar vermis, while neuropsychological tests implicate dysfunction of the frontal lobes. These are recent investigative areas with a rapidly evolving technology, and the field has not yet produced a large body of data from a variety of centres.

Conclusion

Since the 1980s, child psychiatry has made phenomenal advances. It has come of age and joined the modern era of systematic study of multiple concerns pertaining to differential diagnosis, treatment, biology, and risk factors, utilising state-of-the-art methodology. At the same time, it is clear that the work has just begun, and that the best is yet to come.

THE INVOLVEMENT OF SERVICE USERS

by Jennifer Newton & Karen Campbell

The theme of user involvement in psychiatry has become a subject about which a great deal is now written. In fact, it is now a legislated duty in Britain to consult users and carers about community care plans, with the result that no mental health strategy, health needs assessment, quality assurance strategy, conference, professional training course, or research application to evaluate services, is wholly credible without some input from the users concerned. Both British government policy documents and professional guidance reports place an emphasis on the value of the user view that would gratify and probably surprise campaigners of even 20 years ago. Similar developments have occurred in other countries.

In the mid-1980s, there were barely 12 independent user-led action groups in Britain, but 10 years later, roughly 350 local, regional, or national bodies were active. This development was stimulated partly by the realisation after a conference of the World Federation for Mental Health organised by MIND (the National Association for Mental Health) in 1985 that users in other countries, particularly Holland, the USA, and Italy, were achieving considerable success in moves to reform or provide alternatives to existing services. International networks of users have continued to help support each other and foster development.

Much of the activity toward greater user involvement initiated by professionals, planners, and managers can be seen to be explainable in terms of changes to the general management of services. There has been an increasing need to be accountable as economic, efficient, and effective. Throughout Western economies, a gradual shift has taken place in public sector services toward 'new managerialism' and the methods used by successful commercial organisations. Amongst the central themes is the premise that providers should be responsive to customers' preferences.

Many of the methods of consultation which resulted have been no more than tokens, however. Inviting one service user to attend a planning meeting to 'represent' the views of service users can provide only limited information. While their view is a valid and valuable perspective, they can rarely claim to represent others in the sense of having been voted into their position by a group of service users whose views they will have canvassed and to whom they will report back. Even if a long-standing service user, with sufficient involvement in local, regional, or national groups to have knowledge of wider views takes part, their voice is one amongst many others. It may well be ignored, if differing substantially from more influential members. However, more sophisticated methods of consultation have gradually evolved, and user groups have capitalised on this for communicating their views.

On an individual level, some methods of service delivery such as care/case management have developed. These aim to increase the level of participation of the individual patient or 'client' in determining the most appropriate long-term support arrangements, or 'package' of community care services. Yet the power to actually leave a service and find another one better suited to one's needs is not the one most often sought by individual writers and lobby groups. Over the period in which there has been a move for increased consumer rights for service users, users themselves have tended to campaign on a rather different level — for recognition for their needs as people. A number of recurring themes are identifiable, all of which can be linked to the need for people to regain a sense of control over their own lives. Psychiatric services are often experienced as compounding feelings of helplessness, and to help counter this, people argue for service providers to treat them:

- *With respect, and in a dignified manner* — e.g. to be interviewed in private, introduced on wards, treated in acceptable surroundings, looked on as a partner in determining the care plan, and for their informed consent to be obtained for treatments proposed;
- *As participants* — in case conferences on their own care, but also through advocacy schemes, patients' councils, and other user groups in evaluating service provision and in planning;
- *As individuals* — needing a service tailored to their particular circumstances in respect of therapy provided, times of availability, location of service delivery, and religious, cultural, or gender needs;
- *As needing to be properly informed* — about the treatment that is advised (particularly when admitted to hospital), general procedures, the medication, their legal rights, the role of the different professionals, and the help that is available after discharge;
- *As capable of making choices and wanting to be offered choices* — between different types of treatment, to negotiate to change their keyworker, to withdraw from medication, seek a second opinion, or be treated by a worker of the same gender.

The need for three types of services or support still features prominently in lobbying activity by the user movement. First, available through nights and at weekends as well as week days — someone to talk to, perhaps somewhere to go. Second, the possibility of talking to others coping with similar mental health problems, and development of mutual-aid. Third, recognition that people with mental health problems have the same aspirations as anyone else, including a desire to find open employment and be a full participant in society, and need help to do so.

In the jargon of the empowerment literature, mental health service users could be seen as being more concerned to have power through having a 'voice', rather than merely the power of 'exit'. However, the very pragmatic nature of most user movements in the 1980s and later has not always been the dominant characteristic. There are concerns amongst those who have retained a more separatist position and anti-psychiatry stance that by incorporating the user view into its own approach, the current managerial agenda has considerably weakened the ability of users to challenge mainstream psychiatry.

'Abolitionists' and 'reformists'

Prior to their expansion in the mid-1980s, user groups could be described very broadly as falling into two groups: abolitionists and reformists. The first were those who saw psychiatry as oppressive, whose members felt they had been mistreated, who saw themselves as survivors rather than patients or users, and who rejected the terminology of psychiatry, as well as many of the treatments used. Also, like many people with physical disabilities, they saw much of their difficulty as resulting from society's response to their distress, rather than the distress itself. For some activists, the goal was patient-controlled facilities of the sort established by Judi Chamberlin in the USA, and which continue to provide a range of services. Not all radical groups were patient-led, however. In Italy there was more of a partnership between users and professionals such as Basaglia (Chapter 8, p. 270). Internationally, some of the most radical proponents of anti-psychiatry came from professionally dominated organisations.

Reformists, on the other hand, were more likely to be people who wished to use psychiatric services, and who might see themselves as having psychiatric problems, but who wished to see an improvement in those services, and a changed relationship between user and provider. The latter would be willing to collaborate with professionals who were also interested in reform (often described as 'allies'), while the former would see such workers as part of the oppressive system. One of the benefits to participants in all these movements was the opportunity to talk with other people likely to be sympathetic to them, and these contributed to the development of self-help groups of various kinds.

The more ideological and radical user groups were developing in the 1960s and 1970s alongside the civil rights movements for women, black people, and gay and lesbian people. They were challenging even in the names they adopted. Some of those in the USA for instance called themselves the Insane Liberation Front, or the Network Against Psychiatric Assault, while Britain had a Campaign Against Psychiatric Oppression. It was not unusual for such groups to feel that their cause was part of a wider civil rights campaign, and to make connections with anti-war and anti-nuclear movements, feminist campaigners, and trade unions. Many were influenced by the writings of sociologists and radical psychiatrists such as RD Laing, David Cooper, Thomas Scheff, and Thomas Szasz (Chapter 7, p. 202). There was a critical analysis of social structure as a whole, and psychiatrists were seen to be in a particularly powerful position of social control, under whose authority large numbers of people who were considered deviant were 'warehoused', secluded, heavily sedated, and exposed to other harsh treatments. Some groups organised angry public demonstrations campaigning against psychosurgery, ECT and aversion therapy, and sometimes organised 'jailbreaks' of friends committed involuntarily to mental hospitals.

Of course, it was not difficult to find evidence to illustrate injustices — of excessive use of seclusion, restraint, medication, or more commonly, confinement in sometimes appalling conditions with no treatment at all, which litigation in the USA helped to publicise and change. These legal actions were instigated by individuals and/or their professional advocates, rather than the patient liberation movement itself, but were encouraged initially by the increase in civil liberties activism, and the growing prominence of the patient movement. There were some landmark cases, largely in support of two main propositions — that the patient has a right to treatment in the least restrictive alternative suitable to their needs, and that the patient who was deprived of his liberty for the purpose of treatment had a constitutional right to receive it. Litigation was a potent force for change in the USA in the 1960s and 1970s, and in Spring 1976, at least 10 States had court orders pending requiring the provision of services in the least restrictive setting.

As psychiatry gradually moved toward a more community-based service, and the user demand for greater involvement became a reality, a tactical dilemma for the more radical groups emerged — cooperation or confrontation? Discussions in consultation meetings tend to feature a reliance on psychiatric terminology and diagnosis, as well as an assumption that people may face a lifetime of dependency (a stance described as 'mentalism' by some patient groups). But such objections could be interpreted as disruptive, hostile, and unhelpful, or aimed at polarising the discussion. By contrast, those willing to take a more conciliatory stance have been more likely to be successfully engaged in the debate. Perhaps not surprisingly, the reformists are now dominating, and even the more militant organisations have less challenging identities — e.g. the National Alliance of the Mentally Ill (NAMI) in the USA.

When campaigners have found powerful allies within the psychiatric profession, their action has often been diverted toward a reformist agenda. The earliest and possibly best known reformer this century was Clifford Beers, who published in 1908 *A Mind that Found*

Itself, about his experiences and maltreatment during two hospital stays in Connecticut. His work attracted the support of Adolf Meyer, one of the foremost psychiatrists of his day, as well as the philosopher William James, who wrote an introduction. Originally intending to stimulate public feeling against mental hospitals, Meyer's influence led Beers instead toward organising the Connecticut Society for Mental Hygiene in 1908, and a National Committee the following year. The aims were to reform mental hospitals, improve facilities for the mentally ill, and increase understanding of the problem. Later, they focused on possibilities for prevention, and were instrumental in the establishment of child guidance clinics. They were influential in numerous other countries, including Britain, where a sister organisation was established in 1927. In both countries, they merged over time with other groups with similar aims and became part of a respected voluntary sector lobby. These organisations were mostly dominated by non-users and retained powerful professional allies.

Conclusion

In the 1990s, there seems to be a move for users to take back some measure of control in these well-established reformist organisations. The numbers of paid staff who are also service users (and able to make this known) has been increasing, particularly at senior levels. The proportion of their Trustees or Councils of Management (such as at MIND in England) who identify as service users has also increased. Lobby groups for other groups of users — most notably those for people with physical disabilities — are again leading the way by changing from identifying as being *for* a particular group to organisations *of* that group. Despite the frequency with which their views are now sought, many service users argue that the changes they hoped for have not fully materialised. Consultation has often been on plans that were already formulated, and as part of information gathering, rather than decision-making. In fact, there are now some indications that policy makers are retreating from full commitment to community care, that biological advances in psychiatry are again gaining prominence, and that the general public and profession are seeing more need for custodial options and compulsory powers to treat. History suggests that we may expect to see the user movement becoming less conciliatory and more radical and separatist again in the early years of the new century.

FURTHER READING

Psychiatric epidemiology

Anthony JC, Eaton WW, Henderson AS. Introduction: psychiatric epidemiology (Special Issue of Epidemiologic Reviews). *Epidemiologic Reviews*. 1995; **17**:1–8.

Brown GW, Harris T. *The Social Origins of Depression: A Study of Psychiatric Disorder in Women*. London: Tavistock; 1978.

Dohrenwend BP, Dohrenwend BS. *Social Status and Psychological Disorder: A Causal Inquiry*. New York: Wiley-Interscience; 1969.

Eaton WW. The epidemiology of schizophrenia. *Epidemiologic Reviews*. 1985; **7**:105–126.

Geddes JR, Lawrie SM. Obstetric complications and schizophrenia: a meta-analysis. *British Journal of Psychiatry*. 1995; **167**:786–793.

Kety SS, Rosenthal D, Wender PH, Schulsinger F, Jacobsen B. Mental illness in the biological and adoptive families of adopted individuals who have become schizophrenic: a preliminary report based on psychiatric interviews. In: Fieve RR, Rosenthal D, Brill H, eds. *Genetic Research in Baltimore Psychiatry*. Baltimore: Johns Hopkins University Press; 1975: 147–165.

Kramer M. Cross-national study of diagnosis of the mental disorders: origin of the problem. *American Journal of Psychiatry*. 1969; **125**(Suppl. 10).

Mrazek PJ, Haggerty RJ. *Reducing Risks for Mental Disorders*. Washington, DC: National Academy Press; 1994.

Robins LN, Regier DA, eds. *Psychiatric Disorders in America – The Epidemiologic Catchment Area Study*. New York: The Free Press; 1991.

Sartorius N, Jablensky A, Korten A, Ernberg G, Anker G, Cooper J et al. Early manifestations and first-contact incidence of schizophrenia in different cultures. *Psychological Medicine*. 1986; **16**:909–928.

Scheff T. Schizophrenia as ideology. *Schizophrenia Bulletin*. 1970; **2**:15–19.

Szasz T. *The Myth of Mental Illness: Foundations of a Theory of Personal Conduct*. New York: Dell; 1961.

Tsuang M, Tohen M, Zahner G. *Textbook in Psychiatric Epidemiology*. New York: Wiley-Liss; 1995.

Wing J, Birley J, Cooper J, Graham P, Isaacs A. Reliability of a procedure for measuring and classifying 'present psychiatric state'. *British Journal of Psychiatry*. 1967; **113**:499–515.

World Health Organization. *Schizophrenia: A Multinational Study*. Geneva: World Health Organization; 1975.

Leros

Bouras N, Webb Y, Clifford P, *et al*. A needs survey among patients in Leros Asylum. *British Journal of Psychiatry*. 1992; **161**:75–79.

European Commission, Directorate General. *V/B/2 Policy Coordination and Information. Final Report on the Implementation of Council Regulation (EEC) 815/84 on Exceptional Financial Support in Favour of Greece in the Social Field. D 6891/V/95*. Brussels: European Commission, Directorate General; 1995.

Mitrossili M. *Study on the Social and Legal Status of Patients in the Leros State Mental Hospital. V/B/2 Policy Coordination and Information*. Brussels: European Commission, Directorate General; 1995.

Tsiantis J. The children of Leros PIKPA. *British Journal of Psychiatry*. 1995; **167**(Suppl. 28):1–79.

Drugs and AIDS

Advisory Council on the Misuse of Drugs. *AIDS and Drug Misuse, Part 1*. London: HMSO, DHSS report; 1988.

Anderson W. The New York needle trial: the politics of public health in the age of AIDS. In: Berridge V, Strong P, eds. *AIDS and Contemporary History*. Cambridge: Cambridge University Press; 1993: 157–181.

Berridge V. *AIDS in the UK: The Making of Policy, 1981–1994*. Oxford: Oxford University Press; 1996.

Blaxter M. *AIDS: Worldwide Policies and Problems*. London: Office of Health Economics; 1991.

Reuband K-H. Drug use and policy in Western Europe. Epidemiological findings in comparative perspective. *European Addiction Research*. 1997; **3**:32–41.

Robertson R. The Edinburgh epidemic: a case study. In: Strang J, Stimson G, eds. *AIDS and Drug Misuse*. London: Routledge; 1990: 86–94.

Strang J, Stimson G, eds. *AIDS and Drug Misuse*. London: Routledge; 1990.

Waal H. Overstating the case. Methodological comments on 'The effects of harm reduction in Amsterdam' by Buning and van Brussel. *European Addiction Research*. 1997; **3**(4):199–204.

Waal H. *Patterns on the European Drug Scene. An Exploration of Differences*. Oslo: National Institute of Alcohol and Drug Research; 1998.

ICD–10: mental disorders chapter of the International Classification of Diseases, tenth revision

Cooper JE. On the publication of the Diagnostic and Statistical Manual of Mental Disorders: fourth edition (DSM–IV). *British Journal of Psychiatry*. 1995; **166**:4–8.

Cooper JE, ed. *Pocket Guide to the ICD–10 Classification of Mental and Behavioural Disorders*. London: Churchill Livingstone; 1994.

Jablensky A. An overview of the prospects for ICD–10. In: Mezzich JE, von Cranach M, eds. *International Classification in Psychiatry: Unity and Diversity*. Cambridge: Cambridge University Press; 1988.

Janca A, Kastrup M, Katschnig H, Lopez-Ibor JJ Jnr, Mezzich JE, Sartorius N. The ICD–10 multiaxial system for use in adult psychiatry; structure and applications. *Journal of Nervous and Mental Disease*. 1996; **184**:191–192.

Janca A, Sartorius N. The World Health Organization's recent work on the lexicography of mental disorders. *European Psychiatry*. 1995; **10**:321–325.

Janca A, Ustun B, Early T, Sartorius N. The ICD–10 Symptom check list. A companion to the ICD–10 classification of behavioural and mental disorders. *Social Psychiatry and Psychiatric Epidemiology*. 1993; **28**:239–242.

Sartorius N. *Understanding the ICD*. London: Science Press; 1995.

Sartorius N, Jablensky A, Cooper JE, Burke JD. Psychiatric classification in an international perspective. *British Journal of Psychiatry*. 1988; **152**(Suppl. 1):3–52.

Sartorius N, Kaelber C, Cooper JE, Roper M, Rae D, Gulbinat W, *et al*. (on behalf of the collaborating investigators). Progress towards achieving a common language in psychiatry; results from the field trials of the Clinical Guidelines accompanying the WHO classification of Mental and Behavioural Disorders. *Archives of General Psychiatry*. 1993; **50**:115–124.

Ustun TB, Goldberg D, Cooper JE, Simon GE, Sartorius N. A new classification of mental disorders with management guidelines for use in primary care. *British Journal of General Practice*. 1995; **45**:211–215.

Westermeyer J, Janca A, Sartorius N. *Lexicon of Cross-Cultural Terms in Mental Health*. Geneva: WHO; 1995.

World Health Organization. *The ICD–10 Classification of Mental and Behavioural Disorders: Clinical Descriptions and Diagnostic Guidelines*. Geneva: WHO; 1992.

World Health Organization. *The ICD–10 Classification of Mental and Behavioural Disorders: Diagnostic Criteria for Research*. Geneva: WHO; 1993.

World Health Organization. *Lexicon of Alcohol and Drug Terms*. Geneva: WHO; 1994a.

World Health Organization. *Symptom Glossary for Mental Disorders*. Geneva: WHO; 1994b.

World Health Organization. *Diagnostic and Management Guidelines for Mental Disorders in Primary Care: ICD–10 Chapter V Primary Care Version*. Seattle: Hogrefe and Huber; 1996a.

World Health Organization. *Multiaxial Classification of Child and Adolescent Psychiatric Disorders: the ICD–10 Classification of Mental and Behavioural Disorders in Children and Adolescents*. Cambridge: Cambridge University Press; 1996b.

World Health Organization. *The Multiaxial Presentation of ICD–10 for Use in Adult Psychiatry*. Cambridge: Cambridge University Press; 1996c.

World Health Organization. *Multiaxial Classification of Psychiatric Disorders in Mental Handicap*. Geneva: WHO; 1998.

Neuro-imaging

Brown R, Colter N, Corsellis N, *et al*. Postmortem evidence of structural brain changes in schizophrenia. *Archives of General Psychiatry*. 1986; **43**:36–42.

Bucknill JC, Tuke DH. *A Manual of Psychological Medicine*. Philadelphia: Blanchard and Lee; 1858.

Farde L, Wiesel F-A, Halldin C, *et al*. Central D2-dopamine receptor occupancy in schizophrenic patients treated with antipsychotic drugs. *Archives of General Psychiatry*. 1988; **45**:71–76.

Hounsfield GN. Computerised transverse axial scanning (tomography): Part I: Description of the system. *British Journal of Radiology*. 1973; **46**:1016–1022.

Ingvar DH, Franzen G. Abnormalities of cerebral blood flow distribution in patients with chronic schizophrenia. *Acta Psychiatrica Scandinavica*. 1974; **50**:425–462.

Jacobi W, Winkler H. Encephalographische studien an chronisch schizophrenen. *Archiv fur Psychiatrie Nervenkrankheiten*. 1927; **81**:299–332.

Johnstone EC, Crow TJ, Frith CD, *et al*. Cerebral ventricular size and cognitive impairment in chronic schizophrenia. *Lancet*. 1976; *ii*:924–926.

Johnstone EC, Crow TJ, Frith CD, *et al*. The dementia of dementia praecox. *Acta Psychiatrica Scandinavica*. 1978; **57**:305–324.

Johnstone EC, Crow TJ, Macmillan JF, *et al*. A magnetic resonance study of early schizophrenia. *Journal of Neurology, Neurosurgery and Psychiatry*. 1986; **49**:136–139.

Lawire SR, Abukmeil SS. Brain abnormality in schizophrenia. *British Journal of Psychiatry*. 1998; **172**:110–120.

Lawrie SR, Whalley H, Kestelman J, *et al*. Magnetic resonance imaging of the brain in subjects at high risk of developing schizophrenia. *Lancet*. 1999; in press.

McGuire PK, Silbersweig DA, Wright I, *et al*. Abnormal monitoring of inner speech: a physiological basis for auditory hallucinations. *Lancet*. 1995; **346**:596–600.

Schneider K. *Klinische Psychopathologie* (translation of 5th edition by MW Hamilton). New York: Grune and Stratton; 1959.

Smith RC, Calderon M, Ravichandran GK, *et al*. Nuclear magnetic resonance in schizophrenia: a preliminary study. *Psychiatry Research*. 1984; **12**:137–147.

Weinberger DR, Torrey EF, Neophytides N, *et al*. Lateral cerebral ventricular enlargement in chronic schizophrenia. *Archives of General Psychiatry*. 1979; **36**:735–739.

The coming of age of expressed emotion

Brown GW. The discovery of expressed emotion: induction or deduction? In: Leff JP, Vaughn CE, eds. *Expressed Emotion in Families*. New York: Guilford Press; 1985: 7–25.

Brown GW, Birley JLT, Wing JK. Influence of family life on the course of schizophrenic disorders: a replication. *British Journal of Psychiatry*. 1972; **121**:241–258.

Brown GW, Monck EM, Carstairs GM, Wing JK. Influence of family life on the course of schizophrenic illness. *British Journal of Preventive and Social Medicine*. 1962; **16**:55–68.

Butzlaff RL, Hooley JM. Expressed emotion and psychiatric relapse: a meta-analysis. *Archives of General Psychiatry*. 1998; **55**:547–552.

Kavanagh DJ. Recent developments in expressed emotion and schizophrenia. *British Journal of Psychiatry*. 1992; **160**:601–620.

Lam DH. Psychosocial family intervention in schizophrenia: a review of empirical studies. *Psychological Medicine*. 1991; **21**:423–441.

Leff JP, Vaughn CE. *Expressed Emotion in Families*. New York: Guilford Press; 1985.

Miklowitz DJ, Goldstein MJ, Nuechterlein KH, Snyder KS, Mintz J. Family factors and the course of bipolar affective disorder. *Archives of General Psychiatry*. 1988; **45**:225–231.

Vaughn CE, Leff JP. The influence of family and social factors on the course of psychiatric illness: a comparison of schizophrenic and depressed neurotic patients. *British Journal of Psychiatry*. 1976; **129**:125–137.

Vaughn CE, Leff JP. The measurement of expressed emotion in the families of psychiatric patients. *British Journal of Social and Clinical Psychology*. 1976; **15**:157–165.

Child psychiatry since the 1980s

Berquin PC, Giedd JN, Jacobsen LK, Hamburger SD, Krain AL, Rapoport JL, *et al*. The cerebellum in attention deficit/hyperactivity disorder: A morphometric MRI study. *Neurology*. 1998; **50**:1087–93.

> This latest report of brain imaging in children with ADHD is the largest to date. It reports abnormality in the cerebellar vermis and reviews findings from previous studies.

Hinshaw S, Klein RG, Abikoff H. Childhood attention deficit hyperactivity disorder: Nonpharmacological and combination treatments. In: Nathan PE, Gorman JM, eds. *Treatments that Work*. Oxford: Oxford University Press; 1998: 26–64.

> Reviews current knowledge concerning the value of parent training, behaviour therapy, and other psychotherapeutic interventions in children with ADHD.

Kazdin AE. Psychosocial treatments for conduct disorder in children. In: Nathan PE, Gorman JM, eds. *Treatments that Work*. Oxford: Oxford University Press; 1998: 65–89.

> A comprehensive overview of the therapeutic literature in children with conduct disorder.

Pine DS, Cohen P, Gurley D, Brook J, Ma Y. The risk for early-adulthood anxiety and depressive disorders in adolescents with anxiety and depressive disorders. Archives of General Psychiatry. 1998; **55**:56–64.

> Anxiety disorders in adolescence predicted the same disorders in adulthood. Of the anxiety disorders, only overanxious disorder predicted depression in adulthood. The others were only associated with later depression. The findings support the distinction made between anxiety and depressive disorders, and suggest that overanxious disorder is a relatively heterogeneous diagnosis.

Rutter M. Family, area and school influences in the genesis of conduct disorders. In: Hersov LA, Berger M, Shaffer D, eds. *Aggression and Anti-Social Behavior in Childhood and Adolescence*. Oxford: Pergamon Press; 1978.

A large-scale investigation that supports the notion that family adversity and poor quality of school environment contribute to the presence of psychiatric disorders in children.

Rutter, M. *Changing Youth in a Changing Society*. Cambridge, MA: Harvard University Press; 1980.

The longitudinal course of the children from the Isle of Wight study who were reassessed at ages 16 and 26. It demonstrates continuities in neuroticism, and conduct problems, and reports on features of the individual and environment associated with stability of dysfunction.

Rutter M. Temperament: concepts, issues and problems. *Ciba Foundation Symposium*. 1982; **89**:1–19.

Provides a historical overview of the relevance of temperament in child development and child psychiatry.

Rutter M, Tizard, J, Whitmore K. *Education, Health and Behaviour*. London: Longman; 1970.

The book summarises the results of the first modern epidemiological study of childhood disorders from a population of 9–11 year olds on the Isle of Wight. It not only reports on rates of dysfunction, but also social and other factors that are related to them.

Ryan ND, Puig-Antich K. Neurobiologie de la dépression chez l'enfant et l'adolescent. In: Mouren-Siméoni M-C, ed. *Les dépressions chez l'enfant et l'adolescent*. Paris: Expansion Scientifique Publications; 1997: 215–233.

A recent chapter on the literature concerning the psychobiology of depression in children and adolescents, from two pioneers in the area.

Sagvolden T, Sergeant, JA, eds. Attention deficit/hyperactivity disorder. *Behavioural Brain Research* (Special Issue). 1998; **94**:1–224.

This special issue presents current models of brain function in ADHD. Discussions are presented on impaired response to reinforcement, neurobiology, and neuroanatomy.

The involvement of service users

Barker I, Peck E. *Power in Strange Places: User Empowerment in Mental Health Services*. London: Good Practices in Mental Health, available from the first author upon request; 1987.

Barnes M. *Care, Communities and Citizens*. London: Longman; 1997.

Brown P. The mental patient's rights movement, and mental health institutional change. In: Brown P, ed. *Mental Health Care and Social Policy*. Boston: Routledge; 1985.

Campbell P. The history of the user movement in the United Kingdom. In: Heller T, Reynolds J, Gomm R, Muston R, Pattison S, eds. *Mental Health Matters: A Reader*. London: Macmillan in association with the Open University; 1996.

Chamberlin J. *On Our Own: Patient Controlled Alternatives to the Mental Health System*. London: MIND; 1988.

Levine M. *The History and Politics of Community Mental Health*. New York: Oxford University Press; 1981.

Read J, Reynolds J, eds. *Speaking our Minds: An Anthology of Personal Experiences of Mental Distress and its Consequences*. London: Macmillan; 1996.

1991–2000

1991–2000 CHAPTER 10

Major world events
1991 Gulf War (Iraq)
1993 Yasser Arafat and Yztak Rabin signed the Washington agreement
1997 Hong Kong handed back to China by Great Britain

Major events in psychiatry
1992 The False Memory Syndrome Foundation formed in the United States
1992 Publication of the World Health Organization's *ICD–10 Classification of Mental and Behavioural Disorders*
1993 Risperidone — an atypical neuroleptic — introduced clinically for the treatment of schizophrenia
1994 DSM–IV published
1994 Efficacy of olanzopine in schizophrenia demonstrated
1994 In France, a new Penal Code finally removed Article 64 of the Napoleonic Penal Code of 1810
1997 Proposals for the compulsory treatment of sex offenders approved in France
1998 Pierre Deniker died

EATING DISORDERS

by Paul E Garfinkel

While anorexia nervosa was described more than 300 years ago, it has been in the last three decades that it has assumed an increased importance, as clinicians and investigators have recognised its prevalence and its alarming rates of morbidity and mortality. Bulimia nervosa was not documented as a distinct but related syndrome until Russell's clinical description in 1979. This section will review some of the important themes in the evolution of the concepts related to these syndromes.

The early years

From its earliest description, anorexia nervosa was recognised to resemble, but also to be distinct from entirely somatic disorders. Thus, in 1694 Richard Morton, the English physician described two patients whom he differentiated from other tubercular individuals as having 'nervous consumption'. Since then, the history of the concept of anorexia nervosa in relation to primary somatic illness can be divided into three phases. Initially, it was described as a psychological disturbance in which starvation was considered to be responsible for many of the prominent symptoms. Then, after the description of pituitary insufficiency in the early part of the twentieth century, there was a period of 25 years of confusion between these disorders. This was followed by a clarification of the differences between primary pituitary illness on the one hand and the hypothalamic–pituitary manifestations of anorexia nervosa on the other, as well as the associated mechanisms involved in their production.

William Gull, Physician to Guy's Hospital, London, gave an Address at Oxford in 1868 containing a short reference to the disorder which he would later name anorexia nervosa. Gull's method of diagnosing what he first called 'hysteric apepsia' included the criteria of both its clinical manifestations and the exclusion of somatic causes of weight loss. Six years later, Gull began to use the term 'anorexia nervosa', and discussed factors he felt were important in the pathogenesis: the 'morbid mental state' and a perversion of the 'ego' relating to a disturbed nerve force. At about the same time, the Paris physician

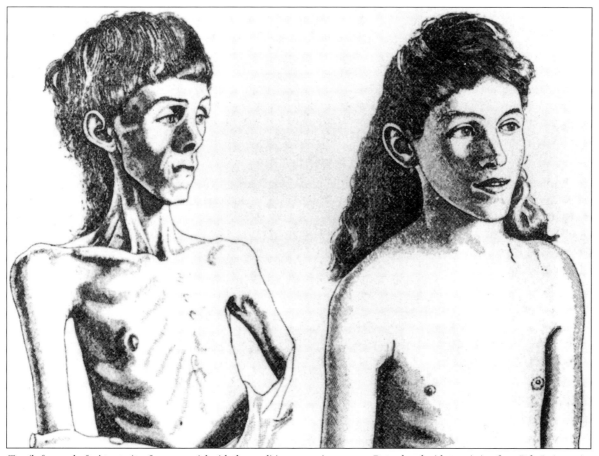

Two 'before and after' portraits of a young girl with the condition anorexia nervosa. Reproduced with permission from Ryle J. Anorexia nervosa. Lancet. *1936; Oct. 17:893–896. © by The Lancet Ltd. Photo courtesy of the Wellcome Institute Library, London.*

Lasegue independently described the disorder. In addition to his detailed clinical descriptions, Lasegue stressed that the patient's active psychological disgust for food leads to the weight loss, and he noted familial involvements in the disorder. Hysterical symptoms were described in seven of the eight patients on whom his reports were based. He termed the disorder 'anorexie hysterique' and, like his contemporaries, viewed hysteria as a predominantly hereditary disturbance of the central nervous system.

During the next few years, anorexia nervosa was clearly defined in the literature. For example, in 1910 Sir Clifford Allbutt described a 'typical' case in his *System of Medicine*, while Dejerine and Gauckler described patients with 'mental anorexia', whose origin was presumed to be purely emotional. In 1895, Stephens had published an autopsy report of an anorexic patient; the brain was described to be 'normal throughout'. Thus, the initial period of attention to anorexia nervosa was characterised by description of the syndrome, of its clinical manifestations, and of its distinction from primary somatic illness.

In 1914, the German pathologist Morris Simmonds described a patient in whom cachexia was associated with destruction of the adenohypophysis. He amplified these observations in papers between 1916 and 1918 which described four more cases, and the condition began to be called Simmonds' disease. In 1930, Smith found that removing the anterior lobe of the rat's hypophysis without injury to adjoining portions of the brain produced an experimental model of Simmonds' disease. He also showed that the hormonal deficiency could be relieved by implanting the pituitary gland. Throughout the 1920s and 1930s, many articles were written on Simmonds' disease, although it seems in retrospect that in a number of instances, these were cases of anorexia nervosa. For example, in 1939 Sheldon estimated that "there are over 80 instances of this misreporting and approximately half of the published cases of anorexia nervosa are indexed under other names", and he described Kylin's 1935 monograph as "a monograph on Simmonds' disease which will always be one of the more important papers on anorexia nervosa". What occurred in the 1930s was a steady rediscovery and ultimately a renaming of the disorder.

Not surprisingly, in view of the confusion between anorexia nervosa and Simmonds' disease, a number of hormonal preparations were recommended as treatment for anorexia nervosa. Because the condition was thought to be due to hypothyroidism, some recommended thyroid hormone. But by the late 1930s, there were reports of alarming degrees of weight loss that resulted from this. Several European investigators attributed anorexia nervosa to 'shrinkage' of the adrenal cortex or to adrenal insufficiency, and this led Reiss to try treatment with corticotrophic hormone; he even based the efficacy of the treatment on a rising output of ketosteroids after its administration. Others recommended as treatment the implanting of a calf's hypophysis in the omentum.

The clear distinction between Simmonds' disease and anorexia nervosa was made in a series of papers beginning in the late 1930s. Ryle, Richardson, and Sheldon independently published reports reintroducing the work of Gull. For instance, Sheldon wrote in 1939:

> "How is it that so many observers — men like ourselves except that so far as they are concerned, Sir William Gull might never have existed — how is it that they universally regard the condition as organic and with almost complete unanimity incriminate the anterior pituitary as the cause of the disease?".

In North America at about the same time, Farquharson and Hyland and McCullah and Tupper wrote on the psychogenic nature of anorexia nervosa and its distinction from Simmonds' disease. In 1948, Berkman summarised his extensive experience with anorexia nervosa and pituitary insufficiency at the Mayo Clinic, while Sheehan and Summers provided a detailed review of pituitary insufficiency, based on pathological diagnosis, and differentiated it from other disorders, including anorexia nervosa. These articles significantly clarified the diagnostic confusion that had existed. In fact, Berkman concluded that the clinical differentiation of anorexia nervosa from pituitary insufficiency was quite easy. While the two disorders shared some features – amenorrhoea and a low basal metabolic rate — there were many differences, not the least of which is the lack of extreme weight loss in most cases of pituitary insufficiency. Moreover, in contrast to the lassitude of the patient with Simmonds' disease, the anorexic patient is frequently active both physically and mentally.

The watershed

To begin to appreciate the vast recent changes in our understanding, we need only to turn to the late 1960s. Recognition of the psychopathology of anorexia nervosa was poor; there had even been questions raised about the discreteness of the syndrome. The endocrine abnormalities were confined to knowledge of the amenorrhoea and the changes in adrenal steroid excretion. Awareness of the complications was minimal. Treatment approaches were split into distinct psychoanalytic or somatic therapy views, and generally, neither of these took into account the special needs of these patients.

At that point, two important influences emerged from different aspects of psychiatry. The first was that of Hilde Bruch. Based on her clinical experience and on the theoretical underpinnings of Harry Stack Sullivan, Bruch became very critical of traditional psychodynamic approaches to the treatment of people with eating disorders. She thought that when these patients received interpretations in a traditional setting, this might recreate a painful re-experiencing of being told what to feel and think; this would reconfirm their sense of inadequacy and interfere with the development of self-awareness and trust in their own psychological abilities. In the early 1960s, she therefore set out to treat these patients in a way that encouraged the anorexic to seek out autonomy and self-directed identity. The framework involved a setting in which what the patient said was listened to, and made the object of repeated exploration. However, this had little to do with restoring patients' nutritional state. When Bruch's therapy was applied to hospitalised emaciated patients, prolonged admissions and continued starvation were the result.

At about this time, a number of articles began to appear on the value of operant conditioning and of multifaceted treatments in hospital. Mickey Stunkard in Philadelphia suggested that a variety of reinforcements might be considered for weight restoration in anorexia nervosa. This approach had a number of advantages: patients did gain weight and at times, they felt actively involved in their treatment. However, often, the details of the operant approach became the focus of treatment, rather than just one aspect of it. Further, the operant programme might be applied at times without sensitivity to a particular patient's psychopathology. Across the Atlantic, at about the same time, Gerald Russell and Arthur Crisp independently began to describe the benefits of multifaceted hospital treatment — consisting of bedrest, with gradual periods of increasing activity, depending on nutritional recovery, intensive nursing support, and high-calorie diets.

Since then, a number of developments have furthered our understanding of these disorders. Amongst the most significant have been: the understanding of them as multidimensional illnesses — rather than being the result of a single factor; knowledge of the effects of starvation and how this can perpetuate the illness; knowledge of the psychopathology of eating disorders; understanding of the differences between bulimics and pure dietary restrictors; and the effects these, and other developments have had on treatment and outcome. There has also been considerable interest in the possible changing frequency of these disorders.

Changes over time

Anorexia nervosa and bulimia nervosa have been considered to be influenced by forces in the broad culture and as these change, there is speculation that the disorders themselves are altered. Whether the eating disorders have increased in frequency and may continue to do so, is open to debate. The literature on this subject is fraught with many methodological problems including: the methods of subject sampling, the definition of a case, the methods of case detection, and response rates.

Over 50 epidemiological studies have been carried out on bulimia nervosa in the past 15 years. Those which permit a longitudinal comparison have found a cohort effect, with an increased frequency of the disorder in individ-

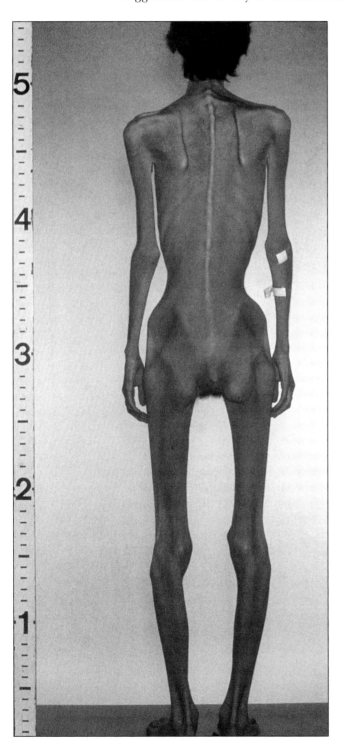

Anorexia nervosa, c. 1985. Reproduced with permission from the Wellcome Institute Library, London.

uals born after 1960 and a younger age of onset in this time period. It is probable that the high rates for bulimia nervosa reflect the onset in vulnerable people who now develop the disorder because of the impact of various cultural pressures that began to be magnified in the 1960s. In other or previous cultures, these emotional vulnerabilities may have remained latent or manifested themselves in other forms. The pressures include the dramatic idealisation of a thin female body form leading to bodily preoccupation and excessive dieting amongst young women, as well as the changing roles for women leading to multiple and at times, conflicting demands as well as high levels of performance expectations.

The evidence for a change in anorexia nervosa is less clear. It is suggestive of an increase based on clinical populations, but it has not been clear how much of this reflects improved recognition alone. The most thorough review of this topic, by Fombonne in 1995, concluded that there was insufficient evidence to support a definitive change in frequency. Nevertheless, reports from at least five different geographical sites (Monroe county, northeast Scotland, Sweden, Rochester, Minnesota, and Switzerland) have noted increases in the cases of anorexia nervosa in the time period from 1930 to 1990.

Conceptual model of pathogenesis

One important development has been the recognition of the eating disorders as multidimensional in nature, the product of a variety of forces in our cultures and families, and within ourselves. A number of risk factors have since been identified. Such a model has not only helped to encourage a more individualised treatment for each person with an eating disorder, but also to dispel a variety of myths regarding eating disorders which include: that they are due to a single traumatic event; that they are the patient's or family's fault; or that they are entirely due to a particular culture.

Psychopathology

After the period of attributing anorexia nervosa to an endocrine disorder, a number of drive-related disturbances were thought to be pathogenic; for example, conflicts regarding oral impregnation were considered to be important in the 1950s. Then, Bruch shifted the emphasis from drives to ego deficits and viewed anorexia nervosa as a disorder of self-regulation. She considered the fundamental psychopathology in both anorexia nervosa and bulimia nervosa to relate to the individual's intense need to maintain her self-worth through undue self-control in the area of weight regulation. This underlying fear of loss of personal control was said to be linked to feelings of helplessness. Rather than experiencing pleasure from their bodies, anorexic and bulimic women were thought to fear the body, as if it were something that must be artificially controlled. In the mid-1960s, a common view of anorexia nervosa was that of Arthur Crisp, who proposed a central role for the retreat from the responsibilities of adulthood; empirical studies confirm this, but such fears of maturity are secondary to the helplessness and intense need to maintain bodily control that these people experience. The 1980s and 1990s have added concepts of deficits in self-esteem regulation and critical abnormalities in cognitive style to our understanding of the psychopathology.

The role of starvation

Since the publication of the Minnesota studies of the late 1940s on semi-starvation, there has been an accumulation of information on the effects of chronic semi-starvation on thinking, feeling, and behaviour. Ancel Keys highlighted these changes in the Minnesota studies, since they were undertaken on men who were psychologically normal at the onset of the starvation. Over a period of months, these men developed many symptoms that at times have been thought to be characteristic of anorexia nervosa. For example, these starving men experienced many food-related symptoms: they were preoccupied with food and many dreamed of food. A few had episodes of bulimia. Cognitively, they displayed poor concentration and indecisiveness. Their moods were characterised by irritability, anxiety, and lability, while sleep became fragmented. Social withdrawal and a narrowing of interests were common. These data were 'rediscovered' in the 1980s. Knowledge of the effects of starvation has been important in helping to explain why anorexia nervosa frequently develops into a self-perpetuating problem: when the anorexic patient experiences these starvation effects, she feels more out of control and then increases her dieting.

Classification and diagnosis

Many earlier sets of criteria for anorexia nervosa lacked reliability. Bruch, for example, stated that there were three characteristic features: a disturbance in body image, a disturbance in recognition of affective and visceral feelings, and an overall sense of ineffectiveness. However, these were hard to define and there were significant overlaps with non-anorexic women in certain aspects.

The first criteria for anorexia nervosa that have a good level of reliability were proposed by Gerald Russell in 1970. He emphasised the need for a behavioural disturbance, a psychopathology, and an endocrine disorder. The behavioural problem leads to a marked loss of body weight; the psychopathology is characterised by a morbid fear of getting fat; and the endocrine disorder manifests itself clinically by amenorrhoea in females. These criteria have gradually been modified in the current DSM–IV and ICD–10, which provide significant advances in the diagnosis of anorexia nervosa. There are, however, some difficulties with them. For example, the amount of weight loss necessary for the diagnosis is not known. Ideally, the point at which an individual becomes caught in the biological syndrome of starvation would be the defining point; this level, however, is still unknown. The other significant problem with our current diagnostic criteria for anorexia nervosa relates to the presence of amenorrhoea. An epidemiological study by the Toronto group found no differences in severity, comorbidity, or family history between anorexics with or without amenorrhoea.

Russell described bulimia nervosa in 1979 and again provided valuable diagnostic criteria. He described the powerful intractable urges to overeat, the compensatory behaviour, and the underlying psychopathology as a morbid fear of fat. Newer criteria have refined this by defining a binge in terms of the amount of food consumed, discrete eating, and a sense of loss of control, as well as setting minimal frequency levels for the diagnosis. While this has been a significantly improved set of diagnostic criteria, the optimal frequency level of the relevant behaviour is not known.

Subtypes

Attempts at distinguishing subtypes of anorexia nervosa date back to Janet, early in this century, who recognised hysterical and obsessional types. This was ignored, however, until Dally in London utilised this approach in the late 1960s. Shortly after, Beumont in Australia began to subtype anorexia nervosa by the presence or absence of vomiting. This was refined a few years later to distinguish subtypes based on the presence or absence of bulimia. Major differences have been described between these two groups.

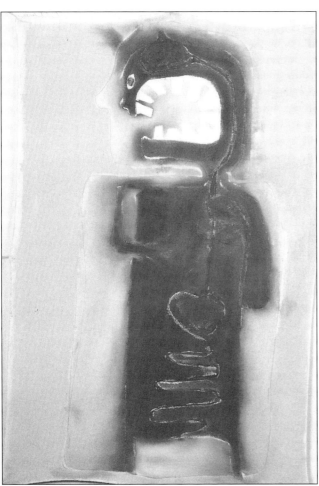

The Anger Within: a painting by Elise Warriner, 1993. The artist suffered from anorexia nervosa for 10 years. Reproduced with permission from E. Warriner.

Bulimic anorexics have weighed more in the early part of their lives and have more frequently been obese premorbidly. They often come from heavier families with more frequent familial obesity. They are also the group who rely on additional methods of weight control — vomiting or laxative abuse — and they more frequently display other impulsive behaviour such as alcohol (Chapter 7, p. 218), street drug use, stealing, and self mutilation. They also display different personality types.

The DSM, in its most recent form, has also separated bulimia nervosa into purging and non-purging types, and there are significant differences here — with more body image disturbance, self-harm behaviour, and general psychopathology in the purging type. Purging bulimics also tend to have an early age of onset, much more frequent comorbidity, and a greatly increased frequency of earlier sexual abuse.

DSM–IV has described two forms of anorexia nervosa and two of bulimia nervosa; it has also added binge eating disorder as a related subject to be studied further. The evidence to date, though, does not provide any distinction between non-purging bulimia nervosa and binge eating disorder.

Treatment

Treatments for the eating disorders are hardly recognisable from 30 years ago. In the 1960s, it was common in some countries to have treatment based on a long-term psychoanalytic model, which was ineffective, or on combinations of potentially harmful medication — for example, Dally and Sargant at St Thomas' Hospital, London, popularised the use of chlorpromazine and insulin, together with bed-rest.

However, work of the past decade has resulted in treatment being more likely to be individualised according to the patient's needs, though there is also general acceptance of the value of nutritional restoration or stabilisation before people can meaningfully benefit from psychotherapy. The types of psychotherapy that are useful vary. Work from the Maudsley Hospital, London has documented the value of family therapy for the young restricting anorexic. Older anorexic patients and bulimics benefit from cognitive–behavioural therapy, but this has been much more carefully described in the case of bulimia nervosa, and the latter group have also been shown to benefit from interpersonal therapy. The antidepressant drugs, including the serotonin reuptake inhibitors, have also been found to be useful for bulimic patients, although in controlled studies they have not been found to be as useful as the psychological treatments. Other work of the past decade has emphasised the complications of the syndromes, and how to approach these. As a result of these advances in understanding and in care, the mortality of anorexia nervosa has been reduced by 50% and more patients are completely well at follow-up. In comparison, bulimia nervosa has a much lower mortality, and a more variable course.

COMMUNITY PSYCHIATRIC NURSING

by Peter Nolan

Although community psychiatric nursing exists in many countries such as the USA, Australia, New Zealand, South Africa, Sweden, Russia, Japan, France, and Germany, its development is perhaps best documented in the UK. There, community psychiatric nurses (CPNs) came into being in the 1950s in an attempt to improve the care of people suffering from severe psychiatric illnesses following their discharge from hospital. The first CPN was Lena Peat whose post at Warlingham Park Hospital in Surrey in 1954 was established with the support of Dr TP Rees, the Physician Superintendent. Three years later, post-discharge community nursing was initiated at Moorhaven Hospital in Devon. The early CPNs had no specific training and no specific title, being variously referred to as out-patient nurses, psychiatric community nurses, after-care nurses, domiciliary nurses, or

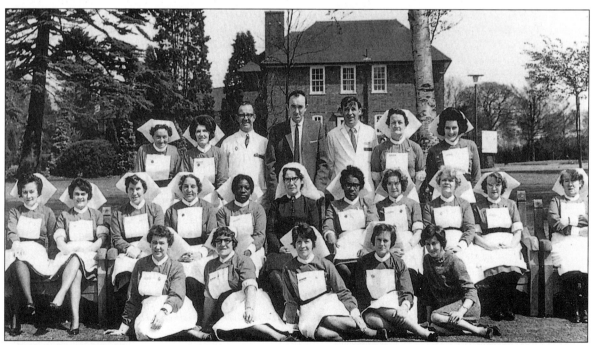

Retirement of Miss K Brennan, Matron, April 1967, with ward sisters and charge nurses, Warlingham Park Hospital. Lena Peat is seated middle row, 4th from left. Reproduced with permission from Bethlem Royal Hospital Archives and Museum (archives of Warlingham Park Hospital).

members of the extra-mural service. By 1966, there were approximately 225 full- and part-time nurses employed by 42 psychiatric hospitals to work in the community, although it was not until the early 1970s that special training became available and the term 'community psychiatric nurse' was generally recognised in Britain.

In the early years, the principal tasks of CPNs were to administer medication and assist with ECT, although the importance of establishing therapeutic relationships with patients was gradually recognised. With the disappearance in Britain of the specialised psychiatric social worker and the introduction of generic social work, the numbers of CPNs increased dramatically, such that by 1990 approximately 4500 were employed in England, Scotland, and Wales. There was no uniformity, however, in the work they were doing, since their jobs were variously defined by different health authorities. In the 1980s, the work of the CPN diversified further as referrals from general practitioners of patients with depression and anxiety became increasingly common, thereby shifting the original emphasis of the work of the CPN away from patients with serious mental illnesses. It may be that CPNs actively encouraged this move towards primary care in order to escape the control of consultant-based medical treatment and to assert their own autonomy. The title of 'community mental health nurse', which has more recently come into favour, may be a further indication that CPNs' involvement with people with severe mental illnesses is diminishing.

Their work in primary care seems set to expand, as evidence accumulates of the possible effectiveness of CPN intervention at this level. CPNs can offer a number of treatment methods to their patients, including anxiety management, cognitive–behavioural work, problem-solving, systematic desensitisation, and counselling; additional specialised training is needed for some of these techniques. They can also provide basic care such as assisting with hygiene and nutrition, and advising on financial matters such as applications for State benefits and welfare rights. They introduce patients to social activities, and carry on health education to ensure mental and physical well-being.

However, in an increasingly competitive health care environment where policies may be driven more by political and economic agendas than by the needs of patients, community psychiatric nursing is in danger of finding the services it offers taken over by other health care workers, by social services, or by new non-nursing agencies. The responsibilities of CPNs remain as uncertain today as was the role of the attendant in the Victorian asylum, perpetuating a long history of insecurity and ambiguity within the mental nursing profession. A British Government review of mental health nursing in 1994 expressed concern that CPNs had lost sight of their original mission to care for the long-term mentally ill, and urged them to refocus their activities accordingly. More recently, it was reported that 80% of people with schizophrenia had no contact with a CPN, and that better training was still needed for these nurses.

Other studies have also reflected the role uncertainty being experienced by CPNs. While the British Mental Health Foundation in 1994 concluded that CPNs allocating their time to people experiencing 'general stress' was not a good use of a valuable resource, another study reported that CPNs were as effective in dealing with anxiety, depression, and phobic disorders as general practitioners. While some would argue that CPNs are essentially primary health care professionals who should be working closely with GPs, others would prefer to see them attached to mental health centres, providing support to those with long-term mental health problems and their families.

CPNs and their equivalents in other countries may feel that they have a legitimate part to play in the care of mentally ill clients. Yet they still need to convince others that they fully understand 'evidence-based care', and that they are part of a new culture which can replace the outdated wisdom of the institutions. Just as nurses working in the nineteenth-century asylums had no clearly defined agenda to guide their practices, so community care has been inaugurated before the needs of community-based patients have been properly identified. Worldwide, there are scattered writings on current developments in community psychiatric nursing in several languages, but lack of translation has meant that they are not accessible outside their country of origin.

Community psychiatric nursing has still to find its feet in a constantly changing world of health care. While, in these circumstances, it may be impossible to define roles precisely, the repeated failure of mental health nursing to attempt such a definition is a serious problem for the profession. Those who pay for mental health services have to be convinced that mental health nurses are an efficient and cost-effective resource for the care of the most vulnerable people in our society. Otherwise the profession — in those countries where it has developed strongly — may eventually disappear along with the institutions in which it was born.

MULTIPLE PERSONALITY DISORDER

by Harold Merskey

'Multiple personality disorder' was renamed by the American Psychiatric Association in its *Diagnostic and Statistical Manual*, Fourth edition (DSM–IV) as '300.14 Dissociative Identity Disorder [DID] (formerly Multiple Personality Disorder)'.

In individuals who are not subject to the physiological effects of substance abuse, alcohol, or drugs, or other medical or organic conditions that might mimic the disorder, the principal features are as shown in the table below.

The name was changed because the concept of multiple personality had been much criticised, but the new criteria only differ in two words. First, *presence* was substituted for the word *existence*. According to David Spiegel, the change was intended to indicate only that patients experience themselves in that way, not that there are a number of real people in one body. Second, *full* was removed from in front of *control*. Thus, the definition allows that a personality may take partial control, or two or more personalities might share control. How this can happen while memory is lost may puzzle the thoughtful. Because the term 'multiple personality' or 'multiple personality disorder' reflects the main growth period of DID, it is referred to here as MPD.

Origins

The founding case of MPD, Mary Reynolds of Pennsylvania, was said to show two forms of consciousness — one very depressed and the other cheerful, bold, overactive and mischievous. We would now call such a condition rapid cycling bipolar affective disorder, but for most of the twentieth century, it has been known as manic–depressive illness.

Another pattern of dual consciousness also began to be identified in the nineteenth century, arising from hypnotism. In 1875, Eugène Azam, a prominent French surgeon, began to think of dual consciousness in terms of states produced under hypnosis. In cases, reported by Janet in Paris from 1887 onwards, different states of the same individual were given different first names. The first use of the term 'multiple personality' was in English by AT Myers in 1886 in an English description of a French report on 'Louis V.', who was said to have had eight personalities. Ian Hacking observes correctly that to science and medicine, this case is nonsense. In his view, the interest in memory and multiple personality in 1875 was largely based on the positivist philosophical movement in France, and came from its neurological and anticlerical allies, who sought to re-interpret ideas of the soul in terms of natural phenomena.

Growth

MPD originated in the misdiagnosis or misapprehension of a well-known psychiatric illness. It expanded through the creation of personalities by hypnosis or allied suggestive effects.

Previously, MPD was considered to be rare. In 1944, 76 such cases were identified, occurring over 128 years, but increased numbers of patients appeared after a prominent case was described. This was noticeable after CH Thigpen and H Cleckley described a case of MPD, followed by their book in 1957 entitled *The Three Faces of Eve*. Films were made of that, and of another book, *Sybil* in 1973. The 1973 Child Abuse Prevention Act — the Mondale Act — was passed by the US Congress in response to growing evidence

---

Multiple Personality Disorder

(a) The presence of two or more distinct identities or personality states (each with its own relatively enduring pattern of perceiving, relating to, and thinking about the environment and self).

(b) At least two of these identities or personality states recurrently take control of the person's behaviour.

(c) Inability to recall important personal information that is too extensive to be explained by ordinary forgetfulness.

of serious childhood abuse, particularly physical. *Sybil* linked a case of a girl with 16 personalities to a history of horrible early childhood treatment. From that point on, childhood abuse was quickly added to the idea of MPD, both conditions began to be described with increasing frequency, and physical abuse — partly in response to radical feminist propaganda — was linked with child sexual abuse.

More and more cases of MPD were described. By 1982, Richard Kluft mentioned 130 patients and had treated 70. In 1980, the third edition of the *Diagnostic and Statistical Manual* of the American Psychiatric Association, DSM–III, established a specific category for MPD. The growth of reported cases subsequently was enormous, and Colin Ross claimed that MPD probably represented about 5% of the normal population.

The numbers of personalities per patient also increased tremendously. The initial cases of dual consciousness rarely had more than three personalities. Some dramatic instances appeared, like Louis V above and Molly Fancher who had at least five personalities, about whom Janet pointed out "...[they] have very poetical pet names 'Sunbeam, Idle, Rosebud, Pearl, Ruby....'" In the 1980s, DSM–III and DSM–III–R both allowed that as many as 100 personalities, or fragments of personality, might exist within the same individual. Kluft described 33 patients with an average of 13.9 'alters' (alternative personalities) in 1984. By 1988, Kluft laid claim to two patients with more than 4000 personalities or personality fragments. This *reductio ad absurdum* of the concept wrecked whatever of its face validity still remained.

MPD was brought into further disrepute by its strong association with false memories (this chapter, p. 336). If individuals were to go through such a radical change as splitting of the personality, it became necessary to explain why they had split. Allegedly the explanation was childhood abuse, but what if the person did not remember abuse? The theory developed that child abuse had resulted in dissociation, that dissociation involved 'splitting', and that adequate work looking for recovered memories (RM) would produce proof of the abuse at the heart of the disorder. Therapists set about recovering memories and readily produced patients (or clients) with recollections of abuse as early as the first year of life, when the brain is not sufficiently mature to register impressions that can be reliably reconstructed pictorially or verbally by the adult. Thus, 'brilliant' therapy was producing impossible results. Similarly, patients with RM, and often with personality disorder, quite frequently 'discovered' they had been involved in extraordinary processes of Satanic ritual abuse. Others were regressed under hypnosis to experience or recall past lives, or determined that they had suffered temporary abduction by aliens who took genital material from them during nocturnal anaesthesia.

The problems of RM are not solely linked with MPD; they occur in countries and places where MPD is rarely found. However, MPD is one of those phenomena which have gone hand-in-hand with the RM campaign, particularly in the United States and Canada, and have raised pointed questions both about the value of the diagnosis and of memory recovery processes.

By the start of the 1990s, MPD was at its peak. The International Society for the Study of Multiple Personality and Dissociation flourished, but mainly in the United States and Canada. Small numbers of psychiatrists diagnosed large numbers of patients as having MPD, while most of the rest of the psychiatric profession looked on without seeing such cases. Psychologists too were making these diagnoses and less well qualified therapists tended to bring them to psychiatrists or psychologists for an imprimatur. In the Netherlands, Norway, and Turkey, a few psychiatrists diagnosed cases of MPD, but otherwise, they were rare worldwide, without even one in Japan. Thus, a pattern of diagnosis, which had evolved in the United States, Britain, and France during the nineteenth century, became primarily an American activity.

Decline

Several factors contributed to the decline of MPD. Strong reasoned critiques and a systematic challenge began with Michael Kenny in 1986, Tom Fahy in 1988, and Ray Aldridge-Morris in 1988. Nicholas Spanos, an experimental social psychologist, illustrated the artificial production of multiple personality symptoms. He demonstrated the features of an interview which could produce 'alters', and concluded that MPD was the enactment of a social role. By 1994, however, the majority of psychiatrists in Canada and presumably also in the United States still accepted the diagnosis of MPD and it persisted in DSM–IV. Francois Mai showed in three centres in Ontario that between 54 and 74% of psychiatrists believed in the diagnosis. In 1999, no published estimates of current views in the United States and Canada are available, but public reaction is commonly sceptical and lawsuits against therapists have resulted in large awards to individuals who were 'given' MPD. The highest so far has been

$10.7 million. It may be an understatement to say that MPD is now in a state of decline, but it is likely, as Ian Hacking has suggested, that it will reach the state of spiritism at the end of the last century, i.e. it will linger on, still affirmed by some who cling to it here and there, but otherwise regarded as a fact that has had its day.

FALSE MEMORIES

by Harold Merskey

In the 1960s, paediatricians and radiologists came to recognise that a number of children who suffered fractures in early life had been violently abused by their parents. From this starting point of increased awareness of physical abuse in childhood, measures were developed in several countries to inhibit the abuse of children and punish offenders. In the United States the Mondale Act (1973) provided federal funds for the discovery and prosecution of abuse. However, interest in abuse was not confined to beatings or fractures alone. Increasing recognition that the frequency of rape had been neglected led to a considerable emphasis on the need to recognise and prevent the sexual abuse of women. These changes were accompanied by the gradual growth of a popular belief that many women had been sexually abused in childhood, usually by members of their families, had forgotten all about those experiences, and could have them revived by suitable psychotherapy. Those who adopted this point of view became known as 'believers' in recovered memory. Their ideas, as just outlined, derived from one aspect of orthodox Freudian theory.

The women's movement spread the message that sexual abuse was frequent and that memory of sexual abuse, later recovered, could also be frequent. Enthusiasts began to look for recovered memories in psychotherapy, without imposing restraints that had been *de rigueur* in psychiatry for most of the previous 100 years, ever since it became recognised that the attitudes and interests of psychotherapists were liable to shape the ideas and reported experiences of their patients. The theme of recovered memory was pursued by psychiatrists, psychologists, and licensed therapists such as marriage guidance counsellors, particularly in the United States. Poorly trained, untrained, and unlicensed individuals helped to swell this crowd who were offering 'therapy'. A number operated out of rape crisis centres and women's counselling centres, adopting the approach of a creative writer, Ellen Bass, and her partner Laura Davis, who in 1986 jointly authored the first version of *The Courage to Heal*. This was followed not long afterwards by *The Courage to Heal Workbook* (by Davis only) which described, with an air of authority, the way in which many women had lost memories of abuse they had experienced and how these could be recovered. This had to be done with suitable patience and determination, by putting together fragments of 'memories', and building on them until the whole picture of childhood abuse could be 'recovered' from under the restraints of Freudian repression.

A series of other books followed, based on self-help notions and the principles of the self-help recovery movement in mental health, which often shared similar notions of personal growth through recollection of the evil done to the patient (or client). Survivor status became increasingly popular amongst troubled individuals, a 'consumer/survivor' movement emerged in North America and elsewhere throughout the English-speaking world, and the stage was set for an epidemic of false memories. Many therapists rushed into the recovery of such memories and prominent clinics and departments in North America from Harvard to Seattle and from Manitoba, generated patients whose main identifying feature seemed to be the recovery of memories of abuse ranging from the age of birth onwards.

The individuals who first fell under the spell of this bewitching process were frequently well educated. They were attending or had attended universities, knew about psychotherapy, and were seeking the help of psychotherapists for problems in living, mild depression, marital conflicts, problems with anorexia or weight-gain, mild puerperal states, etc. In the hands of therapists with varying levels of qualification, they were frequently told that their symptoms were suggestive of sexual abuse in childhood, and submitted to hypnosis, 'guided imagery', dream interpretation, art work with interpretation, narcoanalysis, and group participation with others claiming to have been sexually abused. They also received simple strong suggestion that they should go digging for memories in order to find them, or build upon little scraps of memory that might be available to them already. By the start of the 1990s, it appeared that an epidemic of false memories and false accusations had resulted.

Recognition of false accusations

In 1991, four American psychiatrists, Emily and Martin Orne, Harold Lief, and Paul McHugh in particular recognised the occurrence of numerous false accusations levelled at otherwise blameless parents. In November 1991, Darrel Sifford, a journalist with the *Philadelphia Inquirer*, published an article describing the problem of a couple who said that their adult daughter, after entering therapy, suddenly claimed to recover 'repressed memories' of incest. She then terminated all contact with anyone who would not validate her new identity as an incest survivor. In the week following the publication, Dr Harold Lief, who had been quoted in the column, received close to 100 calls from affected families. A group of families and professionals affiliated with the University of Pennsylvania in Philadelphia, and Johns Hopkins University in Baltimore, then formed the False Memory Syndrome Foundation (FMSF) as a charitable organisation in March 1992. The Foundation aimed to find out more about the phenomenon of the false memory syndrome, bring help to the primary victim (the accuser), assist accused families, and encourage research into the spread and the prevention of false memories. Within two years of its establishment, the Foundation had received more than 20,000 enquiries and became aware not only of accused persons, but also of accusers who had begun to doubt or retract their accusations.

Criminal trials

At the time when the FMSF was established, criminal trials for abuse based on 'recovered memories' were spreading through North America. Hundreds of convictions appear to have been registered against individuals, although the only evidence for the accusations was long-forgotten memories of supposed abuse, recovered in therapy. Lawsuits had also been commenced against parents on a similar basis for the damage done to their children. Similar phenomena also were spreading throughout the United Kingdom, Australia and New Zealand, France, Scandinavian countries, Ireland, the Netherlands, and Israel. In most of these countries, the pattern was the same as in North America, except that the emphasis on an association of abuse and multiple personality disorder was less (apart from the Netherlands). Certain types of moral panics also appeared in association with the recovered memory phenomenon. One was widespread allegations of Satanic ritual abuse, i.e. suggestions that there had been organised bodies operating from generation to generation, carefully hidden in society, involving high-level professional people (doctors, lawyers, judges, police amongst others) and skillfully concealing nefarious activities. These included sexual orgies, the breeding of foetuses or tiny children for sacrifice at those orgies (with cannibalism), rituals and torture of the younger participants, and of course varied forms of sexual and other abuse. Such organisations have never actually been found in any of the countries mentioned despite numerous 'recollections' of them in therapy. There were also individuals who claimed to have recovered their past lives or to have been abducted by aliens in spaceships, sexually investigated surgically, sewn up again, and returned to their beds. Slightly more prosaically, a significant number had memories from before the age of three, when the brain cannot establish adequate episodic memories for long-term retention in semantic or pictorial form.

Children's homes

Another concomitant phenomenon evolved in children's homes. In essentially the same countries, tiny children were found to give evidence of improbable organised events. The first case seems to have been the McMartin Day-Care scandal in Los Angeles in August 1983, when a mother, later diagnosed as having paranoid schizophrenia, noted that her two-year-old's bottom was red and decided that he had been sexually abused. Soon, after repeated questioning of the child, the police decided that the 'offender' was a day-care teacher at the McMartin Pre-School. The local police sent a letter to 200 parents, warning of 'possible criminal acts' such as "oral sex, fondling of genitals, buttocks or chest area and sodomy, possibly committed under the pretense of taking the child's temperature". Within three months, many parents had taken their children away from the pre-school and many had been questioned. Strongly suggestive repeated questions to young children who were never properly cross-examined, led in the end to prolonged court cases in various countries, sometimes with convictions, the loss of livelihoods and reputations, and enormous financial costs in defence before final acquittal. Some were not so lucky and are still in jail. Events of this sort occurred widely in the United Kingdom. In Cleveland, England, large numbers of children were removed temporarily from their homes on the basis of repeated medical assumptions that anal abuse had occurred, based on misinterpretation of the anatomical state of the anus.

Amongst other organisations set up to deal with the matter, the British False Memory Society was founded in the United Kingdom in 1993, Casualties of Sexual Allegations (COSA) in New Zealand, and the False Memory Society in Australia.

Successful defence

The responses of accused people varied. Some hid their shame and kept to themselves; many organised where they could, but kept relatively quiet. Only one in twelve of the families known to the FMSF actually experienced some threat of legal proceedings. As time went by, more and more cases were defended successfully, the basis for the defence usually resting on four pillars. First, the unreliability of memory from long ago was recognised, as well as the difficulty in finding disconfirming information so many years later. Second, scientific challenges led to the conclusion that recovered memories had never been properly demonstrated to occur in scientific investigations. Third, David Holmes pointed out that repression had never been proven experimentally, while Elizabeth Loftus demonstrated that false memories (albeit harmless ones) could be induced in susceptible subjects. Lastly, it became evident that highly suggestive procedures were commonplace with false memory claims. Recovered memory became the 'kiss of death' in court proceedings and a change appeared in the pattern of false accusations and their outcome. Initially, in the United States, most cases dealt with parents being accused in criminal courts or being sued. Later, the number of criminal cases reported fell drastically, and experienced criminal lawyers said that no-one should be convicted in Canada or the United States on the basis of recovered memory allegations alone. Instead, the lawsuits currently being reported in 1998 in the United States reflect awards against therapists. This began with the Ramona case in California in 1994 and reached a level of settlement for $10.6 million in an Illinois case.

Repression and dissociation

There is another unexpected consequence of the false memory syndrome story. The blatant production of alleged repressed memories brought about much closer attention to the whole question of the reality of repression and dissociation. Critics pointed out that there have been hundreds of thousands, indeed millions of cases of one type of abuse or another, and yet we still lack even a single fully proven case of the recovery of a repressed memory. In theory, repressed memories might occur, but since so many instances are known of true abuse, and so few of true proven recovered memory, their value, or importance, or their likelihood of occurring seems to be minimal. This in turn leads to questioning of the theoretical basis for the notion of repression and dissociation.

Coincidentally, but largely ignored by psychiatrists, a radical revision of views of Freudian psychodynamic theory has been going on in the cultural, biographical, and historical literature. The new Freud scholarship demonstrates gross inconsistency in Freud's own work between what he claimed and what he did. In particular, careful study of Freud's own writing indicates that he almost never claimed to have recovered actual memories. Rather, he asserted that psychoanalytic knowledge led him to the inevitable interpretation that something or other had happened in his patients' lives. In other words, he determined the answer and then told the patient. This is not what had been understood from a more trusting reading of psychoanalytic articles. Psychiatry as a whole has been slow to recognise the growth of this literature and its relevance to existing theory. In the second half of this century, psychiatry has been marked by great biological advances in the understanding and treatment of severe psychiatric illness. Until recently, the acceptance of psychodynamic theories went relatively unchallenged, although some diminution and loss of prestige occurred, largely because of the failure to prove that formal dynamic treatment on traditional psychoanalytic lines is any more effective than any other type of psychotherapeutic treatment. However, notions of repression and dissociation continued to be accepted by most psychiatrists. A call for change has begun, however, and is likely to grow very quickly as more and more psychiatrists come to realise the flimsy basis of the information currently held to support overt dissociative states and mechanisms of repression.

NON-WESTERN PSYCHIATRY

by David Mumford

It is a matter of history that psychiatry as we know it now has developed as a branch of Western medicine. The theory and practice of modern psychiatry have been shaped by Western cultural concerns and assumptions as well as by Western social history.

Any nineteenth-century psychiatrist looking beyond his own culture would have been unconsciously influenced by the legacy of Jean-Jacques Rousseau and the notion of a primal idyllic existence which preceded Western civilisation. The pioneering American psychiatrist and epidemiologist Edward Jarvis (1851) claimed that "insanity is a part of the price we pay for civilisation. The causes of the one increase with the developments and results of the other". In the present century, Sigmund Freud echoed this idea in *Civilisation and its Discontents* (1930): "Primitive man was better off, for he knew nothing of any restrictions on his instincts. Civilised man has exchanged some part of his chances of happiness for a measure of security".

By the end of the nineteenth century, Western psychiatrists were beginning to make clinical observations in the non-Western world. Emil Kraepelin visited Java in 1896, and pronounced that dementia praecox (schizophrenia) could be diagnosed in patients he encountered there. In the present century, though, the opinion grew that depression was very rare in non-Western populations of Asia and Africa.

This section summarises the clinical and epidemiological findings that have emerged in recent years from studies in non-Western cultures, and surveys the growing distinctive contributions of non-Western psychiatrists in terms of treatment approaches and academic activity.

Clinical and epidemiological findings

Schizophrenia

It is now some 30 years since the publication of the International Pilot Study of Schizophrenia by the World Health Organization (WHO), which established that the core symptomatology of schizophrenia was similar in the nine participating countries worldwide. The content of delusions and hallucinations and causal attributions (e.g. to witchcraft, spirits, extra-terrestial beings, etc.) vary between cultures, but the form of schizophrenic phenomena appears to be constant.

Schizophrenia has been found in every culture which has been investigated: itself an interesting and important observation. (Bipolar disorders, or manic–depressive illness, have been studied less intensively than schizophrenia, but they also appear to exist in all cultures.) Estimates of the incidence and prevalence of schizophrenia depend on whether a broad or narrow definition is used. However, the overall conclusion from a very large number of epidemiological studies is that, with rare exceptions, the prevalence of schizophrenia varies between 2 and 5 per 1000 population around the globe. The lifetime risk of schizophrenia for any individual is probably about 1% in all cultures.

Yet the course and outcome of schizophrenia seem to be more favourable in non-Western countries. In a five-year outcome study conducted by WHO, 42% of Indian patients and 33% of Nigerian patients had the 'best' outcome; in England, Denmark, and Russia it was only 5–6%. By contrast, only 10% of Indian and Nigerian patients had the 'worst' outcome, whereas in Denmark it was 40%, and over 20% in Russia, Czechoslovakia, and the United States.

The reason for this better prognosis in non-Western societies is assumed to be the family and social environment, although the precise factors involved have yet to be established. If these social factors could be identified, it might suggest some new forms of social intervention which could benefit patients with schizophrenia in Western industrialised countries.

Depressive and anxiety disorders

The presentation of non-psychotic psychiatric illness in non-Western cultures is often quite different from that in the Western; most people there with depressive illnesses or anxiety disorders present with somatic symptoms — the 'somatisation' of emotional distress. This phenomenon has been studied extensively in the Indian subcontinent, China, and Africa. Though the repertoire of somatic symptoms — head, chest and heart, abdomen, whole body symptoms — appears to be largely constant across the world, regional variations in symptomatology reflect local cultural beliefs, e.g. complaints of insects crawling under the skin or through the head which are found in Africa.

There is still a pervasive view in the West that depressive illnesses and anxiety disorders are less common in rural non-Western societies. Yet several major epidemiological studies in Africa and south Asia documenting high rates of psychiatric morbidity in rural populations, especially amongst women, ought by now to have laid this myth to rest. In a study of two rural villages in Uganda, Orley and Wing found 27% of the women and 24% of the men to have a psychiatric disorder. Mumford *et al.* surveyed two mountain villages in the Hindu Kush, northern Pakistan, and reported that at least 46% of the women and 15% of the men suffered from anxiety and depressive disorders. Another similar study

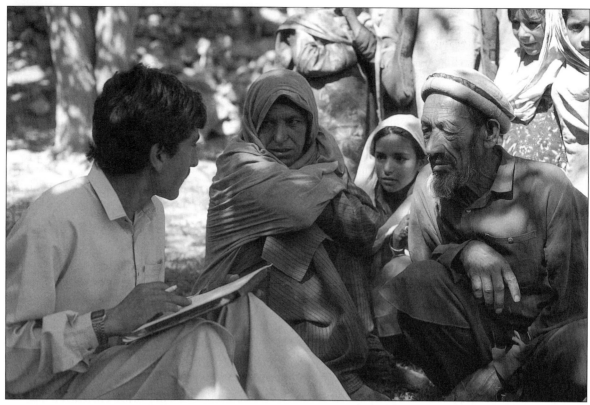

Community survey of mountain villages in Chitral, Pakistan.

in the Punjab estimated rates of 66% for the women and 25% for the men. These rates of psychiatric disorder are considerably higher than found in most epidemiological studies in the Western world.

Both these studies found that lower socio-economic status and illiteracy were associated with higher levels of emotional distress. Multiple social and economic stresses and poor physical health inevitably take their toll on psychological well-being, so it should not be surprising to find high levels of psychiatric ill-health in these populations.

Other neuroses

Some psychiatric disorders which have become infrequent in the West remain common in the non-Western world. Hysterical conversion is still a very common presentation of emotional distress in the Indian subcontinent: pseudo-epilepsy, aphonia, and paralyses are all very familiar to psychiatrists practising in these cultures. For example in Chandigarh, north India, hysteria accounts for just under 10% of all in-patient admissions and out-patient contacts.

On the other hand, some psychiatric disorders which are common in the West are rare in non-Western cultures. Eating disorders have been found infrequently in epidemiological surveys conducted in Malaysia, Hong Kong, and rural Pakistan. However, several studies in Japan and a recent survey of English-language secondary schools in the city of Lahore, Pakistan, suggest that the prevalence of eating disorders may be increasing in young women who are coming under the influence of fashionable Western models of female beauty.

In the Western world, deliberate self-harm (parasuicide) has become a very frequent reaction to acute, distressing life-events. Until recently, this phenomenon was completely unknown in most non-Western societies. But once again, there is evidence that deliberate self-harm is beginning to occur in urban non-Western populations that are undergoing rapid modernisation.

Alcohol and drug abuse

Alcohol and drug abuse are worldwide phenomena. Almost every society has its 'recreational' substances — alcohol, cannabis, khat, opium, and others — and all are capable of abuse, especially where traditional social constraints on their usage are breaking down. It is difficult to measure the extent of the problem of alcohol abuse, but death rates from cirrhosis of the liver are a useful indicator. Amongst the countries of North and South America, death rates from cirrhosis are five times higher in Mexico and Chile than in Canada; Puerto Rico, Ecuador, and Venezuela also have high rates, whereas Panama, Uruguay, and the United States report low rates. Male mortality from liver cirrhosis is consistently 2–3 times higher than amongst females in all cultures.

Other drug abuse can result from severe social dislocation, e.g. large-scale migration to the cities from rural areas, and local availability of drugs. During recent civil wars, Ethiopia and Somalia have experienced a sharp rise in the abuse of khat, an amphetamine-like substance found in leaves which are chewed. In the last 20 years, Pakistan has suffered a huge increase in opiate addiction as an indirect consequence of the Russian occupation of Afghanistan. Opium poppies were then grown freely in Afghanistan and traded for armaments through Pakistan; tougher international policing of the export trade from Pakistan obliged the drug barons to exploit the local Pakistan market instead, with disastrous results.

Suicide

Suicide occurs world-wide, but its frequency varies greatly between cultures and at different times in their history. In some non-Western cultures such as Japan, suicide has been regarded as an honourable act; in others, it is strongly against religious and ethical norms.

The WHO league tables of suicide rates by country (1985 to 1991) reflect this cultural variation. The countries with the highest reported suicide rates are Hungary (39 per 100,000 per year), Sri Lanka (33), USSR (21), China (17), and Japan and West Germany (16). The countries with the lowest reported suicide rates include Costa Rica, Thailand, and Chile (6 per 100,000), Venezuela (5), and Mexico (2). However, there may be substantial under-reporting in countries where suicide carries great shame and stigma.

Studies of specific 'causes' of suicide have reported findings which reflect domestic concerns in that particular culture. In one Indian study, serious physical illness headed the list of known causes (13%), followed by quarrels with in-laws (6%) or spouse (6%), illicit love affairs (5%), insanity (3%), and poverty (2.5%).

Organisation of psychiatric services

Non-Western countries with a history of colonialism have often inherited state-run mental asylums, which have become increasingly neglected in the post-colonial era. Modern psychiatry on the Western model has spread from the university teaching hospitals, and is also often available in privately run clinics in the major cities.

In most non-Western countries, though, there is a great shortage of psychiatrists, and the few that they have are largely based in the cities. For example, Kenya has only 60 psychiatrists to serve a population of 30 million, and amongst the countries of the Pacific Rim, China and Malaysia have a similar ratio. The ratio of psychiatrists to population is substantially lower in the Philippines and Vietnam, but higher in Hong Kong, Korea, and Singapore (12–16 psychiatrists per million population), and much higher in Japan (70 psychiatrists per million), which equates to most Western countries. In most non-Western countries, there is an even greater shortage of trained psychiatric nurses.

Community-based intervention is often seen as the best way forward in societies where severe mental illness is not identified as medically treatable and is not brought to medical attention. In many countries world-wide, WHO has sponsored projects using existing primary health centres, training village health workers to recognise and treat psychiatric disorders. However, there are difficult issues around providing support for these primary health workers, and it is likely that these projects are sustainable only with consistent back-up by psychiatrists and a secondary mental health centre.

Public health education is seen as an important component of community intervention, to help in the recognition and treatment of severe mental illness. As one example, the WHO collaborating centre at Rawalpindi, Pakistan, has made health education in secondary schools its priority. School children are informed about major mental illness and encouraged to report the names of people in their village who show signs of mental illness to the local primary health centre.

In some places, psychiatrists have been willing to go into partnership with traditional indigenous healers such as herbalists, hakim, or local spiritual leaders. Some psychiatric centres have offered training to local traditional healers to help them to recognise and refer on cases of severe mental illness where medication would be effective. At the same time, they respect the ability of traditional healers to handle minor neurotic and behavioural disorders in time-honoured and culturally congruent ways.

Treatment approaches

The most striking feature of the practice of psychiatry in non-Western countries is the prominent role of the family in the management of psychiatric illness. With very restricted mental health facilities, most patients with major mental illness are looked after by their families. The families provide nursing care at home during psychotic episodes and try to ensure compliance with medication. The psychiatrist often works as much with the family as with the patient him/herself.

In the 1960s, there were pioneering developments in Nigeria, West Africa, with the Aro Village community system. Mentally ill people, accompanied by one or two family members, moved into a village near a mental health facility, and remained there until they were able to return to the community. Mental health workers from the nearby hospital visited daily and gave appropriate treatment, such as psychotherapy or drugs.

Formal psychotherapy is not widely practised in non-Western psychiatry, for a variety of reasons. It is labour-intensive, requiring skilled practitioners, and is therefore expensive compared with medication. Doubts have often been expressed about the cultural applicability and relevance of psychological treatments developed in the Western world. In psychologically unsophisticated populations, compliance with 'talking cures', which are not culturally embedded, may be poor.

Some centres of psychiatry in India have for many years used forms of Yoga in place of Western relaxation techniques. Yoga is seen as a culturally more acceptable and congruent treatment modality; evidence for its efficacy in the treatment of anxiety disorders has been established in comparative trials.

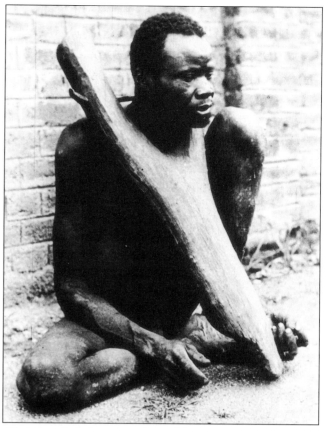

Primitive method of restraint. A homicidal psychotic patient, Sudan, 1947 — Dr N Corkill. The wooden stake was embedded in the ground and broken off by the patient; he arrived at the hospital with the remainder around his neck. Reproduced with permission from the Wellcome Institute Library, London.

Academic activity

If we judge by rates of publication in international medical journals, the most active country in academic psychiatry outside Europe and North America is Japan; South Africa, Taiwan, Hong Kong, India, China, and Brazil all follow some way behind. Much of the research activity in Japan and elsewhere is in biological psychiatry, and belongs to the mainstream of biomedical research world-wide.

To discover what is distinctive in non-Western academic psychiatry, we need to look instead to clinical psychiatry, and to social psychiatry and epidemiology. Here, a number of themes emerge. Non-Western psychiatrists tend to argue for a holistic approach to psychiatry, less materialistic and physically orientated than in the Western world. They generally give a more prominent place to religious and moral concerns. In the clinical setting, non-Western psychiatrists are more ready than their counterparts in the Western world, with its predominant secular ideology, to recommend culturally congruent religious observance and practice.

Non-Western psychiatrists are increasingly engaged in debates about diagnostic issues. Amongst the new generation of psychiatrists, there is less willingness to accept the dominant Western-based diagnostic systems, which may not fit their clinical experience. For example, in Hong Kong, Sing Lee has raised questions about the universal applicability of Western diagnostic criteria for eating disorders, specifically 'weight phobia', which he does not find amongst Chinese patients who otherwise meet the criteria for anorexia nervosa.

Psychiatric syndromes which are well-established diagnostic categories in certain parts of the world are now receiving the attention of empirical researchers: for example, *neurasthenia* in China, *ataque de nervios* in Latin America, and *brain fag syndrome* in southern Africa. These diagnostic categories are somewhat distinct from the classic 'culture-bound syndromes' such as *amok* or *latah*, in that they are probably different ways of characterising common symptom clusters, found universally.

Whether the concept of 'culture-bound syndrome' continues to be useful is still debated. This is one aspect of the whole issue of culture and psychiatric phenomenology (Chapter 7, p. 211). In recent years, Western psychiatrist–anthropologists such as Arthur Kleinman at Harvard and Roland Littlewood in London have questioned the assumption that Western illness categories are universally valid in non-Western cultures. In spite of this debate, psychiatric illness categories used by psychiatrists in the non-Western world are still dominated by Western models.

Cross-cultural psychiatry offers a natural 'laboratory experiment', which can help to tease out the contrasting roles of biology and culture in the pathogenesis of psychiatric disorder. It can help to throw psychiatric illness into relief from its social and cultural context, and illuminate the issue of universality and cultural relativity in the conceptualisation of mental illness.

The worldwide burden

From the perspective of the non-Western psychiatrist, the overwhelming finding of recent years is the enormous extent of psychiatric morbidity throughout the world. It has been estimated that by the year 2000, there will be 24.4 million people suffering from schizophrenia. The more we learn about psychiatric illness world-wide, the greater seems to be the prevalence of mental ill-health and its resulting social and personal disability.

Mental health problems impose a heavy burden of suffering at many levels — the individual, their families, their communities, and the health services. A report by the World Bank in 1993 concluded that mental health problems world-wide accounted for 8.1% of the global burden of disease (as measured by disability-adjusted life years). The loss of productivity and the economic costs of psychiatric disorder are enormous, as was illustrated, for example, in a survey of villages in Laos by Westermeyer. Despite this immense burden of psychiatric ill-health, mental health services are often neglected and poorly resourced.

The WHO slogan 'Health for all by the Year 2000' was always an impossibly ambitious dream; especially as it defined health in very broad terms — physical, psychological, and spiritual. A recent book, *World Mental Health*, which focuses on the mental health problems of non-Western countries, highlights the scale of this huge challenge. The burden of psychiatric disorders world-wide has hardly begun to be quantified, let alone taken up.

PSYCHIATRIC GENETICS

by Alastair Cardno & Peter McGuffin

The foundations of psychiatric genetics were laid around the turn of the nineteenth century by landmark developments in the fields of genetics and the classification of psychiatric disorders. Fundamental progress in the early development of genetics had been made by Sir Francis Galton, an English, largely self-taught scientist, during the latter half of the nineteenth century. Impressed by the theory of natural selection proposed by his cousin, Charles Darwin, Galton investigated the influence of hereditary factors on behaviour. He performed pioneering studies of families and twins, and first proposed the statistical techniques of correlation and regression in order to measure resemblance amongst relatives. His studies of men with high ability were published in *Hereditary Genius: An Inquiry into Its Laws and Consequences* in 1869. He also coined the term 'eugenics' to describe his ideas of improving mankind through selective reproduction. His views gained popularity amongst intellectuals across the whole political spectrum at the time.

Galton's work proceeded without knowledge of the laws of inheritance, which had been discovered by Gregor Mendel in 1866, based on cross-breeding of pea plants in his monastery garden in Moravia. The significance of Mendel's work was initially lost on the scientific community. However, his studies were rediscovered independently by the botanists Correns, de Vries, and Tschermack in 1900, and brought to world attention as fundamental to genetics. Initially, Mendel's laws for the inheritance of qualitative characteristics by hereditary elements (later to be termed *alleles*, the variant forms of a gene) were viewed as conflicting with the legacy of Galton's work on continuous variation, which developed into the discipline of quantitative genetics. However, after much bitter argument, the two approaches were integrated by the English scientist RA Fisher, who demonstrated that the inheritance of continuous variation would result from the combined effects of multiple genes, each of which was individually inherited in a mendelian fashion.

Meanwhile, a workable classification of the major psychiatric disorders was being developed by Emil Kraepelin, Professor of Clinical Psychiatry in Munich (Chapter 2, p. 49). This was based on meticulous clinical observation and the sorting and resorting of cards containing the clinical descriptions of his patients. In 1896, he first described dementia praecox, which he regarded as a separate disorder from manic–depressive psychosis, paranoia, and organic psychosis. He believed that genetic factors were generally important in the aetiology of psychiatric disorders. In his initial description of dementia praecox, Kraepelin stated that "an inherited predisposition occurred in about 70 per cent of cases". Later in his career, encouraged by the work of his junior colleagues in Munich, he wrote that "an understanding of the symptomatology of an illness will, we hope, result above all from genetic research".

The Munich school

Kraepelin began work in Munich in 1904, and in due course established the first 'research institute' for psychiatry. Amongst its members was Ernst Rüdin, who headed the Department for Genealogical Demography, and carried out the first systematic family studies of schizophrenia. Other members of the Institute, such as Hans Luxenburger and Bruno Schulz, also carried out pioneering research in quantitative psychiatric genetics. Since Galton had first proposed the study of twins for genetic research, the 'twin method' of contrasting the degree of resemblance for a characteristic in identical versus non-identical twins had been developed independently by Curtis Merriman in the USA, and Hermann Siemans in Germany, both in 1924. Luxenburger used Siemans's approach to perform the first systematic twin studies of schizophrenia and manic–depressive disorder. The Munich institute was also an important centre for the training of psychiatrists from elsewhere who would later establish programmes of psychiatric genetic research in their own countries. This process was fundamental to the international development of the discipline. Such visiting psychiatrists included Erik Strömgren from Denmark, Hans Essen-Möller from Sweden, and Eliot Slater from the UK.

The situation changed drastically when the Nazis came to power in Germany in 1933 and began to implement eugenic policies (Chapter 4, p. 86). Luxenburger and Schulz opposed these policies on both moral and scientific grounds. However, Rüdin supported the development of laws that introduced 'eugenic courts' to oversee programmes of compulsory sterilisation for the prevention of hereditary diseases. The diseases concerned included schizophrenia, manic–depressive insanity, Huntington's chorea, and severe alcoholism. Later on, the Nazis regarded the sterilisation laws as insufficient for their eugenic requirements, and many long-term psychiatric patients were exterminated, along with others deemed to be of low genetic worth. After the war, Rüdin was tried by the Allies and found guilty of being a 'fellow traveller', rather than a major contributor to war crimes, though the extent of his involvement remains a subject of heated debate.

After the Second World War

Immediately following the war, psychiatric genetic research virtually ceased in Germany. However, it was carried on elsewhere, notably by pre-war visitors to the Munich School. In England during the war, Slater worked in a hospital for military psychiatric casualties. This experience led to the formulation of the diathesis-stressor model of neurosis, with multiple genes (polygenes) contributing to the diathesis, or predisposition. After the war, he re-started a twin study of adult psychiatric disorders which he had begun on his return from Munich in 1935. In 1959, he was appointed director of the Medical Research Council's new psychiatric genetics unit, at the Maudsley Hospital and Institute of Psychiatry in London, based in a temporary building, which came to be known as 'the Genetics Hut'. Slater's senior scientific staff were few, consisting, for most of the Unit's existence, of James Shields, a former social worker turned geneticist, and Valerie Cowie, the Unit's deputy director, a psychiatrist and expert in the genetics of mental retardation. However, the unit also attracted overseas scholars and students such as the Taiwanese psychiatrist Ming Tsuang. One of the unit's particular assets was the Maudsley Hospital Twin Register, initiated by Slater in 1948 and providing a complete listing of every patient who had attended the Bethlem and Maudsley Hospitals and who was born one of a twin pair. The twin register became the starting point for a number of important studies carried out by visiting researchers, most notably that of schizophrenia by a then young post-doctoral fellow from the United States, Irving Gottesman, in collaboration with James Shields.

At the same time, psychiatrists in Scandinavia were taking advantage of the comprehensive system of parish registers, and subsequently national population registers, to perform meticulous family, twin, and adoption studies. Examples amongst many include the Swedish twin study of schizophrenia by Essen-Möller, who had immediately preceded Slater as a visiting fellow in Munich; the Norwegian twin study of all functional psychoses by Kringlen, who had been a visitor to Slater's unit in London; and the pioneering adoption studies of schizophrenia conducted by Rosenthal, Kety, *et al.* in Denmark. Earlier in the USA, large family and twin studies of schizophrenia were carried out by Franz Kallman. He was German by birth, and had worked in Munich but, being half-Jewish, had emigrated in 1933 soon after the Nazis came to power. Further work in the USA included the first adoption study of schizophrenia by Leonard Heston, and the study of army veteran twins with schizophrenia and affective illnesses by Pollin, Allen *et al.*

These and other studies both in Europe and the USA provided the main body of evidence that convincingly established the importance of genetic effects in the aetiology of severe psychiatric disorders. They did much to dispel the influence of the 'anti-psychiatry movement' (actually a rather disparate set of authors) that schizophrenia should not be regarded as an illness, and that psychiatric disorders generally were socially determined or might even be regarded as artificial, socially manufactured myths (Chapter 7, p. 202). In a response to such views, Kety famously remarked that "if schizophrenia is a myth, it is a myth with a strong genetic component!".

Decline, but not fall

A landmark in the history of psychiatric genetics was the publication of the first major textbook in English, Slater and Cowie's *The Genetics of Mental Disorders* in 1971. In addition to reviewing the genetics of the major psychiatric disorders and mental retardation, these authors provided a technically sophisticated approach to the field. They observed that "genetics, in fact, is one of the unifying disciplines which emphasises relationships between biological fields of study, and helps to create channels of communication between psychiatry and the medical sciences".

Ironically, around this time, psychiatric genetics in the UK entered a period of severe decline. In 1969, Slater retired, social psychiatry was the fashionable area amongst British academics, and the MRC closed the psychiatric genetics unit. Cowie left the Maudsley, and only Shields remained with a minimum of research support. However, at the same time, the subject was developing strongly in the USA, with some of the key players being past visitors to centres in the UK. For example, Irving Gottesman returned to work at the University of Minnesota, where he helped to establish one of several important centres for behavioural genetics in the USA. Ming Tsuang established himself in Iowa, where the department of psychiatry headed by George Winokur had a wide range of biological research interests, including genetics. In St Louis, Ted Reich, who had trained in quantitative genetics under DS Falconer at the Institute of Animal Genetics in Edinburgh, established one of the largest and most active psychiatric genetics research groups with colleagues such as Cloninger and Rice. At around the same time, a successful group was being set up by Elliot Gershon and colleagues at the US National Institute of Mental Health (NIMH). These and other developments led to the building up of a very strong psychiatric genetics community in the USA.

It was not until the very end of the 1970s that psychiatric genetics in the UK began to rejuvenate. James Shields died in 1978 and with no obvious successor, Sir Denis Hill, the professor of psychiatry at the Institute of Psychiatry asked Robin Murray to advise him on whether the genetics section had a viable future. Murray was a biological psychiatrist who, although not specifically trained in genetics, had an interest in the area and had the benefit of having just returned from a fellowship at NIMH. He found an ally in David Fulker, a psychologist and statistical geneticist who was director of the psychology department's animal laboratories at the Bethlem Royal Hospital. Murray convinced Hill that genetics was still worth pursuing at the Institute, and the genetics section therefore continued, with Murray as its head.

Murray and Fulker then began to encourage and train a new generation of researchers who once more exploited the Maudsley's twin registers and embarked on a new era of studies. These used biological markers and took some of the first faltering steps in the search for genetic linkage and association. By good fortune, the nearby MRC Social Psychiatry Unit was at that time employing as a statistician Elizabeth Sturt who had worked on linkage analysis under a doyen of statistical genetics, Cedric Smith at University College London. It is a measure of how unfashionable the subject then was in England that a first-rate statistical geneticist should have been forced to work as a general statistician at that time.

Against this background, quantitative studies continued to support a genetic contribution to psychiatric disorders. This was facilitated by more precise and reliable research interviews and operational diagnostic systems which twin studies went some way towards validating. On the basis of the accumulating quantitative genetic evidence, molecular genetic studies that aimed to locate susceptibility genes for disorders within the human genome began to be performed. Initially, the range of genetic markers available for such studies was very limited; it consisted mainly of blood groups such as the ABO and rhesus systems, and the HLA system. The early linkage and association studies that employed these kinds of marker were generally inconclusive, but they paved the way for future work.

Revolution in molecular biology

The prospects for identifying susceptibility genes for complex disorders improved dramatically as a consequence of ground-breaking developments in techniques for studying DNA molecules directly. Outstanding discoveries included the enzyme, reverse transcriptase, in 1970, which allowed the creation of genetic probes to identify specific sequences of genomic DNA. Following this, other enzymes, the restriction endonucleases, were used to create a large number of new genetic markers — 'restriction fragment length polymorphisms' (RFLPs). Also, the rate at which molecular analyses could be performed was substantially increased by the polymerase chain reaction (PCR), first described in 1985. These and other subsequent innovations have greatly increased the power of molecular genetic studies to identify susceptibility genes and study their function; the resulting techniques have been applied to the study of a wide range of medical conditions.

Recognition of the potential for applying such techniques to psychiatric disorders enhanced the standing of psychiatric genetics both in the USA and in the UK and continental Europe. It helped to turn the discipline from being relatively unfashionable to one whose great potential was widely recognised in psychiatric and other medical circles. As part of this process the European Science Foundation set up an initiative, for the molecular biology of mental illness, that facilitated research collaboration between centres in Europe. By 1989, the discipline had grown sufficiently to hold the first World Congress of Psychiatric Genetics, under the chairmanship of TJ Crow, now in Oxford. By the end of the century, there will have been eight such congresses, sponsored by a flourishing new association, the International Society of Psychiatric Genetics.

The impact of the new genetics

The application of DNA technology to psychiatric disorders began to pay dividends during the 1990s. To date, most progress has been made for disorders where a single gene is involved, or where there are single-gene subforms. For example, the genetics of fragile X syndrome and Huntington's disease have been shown to involve the unstable expansion of repeat sequences of three DNA bases (trinucleotide repeats) at sites on the X chromosome and chromosome 4, respectively. Three rare genetic mutations have been found to cause some cases of early-onset familial Alzheimer's disease, and a more general Alzheimer's disease risk factor, possession of the e4 allele of apolipoprotein E (APOE), has been identified.

However, quantitative genetic studies suggest that most common psychiatric disorders are genetically more complex. Predisposition is probably caused by the combined effect of multiple genes, and these may interact with environmental factors in still more complex ways. Recent studies aiming to detect and locate susceptibility genes have attempted to accommodate these complexities. Genetic studies increasingly involve collaboration between research centres, frequently on an international basis. Linkage studies often require screening the entire genome, with many DNA markers spaced along each chromosome. Such studies have been carried out, for example, in schizophrenia, bipolar disorder, autism, and alcohol dependence. The complexity of these disorders has made replication of findings inconsistent to date, but the pace of progress suggests that the molecular genetic basis of the common psychiatric disorders should be established early in the twenty-first century.

Conclusion

The history of psychiatric genetics during the twentieth century has been characterised by the gradual building up of solid scientific evidence through perseverance and the sharing of knowledge internationally, interspersed with episodes of spectacular discovery. It also suggests that there are going to be major implications for current and future discoveries in the field. Since psychiatric geneticists need to remain aware of past misuses, the ethical implications of advances in this knowledge require careful consideration. To the extent that misinterpretation of genetic findings can be a factor in their misapplication, researchers need to be open about their work and to have a role in public education. Beyond this, the application of genetic knowledge is politically important. Societies need to take a stance on a range of issues, including genetic testing, cloning, and the disclosure of genetic information.

One of the consequences of psychiatric genetic research during the second half of this century has been to firmly establish psychiatric disorders as having a biological basis, rather than being merely 'social constructs'. It is very likely that this has facilitated a wide range of research into the causes and treatment of these disorders. It has also relieved a generation of parents from guilt-laden theories of causation to do with the way they brought up their children. The complex interplay between genetic and environmental influences is also becoming more apparent. For example, there is probably a genetic contribution to the experience and perception of some traditionally environmental factors, such as life events.

Finally, there are many potential benefits whose realisation awaits a fuller understanding of genetic susceptibility to psychiatric disorders at the molecular level. It is hoped that this will lead to a clearer understanding of the pathophysiology of these disorders and of the relationships between biological and environmental influences. From this, it may be hoped that improved diagnosis and treatment, both biological and non-biological, will be devised. People at high genetic risk may then benefit from early intervention if they develop symptoms, as well as having the option of prophylactic treatment if they wish to reduce their risk of becoming ill.

PSYCHONEUROENDOCRINOLOGY

by Brian Harris & César Carvajal

The modern, highly sophisticated science of psychoneuroendocrinology may be traced back to a link between the physical and the emotional aspects of the human organism which was recorded in the literature of the Ancient World. From an endocrine perspective, a typical modern counterpart of this tradition is that of primary depression resulting in abnormal thyroid function (a blunted response to the TRH test), while abnormal thyroid function results in a mood disorder. The Biblical figure, Job, who clearly had a major skin disorder with comorbid depression, cried out to his 'miserable comforters' to look at his leanness (weight loss) as a proof of his emotional distress. Much later, in the fifth century BC, Hippocrates described hysteria as due to the wandering of the uterus around the woman's body, which was somehow the cause of the variety of symptoms experienced with that disorder. His theory might be considered a crude prediction of an aspect of the modern position that sex hormones (symbolised for Hippocrates by the uterus) have an effect on behaviour and emotions; some very precise associations between these have now been identified. It is known that androgens are linked to aggression in deer stags during the rutting season, and that oestradiol patch therapy is useful, both alone and as an adjunct to specific antidepressants in the treatment of women with post-natal depression. An anticipated link of mood states with personality and immunological status, might even be found in the writings of Galen, in the second century AC. He felt that the melancholic woman had more possibility of contracting cancer than the sanguine woman, which is possibly an historical prediction of the modern psychoimmunological perspective, linking mood states with the status of the immune system.

Origins

Psychoneuroendocrinology has two main origins. The first of these is the clinical observation that there are psychological and emotional repercussions of endocrine disorder, while the second is its basic science, which is neuroendocrinology. Together with the current progress in immunology, the modern position represents an amalgam of these two concepts. The term 'psychoneuroimmunoendocrinology' describes a discipline whose main goals are to study the aetiology and pathogenesis of psychiatric disorders, as well as to identify and develop endocrine markers in psychiatry.

In 1849, Berthold published a description of the changes which occurred in gelded roosters — atrophy of the comb, reduced aggressiveness, and lowered interest in hens. Although it is sometimes suggested that he was thus the father of modern neuroendocrinology, castration and its resultant eunuchoidism had been known for centuries. Examples published in the nineteenth century and relating to other endocrine glands included the attribution of Graves' disease to adverse experiences; this was when Caleb Parry, in 1825, linked its development in a young woman to an accident in a runaway wheelchair. The concept that stress could result in Graves' disease was to persist for almost 150 years, be discounted in the 1960s, and then re-emerge in the 1990s.

The reverse had also been described; in 1888, the fact that the clinical consequence of myxoedema included mental disorder was recorded at a meeting of the Clinical Society of London. However, it was not until 1908, at a psychiatric congress held in Dijon, France, that Laignel-Lavastine first used the term 'endocrinological psychiatry'. He hoped that this would encourage the study of alterations of personality in relation to the endocrine system. Whilst the linking of mental disorders and endocrine dysfunction had thus been firmly established, it was not until several decades later that further progress was made. In 1931, Von Euler and Gaddum identified substance P in the brain; the importance of this was not fully appreciated at the time, but it was the beginning of the identification of the neuropeptides.

At about the same time, Hans Selye began his investigations into the effects of stress; these were embodied in his classic publications of 1941, where he described the effects of injecting various steroids into rats. Progesterone in particular caused the rat to fall asleep — a discovery which was followed by the development of the pregnane anaesthetic agents, now known to be effective via gabaminergic mechanisms. Selye also made the suggestion that substances might be endogenously produced by the body to protect it in times of stress. In later years, these findings led to considerable research into the aetiology of post-natal depression. It was proposed that the fall in progesterone after delivery might be causative of depression, but this view has not so far been substantiated. Another avenue of research opened when Gjessing in Norway (1938) reported the use of thyroid extract in high doses to treat 'periodic catatonia' (Chapter 5, p. 133). This continued a development of hormonal treatments in psychiatry, which had started a few years earlier with insulin therapy.

At the end of the 1940s, neuroendocrine functioning began to be understood more clearly, and in 1948, the British physiologist George Harris proposed the concept that the hyothalamus played a primary role in the regulation of the pituitary-adrenocortical axis. He also regarded the pituitary as the master gland of the endocrine system, and these concepts were reinforced by the discovery that hypothalamic extracts stimulated the liberation of other hormones. In subsequent years, 'releasing factors' produced by the hypothalamus were isolated; investigators like Samuel McCann, Roger Guillemin, and Andrew Schalley played an important part in these discoveries, the latter two winning the Nobel Prize for physiology in 1977. They also shared a Nobel Prize with Rosalyn Yalow for their significant contributions to the development of radioimmunoassays, enabling more precise and rapid hormonal assays to be performed.

Progress

Various strands of progress which have contributed to the advance of psychoneuroendocrinology included the concept of the synapse, elaborated by Sherrington at Oxford in the 1930s, together with the discovery of chemical neurotransmission, 'modulated' by hormones and even by other neurotransmitters. Further progress included the identification of hypothalamic hormones, and the ability to measure these and others accurately in a variety of body fluids such as plasma, CSF, urine, and saliva. When this could be done over long periods of time, both natural and pathological biorhythms could be detected. Bryson and Martin reported an increase of 17-ketosteroids in the urine of a manic–depressive patient, thus promoting other endocrine measurements in psychiatric patients. These included basal hormone levels, secretion levels, and 'challenge' tests (the latter often with agonists and/or antagonists). The standard examples of challenge procedures are the dexamethasone suppression test (DST) and the TRH (thyrotropin releasing hormone) test. These tests were taken from general medicine and used particularly to examine the hypothalamo-pituitary-adrenal (HPA) and hypothalamo-pituitary-thyroid (HPT) axes in depressed patients.

The dexamethasone suppression test

The DST was first introduced in the 1960s as a test of HPA axis function, and later developed for use in depressed patients by Carroll in the USA. Examination of cortisol levels in patients with major depression, in particular those with 'melancholic' features, showed both hypercortisolaemia and a loss of reduction of secretory rhythm. An abnormal DST result (non-suppression) indicated a dysregulation of the HPA axis, with resistance to glucocorticoid-mediated feedback. Carroll's initial results seemed to indicate the discovery of the first objective test in psychiatry that was of value, and many thousands of scientific papers about it appeared in the literature. However, the specificity of the test was later questioned, e.g. when it was shown to be abnormal in other psychiatric disorders such as alcoholism, anorexia nervosa, and dementia.

In spite of this, the HPA axis continued to receive intensive study in depressed patients, attention turning to CRF (corticotropin releasing hormone), in terms both of a challenge test and of its production and levels in the brain. Studies such as those of Gold *et al.* in 1984 demonstrated hypersecretion of CRF in depression, with down-regulation of CRF receptors and adrenal hypertrophy. In response to CRF, depressed patients show a blunted secretion of ACTH from the pituitary gland — probably a reflection of the effect of negative feedback on the pituitary of higher levels of circulating cortisol. These findings have led to speculation into therapeutic possibilities. For instance, in refractory depression with hypercortisolaemia, the use of ketokonazol — an antisteroidal agent — can have antidepressant effects, though this is still experimental as a treatment. Similarly, neurosteroids (steroid hormones produced in the brain) such as dehidroepiandrosterone (DHEA) may also be shown to have an antidepressant effect, through their antiglucocorticoid activity. Another possibility for the future is the development of antagonists to CRF, since the latter have been shown in some studies to be increased in depressed patients.

The thyrotropin releasing hormone test

Studies of the HPT axis began with the observation by Prange in the USA that tri-iodothyronine (T_3) was useful as an adjunct to imipramine for depression. Much later, this effect was explained as possibly due to the action of T_3 on noradrenergic receptors, and it remains as both a useful strategy and an adjunct in resistant depression. Several years later, Prange reported a blunted response to TRH test in about 25% of patients: when the levels of plasma TSH were measured following a morning intravenous bolus of TRH, a blunted response was recorded, compared to normal subjects. The test was refined by Duval *et al.*, resulting in a 75% sensitivity. Though highly sensitive measurements of TSH have displaced the TRH test, some depressive patients continue to show an abnormal TRH test even after recovery, and this is possibly an acquired marker, indicating vulnerability to early relapse. The detection of sub-clinical hypothyroidism (normal plasma thyroid hormones with elevated TSH) by means of the TRH test or by accurate estimation of TSH has been of value in patients with refractory depression, as well as in those on lithium.

Estimation of thyroid antibodies together with thyroid hormones allows risk factors to be identified in refractory depression, in bipolar disorder (in particular, the refractory type), and in a sub-group of post-partum depression. The account of the latter is fascinating, in that in 1948, Robertson had described from his New Zealand general practice a number of women who showed signs of mild hypothyroidism in the post-partum period. Over three decades later, Amino *et al.* recorded the same, and linked the condition to the presence of thyroid antibodies in the women. They reported that some of these women showed signs of 'depressive psychosis', later establishing an association of post-natal depression with thyroid antibody status. However, the depressive state seems to be independent of the actual thyroid status, and may be linked to the general malaise which accompanies post-partum thyroiditis, due to release of cytokines, which themselves produce depressed mood. Recently, a decrease of transthyretin, the carrier protein which transports T_4 to the brain to be transformed to T_3 (i.e. the active form), has been detected in depression. This protein could therefore represent a new model on which the synthesis of a new type of antidepressant might be based.

Work on the hypothalamo-pituitary-gonadal axis has included the observation that women are apparently more susceptible to stress-related disorders than men, and that depressive symptoms appear to be associated with menarche, the menstrual cycle, the post-partum period, and the menopause. Yet no firm hormonal correlates have so far been demonstrated for any of these. Though the premenstrual syndrome appears to be a mood disorder, no definitive hormonal associations have been established with it. In spite of this, early evidence indicates that hormonal therapies can benefit the patient; oestradiol patch therapy and monthly progestogen can alleviate both the premenstrual syndrome and post-natal depression. The use of leuprolide, a congener of gonadotropin releasing hormone (GnRH), has also been demonstrated to be effective in producing a hypogonadal state, obliterating the hormonal changes which accompany the menstrual cycle, and alleviating severe premenstrual dysphoria.

Conclusion

Psychoneuroendocrinology has thus evolved from a stage of classical descriptions and anecdotal cases to a strict scientific discipline within biological psychiatry. Although tests of diagnostic value do not exist, hormonal studies appear to be leading to the differentiation of subgroups of psychiatric disorders which have a biological basis. Similarly, the development of hormonal therapies represents an exciting challenge for the future of psychoneuroendocrinology.

INTERNATIONAL PSYCHIATRY AND THE WORK OF THE WPA

by Ahmed Okasha

Towards the end of the twentieth century, the World Psychiatric Association (WPA) has come a long way between the objectives of its initial establishment and what it contributes to the promotion of the psychiatric profession and the welfare of mental patients. The beginnings of the WPA in 1950, as an association for the Organization of World Congresses of Psychiatry, with the French psychiatrist Jean Delay as its President and Henry Ey as its Secretary General, must be understood within the context of world events and of developments in the health field.

To date, the WPA incorporates 107 member societies, representing 94 countries from all around the globe, 50 scientific sections in an array of diverse disciplines, and a worldwide distribution of membership. There are also standing committees and taskforces which focus on particular areas of interest, providing a forum for cross-societal and cross-sectional interdisciplinary collaboration.

Scientific and cultural collaboration

It was during the years of the first two World Congresses of Psychiatry, held in Paris in 1950 and Zurich in 1957, that the international psychiatric community recognised that its field was in a state of flux. It was experiencing radical and unprecedented changes in both its conceptual framework and patterns of practice. The advent of psychotropic medication for mental disorders, the expanding frontier of knowledge on brain functioning, substantial efforts at deinstitutionalising psychiatric patients, and awareness of the value of a sociocultural framework to understand illness and help-seeking behaviour, all contributed to these changes. This meant that psychiatrists could no longer function in isolation behind closed doors.

The formal founding of the World Psychiatric Association in 1961 signified a move toward a professional identity, together with an effort to respect diversity and use it effectively to attain unity in purpose. By accommodating under the same roof all psychiatrists of different national and cultural origins, of different schools of thought, of various areas of interest, and of diverging ideological proclivities, the WPA aspired to establish a worldwide front of professionals. This was to be united in the pursuit of increased knowledge in the field and of increased potential for the care of mental patients.

Attentive to world political and social changes, the WPA has incorporated in the last decade virtually all the psychiatric societies of Eastern Europe. Its recently established 18 zones, across five world regions, intend to support the interaction of Member

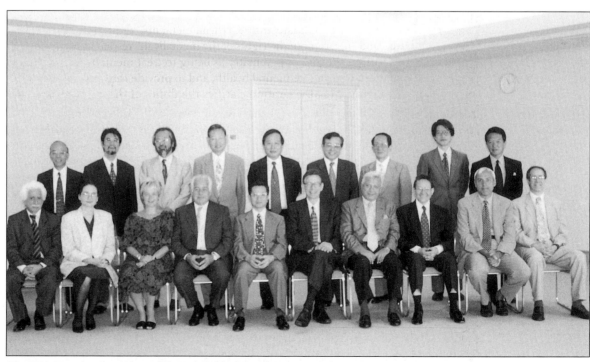

The WPA Executive Committee and the Board of the Japanese Association for Psychiatry and Neurology.

1991–2000

International psychiatry and the work of the WPA

Societies with the governing bodies of the WPA and their fuller participation in all aspects of institutional life.

Twenty-seven years after its establishment, a WPA survey, undertaken to develop the organisation on the basis of the suggestions of its membership, has reinforced the relevance of the initial mandate for which the organisation was established: this is primarily to foster communication amongst both psychiatric professionals and organisations.

A critical factor for ensuring the continuity of vitality and productivity in the WPA between and during congresses, has been the establishment of scientific sections. To date, the WPA contains 50 sections that cut across the different disciplines and schools of psychiatric thought and technological advances. Five interdisciplinary taskforces integrate the common areas of interests of the different sections: the future of psychiatry and neuroscience, education, psychosocial rehabilitation of psychiatric patients, violence, and bioethics. The clustering of sections with common interests for collaborative taskforces is another major initiative of the WPA.

A major task according to the new bylaws is to issue consensus statements on the WPA's various areas of interest and on the concerns of its disciplines. Several have already been proposed regarding: ethical issues and problematic situations; assessment, measurement and informatics; psychosocial intervention; and specific psychiatric disorders. Formulation of those statements regarding the vast array of issues covered by the scientific sections of the WPA will constitute an important contribution of the WPA to the field at large.

Educational activities

Since 1990, the WPA has been paying increased and more systematic attention to educational activities, often in coordination with the World Health Organization. Educational programmes have been developed in various aspects of the psychiatric field: teaching and learning about schizophrenia, the WPA Bulletin on Depression, the WPA/PTD (Prevention and Treatment of Depression) educational programme on depression, the ICD–10-related educational programmes, and the educational programme on ICD–10 anxiety and panic disorders, dysthymia, and social phobia. A WPA General Survey in 1998 to assess the impact of the WPA and monitor its value as an organisational and collaborative tool revealed 53.8% 'good' and 10% 'excellent' assessments of the quality of those programmes, as evaluated by member societies and WPA sections. As many as 81% reported that they perceived the purpose "to increase knowledge and skills for mental health care".

Professional ethics

Stimulated by years of reports of the political abuse of psychiatry in certain countries, the WPA General Assemblies have consistently formulated ethical guidelines on psychiatric practice, including the Hawaii Declaration of 1977 and its amendment in Vienna in 1983. More recently, there was the Madrid Declaration and the first elements of specific guidelines endorsed by the General Assembly in Madrid in 1996. Members of the WPA recognise the importance of this mandate and its crucial elements "to promote the highest ethical standards" and "to promote the rights of the mentally ill" respectively. Seven general guidelines focus on the aim of psychiatry as being to treat mentally ill patients, to prevent mental illness, to promote mental health, and to provide care and rehabilitation for psychiatric patients. This Declaration clarifies the duties of the psychiatrists, prohibiting any abuse and insisting that no treatment should be provided against the patient's will, unless it is necessary for the welfare and safety of the patient and others. Emphasis is placed on advising the patient or caregiver about all details of management, or the need for confidentiality, and on the ethics of research. Five additional specific guidelines state the ethical position in relation to: euthanasia, torture, death penalty, intra-uterine sex selection, and organ transplantation. The collective principles of professional ethics involved in those documents represent a widely acclaimed response to the present state of psychiatry. However, the development of an ethical stand is not a one-time effort. The continuous advancement of science and changing political and economic patterns all over the world challenge our profession with new dilemmas that call for regular position statements.

Another cluster of elements has been identified for further discussion with the view to formulate a professional ethical stand. An ongoing process of consultation amongst members of the Ethics Committee involves relationships with the pharmaceutical industry, and with the media, gene research and counselling, psychotherapy, managed care, ethnic discrimination, and ethnic cleansing. Throughout its years of activities on the ethical guidelines of the profession, the WPA has been working in close collaboration with the UN and the WHO to protect the human rights of mental patients.

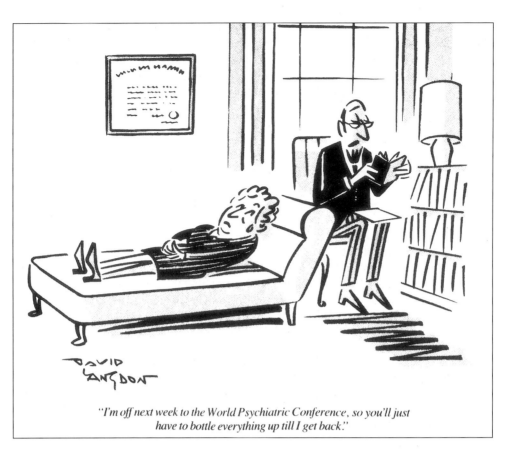

Punch cartoon, 1980s. Reproduced with permission from Punch.

"I'm off next week to the World Psychiatric Conference, so you'll just have to bottle everything up till I get back."

As in its beginnings, WPA has continued to give prominence to the preparation and implementation of World Congresses of Psychiatry as well as to its Regional Meetings in all continents, e.g. 1997 in Beijing, 1998 in India, and 1998 in South Africa. The challenges facing WPA remain great and the tasks ahead formidable. Our only guarantee of success is to nurture the vitality of its foundational spirit, as well as the legacy of those inspired doctors, who recognised the need of psychiatrists to network and exchange experience and expertise in a multicultural, multidisciplinary, professional framework.

PSYCHOPHARMACOLOGY 2000

by David Healy

It is common to hear that there have been no new developments in psychopharmacology since the mid-1960s. It is said that the astonishing decade from the mid-1950s, which saw the introduction of the antipsychotics, the antidepressants, the tranquillisers, and lithium has not been repeated (Chapter 6, p. 169). The agents introduced since the first generation of drugs are said to have been essentially variations on a theme, offering greater selectivity in pharmacological profile, with clinical applications which can perhaps be applied more rationally, but offering little more in terms of efficacy than the original drugs.

There is some truth to this, but nothing unexpected, in so far as in the nature of things, astonishing decades rarely succeed each other. But this view would give a misleading impression if it was therefore assumed that developments in psychopharmacology have not had further impacts on psychiatric theory and practice since the mid-1960s. These impacts have in fact been in four distinct areas. First, in industrialised countries, psychotropic drugs became available on a prescription-only status, when introduced in the 1950s, and are probably still thought to be amongst those that most require that continuing status. A generation of clinicians have grown up so accustomed to these arrangements that they perhaps no longer appreciate the impact this has had on psychiatric thinking. This issue interacts with a second. The methods of evaluating psychopharmacological treatments required operational criteria, rating scales, and randomised controlled trials (RCTs). Developments in this area during the 1970s fed into forces within American psychiatry that have been termed the 'neo-Kraepelinian' school, whose influence led to the creation of DSM–III in 1980 (Chapter 8, p. 233). Third, the psychotropic drugs have been the main stimulus to neuroscientific developments that have taken place in the 1980s and 1990s. These developments are beginning to lead to the emergence of a group of drugs which perhaps blur the boundaries between illness and lifestyle, between disease and dysfunction. Finally, despite popular impressions, there have been a number of significant discoveries, amongst which have been the selective serotonin (5HT) reuptake inhibitors (SSRIs), the specifically antipsychotic effects of clozapine, the role of anticonvulsants in the management of recurrent mood disorders, and the emergence of 'lifestyle' modifiers.

The emergence of selectivity

In the mid-1960s, faced with the then available antidepressants, Paul Kielholz, Professor of Psychiatry at Basel suggested that some of these drugs treat depressed patients by being more drive-enhancing, while others appeared to be doing 'something else'. Faced with this proposal, Arvid Carlsson in Gothenburg (Chapter 6, p. 180) noted that the antidepressants which appeared to be more drive-enhancing had actions on catecholamine systems, whereas those agents that appeared to be doing something else had preferential actions on the 5HT system. This led to the synthesis of the SSRIs, of which the first patented, in 1971, was zimelidine and the first to come into clinical use, in 1978, was indalpine.

At the time of the synthesis of these drugs, monoamine theories of depression had risen to prominence, and according to these, all antidepressants corrected a common lesion. The Hamilton Depression Rating Scale (HDRS) had also begun to be used widely in clinical trials from the end of the 1960s, and on this instrument, all antidepressants effectively looked the same. Both of these factors tended to obscure the differences between the SSRIs and other antidepressants, rather than to highlight them. The marketing of the SSRIs was on the basis that they differed from the tricyclics only in terms of safety in overdose as well as having a more advantageous profile of side-effects. However, most SSRIs have received licenses for use in social phobia, panic disorder, obsessive–compulsive disorder (OCD), and post-traumatic stress disorder (PTSD), in a way that other agents have not. On this basis, it is now clear that Kielholz's and Carlsson's initial supposition that these agents would be different from other antidepressants was correct. The profile of actions of the SSRIs suggests that this includes some promotion of sanguinity, some suppression of emotional reactivity, and some anxiolytic action that is of modest benefit across a wide range of nervous states.

The development of the SSRIs also owed something to the benzodiazepine dependence crisis that hit Western clinical psychopharmacology in the 1980s. A series of reports then implicated the benzodiazepines in the production of physical dependence in patients. Allied to the fact that these drugs had on occasions appeared to be marketed to assist in 'problems of living', rather than for the management of disease, these reports led to vigorous public debate, especially in the United Kingdom. While alprazolam was successfully introduced for panic disorder during the 1980s, no other benzodiazepine has been developed for any anxiety indication since 1980. This impacted on the development of the SSRIs, in that these agents could have been developed either for anxiety or mood disorder indications, but the period was one in which it was more attractive to emphasise their action on mood.

However, from a global perspective, this development was essentially a Western one. Benzodiazepine dependence has not proved to be a problem in Japan, and through the 1990s, the 'conventional' anxiolytic market remained robust, with benzodiazepine derivatives being used more widely than antidepressants. As of 1998, no SSRI had been approved for a mood disorder indication in Japan, although this may also have been related to general difficulties in obtaining a licence in that country. Worldwide, the picture conforms to the Japanese pattern, rather than to the Western one. A WHO survey in 1995 found that for complaints of fatigue and nervousness, a tranquilliser was more likely to be used than an antidepressant and, perhaps surprisingly, that antidepressants were more likely to be used than tranquillisers for anxiety indications. This pattern agrees with the results of two RCTs conducted by Klein and Fink at Hillside Hospital, New York in the 1960s. These investigators randomised all patients to chlorpromazine, imipramine, or placebo. They found that chlorpromazine but not imipramine was useful for psychotic disorders, but also that chlorpromazine and imipramine were equally active for mood disorders, with imipramine only producing selective benefits over chlorpromazine in phobic or anxiety disorders. These results later played a part in the emergence of panic disorder as an important condition, for which SSRIs are now the treatment of choice. This pattern of developments points to the complex mixture of cultural, pharmacogenetic, and pharmaceutical marketing factors that go into drug development. It points also to the complex interplay between those developments and the psychiatric concepts that may either support such developments or arise as a consequence of them.

The period from 1970 through to the present has indeed been one characterised by complex interactions of this type, affecting the 'antidepressants' in particular. In addition to the emergence of panic disorder, OCD was all but rediscovered in some countries. This 'discovery' owed a great deal to a recognition of the superior effects of clomipramine (and by extension the SSRIs) for this condition, in comparison to other agents. Indeed, the increasing recognition of this disabling condition and the ability to produce therapeutic benefits for it with 5HT-selective agents constitutes one of the clearest psychiatric developments since the 1950s. There has also been a recognition of disorders such as social phobia and Gilles de la Tourette syndrome. In all these cases, developments have been driven by the availability of therapeutic agents which offer benefits for the conditions in question. The increasing delineation of such discrete syndromes had a further effect, in that it underpinned the neo-Kraepelinian approach to psychiatry, whose proponents see mental disorders as medical illnesses entirely comparable to disease states found elsewhere in medicine. This approach has been enshrined in DSM–III, which as a research manual marks a revolution in psychiatry and one of the major achievements of the period (Chapter 8, p. 233).

DSM–III and IV are more than research manuals, however. The DSM is linked to the development of rating scales and RCT methods, which have been amongst the triumphs of modern psychiatry. They have permitted convincing demonstrations of efficacy to be achieved in conditions that often show large spontaneous variability, set against the background of diverse constitutional types and psychosocial settings. However, at the end of the century, this triumph risks becoming a trap. As pressure mounts to limit the rise in health care costs, particularly in the USA, the DSM manuals have become the basis for insurance and reimbursement and a tool of health care policy. This is a development that the originators of DSM–III for the most part see as premature and unfortunate. In some instances in the USA, health maintenance organisations will only reimburse for DSM-defined conditions and in addition, will only reimburse for treatments which have been demonstrated scientifically to work for these conditions. In the case of psychiatrists, this often means that reimbursement is restricted to the act of prescribing. Time spent supporting patients or assessing their psychosocial situations is not paid for, so doctors risk becoming prescribers rather than therapists.

The retreat from selectivity

The development of chlorpromazine, reserpine, and haloperidol in the 1950s led to the idea that the agents of benefit in psychoses were neuroleptics, i.e. drugs which had effects on striatal systems and potentially produced extra-pyramidal reactions. In other words, in order to produce benefits in psychotic states, drugs which might be effective would have to have these effects. The basis of these effects was first elucidated in 1963 by Carlsson in Gothenburg (Chapter 6, p. 180), who showed that the neuroleptics had effects on catecholamine systems. Further studies localised these effects to dopamine systems in 1966, and specifically to dopamine D_2 receptors in 1972. These discoveries gave rise to the dopamine hypothesis of schizophrenia, which along with the monoamine hypothesis of affective disorders, provided a rallying point for biological psychiatrists and ultimately a new language for psychiatry. The dopamine hypothesis also led to the quest to produce D_2-selective antagonists, in the belief that agents devoid of effects on other receptors would have greater efficacy and a 'cleaner' profile of side-effects. The quest for pharmacological specificity in both the antipsychotic and antidepressant domains, therefore, dominated psychiatric and psychopharmacological thinking from the mid-1970s through to the early 1990s.

In the meantime clozapine, an agent first synthesised in 1958 and first tested clinically in 1962 but only brought into further clinical development from 1965, appeared to have an unorthodox antipsychotic effect. It was claimed that it could be of benefit without producing extra-pyramidal reactions, and that it was therefore an antipsychotic without being a 'neuroleptic', as strictly defined. This profile, which was at odds with the dominant notions of the day, led to a slow clinical development, which was suspended following the emergence of a series of fatal cases of agranulocytosis in Finland in 1975.

The apparent demise of clozapine then left the field free for the continued development of D_2-selective agents. Some of these that were brought in to clinical use — sulpiride, amisulpride, and remoxipride — did indeed seem to have fewer side-effects. They were not, however, any more efficacious and this, amongst other things, led many of the original proponents of the hypothesis to conclude that while neuroleptics may act preferentially on dopamine systems, the dopamine hypothesis of schizophrenia was wrong. In addition, by the time remoxipride and amisulpride were released in the 1990s, it had become clear that clozapine offered benefits that agents which were highly selective for D_2 receptors did not appear to produce.

Clozapine was resurrected in the mid-1980s, when it was studied in an American clinical trial for treatment-resistant schizophrenic disorders. The methodology of that trial can be questioned, in that the comparative group were on high doses of other neuroleptics, and so the benefits of clozapine might have stemmed as much from a more favourable side-effect profile as by virtue of a greater antipsychotic effect. Nevertheless, the results were clear-cut and have since been consistently replicated. Clozapine re-emerged with a licence in several countries for treatment-resistant schizophrenia and a considerable reputation that led to it become the largest selling antipsychotic worldwide in the mid-1990s.

More importantly, its success led to a revision of the concept of an 'antipsychotic'. It had become clear that actions on other than D_2 receptors were potentially of benefit. The fact that clozapine had an action on $5HT_2$ receptors favoured the development of a number of $5HT_2/D_2$ receptor blockers (serotonin–dopamine antagonists: SDAs). A number of other agents have been developed with effects on $5HT_2$, D_2, and adrenergic receptors, while a series of D_4 receptor antagonists have also been developed in the hope that the peculiar benefits of clozapine might stem from its action on D_4 receptors. To date, none of the newer compounds appears to be the 'clozapine without agranulcytosis' that people have been hoping for. The majority appear to have receptor and clinical profiles which are closer to those of chlorpromazine than those of clozapine. In this sense, none of these latter developments represent the creation of a different therapeutic principle, in the way that the development of the SSRIs did. All of the newer agents are potent D_2 receptor blockers and as such, are conventional neuroleptics, but by virtue of actions on other systems, they are much less likely to cause extra-pyramidal effects. In this sense, they are closer to being antipsychotics like clozapine.

Worldwide, developments in the antipsychotic field have varied considerably, both as regards thinking about antipsychotics and the availability of different compounds. In the United States, all neuroleptics were viewed before clozapine in terms of chlorpromazine-equivalents: all were seen as essentially the same, differing only in their side-effect profile. In contrast, in France, agents such as chlorpromazine, haloperidol, and sulpiride were seen as having quite different therapeutic benefits, rather than simply different side-effect profiles, even though all were characterised as 'neuroleptics'. Some agents such as thioridazine were seen as beneficial by virtue of a more sedative effect, while others such as sulpiride were seen as more alerting or drive enhancing. The French view would appear to have been borne out by developments with clozapine. Just as there has been no uniformity of psychiatric thinking on the nature of the antipsychotics, so also during the period from 1960 to 1990, little uniformity across global markets has been seen in terms of the availability of different compounds. A significant development in the 1990s has been the emergence of a globalisation in drug development. This means that new agents which become available in one part of the world almost invariably become available in all other parts, and do so more or less at the same time. Hitherto, this process has applied to the antipsychotics in a way that so far has not applied to the antidepressants.

Interface between evidence and efficacy

Lithium has had a unique place in psychiatry for a number of reasons. First, no large corporation has promoted its use. Second, its profile of effects differs from that of other agents, in that it has been claimed to have distinctive prophylactic benefits and to be of most benefit when used chronically, whereas all other agents demonstrate their benefits most clearly in the acute management of mental disorders. Third, although it is in widespread use for prophylactic purposes, proving that lithium clearly possesses a prophylactic effect requires large-scale studies that have been almost impossible to carry out to the satisfaction of all.

In the mid-1960s, a further agent was noted to produce benefits in the long-term regulation of mood. This was sodium valproate, whose psychotropic effect was first described in France by Pierre Lambert in 1965. He proposed that this would be useful in disorders within the affective spectrum, largely of the bipolar type, although also suggesting that it acted by being in some way 'personality-strengthening'. (The anticonvulsants appear to help by reducing irritability, in a manner that remains unspecified to this day.) The use of sodium valproate for mood disorders went unnoticed until the 1990s, largely because of reasons to do with the patent on the drug. By then, however, another anticonvulsant had also been shown to have benefits in this area. In 1973, Okuma *et al.* in Japan reported the beneficial effects of carbamazepine in recurrent mood disorders. Unlike valproate, carbamazepine was adopted rapidly, particularly in the United States. The benefits of both these agents have furthermore underpinned efforts to develop lamotrigine and gabapentin for the management of chronic mood disorders.

In recent years, the anticonvulsants have become used widely for these disorders, particularly in the United States, where they have almost supplanted lithium. But there are formidable difficulties in 'proving' that they work. Clinicians witnessing their effects are convinced of this, but proving it to the satisfaction of pharmaceutical regulators involves recruiting hundreds of patients, keeping them on treatment for several years, and keeping many of the most severely ill psychiatric patients on placebo for lengthy periods of time. This is a situation where the complexities of psychiatric practice push up against the boundaries of our evaluative capacities. It is a situation that has arisen at a time when evidence-based medicine is trumpeted as not only a good thing, but a very necessary development. At the turn of this century, however, it remains unclear whether we have been misled to some extent by the relative ease with which evidence can be generated in short-term acute studies.

The story of bipolar disorder is not the only one where the interface between evidence and practice is problematic. While antipsychotics have been given to children with psychotic disorders from the time of their introduction, for the most part, other psychotropic agents were not prescribed for them until the 1980s. However, the increasing prescription of psychotropic drugs to children has led to considerable controversy. Several million prescriptions are issued annually for antidepressants to children in North America, despite the fact that almost all randomised controlled trials in adolescents have failed to demonstrate a benefit. But this clinical use of drugs in the absence of evidence would appear to be balanced by a failure, outside North America, to prescribe stimulants for childhood attention deficit hyperactivity disorder (ADHD), despite what has been portrayed as the most compelling evidence of efficacy in all of medicine.

The period of early discovery in psychopharmacology symbolically closed with the student unrest that occurred worldwide in 1968–1970. Psychiatry, and biological psychiatry in particular, was a target for the students. The disturbances led to the retirement of Jean Delay, one of the discoverers of chlorpromazine, while in Utrecht, Herman van Praag received death threats and had to have a police escort. The Tokyo University department of psychiatry, which was very biologically orientated, was occupied by students for 10 years. While nothing quite like this has happened since, the vigour of the debates surrounding the prescription of psychotropic drugs to children indicates that issues of ideology have not been completely eliminated from psychiatry.

'Lifestyle' drugs

In the 1960s and 1970s, the benzodiazepines had been marketed in some quarters as agents to help with problems of living, and this aspect of their promotion was the subject of considerable criticism. In 1980, the adoption of DSM–III in the United States led to a more explicit focus on disease models in psychiatry, with an attempt to pull back from the mass detection and treatment of community distress. These moves have only been partly successful, however, in that a series of epidemiological studies in the United States, Europe, and elsewhere have pointed to high levels of psychiatric symptoms in the community that can be interpreted as disease-based. As a result, during the 1990s, many psychotropic drugs have been used much more widely than might have been expected in 1980. There has been no reluctance on the part of pharmaceutical companies to market their drugs for milder nervous conditions in the community. But until recently, they had a distinct reluctance to be associated with conditions that might be characterised as not part of the domain of serious medicine, such as sexual dysfunction.

In the case of drugs active on the 5HT system, the benefits of such agents in the management of premature ejaculation were discovered as early as 1973. Indeed, the treatment effect size of the SSRIs for premature ejaculation is greater than their effect size for depression. There is, in addition, a very considerable problem with premature ejaculation in the community, with some estimates that up to one-third of men may be affected by this condition. Nevertheless, pharmaceutical companies were reluctant to be involved in this area. The issue of sexual functioning was only confronted by the sponsors of a post-SSRI generation of drugs, which had different effects on sexual functioning. But their efforts to establish and market the evidence of the frequency with which SSRIs brought about sexual 'dysfunction' also made it clear that by the mid-1990s, this area was no longer subject to taboo, in the way that it had been.

This laid the basis for the market development of a series of treatments for impotence, culminating with the release of sildenafil (Viagra), which marks an important point in the development of psychopharmacology for a number of reasons. First, despite regulatory efforts to contain this agent within a disease framework, company executives and many others are talking openly about a new generation of lifestyle drugs. These will include agents to enhance sexual functioning, reverse skin ageing, and tackle obesity. In the process, there will inevitably be a blurring between the boundaries of illness and normality, which will impact on the mental illness domain in so far as behaviour is the target of these agents. The development of the Internet, in addition, has created a capacity for the use of supposedly prescription-only agents outside a medical framework. Anyone can now order any of these newer agents by this means, without having to consult a doctor.

This will have an impact on notions of mental illness for the following reason. Many of the SSRIs are approaching the end of their patents. One possibility is for them to become available over-the-counter (OTC), as a number of H_2-antagonists are already available for stomach disorders. Both groups of drugs would seem to pose the same level of risk — much lower than with aspirin or paracetamol. Given the new climate of lifestyle modification with pharmacological agents, it is probable that an SSRI will become available for an indication like premature ejaculation. Alternatively, it may become available on the Internet for this purpose. If used in this way, however, these agents would also have anti-anxiety properties and would most probably be used by some people for this purpose. In all probability, such use of an SSRI would follow the profile associated with the use of St John's Wort herb. This has anti-nervousness properties that are sufficiently robust to come through the critical scrutiny of an RCT. St John's Wort, however, is portrayed as being helpful for stress, burnout, and problems of living, rather than for a disease. On the basis that lay-models of nervous disorders differ from medical models, an OTC SSRI would almost certainly be portrayed in a similar manner.

It is unclear how far psychiatric thinking about disease entities controls and regulates drug development. Nor is it clear how much psychiatric thinking is in turn controlled by the availability of certain compounds and markets, as well as the regulatory framework within which these compounds are brought to the market. A pharmaceutical company's support for particular viewpoints is a potent element in selecting the opinion that will be aired at international and in other scientific forums. We have been living through a period when the regulatory framework of psychopharmacology has put a premium on disease models, in the hope that the restriction of agents to those who stand to benefit most will lead to a favourable risk–benefit ratio in the use of pharmaceuticals. Restricting new agents to prescription-only arrangements has encouraged companies to develop drugs for specific disease indications, and to endorse medical models. But many of these agents can produce benefits as significant to lifestyle as for diseases, and even in the West, they are becoming available outside the medical framework.

The emergence of Viagra and the anti-obesity agent Xenical also appears to have brought the question of health care rationing into the realm of public debate. There is no contest about the efficacy of some of these newer agents, and little basis to proscribe them in the way the hallucinogens and drugs of abuse have been proscribed. But there can be legitimate concerns about making them available through tax-payers' money or health care insurance schemes for purposes other than the treatment of 'genuine' disease. Diseases were first defined as states of distress or illness, but with the rise of the biological sciences in the late nineteenth century, they began to be defined in terms of a biological lesion. We may be entering a period where they will be defined economically, in terms of what third-party payers will reimburse.

The impact of neuroscience

When the psychotropic drugs first emerged, there was no understanding as to how they might work. It was not even accepted that chemical neurotransmission had a role in brain functioning. Since then, efforts to develop new agents have led to an increasing understanding of how the brain functions, and these efforts in turn have expanded into neuroscience. This is now a vast endeavour whose realms of research extend far beyond questions to do with the mechanism of action of psychotropic drugs. Its development goes beyond therapeutics to embrace hitherto undreamt of biopsychoengineering possibilities. Until the 1990s, neuroscientific developments played very little part in driving drug development. At present, however, changes in the neuroscientific knowledge base are fuelling changes in psychopharmacology in a number of ways. One has to do with the imminent emergence of a number of truly different psychotropic agents. These include substance P antagonists, sigma-2 antagonists, and a range of other drugs with no direct effects on the monoamine systems that have hitherto been the conventional targets of psychotropic drug development. It is not immediately clear that the psychotropic properties of these new agents will fit the traditional framework of antidepressants, anxiolytics, and antipsychotics.

At least as important are developing capacities within pharmacogenetics and neuroimaging. Hitherto, these capacities have been rudimentary. The resolution of neuroimaging technologies to date has been so modest that the handheld post-mortem brain can reveal as much. In the near future, however, a new generation of machines will be capable of far greater resolution, and this will permit *in vivo* functional histology. Clinicians will be able to see if their treatments are working in the expected manner, particularly when they are not producing the expected clinical change.

There have been clear indications for over three decades that responses to psychotropic drugs breed true in families. Within five years, simple blood tests will be available to predict the likelihood of adverse effects to particular therapeutic agents. Once these tests become available, legal and financial considerations will drive their early and comprehensive use. This implementation in turn will necessarily reveal differences in constitutional types, pushing us back from our current highly categorical views of nervous disorders toward a more dimensional framework.

Combined, these developments will allow a significant increase in the quality of the outcomes following clinical interventions — where quality is defined in industrial terms as reliable reproducibility. This will present us with a hitherto hidden aspect of the disease model, which is that in terms of quality, defined in this way, it is 'forgiving'. Up to now, because patients have so much to lose when left untreated, doing something has been better than doing nothing, even though the treatment itself may be risky or carry a heavy burden of side-effects. We may be on the verge of a substantial increase in the reliability with which outcomes may be brought about, which would tend to shift practice from a disease model to something closer to a bio-engineering model. In addition, the availability of effective agents and neuroscientific knowledge, which have so far underpinned medical and categorical models of nervous disorders, may in the near future favour more dimensional models and the OTC availability of many psychotropic agents. The clinical and regulatory models that have been the basis of therapeutic practice in the second half of the twentieth century, therefore, may be set for a dramatic change in the early years of the new millennium.

FURTHER READING

Eating disorders

Bruch H. *Eating Disorders: Obesity, Anorexia Nervosa and the Person Within*. New York: Basic Books; 1973.

Dancyger IF, Garfinkel PE. The relationship of partial syndrome eating disorders to anorexia nervosa and bulimia nervosa. *Psychological Medicine*. 1995; **25**:1019–1026.

Fombonne E. Anorexia nervosa. No evidence of an increase. *British Journal of Psychiatry*. 1995; **166**:462–471.

Garfinkel PE, Goldbloom D. Bulimia nervosa: A review of therapy research. *Journal of Psychotherapy Practice and Research*. 1993; **2**:38–50.

Garfinkel PE, Walsh BT. Drug therapies for the eating disorders. In: Garner DH, Gafinkel PE, eds. *Handbook for Treatment of Eating Disorders*. New York: Guilford Press; in press.

Garfinkel PE, Kennedy S, Kaplan AS. Diagnosis and classification of the eating disorders. *Canadian Journal of Psychiatry*. 1995; **40**:445–456.

Kendler KS, MacLean C, Neal M, *et al*. The genetic epidemiology of bulimia nervosa. *American Journal of Psychiatry*. 1991; **148**:1627–1637.

Russell GFM. Bulimia nervosa: an ominous variant of anorexia nervosa. *Psychological Medicine*. 1979; **9**:429–448.

Woodside B. Bulimia nervosa in a Canadian community sample: prevalence and co-morbidity. *American Journal of Psychiatry*. 1995; **152**:1052–1058.

Community psychiatric nursing

Bowers L. Community psychiatric nurse caseloads and the 'worried well': misspent time or vital work? *Journal of Advanced Nursing*. 1997; **26**:930–936.

Brooker C, White E, eds. *Community Psychiatric Nursing*. London: Chapman and Hall; 1995.

Department of Health. *Working in Partnership: Report of the Mental Health Nursing Review Team*. London: HMSO; 1994.

Gournay K, Brooking J. The community psychiatric nurse in primary care: an economic analysis. *Journal of Advanced Nursing*. 1995; **22**:769–778.

Mental Health Foundation. *Creating Community Care: Report of the Mental Health Foundation Inquiry into Community Care for People with Severe Mental Illness*. London: Mental Health Foundation; 1994.

Nolan P. *A History of Mental Health Nursing*. London: Chapman and Hall; 1993.

Skidmore D, ed. *Community Care*. London: Arnold; 1997.

Webster C. Nursing and the early crisis of the National Health Service. *The History of Nursing Group at the RCN, Bulletin*. 1985; **7**:12–24.

White E, Brooker C. The care programme approach. *Nursing Times*. 1990; **87**:66–67.

Wilson HS, Kneisl CR. *Psychiatric Nursing*, 3rd edn. California: Addison-Wesley Publishing Company; 1988.

Multiple personality disorder

Hacking I. *Rewriting the Soul*. Princeton, NJ: Princeton University Press; 1995.

Merskey H. The manufacture of personalities. The production of multiple personality disorder. *British Journal of Psychiatry*. 1992; **160**:327–340.

Piper A, Jr. *Hoax and Reality. The Bizarre World of Multiple Personality Disorder*. Northvale, NJ: Jason Aronson; 1997.

False memories

Loftus E, Ketcham K. *The Myth of Repressed Memory. False Memories and Allegations of Sexual Abuse*. New York: St Martin's Press; 1994.

Pendergrast M. *Victims of Memory*, 2nd edn. Hinesburg VT: Upper Access Books; 1997. (Paperback edition: London: Harper Collins; 1998.)

Non-Western psychiatry

Desjarlais R, Eisenberg L, Good B, Kleinman A. *World Mental Health: Problems and Priorities in Low-Income Countries*. New York: Oxford University Press; 1995.

Jablensky A, Sartorius N, Ernberg G, Anker M, Korten A, Cooper JE, *et al. Schizophrenia: Manifestations, Incidence and Course in Different Cultures: A WHO Ten-Country Study. Psychological Medicine Monograph Supplement 20*. Cambridge: Cambridge University Press; 1992.

Kleinman A, Good BJ, eds. *Culture and Depression*. Berkeley: University of California Press; 1985.

Lee S. Anorexia nervosa in Hong Kong: a Chinese perspective. *Psychological Medicine*. 1991; **21**:703–711.

Leff J. *Psychiatry Around the Globe: A Transcultural View*. London: Gaskell; 1988.

Mumford DB, Nazir M, Jilani F, Baig IY. Stress and psychiatric disorder in the Hindu Kush: a community survey of mountain villages in Chitral, Pakistan. *British Journal of Psychiatry*. 1996; **168**:299–307.

Murphy HBM. *Comparative Psychiatry: The International and Intercultural Distribution of Mental Illness*. Berlin: Springer-Verlag; 1982.

Orley JH, Wing JK. Psychiatric disorders in two African villages. *Archives of General Psychiatry*. 1979; **36**:513–520.

Patel V. *Culture and Common Mental Disorders in Sub-Saharan Africa. Maudsley Monograph 41*. London: Psychology Press; 1998.

Tsuang MT, Tohen M, Zahner GE. *Textbook in Psychiatric Epidemiology*. New York: Wiley-Liss; 1995.

Westermeyer J. Economic losses associated with chronic mental disorder in a developing country. *British Journal of Psychiatry*. 1984; **144**:475–481.

Psychiatric genetics

Galton F. *Hereditary Genius: An Inquiry into its Laws and Consequences*. London: MacMillan; 1869.

Gottesman II, McGuffin P. Eliot Slater and the birth of psychiatric genetics in Great Britain. In: Freeman H, Berrios GE, eds. *150 Years of British Psychiatry*, Vol. 2: *The Aftermath*. London: Athlone; 1996: 537–548.

McGuffin P, Owen MJ, O'Donovan MC, Thapar A, Gottesman II. *Seminars in Psychiatric Genetics*. London: Gaskell; 1994.

Plomin R, DeFries JC, McClearn GE, Rutter M. *Behavioral Genetics. Mental Disorders*. Oxford: Oxford University Press; 1971. (Reprinted: New York: WH Freeman and Company; 1997.)

Weatherall DJ. *The New Genetics and Clinical Practice*. Oxford: Oxford University Press; 1991.

Psychoneuroendocrinology

Amino N, Miyai K, Onishi T, Hashimoto T, Arai K, Ishibashi K, *et al.* Transient hypothyroidism after delivery in autoimmune thyroiditis. *Journal of Clinical Endocrinology and Metabolism*. 1976; **42**:296–301.

Bryson R, Martin D. 17-Ketosteroid excretion in a case of manic depressive psychosis. *Lancet*. 1954; **2**:365–367.

Carrroll B, Feinberg M, Greden J, Terika J, Albala AA, Haskett RF, *et al.* A specific laboratory test for the diagnosis of melancholia. *Archives of General Psychiatry*. 1981; **38**:15–22.

Duval F, Macher JP, Mokrani MC. Difference between evening and morning thyrotropin responses to protirelin in major depressive episode. *Archives of General Psychiatry*. 1990; **47**:443–448.

Halbreich U. Hormonal interventions with psychopharmacological potential: an overview. *Psychopharmacology Bulletin*. 1997; **33**:281–288.

Kathol R, Jaeckle R, Lopez J, Meller W. Pathophysiology of HPA axis abnormalities in patients with major depression: an update. *American Journal of Psychiatry*. 1989; **164**:311–317.

Licinio J, Gold PW, Chrousos GP, Sternberg EM. Forty years of neuroendocrinology: a tribute to SM McCann (editorial). *Molecular Psychiatry*. 1997; **2**:347–349.

Loosen P. The TRH-induced TSH response in psychiatric patients: a possible neuroendocrine marker. *Psychoneuroendocrinology*. 1979; **4**:227–235.

Loosen P, Garbutt J, Prange A. Evaluation of the diagnostic utility of TRH induced response in psychiatric disorders. *Pharmacopsychiatry*. 1987; **20**:90–95.

Mortola JF, Girton L, Fisher U. Successful treatment of severe premenstrual syndrome by combined use of gonadotropin-releasing hormone agonist and estrogen/progestin. *Journal of Clinical Endocrinology and Metabolism*. 1991; **72**:252A–252F.

Parry CH. Collections from the unpublished writings of the late CH Parry, Volume 2. London: Underwoods; 1825.

Prange A, Wilson I, Rabon A, Lipton MA, *et al*. Enhancement of imipramine antidepressant activity by thyroid hormone. *American Journal of Psychiatry*. 1969; **126**:457–469.

Robertson HEW. Lassitude, coldness and hair changes following pregnancy, and then treatment with thyroid extract. *British Medical Journal*. 1948; **2**(Suppl.):2275–2276.

Selye H. The anaesthetic effect of steroid hormones. *Proceedings of the Society of Experimental and Biological Medicine*. 1941; **46**:116–121.

Wolkowitz OM, Reus VI, Manfredi F, *et al*. Ketoconazole administration in hypercortisolaemic depression *American Journal of Psychiatry*. 1993; **150**:810–812.

International psychiatry and the work of the WPA

Madrid Declaration: Codes of Ethics and Specific Guidelines endorsed by the General Assembly WPA. Madrid; 1996.

World Psychiatric Association. *WPA General Survey Report*, April 1998.

World Psychiatric Association. *WPA Information Folder, 1996–1999*.

Psychopharmacology 2000

Carlsson A. The current status of the dopamine hypothesis of schizophrenia. *Neuropsychopharmacology*. 1988; **1**:179–186.

Carlsson A. The rise of neuroppsychopharmacology: impact on basic and clinical neuroscience. In: Healy D, ed. *The Psychopharmacologists*, Vol. 1. London: Chapman and Hall; 51–80.

Healy D. The marketing of 5HT: anxiety or depression. *British Journal of Psychiatry*. 1991; **158**:737–742.

Healy D. *The Antidepressant Era*. Cambridge, MA: Harvard University Press; 1997.

Hippius H. The founding of the CINP and the discovery of clozapine. In: Healy D, ed. *The Psychopharmacologists*, Vol. 1. London: Chapman and Hall; 187–213.

Kane J, Honigfeld G, Singer J, Meltzer HY and the Clozaril Collaborative Study Group. Clozapine for the treatment-resistant schizophrenic: A double-blind comparison with chlorpromazine. *Archives of General Psychiatry*. 1988; **45**:789–796.

Kielholz P. *Diagnose und Therapie der Depressionem fur Praktiker*. Munchen: JF Lehmanns; 1971.

Lambert PA, Borselli S, Midenet J, Bouchardy C, Marcou G, Bouchardy M. L'action favorable du Depamide sure l'evolution a long terme du psychoses maniaco-depressives. *CR Congres de Psychiatrie et de Neurologie de Langue Francaise*. Paris: Masson; 1968: 489–495.

Okuma T, Kishimoto A, Inoue K, Matsumoto H, Ogura A, Matsuhita T, *et al*. Anti-manic and prophylactic effects of carbamazepine (Tegretol) on manic-depressive psychoses – A preliminary report. *Folia Psychiatrica & Neurologica Japonica*. 1973; **27**:283–297 (in Japanese).

Shorter E. *A History of Psychiatry*. Wiley & Sons; 1996.

Smith MC. *A Social History of the Minor Tranquillisers*. Binghampton, NY: Haworth Press; 1991.

INDEX